FIFTH EDITION

Essentials of Clinical Immunology

Helen Chapel

MA, MD, FRCP, FRCPath
Consultant Immunologist, Reader
Department of Clinical Immunology
Nuffield Department of Medicine
University of Oxford

Mansel Haeney

MSc, MB ChB, FRCP, FRCPath
Consultant Immunologist, Clinical Sciences Building
Hope Hospital, Salford

Siraj Misbah

MSc, FRCP, FRCPath
Consultant Clinical Immunologist, Honorary Senior Clinical Lecturer in Immunology
Department of Clinical Immunology and University of Oxford
John Radcliffe Hospital, Oxford

Neil Snowden

MB, BChir, FRCP, FRCPath
Consultant Rheumatologist and Clinical Immunologist
North Manchester General Hospital, Delaunays Road
Manchester

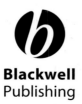

Blackwell
Publishing

Published by Blackwell Publishing Ltd
Blackwell Publishing, Inc., 350 Main Street, Malden, Massachusetts 02148-5020, USA
Blackwell Publishing Ltd, 9600 Garsington Road, Oxford OX4 2DQ, UK
Blackwell Publishing Asia Pty Ltd, 550 Swanston Street, Carlton, Victoria 3053, Australia

First published 1984
ELBS edition 1986
Second edition 1988
Third edition 1993
Fourth edition 1999
Fifth edition 2006

3   2008

Library of Congress Cataloging-in-Publication Data
Data is available

ISBN: 978-1-4051-2761-5

A catalogue record for this title is available from the British Library

Set in 9/12 pt Palatino by Sparks, Oxford – www.sparks.co.uk
Printed and bound in Malaysia by KHL Printing Co Sdn Bhd

Commissioning Editor: Vicki Noyes
Development Editor: Geraldine Jeffers
Production Controller: Kate Charman
Website: Mark Allen, Meg Barton, Shaun Embury

For further information on Blackwell Publishing, visit our website:
http://www.blackwellpublishing.com

The publisher's policy is to use permanent paper from mills that operate a sustainable
forestry policy, and which has been manufactured from pulp processed using acid-free
and elementary chlorine-free practices. Furthermore, the publisher ensures that the text
paper and cover board used have met acceptable environmental accreditation standards.

Contents

Companion website: www.immunologyclinic.com

Preface to the Fifth Edition

At last, after 20 years, *Essentials of Clinical Immunology* is in colour. This has enabled us to increase the number of figures and to include clinical photographs, often alongside the histological drawings for improved clarity. We are grateful to many colleagues who have agreed so willingly for us to use slides from their own collections. In fact we had so many that, despite incorporating over 250 figures, we could not include them all in the book so we have added remaining photographs to the website (www.immunologyclinic.com) to illustrate the cases there.

This new edition has been thoroughly updated in conjunction with new clinical data and the expansion of our understanding of basic immunological concepts. All diagrams have been redrawn for clarity and colour has improved their impact. As before, each chapter concludes with a reference to the website where a short list of key review articles will be updated regularly. The live links to PubMed will enable students to download PDFs easily and quickly. A list of useful immunological web addresses is included as an Appendix to provide additional resources, guidelines and clinical protocols in specific areas. Multiple-choice questions relating to each chapter may be found at the end of the book, with a separate section for the answers. These MCQs and more extensive formative answers are also available on the website, www.immunologyclinic.com, with appropriate cross-linking to illustrative cases.

Essentials of Clinical Immunology is aimed at clinical medical students, doctors in training and career grade doctors seeking refreshment. The key feature remains the continued use of real (but anonymous) case histories to illustrate key concepts. For this edition, more cases have been added to reflect the increasing use of problem-orientated learning in medical school undergraduate curricula. Dealing with real-life patients is the daily work of the qualified doctor; learning in the context of case histories is immediately relevant to training and to continuing professional development in all medical specialties. New cases that illustrate new diseases, treatments or management regimes have also been added to the website.

As ever, we are grateful to our colleagues for keeping us up-to-date with rapid advances in basic and clinical immunology. Professors Lars Fugger and Ian Sargent and Drs David Davies and Graham Ogg provided critical reviews of Chapters 1 and 18.

In terms of copyright to figures, we specifically thank Dr John Axford for use of multiple photographs from *Medicine* (second edition with Dr Chris O'Callaghan) in Chapters 6 and 17, and Drs Roy Reeve and Gordon Armstrong for cellular pathology sections in Chapters 9 and 14. Our thanks also go to the Royal College of Physicians for permission to use illustrations from *Medical Masterclass* in Chapters 10 and 12, and to Science AAAS for permission to reproduce Fig. 19.21.

We also wish to thank Fiona Pattison, Martin Sugden and Vicki Noyes at BPL, Tom Fryer at Sparks and Jane Fallows for their patience and help.

We hope that this new edition will continue to encourage those entering, and those already submersed in clinical medicine, to view clinical immunology as relevant, stimulating and fun and to join the growing ranks of Clinical Immunologists worldwide involved in the care of these interesting patients.

Helen Chapel
Mansel Haeney
Siraj Misbah
Neil Snowden

Preface to the First Edition

Immunology is now a well-developed basic science and much is known of the normal physiology of the immune system in both mice and men. The application of this knowledge to human pathology has lagged behind research, and immunologists are often accused of practising a science which has little relevance to clinical medicine. It is hoped that this book will point out to both medical students and practising clinicians that clinical immunology is a subject which is useful for the diagnosis and management of a great number and variety of human disease.

We have written this book from a clinical point of view. Diseases are discussed by organ involvement, and illustrative case histories are used to show the usefulness (or otherwise) of immunological investigations in the management of these patients. While practising clinicians may find the case histories irksome, we hope they will find the application of immunology illuminating and interesting. The student should gain some perspective of clinical immunology from the case histories, which are selected for their relevance to the topic we are discussing, as this is not a textbook of general medicine. We have pointed out those cases in which the disease presented in an unusual way.

Those who have forgotten, or who need some revision of, basic immunological ideas will find them condensed in Chapter 1. This chapter is not intended to supplant longer texts of basic immunology but merely to provide a springboard for chapters which follow. Professor Andrew Mc-Michael kindly contributed to this chapter and ensured that it was up-to-date. It is important that people who use and request immunological tests should have some idea of their complexity, sensitivity, reliability and expense. Students who are unfamiliar with immunological methods will find that Chapter 17 describes the techniques involved.

Helen Chapel
Mansel Haeney
1984

Acknowledgements to the First Edition

We would first like to acknowledge our debt to Professor Philip Gell FRS and the staff of the Immunology Department at the University of Birmingham, Professor Richard Batchelor and Dr Ron Thompson, all of whom stimulated and sustained our interest in immunology.

We are grateful to everyone who made this book possible. Our sincere thanks are due to Dr John Gillman; without his advice and support, this book would never have been started, let alone completed. Many of our colleagues in Oxford and Salford were particularly helpful; they not only provided case histories but, in many instances, also reviewed relevant chapters and corrected any immunological bias. We wish to thank Professor P. Morris and Drs R. Bonsheck, M. Byron, C. Bunch, H. Cheng, A. Dike, R. Greenhall, A.M. Hoare, J.B. Houghton, N. Hyman, D. Lane, J. Ledingham, M.N. Marsh, P. Millard, G. Pasvol, A. Robson, J. Thompson, S. Waldek, A. Watson and J. Wilkinson. Dr C. Elson kindly checked several chapters and gave constant encouragement, while Dr H. Dorkins was our undergraduate 'guinea-pig' who ensured that the text was comprehensible to clinical students.

Our secretaries, Mrs Elizabeth Henley and Mrs Eileen Walker, were patient and long-suffering, while Mr David Webster, of the Medical Illustration Department at the John Radcliffe Hospital, meticulously prepared the illustrations. We are also grateful to Blackwell Scientific Publications Ltd, especially to Peter Saugman, who provided help and advice promptly, and to Nicola Topham, for her careful subediting of the first edition.

Finally, we owe an enormous debt to our understanding, though overstressed, families for their constant support and acceptance of our bad tempers and the seemingly endless intrusion of clinical immunology into their lives.

1984

User Guide

Throughout the illustrations standard forms have been used for commonly-occurring cells and pathways. A key to these is given in the figure below.

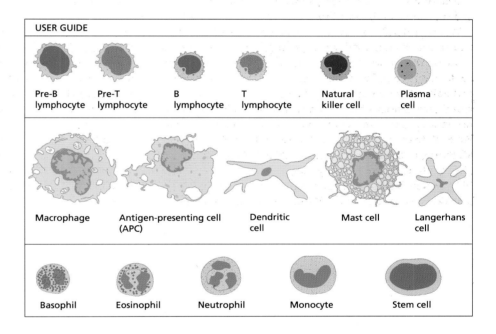

USER GUIDE

Pre-B lymphocyte · Pre-T lymphocyte · B lymphocyte · T lymphocyte · Natural killer cell · Plasma cell

Macrophage · Antigen-presenting cell (APC) · Dendritic cell · Mast cell · Langerhans cell

Basophil · Eosinophil · Neutrophil · Monocyte · Stem cell

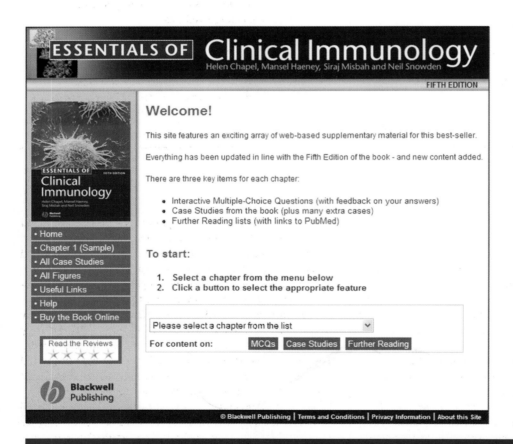

ESSENTIALS OF Clinical Immunology

Helen Chapel, Mansel Haeney, Siraj Misbah and Neil Snowden

FIFTH EDITION

Welcome!

This site features an exciting array of web-based supplementary material for this best-seller.

Everything has been updated in line with the Fifth Edition of the book - and new content added.

There are three key items for each chapter:

- Interactive Multiple-Choice Questions (with feedback on your answers)
- Case Studies from the book (plus many extra cases)
- Further Reading lists (with links to PubMed)

To start:

1. **Select a chapter from the menu below**
2. **Click a button to select the appropriate feature**

Please select a chapter from the list

For content on: MCQs | Case Studies | Further Reading

- Home
- Chapter 1 (Sample)
- All Case Studies
- All Figures
- Useful Links
- Help
- Buy the Book Online

Read the Reviews
★ ★ ★ ★ ★

Blackwell Publishing

© Blackwell Publishing | Terms and Conditions | Privacy Information | About this Site

ESSENTIALS OF CLINICAL IMMUNOLOGY

Visit the companion website for this book at:
www.immunologyclinic.com

For:
- interactive multiple-choice questions for each chapter
- database of images
- additional case histories
- 'Further reading' with links to PubMed

CHAPTER 1

1

Basic Components: Structure and Function

1.1 Introduction

The immune system evolved as a defence against infectious diseases. Individuals with markedly deficient immune responses, if untreated, succumb to infections in early life. There is, therefore, a selective **evolutionary pressure** for an efficient immune system. The evolution to adaptive responses has improved the efficiency of immune responses, though a parallel evolution in pathogens means that all species, plants, insects, fish, birds and mammals, have continued to improve their defence mechanisms over millions of years, giving rise to redundancies.

An immune response consists of **four parts**: an early innate (non-specific) response to invasion by material recognized as foreign, a slower specific response to a particular antigen and a non-specific augmentation of this response. There is also memory of specific immune responses, providing a quicker and larger response the second time that a particular antigen is encountered.

Innate immunity, though phylogenetically older and important in terms of speed of a response, is currently less well defined. Humoral components (soluble molecules in the plasma) and cells in blood and tissues are involved. Such

responses are normally accompanied by inflammation and occur within a few hours of stimulation (Table 1.1).

Specific immune responses are also divided into humoral and cellular responses. Humoral responses result in the generation of antibody reactive with a particular antigen. Antibodies are proteins with similar structures, known collectively as immunoglobulins (Ig). They can be transferred passively to another individual by injection of serum. In contrast, only cells can transfer cellular immunity. Good examples of cellular immune responses are the rejection of a graft by lymphoid cells as well as graft-versus-host disease, where transferred cells attack an immunologically compromised recipient.

Gowans demonstrated the vital role played by **lymphocytes** in humoral and cellular immune responses over 50 years ago; he cannulated and drained rat thoracic ducts to obtain a cell population comprising more than 95% lymphocytes. He showed that these cells could transfer the capacity both to make antibody and to reject skin grafts. Antibody-producing lymphocytes, which are dependent on the bone marrow, are known as B cells. In response to antigen stimulation, B cells will mature to antibody-secreting plasma cells. Cellular immune responses are dependent on an intact thymus, so the lymphocytes responsible are

Table 1.1 Components of innate and adaptive immunity

Features	Innate	Adaptive
Foreign molecules recognized	Structures shared by microbes, recognized as patterns (e.g. repeated glycoproteins)	Wide range of very particular molecules or fragments of molecules on all types of extrinsic and modified self structures
Nature of recognition receptors	Germline encoded—limited	Somatic mutation results in wide range of specificities and affinities
Speed of response	Immediate	Time for cell movement and interaction between cell types
Memory	None	Efficient
Humoral components	Complement components	Antibodies
Cellular components	Neutrophils, macrophages, NK cells, B1 cells, epithelial cells, mast cells	Lymphocytes—T (Tαβ, Tγδ), B, NKT

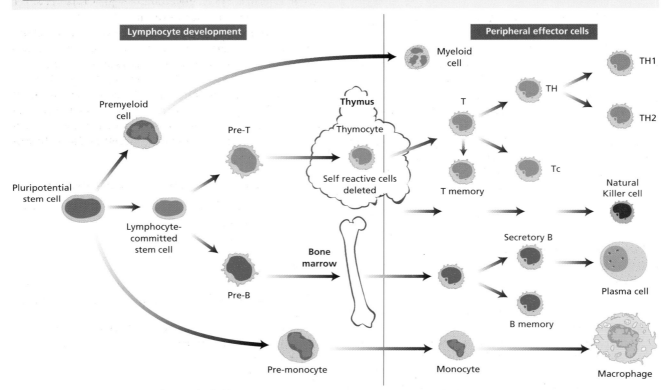

Fig. 1.1 Development of different types of lymphocytes from a pluripotential stem cell in the bone marrow. The developmental pathway for natural killer (NK) cells is shown separately because it is thought NK cells may develop in both the thymus and the bone marrow.

known as thymus-dependent (T) cells. The developmental pathways of both cell types are fairly well established (Fig. 1.1).

All immune responses, innate and adaptive, have two phases. The **recognition phase** involves antigen-presenting cells, in which the antigen is recognized as foreign. In the **effector phase**, neutrophils and macrophages (innate immunity) and antibodies and effector T lymphocytes (adaptive immunity) eliminate the antigen.

1.2 Key molecules

Many types of molecules play vital roles in both phases of immune responses; *some are shared by both the innate and the adaptive systems* (see p. 10). Antigens are substances that are recognized by immune components. Detection molecules on innate cells recognize general patterns of 'foreign-ness' on non-mammalian cells, whereas those on adaptive cells are specific for a wide range of very particular molecules or fragments of molecules. Antibodies are not only the surface receptors of B cells that recognize specific antigens, but, once the appropriate B cells are activated and differentiate into plasma cells, antibodies are also secreted into blood and body fluids in large quantities to prevent that antigen from causing damage. T cells have structurally similar receptors for recognizing antigens, known as T-cell receptors. Major histocompatibility complex (MHC) molecules provide a means of self-recognition and also play a fundamental role in T lymphocyte effector functions. Effector mechanisms are often dependent on messages from initiating or regulating cells; soluble mediators, which carry messages between cells, are known as interleukins, cytokines and chemokines.

1.2.1 Molecules recognized by immune systems

Foreign substances are recognized by both the innate and adaptive systems, but in different ways, using different receptors (see below). The innate system is activated by 'danger signals', due to pattern recognition receptors (PRRs) on innate (dendritic) cells recognizing conserved microbial structures directly, often repeated polysaccharide molecules, known as **pathogen associated molecular patterns (PAMPs)**. Toll-like receptors (receptors which serve a similar function to toll receptors in drosophila) make up a large family of non-antigen-specific receptors for a variety of individual bacterial, viral and fungal components such as DNA, lipoproteins and lipopolysaccharides. Activation of dendritic cells by binding to either of these detection receptors leads to inflammation and *subsequently activation of the adaptive system*.

Phagocytic cells also recognize particular patterns associated with potentially damaging materials, such as lipoproteins and other charged molecules or peptides.

Traditionally, **antigens** have been defined as molecules that interact with components of the adaptive system, i.e. T- and B-cell recognition receptors and antibody. *An antigenic molecule may have several antigenic determinants (epitopes)*; each **epitope** can bind with an individual antibody, and a single antigenic molecule can therefore provoke many antibody molecules with different binding sites. Some low-molecular-weight molecules, called **haptens**, are unable to provoke an immune response themselves, although they can react with existing antibodies. Such substances need to be coupled to a carrier molecule in order to have sufficient epitopes to be antigenic. For some chemicals, such as drugs, the carrier may be a host (auto) protein. The tertiary structure, as well as the amino acid sequence, is important in determining antigenicity. Pure lipids and nucleic acids are also poor antigens, although they do activate the innate system and can be inflammatory.

Antigens are conventionally divided into thymus-dependent and thymus-independent antigens. **Thymus-dependent antigens** require T-cell participation to provoke the production of antibodies; most proteins and foreign red cells are examples. **Thymus-independent antigens** require no T-cell cooperation for antibody production; they directly stimulate specific B lymphocytes by virtue of their ability to cross-link antigen receptors on the B-cell surface, produce predominantly IgM and IgG_2 antibodies and provoke poor immunological memory. Such antigens include bacterial polysaccharides, found in bacterial cell walls. Endotoxin, another thymus-independent antigen, not only causes specific B-cell activation and antibody production but also acts as a polyclonal B-cell stimulant.

Factors other than the intrinsic properties of the antigen can also influence the quality of the immune response (Table 1.2). Substances that improve an immune response to a separate, often rather weak, antigen are known as **adjuvants**. The use of adjuvants in humans is discussed in Chapter 7.

Superantigen is the name given to those foreign proteins which are not specifically recognized by the adaptive system but do activate large numbers of T cells via direct action with an invariant part of the T-cell receptor (see Chapter 2).

Self-antigens are not recognized by dendritic cells of the innate system, so inflammation and co-stimulation of naive T cells (see section 1.4.1) is not induced. There are mechanisms to control adaptive responses to **self-antigens**, by pre-

Table 1.2 Factors influencing the immune response to an antigen, i.e. its immunogenicity

---

1 Nature of molecule:
   Protein content
   Size
   Solubility

2 Dose:
Low dose → small amounts of antibody with high affinity and restricted specificity
Moderate dose → large amounts of antibody but mixed affinity and broad specificity
High dose → tolerance

3 Route of entry:
ID, IM, SC → regional lymph nodes
IV → spleen
Oral → Peyer's patches
Inhalation → bronchial lymphoid tissue

4 Addition of substances with synergistic effects, e.g. adjuvants, other antigens

5 Genetic factors of recipient animal:
   Species differences
   Individual differences

ID, Intradermal injection; IM, intramuscular injection; IV, intravenous injection; SC, subcutaneous injection.

Table 1.3 Markers on dendritic cells

	Immature dendritic cells	Mature dendritic cells
Function	Antigen capture	Antigen presentation to T cells
Co-stimulatory molecule expression, e.g. CD80, CD86	Absent or low	++
Adhesion molecules, e.g. ICAM-1	Absent or low	++
Cytokine receptors, e.g. IL-12R	Absent or low	++
Pattern recognition receptors (PRRs), e.g. mannose receptor	++	−
MHC class II:		
turnover	Very rapid	Persist > 100 h
density	Reduced (approx. 1×10^6)	Very high (approx. 7×10^6)

ICAM-1, Intercellular adhesion molecule-1.

vention of production of specific receptors and limitation of the response if the immune system is fooled (see Chapter 5, Autoimmunity).

1.2.2 Recognition molecules

There are several sets of detection molecules on innate cells: PRRs, such as Toll-like receptors, as well as chemotactic receptors and phagocytic receptors. **PRRs** may be soluble or attached to cell membranes (see Table 1.3). Mannan binding lectin is a protein that binds sugars on microbial surfaces; if attached to a macrophage, it acts as a trigger for phagocytosis and, if soluble, it activates the complement cascade resulting in opsonization. Others belonging to this family are less well defined.

Toll-like receptors (TLRs) are part of this family too. These are evolutionarily conserved proteins found on macrophages, dendritic cells and neutrophils; like other PRRs, the precise structures are as yet undefined. At least ten different TLRs are found in humans, each TLR recognizing a range of particular motifs on pathogens, such as double-stranded RNA of viruses (TLR3), lipopolysaccharides of Gram-negative bacterial cell walls (TLR4), flagellin (TLR5) and bacterial DNA (TLR9), all highly conserved motifs unique to microorganisms. Upon binding to their ligands, TLRs induce signal transduction, via a complex cascade of intracellular adaptor molecules and kinases, culminating in the induction of nuclear factor kappa B transcription factor (NF-κB)-dependent gene expression and the induction of pro-inflammatory cytokines (Fig. 1.2). The clinical consequences of a defective

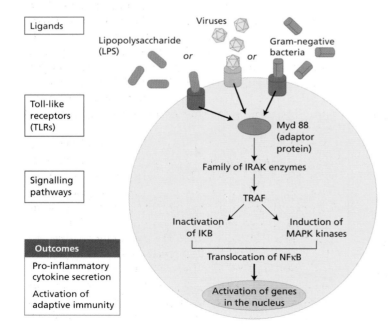

Fig. 1.2 Sequential cellular events induced by engagement of Toll-like receptors by microbial ligands (TRAF, TNF receptor-associated factor; IKB, inhibitor kappa B; MAPK, mitogen-activated protein kinase; IRAK, interleukin-1 receptor-associated kinase).

TLR pathway are discussed in Chapter 3 (see Box 1.1 in this chapter also).

CD1 molecules are invariant proteins (MHC-like and associated with β_2-microglobulin—see below), which are present on antigen presenting cells and epithelia. CD1 combine with lipids, which are poor antigens and not usually well presented to the adaptive immune system, and so act as recognition molecules for the intestine and other microbial rich surfaces. CD1 present lipids to the non-MHC-restricted natural killer (NK) T cells and $\gamma\delta$T cells in the epithelium.

Each T cell, like B cells, is pre-committed to a given epitope. It recognizes this by one of two types of **T-cell receptors (TCRs)**, depending on the cell's lineage and thus its final function. T cells have either $\alpha\beta$TCR [a heterodimer of alpha (α) and beta (β) chains] or $\gamma\delta$TCR [a heterodimer of gamma (γ) and delta (δ) chains]. $\alpha\beta$TCR cells predominate in adults, although 10% of T cells in epithelial structures are of the $\gamma\delta$TCR type. In either case, TCRs are associated with several transmembrane proteins that make up the cluster differentiation 3 (CD3) molecule (Fig. 1.3), to make the CD3–TCR complex responsible for taking the antigen recognition signal inside the cell (signal transduction). Signal transduction requires a group of intracellular tyrosine kinases (designated p56 lck, p59 fyn, ZAP 70) to join with the cytosolic tails of the CD3–TCR complex and become

phosphorylated. Nearby accessory molecules, CD2, LFA-1, CD4 and CD8, are responsible for increased adhesion (see section 1.2.6) but are not actually involved in recognizing presented antigen.

The genes for TCR chains are on different chromosomes: β and γ on chromosome 7 and α and δ on chromosome 14. The structures of TCRs have been well defined over the last 15 years; each of the four chains is made up of a variable and a constant domain. The variable regions are numerous (although less so than immunoglobulin variable genes). They are joined by D and J region genes to the invariant (constant) gene by recombinases, *RAG1* and *RAG2, the same enzymes used for making antigen receptors on B cells (BCRs) and antibodies (see below).* The **diversity of T-cell antigen receptors** is achieved in a similar way for immunoglobulin, although TCRs are less diverse since somatic mutation is not involved; perhaps the risk of 'self recognition' would be too great. The diversity of antigen binding is dependent on the large number of V genes and the way in which these may be combined with different D and J genes to provide different V domain genes. The similarities between TCRs and BCRs have led to the suggestion that the genes evolved from the same parent gene and both are *members of a 'supergene' family.* Unlike immunoglobulin, T-cell receptors are not secreted and are not independent effector molecules.

A particular T-cell receptor complex recognizes a processed antigenic peptide in the context of MHC class I or II antigens (see below) depending on the type of T cell; helper T cells recognize class II with antigen, and the surface accessory protein CD4 (see below) enhances binding and intracellular signals. Suppressor/cytotoxic T cells recognize antigens with class I (see section 1.3.1) and use CD8 accessory molecules for increased binding and signalling. Since the number of variable genes available to T-cell receptors appears to be more limited, reactions with antigen would have low affinity were it not for increasing binding by these **accessory mechanisms**. Recognition of processed antigen alone is not enough to activate T cells. Additional signals, through soluble interleukins, are needed; some of these are generated during 'antigen processing' (see Antigen processing below).

Major histocompatibility complex molecules (MHC) are known as 'histocompatibility antigens' because of the vigorous reactions they provoked during mismatched organ transplantation. However, these molecules also play a fundamental role in immunity by presenting antigenic peptides to T cells. Histocompatibility antigens in humans [known as human leucocyte antigens (HLA)] are synonymous with the MHC molecules. MHC molecules are cell-surface glycoproteins of two basic types: class I and class II (Fig. 1.4). They exhibit extensive genetic polymorphism with multiple alleles at each locus. As a result, genetic variability between individuals is very great and most unrelated individuals

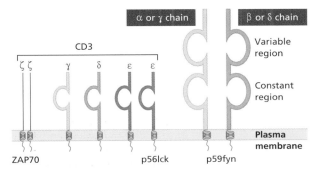

Fig. 1.3 Diagram of the structure of the T-cell receptor (TCR). The variable regions of the alpha (α) and beta (β) chains make up the T idiotype, i.e. antigen/peptide binding region. The TCR is closely associated on the cell surface with the CD3 protein.

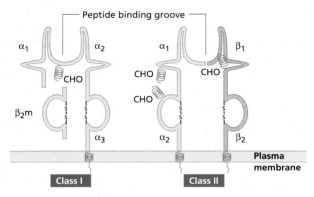

Fig. 1.4 Diagrammatic representation of MHC class I and class II antigens. β_2m, β_2-microglobulin; CHO, carbohydrate side chain.

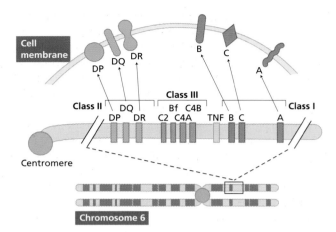

Fig. 1.6 Major histocompatibility complex on chromosome 6; class III antigens are complement components. TNF, Tumour necrosis factor.

possess different HLA molecules. This means that it is very difficult to obtain perfect HLA matches between unrelated persons for transplantation (see Chapter 8).

Extensive polymorphism in MHC molecules is best explained by the need of the immune system to cope with an ever-increasing range of pathogens adept at evading immune responses (see Chapter 2).

The TCR of an individual T cell will only recognize antigen as part of a complex of antigenic peptide and self-MHC (Fig. 1.5). This process of **dual recognition of peptide and MHC molecule** is known as MHC restriction, since the MHC molecule restricts the ability of the T cell to recognize antigen (Fig. 1.5). The importance of MHC restriction in the immune response was recognized by the award of the Nobel

prize in Medicine to Peter Doherty and Rolf Zinkernagel, who proposed the concept on the basis of their studies with virus-specific cytotoxic T cells.

MHC class I antigens are subdivided into three groups: A, B and C. Each group is controlled by a different gene locus within the MHC on chromosome 6 (Fig. 1.6). The products of the genes at all three loci are chemically similar. MHC class I antigens (see Fig. 1.4) are made up of a heavy chain (α) of 45 kDa controlled by a gene in the relevant MHC locus, associated with a smaller chain called β_2-microglobulin (12 kDa), controlled by a gene on chromosome 12. The differences between individual MHC class I antigens are due to variations in the α chains; the β_2-microglobulin component is constant. The detailed structure of class I antigens was determined by X-ray crystallography. This shows that small antigenic peptides (approx. nine amino acids long) can be tightly bound to a groove produced by the pairing of the two extracellular domains (α_1 and α_2) of the α chain. The *affinity of individual peptide binding depends on the nature and shape of the groove*, and accounts for the MHC restriction above.

The detailed structure of **MHC class II antigens** was also determined by X-ray crystallography. It has a folded structure similar to class I antigens with the peptide-binding groove found between the α_1 and β_1 chains (see Fig. 1.4). Whereas most nucleated cells express class I molecules, *expression of class II molecules is restricted to a few cell types*: dendritic cells, B lymphocytes, activated T cells, macrophages, inflamed vascular endothelium and some epithelial cells. However, other cells (e.g. thyroid, pancreas, gut epithelium) can be induced to express class II molecules under the influence of interferon (IFN)-γ released during inflammation. In humans, there are three groups of variable class II antigens: the loci are known as HLA-DP, HLA-DQ and HLA-DR.

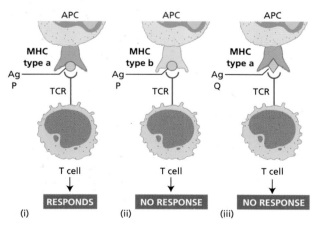

Fig. 1.5 MHC restriction of antigen recognition by T cells. T cells specific for a particular peptide and a particular MHC allele will not respond if the same peptide were to be presented by a different MHC molecule as in (ii) or as in (iii) if the T cell were to encounter a different peptide. APC, Antigen-presenting cell; TCR, T-cell receptor.

In practical terms, MHC restriction is a mechanism by which antigens in different intracellular compartments can be captured and presented to CD4+ or CD8+ T cells. **Endogenous antigens** (including viral antigens) are processed by the endoplasmic reticulum and presented by MHC class I-bearing cells exclusively to CD8+ T cells. Prior to presentation on the cell surface, endogenous antigens are broken down into short peptides, which are then actively transported from the cytoplasm to endoplasmic reticulum by proteins. These proteins act as a shuttle and are thus named 'transporters associated with antigen processing' (TAP-1 and TAP-2). TAP proteins (coded in MHC class II region) deliver peptides to MHC class I molecules in the endoplasmic reticulum, from where the complex of MHC and peptide is delivered to the cell surface. Mutations in either TAP gene prevent surface expression of MHC class I molecules.

In contrast, **exogenous antigens** are processed by the lysosomal route and presented by MHC class II antigens to CD4+ T cells (Fig. 1.7). As with MHC class I molecules, newly synthesized MHC class II molecules are held in the endoplasmic reticulum until they are ready to be transported to the cell surface. Whilst in the endoplasmic reticulum, class II molecules are prevented from binding to peptides in the lumen by a protein known as MHC class II-associated invariant chain. The invariant chain also directs delivery of class II molecules to the endosomal compartment where exogenous antigens are processed and made available for binding to class II molecules.

The **MHC class III region** (see Fig. 1.6) contains genes encoding proteins that are involved in the complement system (see section 1.4.1): namely, the early components C4 and C2 of the classical pathway and factor B of the alternative pathway. Other inflammatory proteins, e.g. tumour necrosis factor (TNF), are encoded in adjacent areas.

Invariant MHC-like proteins, such as CD1 lipid-recognition receptors, are not coded for on chromosome 6, despite being associated with β_2-microglobulin. Other genes for invariant proteins coded here, such as enzymes for steroid metabolism and heat shock proteins, have no apparent role in adaptive immunity.

Antigen receptors on B cells – BCRs – are surface-bound immunoglobulin molecules. As with TCRs, they have predetermined specificity for epitopes and are therefore extremely diverse. *The immune system has to be capable of recognizing all pathogens, past and future.* Such diversity is provided by the way in which all three types of molecules, TCR, BCR and antibody, are produced.

The **basic structure of the immunoglobulin** molecule is shown in Fig. 1.8. It has a four-chain structure: two identical heavy (H) chains (mol. wt 50 kDa) and two identical light (L)

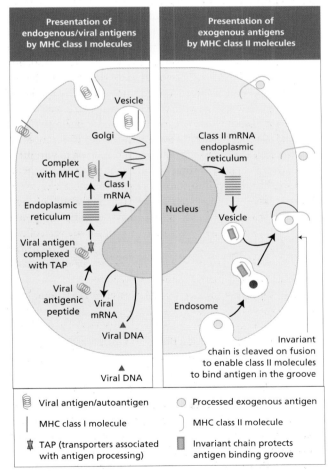

Fig. 1.7 Different routes of antigen presentation.

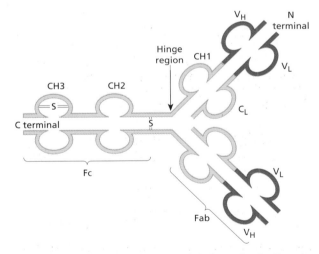

Fig. 1.8 Basic structure of an immunoglobulin molecule. Domains are held in shape by disulphide bonds, though only one is shown. CH_{1-3}, constant domain of a heavy chain; C_L, constant domain of a light chain; V_H, variable domain of a heavy chain; V_L, variable domain of a light chain. =S=, disulphide bond.

chains (mol. wt 25 kDa). Each chain is made up of domains of about 110 amino acids held together in a loop by a disulphide bond between two cysteine residues in the chain. The domains have the same basic structure and many areas of similarity in their amino acid sequences. The heavy chains determine the isotype of the immunoglobulin, resulting in pentameric IgM (Fig. 1.9) or dimeric IgA (Fig. 1.10).

The amino (N) terminal domains of the heavy and light chains include the **antigen-binding site**. The amino acid sequences of these N-terminal domains vary between different antibody molecules and are known as variable (V) regions. Most of these differences reside in three hypervariable areas of the molecule, each only 6–10 amino acid residues long.

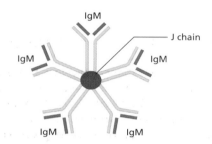

Fig. 1.9 Schematic representation of IgM pentamer (MW 800 kDA).

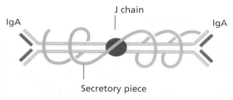

Fig. 1.10 Schematic representation of secretory IgA (MW 385 kDA).

In the folded molecule, these hypervariable regions in each chain come together to form, with their counterparts on the other pair of heavy and light chains, the antigen-binding site. The structure of this part of the antibody molecule is unique to that molecule and is known as the **idiotypic determinant**. In any individual, about 10^6–10^7 different antibody molecules could be made up by 10^3 different heavy chain variable regions associating with 10^3 different light chain variable regions.

The part of the antibody molecule next to the V region is the constant (C) region (Fig. 1.8), made up of one domain in a **light chain** (C_L) and three or four in a **heavy chain** (C_H). There are two alternative types of C_L chain, known as kappa (κ) and lambda (λ); an antibody molecule has either two κ or two λ light chains, never one of each. Of all the antibodies in a human individual, roughly 60% contain κ and 40% contain λ light chains. There are no known differences in the functional properties between κ and λ light chains. In contrast, there are several possible different types of C_H domain, each with important functional differences (Table 1.4). The heavy chains determine the class (isotype) of the antibody and the ultimate physiological function of the particular antibody molecule. Once the antigen-binding site has reacted with its antigen, the molecule undergoes a change in the conformation of its heavy chains in order to take part in effector reactions, depending on the class of the molecule.

The mechanisms for this supergene family are identical in terms of **recombination**, though the coding regions for the α,β,γ and δ chains for the TCRs are obviously on different chromosomes. Immunoglobulin production, whether for BCR or antibody production, is the same. The light and heavy chain genes are carried on different chromosomes (Fig. 1.11). Like those coding for other macromolecules, the genes are broken up into coding segments (exons) with in-

Table 1.4 Immunoglobulin classes and their functions

Isotype	Heavy chain	Serum concentration*	Main function	Complement fixation†	Placental passage	Reaction with Fc receptors‡
IgM	μ	0.5–2.0	Neutralization and opsonization	+++	–	L
IgG_1	γ_1	5.0–12.0	Opsonization	+++	++	M, N, P, L, E
IgG_2	γ_2	2.0–6.0		+	±	P, L
IgG_3	γ_3	0.5–1.0	Opsonization	+++	++	M, N, P, L, E
IgG_4	γ_4	0.1–1.0		–	+	N, L, P
IgA_1	α_1	0.5–3.0	Neutralization at mucosal surfaces	–	–	M, N
IgA_2	α_2	0.0–0.2		–	–	–
IgD	δ	Trace	Lymphocyte membrane receptor	–	–	–
IgE	ε	Trace	Mast cell attachment	–	–	B, E, L

*Normal adult range in g/l.
†Classical pathway.
‡Fc receptors on: basophils/mast cells, B; on eosinophils, E; on lymphocytes, L; on macrophages, M; on neutrophils, N; on platelets, P.

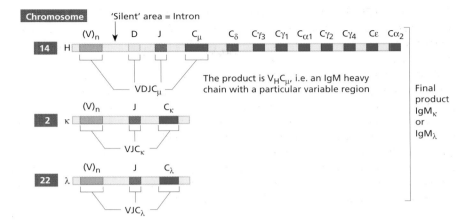

Fig. 1.11 Immunoglobulin genes (see text for explanation).

tervening silent segments (introns). The heavy chain gene set, on chromosome 14, is made up of small groups of exons representing the constant regions of the heavy chains (e.g. mu (μ) chain) and a very large number of V region genes, perhaps as many as 10^3. Between the V and C genes are two small sets of exons, D and J (Fig. 1.11). In a single B cell, one V region gene is selected, joined to one D and J in the chromosome and the VDJ product is joined at the level of RNA processing to C_μ when the B cell is making IgM. The cell can make IgG by omitting the C_μ and joining VDJ to a C_γ. Thus, the cell can make IgM, IgD and IgG/A/E in sequence, while still using the same variable region. VDJ gene recombination is controlled by the same enzymes used for the TCRs, and coded for by two recombination activating genes: RAG1 and RAG2. Disruption of the RAG1 or RAG2 function in infants with mutations in these genes causes profound immune deficiency, characterized by absent mature B and T cells, as neither TCR or BCR can be produced. On a different chromosome in the same cell, a V gene is joined to a J gene (there is no D on the light chain) and then the V product is joined at the RNA level to the C_κ or C_λ (Fig. 1.11).

The wide diversity of antigen binding is dependent on the large number of V genes and the way in which these may be combined with different D and J genes to provide different rearranged VDJ gene segments. Once V, D and J rearrangement has taken place to produce a functional immunoglobulin molecule, further V region variation is introduced only when antibodies rather than BCRs are produced.

Natural killer cells also have recognition molecules. These cells are important in killing virally infected cells and tumour cells. They have to be able to recognize these targets and distinguish them from normal cells. They recognize and kill cells that have reduced or absent MHC class I, using two kinds of receptors [called inhibitory (KIR) and activating (KAR)] to estimate the extent of MHC expression. They also have one type of Fc IgG (Fcγ) receptor, that for low-affinity binding, and are able to kill some cells with large amounts of antibody on their surfaces.

The major purpose of the complement pathways is to provide a means of removing or destroying antigen, regardless of whether or not it has become coated with antibody. This requires that **complement components recognize** damaging material such as immune complexes (antigen combined with antibodies) or foreign antigens. The four complement pathways are discussed in more detail in section 1.4.1.

1.2.3 Accessory molecules

The binding of a specific TCR to the relevant processed antigen–MHC class II complex on an antigen-presenting cell provides an insufficient signal for T-cell activation. So additional stimuli are provided by the binding of adhesion molecules on the two cell surfaces. Accessory molecules are lymphocyte surface proteins, distinct from the antigen binding complexes, which are necessary for **efficient binding, signalling and homing**. *Accessory molecules are invariant, non-polymorphic proteins.* Each accessory molecule has a particular ligand—corresponding protein to which it binds. They are present on all cells which require close adhesion for these functions; for example, there are those on T cells for each of the many cell types activating/responding to T cells (antigen-presenting cells, endothelial cells, etc.) and also on B cells for efficiency of T-cell help and stimulation by follicular dendritic cells.

There are several families of accessory molecules, but the most important appear to be the immunoglobulin supergene family of **adhesion molecules**, which derives its name from the fact that its members contain a common immunoglobulin-like structure. Members of their family strengthen the interaction between antigen-presenting cells and T cells (Fig. 1.12); those on T cells include CD4, CD8, CD28, CTLA-4, CD45R, CD2 and lymphocyte function anti-

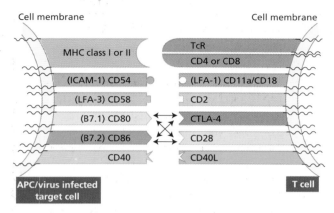

Fig. 1.12 Diagrammatic representation of adhesion molecules on T cells and their ligands on antigen-presenting cells/virus-infected target cells.

gen 1 (LFA-1). For interaction with B cells, CD40 ligand and ICOS are important for class switching (see section 1.4.3). Adhesion molecules, for binding leucocytes (both lymphocytes and polymorphonuclear leucocytes) to endothelial cells and tissue matrix cells, are considered below in section 1.2.6. On B cells, such molecules include CD40 (ligand for CD40L, now named CD154), B-7-1 and B7-2 (ligands for CD28).

1.2.4 Effector molecules

There are humoral and cellular effector molecules in both the innate and the adaptive immune systems (Table 1.5). Several of the same mechanisms are used in both types of immune responses, especially in killing of target cells, suggesting that evolution of immune responses has been conservative in terms of genes, though with much redundancy to ensure the life-preserving nature of the immune systems in the face of rapid evolution of pathogenic microbes.

Antibodies

Antibodies are the best described important effector mechanisms in adaptive immunity. They are the **effector arm of B cells** and are secreted by plasma cells in large quantities, to be carried in the blood and lymph to distant sites. As shown in Table 1.4, there are five major isotypes of antibodies, each with different functions (see also Box 1.2).

IgM is a large molecule whose major physiological role is intravascular neutralization of organisms (especially viruses). **IgM** has five complement-binding sites, resulting in

---

BOX 1.2 IMMUNOGLOBULIN ISOTYPES AND THEIR SIGNIFICANCE

IgM is phylogenetically the oldest class of immunoglobulin. It is a large molecule (Fig. 1.9) and penetrates poorly into tissues. IgM has five complement-binding sites, which results in excellent complement activation.

IgG is smaller and penetrates tissues easily. It is the only immunoglobulin to provide immune protection to the neonate (Table 1.4). There are four subclasses of IgG, with slightly different functions.

IgA is the major mucosal immunoglobulin—sometimes referred to as 'mucosal antiseptic paint'. IgA in mucosal secretions consists of two basic units joined by a J chain (Fig. 1.10); the addition of a 'secretory piece' prevents digestion of this immunoglobulin in the intestinal and bronchial secretions.

IgD is synthesized by antigen-sensitive B lymphocytes, is not secreted, acting as a cell-surface receptor for activation of these cells by antigen.

IgE is produced by plasma cells but is taken up by specific IgE receptors on mast cells and basophils. IgE then provides an antigen-sensitive way of expelling intestinal parasites by increasing vascular permeability and inducing chemotactic factors via mast cell degranulation (see section 1.7).

Table 1.5 Effector molecules in immunity

	Innate	Adaptive
Humoral	Complement components for opsonization or lysis	Specific antibodies for opsonization and phagocytosis or lysis with complement
Cellular	Perforin in NK cells creates pores in target cell membranes	Perforin in cytolytic (CD8) T cells creates pores in specific target cell membranes
	Granzymes in NK cells induce apoptosis in target cells	NKT cells induce apoptosis? by perforin production
	Lysosomes in phagocytic vacuoles result in death of ingested microbes	
	Preformed histamine and related vasoactive substances as well as leukotrienes in mast cells	

excellent complement activation and subsequent removal of the antigen–antibody–complement complexes by complement receptors on phagocytic cells or complement-mediated lysis of the organism (see section 1.4).

IgG is a smaller immunoglobulin which penetrates tissues easily. Placental transfer is an active process involving specific placental receptors for the Fc portion of the IgG molecule, termed FcRn (Fc receptor of the neonate). The FcRn receptor is also present on epithelial and endothelial cells and is an important regulator of IgG metabolism (see section 7.4 and Fig. 7.8). Of the four subclasses, IgG_1 and IgG_3 activate complement efficiently and are responsible for clearing most protein antigens, including the removal of microorganisms by phagocytic cells (see section 1.5). IgG_2 and IgG_4 react predominantly with carbohydrate antigens (in adults) and are relatively poor opsonins.

IgA is the major mucosal immunoglobulin. Attachment of 'secretory piece' prevents digestion of this immunoglobulin in the intestinal and bronchial secretions. IgA_2 is the predominant subclass in secretions and neutralizes antigens that enter via these mucosal routes. IgA_1, the main IgA in serum, is capable of neutralizing antigens that enter the circulation but IgA_1 is sensitive to bacterial proteases and therefore less useful for host defence. IgA has additional functions via its receptor (FcαR or CD89), present on mononuclear cells and neutrophils, for activation of phagocytosis, inflammatory mediator release and antibody-dependent cell-mediated cytotoxicity (ADCC) (see section 1.5).

There is little free **IgD or IgE** in serum or normal body fluids, since both act as surface receptors only.

As mentioned above, mechanisms of recombination in immunoglobulin production, whether for BCR or antibody production, are the same (Fig. 1.11). Once V, D and J region rearrangement has taken place, further variation is introduced when antibodies are made, by the introduction of point mutations in the V region genes. This process, known as **somatic hypermutation**, occurs in the lymphoid germinal centres and is critically dependent on activation-induced cytidine deaminase (AID), an enzyme responsible for deamination of DNA. Somatic hypermutation helps to increase the possible number of combinations and accounts for the enormous diversity of antibody specificities (10^{14}), which by far exceeds the number of different B cells in the body (10^{10}).

Cytokines and chemokines

Cytokines are soluble mediators secreted by macrophages or monocytes (monokines) or lymphocytes (lymphokines). These mediators act as **stimulatory or inhibitory signals** between cells; those between cells of the immune system are known as interleukins. As a group, cytokines share several common features (see Box 1.3). Amongst the array of cytokines produced by macrophages and T cells, interleukin-1 (IL-1) and IL-2 are of particular interest due to their pivotal

BOX 1.3 COMMON FEATURES OF CYTOKINES

- Their half-lives are short.
- They are rapidly degraded as a method of regulation and thus difficult to measure in the circulation.
- Most act locally within the cell's microenvironment.
- Some act on the cell of production itself, promoting activation and differentiation through high-affinity cell-surface receptors.
- Many cytokines are pleiotropic in their biological effects, i.e. affecting multiple organs in the body.
- Most exhibit biologically overlapping functions, thus illustrating the redundancy of the group. For this reason, therapeutic targeting of individual cytokines in disease has had limited success (effects of deletion of individual cytokine genes are listed in Table 1.7).

role in amplifying immune responses. IL-1 acts on a wide range of targets (Table 1.6), including T and B cells. In contrast, the effects of IL-2 are largely restricted to lymphocytes. Although IL-2 was originally identified on account of its ability to promote growth of T cells, it has similar trophic effects on IL-2 receptor-bearing B and NK cells. The considerable overlap between actions of individual cytokines and interleukins is summarized in Table 1.7.

Cytokines that induce chemotaxis of leucocytes are referred to as **chemokines**, a name derived from chemo + kine, i.e. something to help movement. Some cytokines and interleukins have been redefined as chemokines, e.g. IL-8 = CXCL8. Chemokines are structurally similar proteins of

Table 1.6 Actions of interleukin-1

Target cell	Effect
T lymphocytes	Proliferation
	Differentiation
	Lymphokine production
	Induction of IL-2 receptors
B lymphocytes	Proliferation
	Differentiation
Neutrophils	Release from bone marrow
	Chemoattraction
Macrophages	
Fibroblasts	
Osteoblasts	Proliferation/activation
Epithelial cells	
Osteoclasts	Reabsorption of bone
Hepatocytes	Acute-phase protein synthesis
Hypothalamus	Prostaglandin-induced fever
Muscle	Prostaglandin-induced proteolysis

Table 1.7 Clinically important cytokines grouped by effect on immune or inflammatory responses, to show source and site of action

Cytokines	Action	CONSEQUENCES OF GENE DELETION*
(a) Promotion of non-specific immunity and inflammation		
Interleukin-1 (IL-1)	(see Table 1.6)	
Interleukin-6 (IL-6)	Growth and differentiation of T, B and haematopoietic cells Production of acute-phase proteins by liver cells	↓Acute-phase response
Interleukin-8 (now CXCL8)	Chemotaxis and activation of neutrophils, and other leucocytes	
Interferon-α (IFN-α)	Antiviral action by: activation of natural killer (NK) cells, up-regulation of MHC class I antigens on virally infected cells, inhibition of viral replication	
Interleukin-5 (IL-5)	Activation of B cells, especially for IgE production Activation of eosinophils	
Tumour necrosis factor (TNF)	Promotion of inflammation by: activation of neutrophils, endothelial cells, lymphocytes, liver cells (to produce acute-phase proteins) Interferes with catabolism in muscle and fat (resulting in cachexia)	Deletion of gene for TNF receptor leads to ↓Resistance to endotoxic shock ↑Susceptibility to infections
Interferon-γ (IFN-γ)	Activation of macrophages, endothelial cells and NK cells Increased expression of MHC class I and class II molecules in many tissues; inhibits allergic reactions (↓IgE production)	↑Susceptibility to intracellular bacterial infection and mycobacteria
(b) Lymphocyte activation, growth and differentiation, i.e. specific immunity		
Interleukin-2 (IL-2)	Proliferation and maturation of T cells, induction of IL-2 receptors and activation of NK cells	Inflammatory bowel disease
Interleukin-4 (IL-4) and interleukin-5 (IL-5)	Induction of MHC class II, Fc receptors and IL-2 receptors on B and T cells Induction of isotype switch in B cells Facilitation of IgE production (mainly IL-4) Activation of macrophages Proliferation of bone marrow precursors	Deletion of IL-4 gene: ↓IgE production Deletion of IL-5 gene: inability to mount allergic response

Cytokine	Function	Knockout phenotype*
Interleukin-12 (IL-12)†	Synergism with IL-2; regulates IFN-γ production / Activation of NK cells	Deletion of IL-12 gene: ↓IFN-γ production
Interleukin-13 (IL-13)	Actions overlap with IL-4, including induction of IgE production / IL-13 receptor acts as a functional receptor for IL-4	
Interleukin-15 (IL-15)	Similar to IL-12	
Interleukin-16 (IL-16)	Chemotaxis and activation of CD4 T cells	
(c) Colony stimulation of bone marrow precursors		
GM-CSF	Stimulates growth of polymorph and mononuclear progenitors	
G-CSF	Stimulates growth of neutrophil progenitors	
M-CSF	Stimulates growth of mononuclear progenitors	
(d) Regulatory cytokines		
Interleukin-10 (IL-10); also called cytokine synthesis inhibitory factor‡	Inhibition of cytokine production / Growth of mast cells	Inflammatory bowel disease
Transforming growth factor-β (TGF-β)	Anti-inflammatory / Inhibits cell growth	Lethal inflammatory phenotype
(e) Chemokines		
Interleukin-8 (IL-8)	See under section (a)	
RANTES (regulated on activation, normal T cell expressed and secreted)	Chemoattractant for eosinophils, monocytes	
Monocyte chemotactic protein (MCP 1, 2, 3)	Chemoattractant for monocytes	
Eotaxin	Chemoattractant for eosinophils; synergistic with IL-5	↓Recruitment of eosinophils into tissues following antigen challenge

*Evidence from murine models. See appendix for web address for update on knockout mice.
†IL-12 family of cytokines includes IL-23 and IL-27.
‡IL-10 family includes IL-19, IL-20 and IL-22.

small molecule size (8–10 kDa), which are able to diffuse from the site of production to form a concentration gradient along which granulocytes and lymphocytes can migrate towards the stimulus. The migration of leucocytes to sites of inflammation differs from that of differentiating cells moving to a specific site for activation (see section 1.2.5), although chemokines are involved in both. There are therefore two main types: the inflammatory chemokines (CXC) coded for by genes on chromosome 17 and attractants for granulocytes, and the homeostatic chemokines acting as attractants for lymphocytes (CC) and coded by genes on chromosome 4. The corresponding receptors on inflammatory cells are designated CXCR on neutrophils and CCR on lymphocytes; of course, there are exceptions!

Molecules for lysis and killing

The other major sets of effector molecules are the cytolytic molecules, though less is known about their diversity or mechanisms of action. They include **perforin** in CD8 T cells and in NK cells, as well as **granzymes**, enzymes that induce apoptosis in target cells (Table 1.5). Macrophages and polymorphonuclear leucocytes also contain many substances for the destruction of ingested microbes, some of which have multiple actions, such as TNF. The duplication of many of the functions of this essential phylogenetically ancient protein during evolution underlines the continued development of mammalian immunity to keep up with microbial invaders.

1.2.5 Receptors for effector functions

Without **specific cytokine receptors** on the surface of the cells for which cytokines play an important role in activation, cytokines are ineffective; this has been demonstrated in those primary immune deficiencies in which gene mutations result in absence or non-functional receptors, such as the commonest X-linked form of severe combined immune deficiency (see Chapter 3), IL-12 receptor or IFN-γ receptor deficiencies (see Chapter 3). Some cytokines may have unique receptors but many others share a common structural chain, such as the γ-chain in the receptors for IL-2, IL-4, IL-7, IL-9, IL-15 and IL-23, suggesting that *these arose from a common gene originally*. There are other structurally similar cytokine receptors, leading to the classification of these receptors into five families of similar types of receptors, many of which have similar or identical functions, providing a safety net (redundancy) for their functions, which are crucial for both immune systems.

Less is known at present about **chemokine receptors** (see above). These receptors are sometimes called differentiation 'markers', as they become expressed as an immune reaction progresses and cells move in inflammatory responses.

Receptors for the Fc portions of immunoglobulin molecules (FcR) are important for effector functions of phago-

cytic cells and NK cells. There are at least **three types of Fcγ receptors**; FcRγI are high-affinity receptors on macrophages and neutrophils that bind monomeric IgG for phagocytosis, FcRγII are low-affinity receptors for phagocytosis on macrophages and neutrophils and for feedback inhibition on B cells, and FcRγIII on NK cells as mentioned above. There are also FcRn involved in the transfer of IgG across the placenta (see Chapter 18, Pregnancy); these receptors are also involved in IgG catabolism. IgE receptors are found on mast cells, basophils and eosinophils for triggering degranulation of these cells, but the role of IgA receptors remains unsure.

Complement receptors for fragments of C3 produced during complement activation (see section 1.4.b) also provide a mechanism for phagocytosis and are found on macrophages and neutrophils. However, there are several types of **complement receptors**: those on red blood cells for transport of immune complexes for clearance (CR1), those on B cells and dendritic cells in lymph nodes to trap antigen to stimulate a secondary immune response (CR2) (see section 1.4.3), those on macrophages, neutrophils and NK cells to provide adhesion of these mobile blood cells to endothelium, prior to movement into tissues (CR3).

1.2.6 Adhesion molecules

Adhesion molecules comprise another set of cell surface glycoproteins that play a pivotal role in the immune response by **mediating cell-to-cell adhesion**, as well as adhesion between cells and extracellular matrix proteins. Adhesion molecules are grouped into two major families: (i) integrins and (ii) selectins (Table 1.8). The migration of leucocytes to sites of inflammation is dependent on three key sequential steps mediated by adhesion molecules (Fig. 1.13): rolling of leucocytes along activated endothelium is selectin dependent, tight adhesion of leucocytes to endothelium is integrin dependent and transendothelial migration occurs under the influence of chemokines. Cytokines also influence the selectin and integrin-dependent phases.

Integrins are heterodimers composed of non-covalently associated α and β subunits. Depending on the structure of the β subunit, integrins are subdivided into five families (β_1 to β_5 integrins). β_1 and β_2 integrins play a key role in leucocyte–endothelial interaction. β_1 integrins mediate lymphocyte and monocyte binding to the endothelial adhesion receptor called vascular cell adhesion molecule (VCAM-1). β_2 integrins share a common β chain (CD18) that pairs with a different α chain (CD11a, b, c) to form three separate molecules (CD11a CD18, CD11b CD18, CD11c CD18) and also mediate strong binding of leucocytes to the endothelium. β_3 to β_5 integrins mediate cell adhesion to extracellular matrix proteins such as fibronectin and vitronectin.

The **selectin** family is composed of three glycoproteins designated by the prefixes E (endothelial), L (leucocyte) and

Table 1.8 Examples of clinically important adhesion molecules.

Adhesion molecule	Ligand	Clinical relevance of interaction	Consequences of defective expression
β₁ integrin family VLA-4 (CD49d–CD29) expressed on lymphocytes, monocytes	VCAM-1 on activated endothelium	Mediates tight adhesion between lymphocytes, monocytes and endothelium	? Impaired migration of lymphocytes and monocytes into tissue. Defective expression of either β_1 integrins or VCAM-1 has not yet been described in humans
β₂ integrin family CD18/CD11 expressed on leucocytes	ICAM-1 on endothelium	Mediates tight adhesion between *all* leucocytes and endothelium	Defective expression of CD18/CD11 is associated with severe immunodeficiency, characterized by marked neutrophil leucocytosis, recurrent bacterial and fungal infection, and poor neutrophil migration into sites of infection
Selectin family E-selectin (CD62E) expressed on activated endothelial cells	Sialyl Lewis X (CD15) on neutrophils, eosinophils	Mediates transient adhesion and rolling of leucocytes on monocytes	Defective expression of CD15 is associated with severe endothelium immunodeficiency — clinical features similar to CD18 deficiency. Mice deficient in both E- & P-selectin exhibit a similar clinical phenotype
L-selectin (CD62L) expressed on all leucocytes	CD34, Gly CAM on high endothelial venules	L-selectin mediates transient adhesion and rolling of leucocytes in lymph nodes, and also acts as a homing molecule directing lymphocytes into lymph nodes	L-selectin-deficient mice exhibit reduced leucocyte rolling and impaired lymphocyte homing.

VLA, very late activation antigen; VCAM, vascular cell adhesion molecule; ICAM, intercellular adhesion molecule.

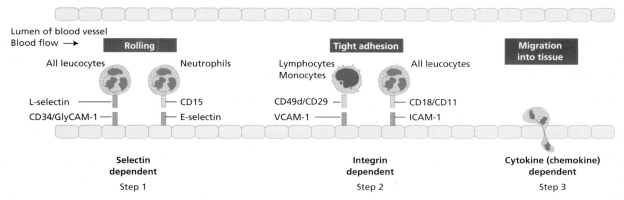

Fig. 1.13 Adhesion molecules and leucocyte–endothelial interactions.

P (platelet) to denote the cells on which they were first described. Selectins bind avidly to carbohydrate molecules on leucocytes and endothelial cells and regulate the homing of the cells to sites of inflammation.

1.3 Functional basis of innate responses

The aim of an immune response is to destroy foreign antigens, whether these are inert molecules or invading organisms. To reach the site of invasion, the components of the immune systems have to know where to go and to how to breach the normal barriers, i.e. the endothelial cells of the vascular system. Humoral factors (such as antibodies and complement) are carried in the blood and enter tissues following an increase in permeability associated with **inflammation**. Immune cells (innate and antigen specific) are actively attracted to a site of inflammation and enter the tissues via specific sites using active processes of adhesion.

Non-specific factors are older, in evolutionary terms, than antibody production and antigen-specific T cells. The major cells involved in the innate system are phagocytic cells (macrophages and polymorphonuclear leucocytes), which remove antigens including bacteria. The major humoral components of the four complement pathways can either directly destroy an organism or initiate/facilitate its phagocytosis. Dendritic cells recognize pathogens (section 1.4.1).

1.3.1 Endothelial cells

The endothelium forms a highly active cell layer lining the inside of blood vessels and thus pervades all tissues. In addition to the critical role in maintaining vasomotor tone, the **endothelium** is closely involved in inflammation, wound healing and the formation of new blood vessels (angiogenesis). Immunologically, endothelial cells are intimately involved in interactions with leucocytes, prior to their exit from the circulation to enter sites of tissue damage (Fig. 1.13). The endothelium also plays an important role in regulating the turnover of IgG, through the presence of FcRn, a receptor that prevents IgG from undergoing lysosomal degradation (see sections 1.2.4 and 7.4). The immunological importance of the endothelium is summarized in Box 1.4.

1.3.2 Neutrophil polymorphonuclear leucocytes

Neutrophils are short-lived cells that play a major role in the body's defence against acute infection. They synthesize and express adhesion receptors so they can adhere to, and

---

BOX 1.4 IMMUNOLOGICAL IMPORTANCE OF THE ENDOTHELIUM

- Expresses a wide range of molecules on the cell surface (E-selectin, ICAM-1, VCAM-1, complement receptors) and thus plays a critical role in leucocyte–endothelial interactions (Fig. 1.13).
- Major site of IgG turnover.
- Forms important component of the innate immune response by expressing Toll-like receptors.
- Capable of antigen presentation.

---

migrate out of, blood vessels into the tissues. They move in response to **chemotactic agents** produced at the site of inflammation; substances include CXCL8, complement-derived factors (such as C3a and C5a), kallikrein, cytokines released by TH1 cells and chemotactic factors produced by mast cells.

Neutrophils are **phagocytic** cells. They are at their most efficient when entering the tissues. Morphologically, the process of phagocytosis is similar in both neutrophils and macrophages. Neutrophils are also able to kill and degrade the substances that they ingest. This requires a considerable amount of energy and is associated with a 'respiratory burst' of oxygen consumption, increased hexose monophosphate shunt activity and superoxide production.

1.3.3 Macrophages

Macrophages and their circulating precursors, monocytes, represent the mononuclear phagocytic system. Lymphocytes and macrophages are derived from closely related stem cells in the bone marrow (Fig. 1.1); each cell lineage has a different colony-stimulating factor and, once differentiated, they have entirely different functions. Whilst most polymorphonuclear leucocytes develop in the bone marrow and emerge only when mature, **macrophages differentiate** in the tissues, principally in subepithelial interstitia and lymphatic sinuses in liver, spleen and lymph nodes, sites where antigens gain entry. Monocytes circulate for only a few hours before entering the tissues, where they may live for weeks or months as mature macrophages. Tissue macrophages are heterogeneous in appearance, in metabolism and also in function; they include freely mobile alveolar and peritoneal macrophages, fixed Kupffer cells in the liver and those lining the sinusoids of the spleen. When found in other tissues, they are called histiocytes.

A major function of the mononuclear phagocyte system is to phagocytose invading organisms and other antigens. Macrophages have prominent lysosomal granules containing acid hydrolases and other degradative enzymes with which to destroy phagocytosed material. The material may be an engulfed viable organism, a dead cell, debris, an antigen or an immune complex. In order to carry out their functions effectively, macrophages must be 'activated'; in this state, they show increased **phagocytic and killing** activity. Stimuli include cytokines (see above), substances which bind to other surface receptors (such as IgG:Fc receptors, Toll-like receptors for endotoxin and other microbial components, receptors for bacterial polysaccharides and for soluble inflammatory mediators such as C5a (see Fig. 1.14). Activation may result in release of monokines (cytokines from monocytes) such as TNF or IL-1, which may cause further damage in already inflamed tissues.

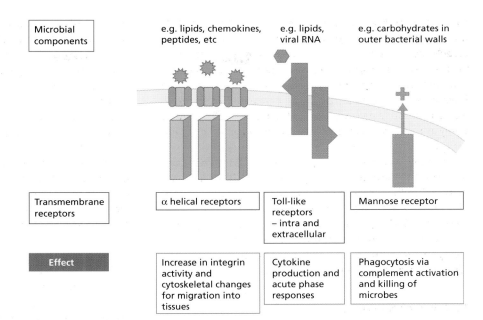

Fig. 1.14 Receptors and functions of mononuclear phagocytic cells.

Monocytes are also the **precursors of dendritic cells**, important for the processing of antigen to other cells of the immune system (section 1.4.1).

1.3.4 Complement

The complement system consists of a series of heat-labile serum proteins that are activated in turn. The components normally exist as soluble inactive precursors; once activated, a complement component may then act as an enzyme (Fig. 1.15), which cleaves several molecules of the next component in the sequence (rather like the clotting cascade). Each precursor is cleaved into two or more fragments. The **major**

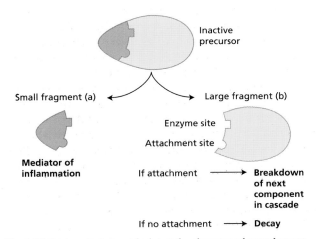

Fig. 1.15 Basic principle underlying the cleavage of complement components.

fragment has two biologically active sites: one for binding to cell membranes or the triggering complex and the other for enzymatic cleavage of the next complement component (Fig. 1.16). Control of the sequence involves spontaneous decay of any exposed attachment sites and specific inactivation by complement inhibitors. **Minor fragments** (usually prefixed 'a') generated by cleavage of components have important biological properties in the fluid phase, such as chemotactic activity.

The history of the discovery of the complement pathways has made the terminology confusing. Several of the components have numbers, but they are not necessarily activated in numerical order; the numbering coincides with the order of their discovery and not with their position in the sequence. Activated components are shown with a bar over the number of the component (e.g. C1 is activated to C1̄) and fragments of activated components by letters after the number (e.g. C3 is split initially into two fragments C3a and C3b).

The major purpose of the complement pathways is to provide a means of removing or destroying antigen, regardless of whether or not it has become coated with antibody (Fig. 1.16). The **lysis** of whole invading microorganisms is a dramatic example of the activity of the complete sequence of complement activation, but it is not necessarily its most important role. The key function of complement is probably the **opsonization** of microorganisms and immune complexes; microorganisms coated (i.e. opsonized) with immunoglobulin and/or complement are more easily recognized by macrophages and more readily bound and phagocytosed through IgG:Fc and C3b receptors.

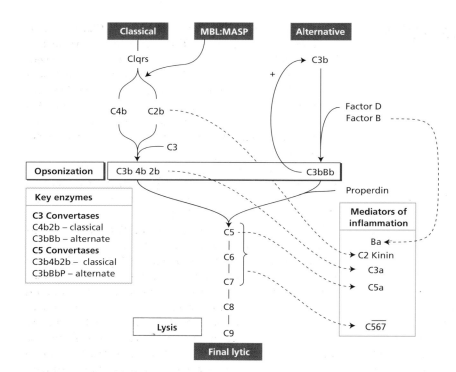

Fig. 1.16 Functions of complement pathways. MBL, Mannan-binding lectin; MASP, MBL-associated serine protease.

Similarly, immune complexes are opsonized by their activation of the classical complement pathway (see below); individuals who lack one of the classical pathway components suffer from immune complex diseases. Soluble complexes are **transported** in the circulation from the inflammatory site by erythrocytes bearing CR1 which bind to the activated C3 (C3b) in the immune complex. Once in the spleen or liver, these complexes are removed from the red cells, which are then recycled (Fig. 1.17).

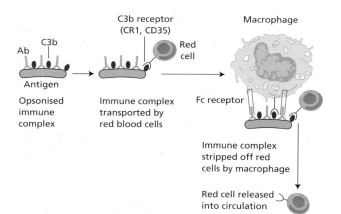

Fig. 1.17 Transport of immune complexes by erythrocytes to macrophages in liver and spleen.

Minor complement fragments are generated at almost every step in the cascade and contribute to the **inflammatory response**. Some increase vascular permeability (C3a), while others attract neutrophils and macrophages for subsequent opsonization and phagocytosis (C5a) (Fig. 1.16). C5a not only promotes leucocytosis in the bone marrow, but mobilizes and attracts neutrophils to the inflammatory site where it increases their adhesiveness; it also up-regulates complement receptors CR1 and CR3 on neutrophils and macrophages to maximize phagocytosis.

Complement **activation** occurs in two phases: activation of the C3 component, followed by activation of the 'attack' or lytic sequence. The critical step is a cleavage of C3 by complement-derived enzymes termed 'C3 convertases'. The cleavage of C3 is achieved by three routes, the classical, alternative and lectin pathways, all of which can generate C3 convertases but in response to different stimuli (Fig. 1.18). The pivotal role of C3 in complement activation is underlined by patients with a deficiency of C3, who cannot opsonize pathogens or immune complexes, predisposing them to bacterial infection as well as immune complex diseases.

The **classical pathway** was the first to be described. It is activated by a number of substances, the most widely recognized being antigen–antibody complexes where the antibody is either IgM or IgG (Fig. 1.18). The reaction of IgM or IgG with its antigen causes a conformational change in the Fc region of the antibody to reveal a binding site for the first component in the classical pathway, C1q. C1q is a re-

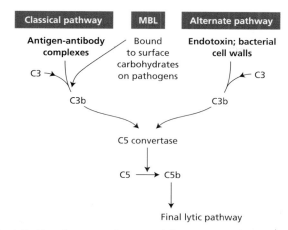

Fig. 1.18 Complement pathways and their initiating factors. MBL, Mannan-binding lectin.

markable, collagen-like protein composed of six subunits, resembling a 'bunch of tulips' when seen under the electron microscope. C1q reacts with Fc via its globular heads; attachment by two critically spaced binding sites is needed for activation. The Fc regions of pentameric IgM are so spaced that one IgM molecule can activate C1q; in contrast, IgG is relatively inefficient because the chance of two randomly sited IgG molecules being the critical distance apart to activate C1q is relatively low. IgA, IgD and IgE do not activate the classical pathway.

Once C1q is activated, C1r and C1s are **sequentially bound** to generate enzyme activity (C1 esterase) for C4 and C2 (see Fig. 1.16), splitting both molecules into a and b fragments. The complex $\overline{C4b2b}$ is the classical pathway C3 convertase. Other fragments released are C4a, C2a and a vasoactive peptide released from C2. $\overline{C4b2b}$ cleaves C3 into two fragments, C3a possessing anaphylotoxic and chemotactic activity and C3b that binds to the initiating complex and promotes many of the biological properties of complement. The $\overline{C4b2b3b}$ complex so generated is an enzyme, C5 convertase, which initiates the final lytic pathway (the 'attack' sequence).

The **alternative pathway** is phylogenetically older than the classical pathway. It is relatively inefficient in the tissues, and high concentrations of the various components are required. The central reaction in this pathway, as in the classical one, is the activation of C3, but the alternate pathway generates a C3 convertase without the need for antibody, C1, C4 or C2. Instead, the most important activators are bacterial cell walls and endotoxin (Fig. 1.18).

The initial **cleavage** of C3 in the alternative pathway happens continuously and **spontaneously** (see Fig. 1.18), generating a low level of C3b. C3b is an unstable substance and, if a suitable acceptor surface is not found, the attachment site in C3b decays rapidly and the molecule becomes inactive. If,

however, an acceptor surface is nearby, the C3b molecules can bind and remain active. C3b is then able to use factors D and B of the alternate pathway to produce the active enzyme 'C3bBb'. This latter substance has two properties. It can break down more C3, providing still more C3b; this is known as the 'positive feedback loop' of the alternative pathway (Fig. 1.16). Alternatively, C3bBb becomes stabilized in the presence of properdin to form the C5 convertase of the alternate pathway.

There are thus two ways of producing **C5 convertase**. In the classical pathway, C5 convertase is made up of C3b, C4b and C2b, while in the alternate pathway it is produced by C3b, Bb and properdin (Fig. 1.16).

The third pathway of complement activation is initiated by **mannan-binding lectin**, MBL (also known as mannan-binding protein), a surface receptor (see Fig. 1.16) shed into the circulation, binding avidly to carbohydrates on the surface of microorganisms. MBL is a member of the collectin family of C-type lectins, which also includes pulmonary surfactant proteins, A and D. MBL is structurally related to C1q and activates complement through a serine protease known as MASP (MBL-associated serine protease), similar to C1r and C1s of the classical pathway. Inherited deficiency of MASP-2 has recently been shown to predispose to recurrent pneumococcal infections and immune complex diseases.

The **final lytic** pathway ('attack' sequence) of complement involves the sequential attachment of the components C5, C6, C7, C8 and C9 and results in lysis of the target cell such as an invading organism or a virally infected cell. The lytic pathway complex binds to the cell membrane and a transmembrane channel is formed. This can be seen by electron microscopy as a hollow, thin-walled cylinder through which salts and water flow, leading to the uptake of water by a cell, swelling and destruction. During the final lytic pathway, complement fragments are broken off. C5a and the activated complex $\overline{C567}$ are both potent mediators of inflammation. C5a, along with C3a, are anaphylotoxins, i.e. cause histamine release from mast cells with a resulting increase in vascular permeability. C5a also has the property of being able to attract neutrophils to the site of complement activation (i.e. it is chemotactic) (see Fig. 1.16).

The **control of any cascade sequence** is extremely important, particularly when it results in the production of potentially self-damaging mediators of inflammation. The complement pathway is controlled by three mechanisms (see Box 1.5).

These mechanisms ensure that the potentially harmful effects of complement activation remain confined to the initiating antigen without damaging autologous (host) cells. Table 1.9 lists some of the clinically important complement regulatory proteins. When considering their role in pathology, there are important caveats (see Box 1.5).

Table 1.9 Proteins controlling classical and alternative complement pathways*

Protein	Function	Clinical consequences of DEFICIENCY
Circulating inhibitors		
C1 esterase inhibitor	Binds to activated C1r, C1s uncoupling it from C1q	Uncontrolled activation of classical pathway leading to hereditary angioneurotic oedema
Factor H	Binds C3b displacing Bb; cofactor for factor I	Acquired C3 deficiency leading to recurrent bacterial infection
Factor I	Serine protease that cleaves C3b; acts synergistically with factor H	As for factor H
Membrane inhibitors		
Complement receptor 1 (CR1; CD35)	Receptor for C3b	Protect mammalian cells. Low CR1 numbers on red cells in SLE is a consequence of fast turnover
Decay accelerating factor (DAF; CD55)	Accelerates decay of C3b Bb by displacing Bb	DAF deficiency alone does not cause disease
Protectin (CD59)	Inhibits formation of lytic pathway complex on homologous cells; widely expressed on cell membranes	In combination with DAF deficiency leads to paroxysmal nocturnal haemoglobinuria (see Chapter 16)

SLE, Systemic lupus erythematosus.
*This is not an exhaustive list.

BOX 1.5 PHYSIOLOGICAL CONTROL OF COMPLEMENT

1 A number of the activated components are inherently unstable; if the next protein in the pathway is not immediately available, the active substance decays.

2 There are also a number of specific inhibitors, for example C1 esterase inhibitor, factor I and factor H.

3 There are, on cell membranes, proteins that increase the rate of breakdown of activated complement components.

These mechanisms ensure that the potentially harmful effects of complement activation remain confined to the initiating antigen without damaging autologous (host) cells. Table 1.9 lists some of the clinically important complement regulatory proteins.

1.3.5 Antibody-dependent cell-mediated cytotoxicity

ADCC is a mechanism by which antibody-coated target cells are destroyed by cells bearing **low-affinity FcγRIII receptors** (NK cells, monocytes, neutrophils) (see section 1.2.4) (Fig. 1.19), without involvement of the MHC. Clustering of several IgG molecules is required to trigger these low-affinity receptors to bind, resulting in secretion of IFN-γ and discharge of granules containing perforin and granzymes, as found in cytotoxic T cells. The overall importance of ADCC in host defence is unclear, but it represents an additional mechanism by which bacteria and viruses can be eliminated.

1.3.6 Natural killer cells

NK cells look like large granular lymphocytes. They can kill target cells, even in the absence of any antibody or antigenic stimulation. The name '**natural killer**' reflects the fact that, unlike the adaptive system, they do not need prior activation but have the relevant recognition molecules on their surfaces already. Non-specific agents, such as mitogens, IFN-γ and IL-12, can activate them further. NK cells form an integral part of the early host response to viral infection (Fig. 1.20). The exact mechanisms by which NK cells distinguish between infected and non-infected cells is not clear

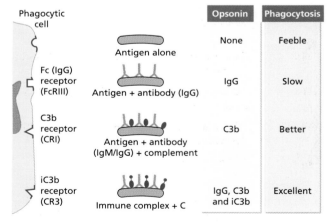

Fig. 1.19 Opsonins and the relationship to phagocytosis.

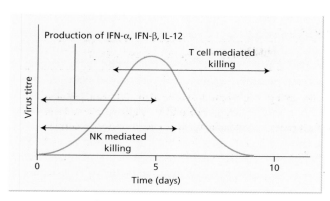

Fig. 1.20 Role of natural killer cells in early immune response to virus infection.

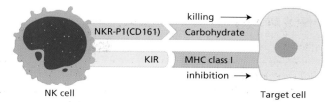

Fig. 1.21 Natural killer (NK) cell recognition of target cells. NK cell killing is mediated by engagement of the receptor NKR-P1 with its carbohydrate ligand on the target cell. This is inhibited by the interaction between the inhibitory receptor (KIR) and MHC class I on the target cell.

but is likely to involve **cell-surface receptors** (Fig. 1.21). NK cells express two types of surface receptor (see section 1.2.2). Expression of MHC class I proteins by most normal cells prevents NK cells from killing healthy cells. Interference with this inhibition, by virally induced down-regulation or alteration of MHC class I molecules, results in NK-mediated killing.

NK cells are not immune cells in the strictest sense because, like macrophages, they are not clonally restricted; in addition, they show **little specificity** and they have no memory. The range of their potential targets is broad. Animals and rare patients with deficient NK cell function have an increased incidence of certain tumours and viral infections. A subset of NK cells, NKT cells, are therefore important in 'immune' surveillance against tumours (see p. 25).

1.4 Functional basis of the adaptive immune responses

Antigen-specific effector lymphocytes are of two types: B cells and T cells. B cells are ultimately responsible for antibody production and act as antigen-presenting cells in secondary immune responses. T cells act as effector cells and have several different functional activities (Table 1.10). Other T cells have a regulatory rather than effector role. T-cell functions of help, killing or regulation may depend on different stimuli resulting in different cytokines being produced with predominantly activating or inhibitory effects.

The factors regulating a normal immune response (see later Box 1.7) are complex and include antigen availability, specific suppression by T cells and the balance of cytokines produced (section 1.4.2)

Table 1.10 Lymphocytes involved in adaptive immune responses

Cell type	Function of cell	Product of cell	Function of product
B	Produce antibody Antigen presentation	Antibody	Neutralization Opsonization Cell lysis
TH2	↑B cell antibody production ↑Activated T_C	Cytokines IL-3, -4, -5, -10, -13	Help B and T_C cells
TH1	Inflammation: initiation and augmentation	IL-2, IFN-γ, TNF	Inflammatory mediators
T_R	↓ B cell antibody production ↓Activated T_C	Suppressor factor(s), e.g. TGF-β	Suppress TH and therefore indirectly B and T_C
T_C	Lysis of antigenic target cells	IFN-γ Perforins	Enhances MHC expression Activates NK cells Disrupt target cell membranes
NKT	Target cell killing	IL-4, IFN-γ	

T_C, Cytotoxic T cell; TH1 and TH2, helper T cell types; T_R, regulatory T cell (see text).

1.4.1 Antigen processing

The first stage of an antigen-specific immune response involves capture and modification of that antigen by specialized cells, prior to presentation to the immune cells. *This is not an antigen-specific process, unlike the subsequent restricted binding of antigen to lymphocytes predetermined to react with that antigen only.* Antigen is processed by specialized cells, known as **antigen-processing cells (APCs)**, then carried and 'presented' to lymphocytes. T cells cannot recognize antigen without such processing; since activation of T cells is essential for most immune responses, antigen processing is crucial. The specialized cells involved are dendritic cells (and some macrophages) for a primary immune response and B cells for a secondary immune response when the antigen has been recognized and responded to on a previous occasion.

Dendritic cells are the only cell type whose sole function is to capture, process and present antigen. They are mononuclear cells derived from bone marrow precursors and closely related to monocytes. Immature dendritic cells are ubiquitous, particularly in epithelia that serve as a portal of entry for microbes, where they capture antigens. Subsequently, these activated dendritic cells migrate to draining lymph nodes and mature to become antigen-presenting cells (Fig. 1.22). Immature and mature dendritic cells have different sets of surface proteins (which act as distinct markers), in keeping with their different functions (see Table 1.3).

The interaction between dendritic cells and T cells is strongly influenced by a group of cell surface molecules which function as **co-stimulators**: CD80 (also known as B7-1) and CD86 (B7-2) on the activated dendritic cell, each of which engages with counter receptors on the T-cell surface referred to as CD28 and CTLA-4. A functional co-stimulatory pathway is essential for T-cell activation. In the absence of a co-stimulatory signal, interaction between dendritic cells and T cells leads to T-cell unresponsiveness (Fig. 1.23). The importance of the co-stimulatory pathway is underlined by the ability of antagonists to co-stimulatory molecules to interrupt immune responses both in vitro and in vivo. This observation has been exploited therapeutically in mice with advanced lupus, in which treatment with a CTLA-4 antagonist leads to significant improvement in disease activity.

Processed antigen is presented to T cells alongside the MHC class II antigens on the APC surface, since T cells do not recognize processed antigen alone. The most efficient APCs are the **interdigitating dendritic cells** found in the T-cell regions of a lymph node (Figs 1.22 and 1.31). Such cells have high concentrations of MHC class I and II molecules, co-stimulatory molecules (CD80, CD86) as well as adhesion molecules on their surfaces (Table 1.3) and limited enzymatic powers, which enable antigen processing but not complete digestion. Being mobile, they are able to capture antigen in the periphery and migrate to secondary lymphoid organs where they differentiate into mature dendritic cells and interact with naive T cells. These cells are known as Langerhans cells when present in the skin.

These cells differ from the **follicular dendritic cells** in the follicular germinal centre (B-cell area) of a lymph node (see Figs 1.22 and 1.31). Follicular dendritic cells have receptors for complement and immunoglobulin components and their function is to trap immune complexes and to feed them

				Present to:
Interdigitating dendritic cells	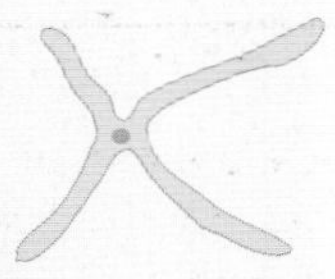	Paracortex of lymph node	Mobile	T cells
Langerhans' cells		Skin	Mobile	T cells
Veiled cells		Lymph	Mobile	T cells
Follicular dendritic cells	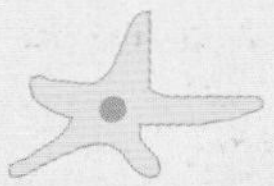	Lymph node follicles	Static	B cells
Macrophages	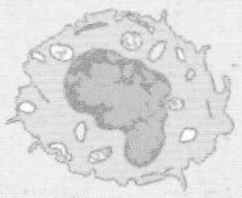	Lymph node medulla Liver (Kupffer cells) Brain (astrocytes)	Mobile Static Static	T and B cells
B cell (especially if activated)	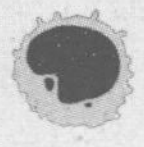	Lymphoid tissue	Mobile	T cells

Fig. 1.22 Antigen-presenting cells and their surface molecules

* Appears on activation

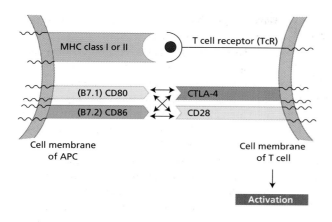

Fig. 1.23 Role of co-stimulatory pathway in T-cell activation.

to B cells in the germinal centre. This is part of the secondary immune response, since pre-existing antibodies are used, accounting for B-cell memory. **Activated B cells** themselves are also able to present antigen (Fig. 1.22).

1.4.2 T cell-mediated responses

T-cell help
T-cell help is always antigen-specific. Only helper T cells, which have responded to antigen previously presented in the context of MHC class II, can subsequently help those B cells already committed to the same antigen (Burnet's clonal selection theory). **Helper T cells** recognize both antigen and MHC class II antigens as a complex on the presenting cells. They then recognize the same combination of antigen and the particular class II antigen on the corresponding B cell. **Co-stimulation** is essential for T-cell activation and accessory molecules are vital (Fig .1.23).

MHC class II molecules play an important role in the activation of helper T cells. T cells from one individual will not cooperate with the APCs and B cells from a different person (i.e. of different HLA type). Certain MHC class II molecules on the presenting cells fail to interact with some antigens (as a prelude to triggering helper T cells) and so fail to trigger an adaptive immune response. This provides a mechanism for the **genetic regulation of immune responses** (originally attributed to distinct immune response genes). The MHC class II molecules thus determine the responsiveness of an individual to a particular foreign antigen, since they interact with the antigen before T-cell help can be triggered.

When helper T cells meet an antigen for the first time, there is a limited number that can react with that antigen to provide help for B cells; these T cells therefore undergo blast transformation and **proliferation**, providing an increased number of specific helper T cells when the animal is re-exposed, i.e. an expanded clone. The immune response

on second and subsequent exposure is quicker and more vigorous.

Two other mechanisms also help to improve efficiency. **Memory T cells** (which bear the surface marker CD45RO) have increased numbers of adhesion molecules (LFA-1, CD2, LFA-3, ICAM-1) (see section 1.2.6) as well as a higher proportion of high-affinity receptors for the relevant antigen. Memory cells are therefore easily activated and produce high concentrations of IL-2 to recruit more helper T cells of both types, TH1 and TH2 (see below). Thus T-cell memory is a combination of an increase of T cells (quantitative) as well as a qualitative change in the efficiency of those T cells.

Antigen-specific cell-mediated effector responses are carried out by T lymphocytes. T cells can lyse cells expressing specific antigens (cytotoxicity), release cytokines that trigger inflammation (delayed hypersensitivity) or regulate immune responses (regulation). **Distinct T-cell populations** mediate these types of T-cell responses: CD8$^+$ T$_C$ cytotoxic cells, CD4$^+$ T$_H$1 cells and CD4$^+$CD25$^+$T$_R$ cells (see below).

T helper cells
Helper T cells are grouped into two distinct subgroups depending on their cytokine profile. T$_H$1 cells secrete TNF and IFN-γ and consequently mediate cellular immunity. In contrast, T$_H$2 cells predominantly secrete IL-4, IL-5, IL-10 and IL-13 (Fig. 1.24) and are responsible for stimulating vigorous antibody production by B cells. T cells expressing cytokine profiles common to **both T$_H$1 and T$_H$2** cells are designated T$_H$0. It is unclear how a naive T cell selects which cytokine profile to secrete, but there is evidence to suggest that exposure to certain cytokines is an important influence. Exposure to IL-4 and IL-6 stimulates development of T$_H$2 cells while IL-12 and IFN-γ result in a developing T cell acquiring T$_H$1 properties. Recent evidence suggests that CD8 T cells are also capable of secreting cytokine profiles typical of T$_H$1 or T$_H$2 cells.

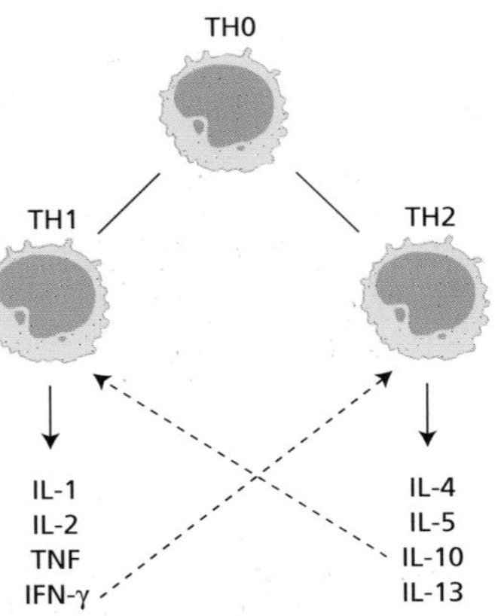

Fig. 1.24 T helper cells and their cytokine profiles; broken arrows indicate inhibition.

In humans, a T_H1 cytokine profile is essential for protection against intracellular pathogens, while a T_H2 cytokine profile is associated with diseases characterized by overproduction of antibodies including IgE. The clinical consequences of inducing a **particular T_H response** are strikingly illustrated in patients with leprosy, an infectious disease caused by Mycobacterium leprae, an intracellular bacterium. Patients who mount a protective T_H1 response develop only limited disease (tuberculoid leprosy), since their macrophages are able to control M. leprae efficiently. In contrast, patients who produce a predominant T_H2 response develop disabling lepromatous leprosy, since antibody is ineffective in tackling an intracellular pathogen.

T cells for inflammation

Delayed-type hypersensitivity (DTH) reactions are mediated by specific T cells that produce T_H1-type cytokines on exposure to antigen. The tuberculin test (Mantoux test) is a good example of a DTH response. Individuals who have previously been infected with Mycobacterium tuberculosis mount a T-cell response that evolves over 24–72 h following intradermal injection of tuberculin. This is clinically manifest as local swelling and induration; biopsy of the site reveals T-cell and macrophage infiltration. The histology of tissue granulomas in tuberculosis and sarcoidosis are further examples of DTH. Like the induction of T-cell help, the induction of **delayed hypersensitivity** varies with MHC polymorphism.

T cell lysis

CD8+ cytotoxic T cells lyse cells infected with virus and possibly those tumour cells with recognizable tumour antigens too. Such cytotoxicity is antigen specific and only cells expressing the relevant viral proteins on their surfaces are killed (see Fig. 1.5), so obeying the rules of the clonal selection theory. Since infected cells express surface viral proteins

prior to the assembly of new virus particles and viral budding, **cytotoxic T cells** are important in the recovery phase of an infection, destroying the infected cells before new virus particles are generated.

In contrast to helper T cells, cytotoxic T cells recognize viral antigens together with MHC class I molecules on both dendritic cells for activation and target cells for effector function. They show exquisite specificity for self-MHC molecules, in that they can lyse only cells expressing the same MHC class I molecules. MHC class I molecules may affect the **strength of the effector cytotoxic T-cell response** to a particular virus, providing a further strong selective stimulus for the evolution of a polymorphic MHC system. All endogenous antigens (including viral antigens) are presented in the context of MHC class I antigens (see Fig. 1.7). This combination on the dendritic cells directly activates CD8+ T cells and provides the appropriate target cells for virally induced T-cell cytotoxicity as well as mechanisms for graft rejection and tumour surveillance. Their relevance to transplantation is discussed in Chapter 8.

Regulatory T cells

After initial scepticism in the 1980s regarding the existence of suppressor T cells (re-named regulatory T cells), there is now good evidence to support the presence of a subset of CD4+ T cells (T_R) with a distinct phenotype (**CD4+, CD25+**) which play a key role in immunoregulation by dampening down a wide range of immune responses, including responses to self-antigens, alloantigens, tumour antigens as well as to pathogens.

Regulatory T cells develop from a **distinct lineage** of thymic T cells and are responsible for the maintenance of peripheral tolerance by actively suppressing the activation and expansion of self-reactive T cells. It is thought that T_R cells act by producing immunosuppressive cytokines such as transforming growth factor-β and IL-10, as well as through direct cell-to-cell contact.

The development of CD4+ T_R cells is under the control of a gene called FOXP3 that encodes a transcription repressor protein specifically in CD4+, CD25+ T cells in the thymus as well as in the periphery. Mutations in the FOXP3 gene result in severe autoimmune disease and allergy (see Box 1.6).

BOX 1.6 EVIDENCE THAT CD4+CD25+ T CELLS ARE IMPORTANT IN IMMUNOREGULATION

Depletion of CD4+CD25+ T cells in humans, due to mutations in the FOXP3 gene, is associated with the rare IPEX syndrome—immune dysregulation, polyendocrinopathy, enteropathy, X-linked syndrome—characterized by autoimmune diabetes, inflammatory bowel disease and severe allergy.

NKT cells

A few T cells express some of the markers of NK cells and are therefore known as NKT cells. These cells are not only CD3[+] but have α chains of TCR, with limited diversity, and are able to **recognize lipids** in conjunction with CD1, MHC class I-like molecules of equally limited diversity. Their precise role in immune surveillance is not yet clear.

1.4.3 Antibody production

Antibody production involves at least three types of cell: APCs, B cells and helper T cells (Table 1.10).

B cells

Antibodies are synthesized by B cells, and their mature progeny, plasma cells. B cells are readily recognized because they express **immunoglobulin on their surface**, which acts as the BCR (see section 1.2.2). During development, B cells first show intracellular μ chains and then surface IgM (μ combined with one light chain—κ or λ). These cells are able to switch from production of IgM to one of the other classes as they mature, so that they later express IgM and IgD and, finally, IgG, IgA or IgE, a process known as isotype switching. The final type of surface immunoglobulin determines the class of antibody secreted; surface and secreted immunoglobulin are identical. This immunoglobulin maturation sequence fits with the kinetics of an antibody response; the primary response is mainly IgM and the secondary response predominantly IgG (Fig. 1.25). **Isotype switching** is mediated by the interaction of several important proteins: for example, CD40 on the B-cell surface engages with its ligand (CD40L) on activated T cells (Fig. 1.26), under the influence of IL-4. Deficiency of either molecule (CD40 or CD40L) in mice and humans leads to a severe immunodeficiency characterized by inability to switch from IgM to IgG production with consequently low serum concentrations of IgG and IgA but a normal or even high serum IgM (hence called a hyper-

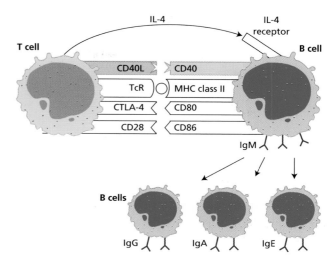

Fig. 1.26 Interaction between CD40L on T cells and CD40 on B cells under the influence of IL-4 leading to isotype switching.

IgM syndrome), poor germinal centre formation and inability to produce memory B cells.

Each B cell is committed to the production of an antibody which has a unique V_H–V_L combination (see section 1.2.4). This uniqueness is the basis of Burnet's clonal selection theory, which states that each B cell expresses a surface immunoglobulin that acts as its antigen-binding site. Contact with antigen and factors released by helper T cells (IL-4, -5, -13) stimulate the B cells to divide and differentiate, generating more antibody-producing cells, all of which make the same antibody with the same V_H–V_L pair. Simultaneously, a population of memory cells is produced which expresses the same surface immunoglobulin receptor. The result of these cell divisions is that a greater number of antigen-specific B cells become available when the animal is exposed to the same antigen at a later date; this is known as **clonal expansion** and helps to account for the increased secondary response.

As well as being quicker and more vigorous (Fig. 1.25), secondary responses are more efficient. This is due to the production of antibodies that bind more effectively to the antigen, i.e. have a higher affinity. There are two reasons for this. First, as antigen is removed by the primary response, the remaining antigen (in low concentration) reacts only with those cells that have high-affinity receptors. Second, the rapid somatic mutation, which accompanies B-cell division in the germinal centre, provides B cells of higher affinity, a process known as '**affinity maturation**'. In the secondary response, these B cells bind preferentially to antigen already bound to antibody and hence the follicular dendritic cell. C3 fragments play a key role in the antibody response by interacting with the co-stimulation receptors on B cells.

A minority subset of B cells will respond directly to antigens called **T-independent antigens** (see section 1.2.1).

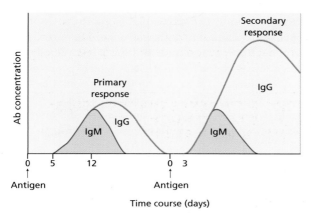

Fig. 1.25 Primary and secondary antibody (Ab) responses.

They have repeating, identical, antigenic determinants and provoke predominantly IgM antibody responses. These responses are relatively short-lived and restricted in specificity and affinity, due to the lack of T-cell involvement. Some T-independent antigens provoke non-specific proliferation of memory B cells and are therefore known as polyclonal B-cell mitogens.

A given B cell is **pre-selected** to produce particular V_H and V_L domains and all the daughter cells of that B cell produce the same V_H and V_L. Initially, the B cell produces intracellular antigen-specific IgM, which then becomes bound to the surface of the cell (surface immunoglobulin) and acts as the antigen receptor for that cell; the B cell is then 'antigen-responsive'. On exposure to that antigen, a committed B cell fixes the isotype (or class) of immunoglobulin that it will produce, and divides; all the progeny produce identical immunoglobulin molecules (known as monoclonal immunoglobulins). Many of these cells then mature into plasma cells, whilst others act as antigen-presenting cells (section 1.4.1) or memory cells.

1.5 Physiological outcomes of immune responses

Once the immune response is initiated, the end result depends on the nature and localization of the antigen, on whether the predominant response has been humoral or cell mediated, on the types of T cells and/or antibodies provoked and whether the augmentation processes have been involved.

1.5.1 Killing of target cells

Target cells killed as a result of an immune response include organisms and cells bearing virally altered or tumour-specific antigens on their surfaces. They may be killed directly by antigen-specific mechanisms such as antibody and complement, ADCC following binding of specific antibody or antigen-specific cytotoxic T cells.

Cytokine production results in activation of NK cells, neutrophils and macrophages and subsequently non-specific killing by mechanisms similar to those in adaptive immunity (see section 1.2.3).

1.5.2 Direct functions of antibody

Although some forms of antibody are good at neutralizing particulate antigens, many other factors, such as the concentration of antigen, the site of antigen entry, the availability of antibody and the speed of the immune response, may influence antigen removal (Box 1.7).

Neutralization is one direct effect of antibody and IgM is particularly good at this. A number of antigens, including diphtheria toxin, tetanus toxin and many viruses, can be neutralized by antibody. Once neutralized, these substances are no longer able to bind to receptors in the tissues; the resulting antigen–antibody complexes are usually removed from the circulation and destroyed by macrophages.

Although the physiological function of IgE antibody is unknown, it may have a role in the expulsion of parasites from the gastrointestinal tract. IgE antibody is normally bound to tissue mast cells. Attachment of antigen to IgE antibodies results in mast cell triggering, and release of a number of mediators of tissue damage (see Fig. 1.27 and Chapter 4).

1.5.3 Indirect functions of antibody

Opsonization is the process by which an antigen becomes coated with substances (such as antibodies or complement) that make it **more easily engulfed** by phagocytic cells. The

---

BOX 1.7 SOME FACTORS AFFECTING IMMUNE RESPONSES

Antigen

- Nature: polysaccharide antigens tend to elicit a predominant IgM + IgG_2 response in contrast to protein antigens, which elicit both cellular and humoral responses.
- Dose: in experimental animals large doses of antigen induce tolerance.
- Route of administration: polio vaccine administered orally elicits a stronger antibody response than intramuscular injection.

Antibody

- Passive administration of antibody can be used to modulate immune responses, e.g. maternal administration of antibodies to the red cell Rh antigen is used to prevent haemolytic disease of the newborn by removing fetal red cells from the maternal circulation.

Cytokines

- Cytokines released by TH1/TH2 lymphocytes influences type of immune response. TH1 cytokines favour development of cellular immunity, while TH2 cytokines favour antibody production.

Genes

- MHC-linked genes control immune responses to specific antigens, e.g. studies in mice have identified strains that are high responders to certain antigens but poor responders to others. This is mirrored in humans by the strong link between certain MHC genes and the development of autoimmune diseases.
- Non-MHC genes may also influence immune responses, e.g. mutations in the recombinase gene responsible for immunoglobulin and T-cell receptor gene rearrangement result in severe combined immunodeficiency in babies.

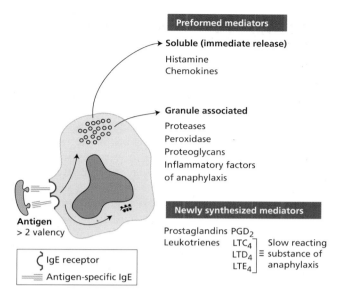

Fig. 1.27 IgE-mediated hypersensitivity.

coating of soluble or particulate antigens with IgG antibodies renders them susceptible to cells that have surface receptors for the Fc portions of IgG (FcRIII) (Fig. 1.19). Neutrophils and macrophages both have these Fc receptors and can phagocytose IgG-coated antigens; however, this process is relatively inefficient if only Fc receptors are involved. The activation of complement by antibody (via the classical pathway) or by bacterial cell walls (via the alternate pathway) generates C3b on the surface of microorganisms and makes them susceptible to binding by several types of C3 receptors on macrophages and neutrophils (see Fig. 1.19). C3 receptors are very efficient in triggering phagocytosis.

1.5.4 Inflammation: a brief overview

Inflammation is defined as increased vascular permeability accompanied by an infiltration of 'inflammatory' cells, initially neutrophil polymorphonuclear leucocytes and later macrophages, lymphocytes and plasma cells. **Vascular permeability** may be increased (resulting in oedema) by a number of agents, which include complement fragments such as C3a, C5a, factor Ba and C2 kinnin. Some fragments (C3a, C5a and $\overline{C567}$) also attract neutrophils and mobilize them from the bone marrow; cytokines generated by activated dendritic cells, T cells and macrophages, such as IL-1, IL-6, TNF and IL-12, have similar properties, as well as activating vasodilation to increase blood flow (resulting in erythema). Inflammatory chemokines also attract a variety of cells to **migrate into tissues**.

The triggering of mast cells via IgE is also a method of causing inflammation, due to release of histamine and leu-

kotrienes (which are quite distinct from cytokines). This is discussed further in Chapter 4.

The inflammatory cytokines (IL-1, IL-6 and TNF) also provoke increased synthesis of particular serum proteins in the liver. The proteins are known as '**acute-phase proteins**' and include proteins that act as mediators (as in opsonization — C3 and C4 complement components, C-reactive protein), enzyme inhibitors (α_1-antitrypsin) or scavengers (haptoglobin); the increased serum concentrations of such proteins are helpful in resolving inflammation. In practical terms, serial measurements of C-reactive protein (CRP) give a useful indication of the extent and persistence of inflammation; since the half-life of CRP is only a few hours, changes in serum levels reflect rapid changes in inflammation (such as after antibiotic therapy) sufficiently quickly to be clinically useful. This is in contrast to fibrinogen [another acute-phase protein and the major factor in the erythrocyte sedimentation rate (ESR)], where changes are much slower.

1.6 Tissue damage caused by the immune system

Unfortunately, the recognition of antigen by antibodies can cause incidental tissue damage as well as the intended destruction of the antigen. Reactions resulting in tissue damage are often called '**hypersensitivity**' reactions; Gell and Coombs defined four types (Table 1.11) and this classification (though arbitrary) is still useful to distinguish types of immunological mechanisms. *Most hypersensitivity reactions are not confined to a single type; they usually involve a mixture of mechanisms.*

Immediate hypersensitivity (type I) reactions are those in which antigen interacts with IgE bound to tissue mast cells or basophils. IgE responses are usually directed against antigens that enter at epithelial surfaces, i.e. inhaled or ingested antigens. IgE production requires helper T cells and is regulated by T-cell-derived cytokines. IL-4 and IL-13 stimulate IgE production, while IFN-γ is inhibitory. The balance between help and suppression depends on many variables, including the route of administration of the antigen, its chemical composition, its physical nature, and whether or not adjuvants were employed and the genetic background of the animal. Following the interaction of cell-surface IgE and allergen, **activation of the mast cell** causes the release of pharmacologically active substances (see Chapter 4). Type I reactions are rapid; for example, if the antigen is injected into the skin, 'immediate hypersensitivity' can be seen within 5–10 min as a 'weal and flare reaction', where the resulting oedema from increased vascular permeability is seen as a weal and the increased blood flow as a flare. In humans, there is a familial tendency towards IgE-mediated hypersensitivity, although the genes related to this 'atopic tendency' do not determine the target organ or the disease. Clinical examples of type I reactions include anaphylactic reactions due to insect venoms, peanuts and drugs, as well as the atopic diseases of hay fever and asthma (see Chapter 4).

Type II reactions are initiated by antibody reacting with antigenic determinants that form **part of the cell membrane**. The consequences of this reaction depend on whether or not complement or accessory cells become involved, and whether the metabolism of the cell is affected (Fig. 1.28). IgM and IgG can be involved in **type II reactions**. The best clinical examples are some organ-specific autoimmune diseases (see Chapter 5), and immune haemolytic anaemias (see Chapter 16) (see Table 1.11).

Although type II reactions are mediated by autoantibodies, T cells are also involved. For example, in Graves' disease, which is known to be due to autoantibodies stimulating thyroid-stimulating hormone (TSH) receptors, specific reactive T cells are present also. It is not clear whether T cells are only instrumental in promoting antibody production (primary effect) or whether sensitization is **secondary to tissue damage**. In contrast, the autoreactive T cells cloned from patients with rheumatoid arthritis and multiple sclerosis have a **primary role** in tissue damage.

Type III reactions result from the presence of immune complexes in the circulation or in the tissues. Localization of **immune complexes** depends on their size, their charge, and the nature of the antigen and the local concentration of complement. If they accumulate in the tissues in large quantities, they may activate complement and accessory cells and produce extensive tissue damage. A classic example is the Arthus reaction, where an antigen is injected into the skin of an animal that has been previously sensitized. The reaction of preformed antibody with this antigen results in high concentrations of local immune complexes; these cause complement activation and neutrophil attraction and result in local inflammation 6–24 h after the injection. Serum sickness is another example: in this condition, urticaria, arthralgia and glomerulonephritis occur about 10 days after initial exposure to the antigen. This is the time when maximum amounts of IgG antibody, produced in response to antigen stimulation, react with remaining antigen to form circulating, soluble immune complexes (Fig. 1.29). As these damaging complexes are formed, the antigen concentration is rapidly lowered; the process only continues as long as the antigen persists and thus is usually self-limiting. Further clinical examples include systemic lupus erythematosus (SLE) (see Chapter 5), glomerulonephritis (see Chapter 9) and extrinsic allergic alveolitis (see Chapter 13).

Type IV reactions are initiated by T cells which react with antigen and release T_H1 cytokines. Cytokines attract other cells, particularly macrophages, which in turn liberate lysosomal enzymes. Histologically, the resultant acute lesions consist of **infiltrating lymphocytes, macrophages** and occa-

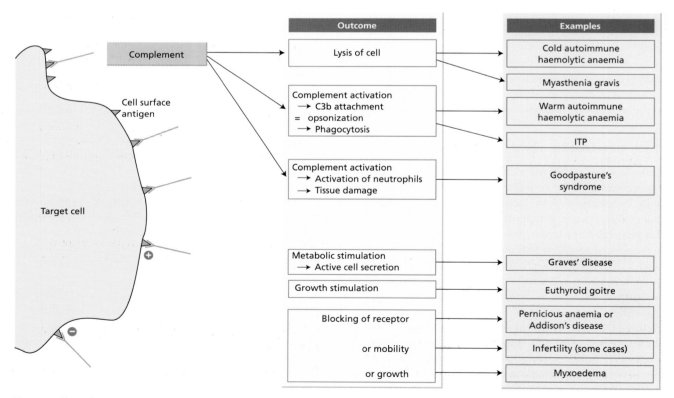

Fig. 1.28 Clinical consequences of cell-bound hypersensitivity.

Table 1.11 Types of hypersensitivity—mechanism, examples of disease and relevant therapy

Types	Mechanism	Therapy	Disease example
Immediate (type I)	IgE production Mast cell degranulation Mediators: 　Histamine 　Leukotrienes 　Granule-associated mediators	Antigen avoidance Mast cell stabilizers (disodium cromoglycate) Antihistamines Leukotriene receptor antagonists Corticosteroids	Anaphylaxis Atopic diseases
Cell-bound antigen (type II)	IgG/IgM autoantibodies: 　Complement lysis 　Neutrophil activation 　Opsonization 　Metabolic stimulation 　Blocking antibodies	Immune suppression and/or plasma exchange Splenectomy/intravenous immunoglobulin Correct metabolism Replace factors missing due to atrophy	Cold autoimmune haemolytic anaemia Myasthenia gravis Goodpasture's syndrome Warm autoimmune haemolytic anaemia Immune thrombocytopenic purpura Graves' disease Pernicious anaemia Myxoedema Infertility (some cases)
Immune complex (type III)	High concentrations of immune complexes, due to persistent antigen and antibody production, leading to complement activation and inflammation	Removal/avoidance of antigen if possible Anti-inflammatory drugs: 　Non-steroidals 　Corticosteroids Immune suppression: 　Cyclophosphamide Plasma exchange to reduce mediator levels	Serum sickness Extrinsic allergic alveolitis Lepromatous leprosy Systemic lupus erythematosus Cutaneous vasculitis Some glomerulonephritides
Delayed-type hypersensitivity (type IV)	TH1 cytokine production Macrophage activation	Block cytokine production: 　Cyclosporin 　Azathioprine Anti-inflammatory: 　Corticosteroids Reduce macrophage activity: 　Corticosteroids Remove antigen	Graft rejection Graft-versus-host disease Tuberculosis, tuberculoid leprosy Contact dermatitis

sionally eosinophil polymorphonuclear leucocytes. Chronic lesions show necrosis, fibrosis and, sometimes, granulomatous reactions. An understanding of mechanisms that lead to tissue damage helps to find relevant therapy (Table 1.11).

1.7 Organization of the immune system: an overview

All lymphoid cells originate in the bone marrow. The nature of

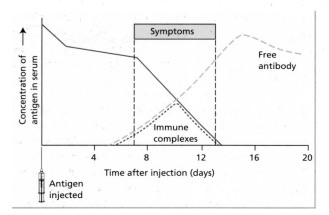

Fig. 1.29 Immune complex formation in acute serum sickness.

the uncommitted lymphoid stem cell is not yet clear (see Fig. 1.1). An understanding of the developmental pathways is important, not only to clarify the physiology of the normal immune response, but because some leukaemias and immunodeficiency states represent maturation arrest of cells in their early stages of development (see Chapter 6) and some forms

of therapy, such as bone marrow transplantation and gene therapy, depend on the identification and use of stem cells.

Lymphoid progenitors destined to become T cells migrate from the bone marrow into the cortex of the **thymus**. Under the influence of stromal cells and Hassalls' corpuscles in the thymic cortex, further differentiation into mature T cells occurs. The passage of T cells from the thymic cortex to medulla is associated with the acquisition of characteristic surface glycoprotein molecules so that medullary thymocytes eventually resemble mature, peripheral T cells. T-cell development in the thymus (Fig. 1.30) is characterized by a process of positive selection whereby T cells that recognize and bind with low affinity to fragments of self-antigen in association with self-MHC proceed to full maturation. In contrast, other T cells which do not recognize self-MHC or recognize and bind self-antigen with high affinity are selected out (negative selection) and do not develop any further. Negatively selected T cells kill themselves by apoptosis (programmed cell death). Deletion of self-reactive, developing T cells in the thymus is an important mechanism by which autoimmune disease is prevented (Chapter 5). The role of the thymus in T-cell selection has been succinctly summarized by Von Boehmer, who stated that the thymus selects the useful,

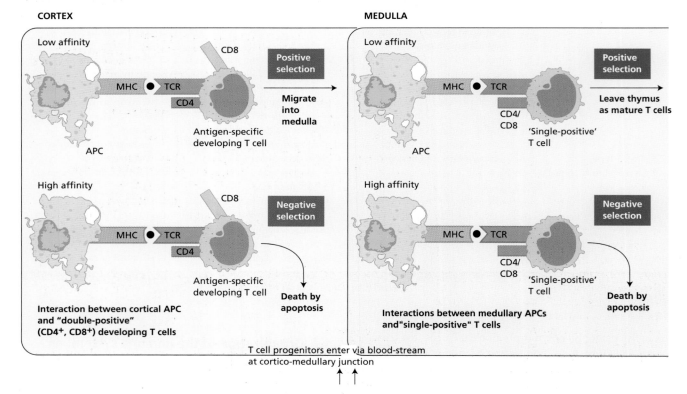

Fig. 1.30 Diagrammatic representation of T-cell selection in the thymus. APC, Antigen-presenting cell; MHC, major histocompatibility complex; TCR, T-cell receptor; ●, peptide fragment of self-antigen.

neglects the useless and destroys the harmful (a reference to autoreactive T cells).

In contrast, B-cell development occurs in the **bone marrow** and is closely dependent upon interaction between a surface glycoprotein on non-lymphoid stromal cells called stem cell factor (SCF) and its receptor on B-cell precursors, Kit tyrosine kinase. Activation of Kit by SCF triggers the early stages of B-cell development; later stages of B-cell development occur under the influence of cytokines secreted by stromal cells, principally IL-7.

The thymus and the bone marrow are **primary lymphoid organs**. They contain cells undergoing a process of maturation from stem cells to antigen sensitivity and restriction. *This process of maturation is independent of antigenic stimulation within the animal.* In contrast, secondary lymphoid organs are those that contain antigen-reactive cells in the process of recirculating through the body. They include lymph nodes, spleen, bone marrow (part) and mucosal-associated lymphoid tissues. Antigenic stimulation changes the relative proportions of the mature cell types in secondary tissues.

Peripheral T and B cells circulate in a definite pattern through the **secondary lymphoid organs** (Fig. 1.31). Most of the recirculating cells are T cells and the complete cycle takes about 24 h; some B cells, including long-lived memory B cells, also recirculate. Lymphocyte circulation is strongly influenced by chemokine receptors on the lymphocyte surface that act as homing agents. There are also adhesion molecules directing cells to their respective ligands on high endothelial venules of lymph nodes and mucosal tissue. For instance, L-selectin is a surface glycoprotein on lymphocytes responsible for homing into lymph nodes (see section 1.2.6 and Table 1.8).

Lymph node architecture is well adapted to its function (Fig. 1.31). The **lymphatic network**, which drains the extravascular spaces in the tissues, is connected to the lymph nodes by lymphatic vessels; these penetrate the lymph node capsule and drain into the peripheral sinus, from which further sinuses branch to enter the lymph node, passing through the cortex to the medulla and hence to the efferent lymphatic vessel. This sinus network provides an excellent filtration system for antigens entering the lymph node from peripheral tissues (Fig. 1.31).

The **cortex** contains primary follicles of B lymphocytes, surrounded by T cells in the 'paracortex'. There is a meshwork of interdigitating cells throughout the lymph node. Antigen is probably filtered and then presented to lymphoid cells by these interdigitating cells. On antigen challenge, the 'primary' follicles of the lymph node develop into 'secondary' follicles. In contrast to primary follicles, secondary follicles contain germinal centres. These comprise mainly B cells with a few helper T cells and a mantle zone of the original primary follicle B cells. B cells in a secondary follicle are an-

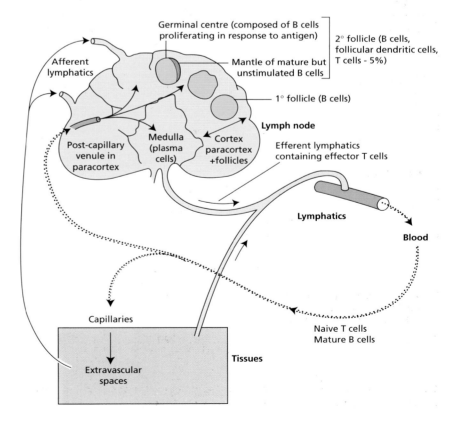

Fig. 1.31 Recirculation pathways of lymphocytes. The majority of naive T cells entering the lymph node cortex from blood will leave the node immediately via efferent lymphatics. Naive T cells that recognize specific antigen differentiate into effector T cells before re-entering the circulation. B-cell recirculation follows a similar route; those B cells that encounter specific antigen proliferate to form germinal centres.

tigen-activated and more mature; most have IgG on their surfaces, whereas those B cells in the primary follicle and mantle zone are less mature, bearing both IgD and IgM. Activated B cells migrate from the follicle to the medulla, where they develop into plasma cells in the **medullary cords** before releasing antibody into the efferent lymph.

The architecture of the spleen is similar. The white pulp around arterioles is arranged into T- and B-cell areas with primary and secondary follicles (Fig. 1.32). Antigen challenge results in expansion of the white pulp with B-cell activation and the development of secondary follicles. Plasma cells migrate to the red pulp.

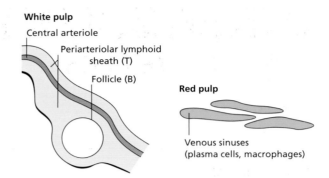

Fig. 1.32 Organization of spleen.

1.8 Conclusions

The aim of this chapter is to give an overview of the normal workings of the immune systems, so that the pathological processes involved in diseases are easily understood. Unlike the subsequent chapters, this one starts with descriptions of the molecules involved, moving onto the role of each in the immune processes rather than the more traditional sequence of anatomical structure, cellular composition and then molecular components. It is hoped that this gives a sense of their relationship in terms of immediacy and dependency as well as the evolution of the two immune systems.

FURTHER READING

See website: www.immunologyclinic.com

2.1 Introduction

Infectious disease is the major cause of morbidity and mortality worldwide. In Africa alone, the World Health Organization estimates that about 100 million people suffer from malaria. New infectious diseases also attract attention in developed countries for several reasons. These include the identification of seemingly 'new' infections, such as Helicobacter pylori, new variant Creutzfeldt–Jakob disease and the latest epidemic of severe acute respiratory syndrome (SARS). There are also changes in clinical practice, which have altered patterns of hospital infection, such as antibiotic resistance. The growth in numbers of iatrogenically immunosuppressed patients at risk from 'opportunistic' infections and an increase in imported diseases accompanying the rising volume of international air travel provide new challenges. There is also an increasing awareness of diseases resulting from self-damaging, host responses to pathogens.

For most infections, a balance is maintained between human defences and the capacity of the microorganism to overcome or bypass them (Table 2.1). A detailed discussion of **virulence** is outside the scope of this book, but disease

Table 2.1 Factors influencing the extent and severity of an infection

Pathogen factors
- Dose (i.e. degree of exposure)
- Virulence of organism
- Route of entry

Host factors
- Integrity of non-specific defences
- Competence of the immune system
- Genetic capacity to respond effectively to a specific organism
- Evidence of previous exposure (natural or acquired)
- Existence of co-infection

will also occur if the host makes an **inadequate** or **inappropriate immune response** to an infection.

2.2 Normal resistance to infection

2.2.1 Non-specific resistance

Non-specific or natural resistance refers to barriers, secretions and the normal flora that make up the external defences (Fig. 2.1), together with the actions of phagocytes and complement.

Mechanical barriers (Fig. 2.1) are highly effective, and their failure often results in infection; for example, defects in the mucociliary lining of the respiratory tract (as in cystic fibrosis) are associated with an increased susceptibility to lung infection. However, many common respiratory pathogens have specific substances on their surfaces (e.g. the haemagglutinin of influenza virus), which help them attach to epithelial cells and so breach physical barriers.

Phagocytic cells ingest invading microorganisms and, in most cases, kill and digest them. There are two types of phagocyte: monocytes/macrophages and polymorphonuclear leucocytes. A prompt response to infection is achieved by concentrating phagocytes at likely sites of infection and having a population of cells that can be rapidly mobilized during an inflammatory response.

The **polymorphonuclear leucocytes** form a large circulating pool of phagocytic cells with reserves in the bone marrow.

Invading microorganisms trigger an inflammatory response with the release of cytokines and chemotactic factors: as a result, circulating polymorphonuclear leucocytes adhere to vascular endothelium, squeeze out of blood vessels and actively migrate towards the focus of infection (Figs 1.13 and 2.2). Phagocytosis then occurs. Severe neutropenia or neutrophil dysfunction is associated with life-threatening infections, usually caused by Staphylococcus aureus, Gramnegative bacteria or fungi (see Chapter 3). Even in normal conditions, polymorphonuclear leucocytes are short-lived; in infection, the increased output from the bone marrow results in a polymorphonuclear leucocytosis in the blood. If a particularly rapid response is needed, immature cells may also be released — described as 'a shift to the left' on a blood film.

Phagocytosis is promoted by serum factors termed '**opsonins**' (see Chapter 1; Fig. 1.19): IgG antibody, complement and mannan-binding lectin are the best opsonins. Non-opsonized bacteria can still be recognized and bound by phagocyte receptors specific for sugars which are present in bacterial cell walls. **Phagocytic receptors and complement** are important for removal of bacteria before antigen-specific immune responses (T cells and antibody) have had a chance to develop.

Macrophages occur in the subepithelial tissues of the skin and intestine and line the alveoli of the lungs. Organisms which penetrate an epithelial surface will encounter these local tissue macrophages (histiocytes). If invasion by microorganisms occurs via blood or lymph, then defence is provided by fixed macrophages lining the blood sinusoids of the liver (Kupffer cells), the spleen and the sinuses of lymph nodes. The interaction of macrophages with certain bacterial components leads to the production of an array of macrophage-

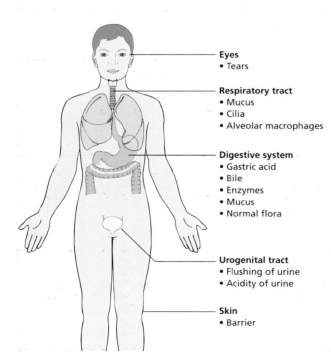

Eyes
• Tears

Respiratory tract
• Mucus
• Cilia
• Alveolar macrophages

Digestive system
• Gastric acid
• Bile
• Enzymes
• Mucus
• Normal flora

Urogenital tract
• Flushing of urine
• Acidity of urine

Skin
• Barrier

Fig. 2.1 Some non-specific defence mechanisms.

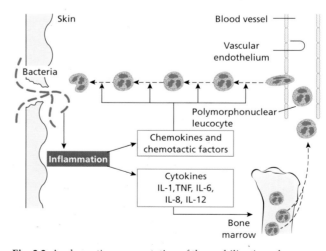

Fig. 2.2 A schematic representation of the mobilization of bone marrow stores of polymorphs following an inflammatory response.

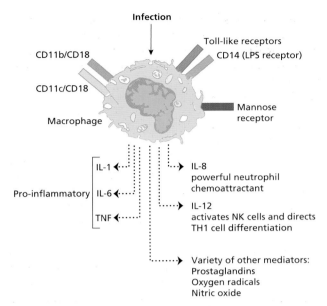

Fig. 2.3 Role of the macrophage in host defence.

derived cytokines, which non-specifically amplify inflammatory reactions (Fig. 2.3). Macrophages are able to engulf opsonized organisms as well as directly bind to certain pathogens by pattern-recognition and other receptors; for example, CD14 acts as a receptor for bacterial lipopolysaccharide (LPS); the integrin molecules CD11b/CD18, CD11c/CD18 recognize several microbes including Leishmania, Bordetella, Candida and LPS; Toll-like receptors (TLR) recognize a range of pathogens (see section 1.2.2).

Most pathogenic microorganisms have evolved methods of resisting phagocytic cells. Staphylococci produce potent extracellular toxins, which kill phagocytes and lead to the **formation of pus**, so characteristic of these infections. Some microorganisms have substances on their cell surfaces which inhibit direct phagocytosis, e.g. the polysaccharide capsule of pneumococci. Under these circumstances, phagocytosis can proceed effectively only when the bacteria are coated (opsonized) by IgG or IgM antibodies or complement. Other microorganisms, e.g. Mycobacterium tuberculosis, are effectively ingested by phagocytic cells but can resist intracellular killing.

2.2.2 Specific resistance

A specific immune response is conventionally classified into humoral and cell-mediated immunity (see Chapter 1). The relative importance of humoral vs. cell-mediated immunity varies from infection to infection. Experimental animal models and naturally occurring immunodeficiency states in humans (see Chapter 3) demonstrate that *certain components of the immune response are essential for controlling particular infections (Fig. 2.4)*.

Individuals with **antibody deficiency** are prone to repeated infections with pyogenic bacteria (see Chapter 3), but replacement therapy with immunoglobulin markedly reduces the frequency of these infections. The course of infections with many viruses (such as varicella or measles) is normal in these patients; however, in the absence of mucosal antibody, there is an increased susceptibility to some enteroviruses (such as polio).

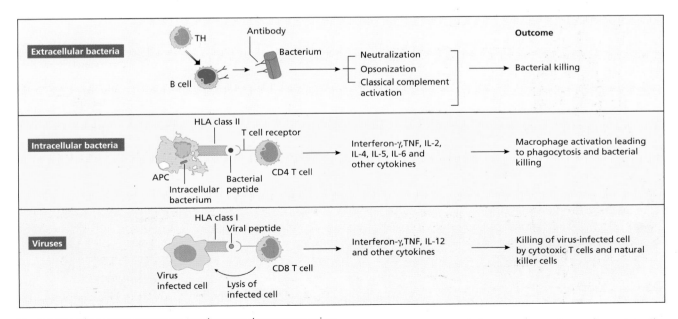

Fig. 2.4 Specific immune responses to microorganisms: an overview.

In viral and bacterial infections with intracellular organisms, T-lymphocyte function is more important than humoral immunity. Patients with **impaired cell-mediated immunity** recover from most bacterial infections but have difficulty in controlling and eradicating infections with viruses such as measles, varicella and herpes. They also show increased susceptibility to mycobacteria, Listeria monocytogenes and some fungi. *Recurrent infections or infection by an unusual organism suggest the possibility of an underlying immunodeficiency.*

Infections are discussed by type of organisms in this chapter. It is impossible to discuss the immune response to all pathogens; illustrative examples are given in each section.

2.3 Viral infection

2.3.1 Epstein–Barr virus infection

Infectious mononucleosis is caused by the Epstein–Barr virus (EBV), a member of the herpes group of viruses. By the age of 3 years, 99% of children in developing countries have been subclinically infected with EBV. In developed countries, clinically recognizable infection most frequently occurs in the 15–25-year age group; the virus is excreted in oropharyngeal secretions for some months, and is responsible for person-to-person transmission.

The pattern of antibody responses to different **EBV antigens** helps in distinguishing acute or subclinical infection from past EBV infection (Table 2.2). IgM antibodies to the viral capsid antigen (VCA) appear early in the course of infection; by the time symptoms of infectious mononucleosis develop, IgG antibody titres to VCA are also high and testing of paired sera for a rise in antibody titre, essential in the diagnosis of many viral infections, is not helpful. Antibodies to EB nuclear antigen (EBNA) develop about 4 months after infection and remain for life. Antibodies to early antigen (EA) appear during primary infection in about 70% of patients and traditionally have been considered an indicator of active infection.

Table 2.2 Patterns of antibodies to Epstein–Barr viral (EBV) antigens

Anti-VCA				
IgM	IgG	Anti-EA	Anti-EBNA	Interpretation
+	+	±	–	Primary infection (with/without symptoms)
–	+	–	+	Past EBV infection (> 4 months)

VCA, Viral capsid antigen; EA, early antigen; EBNA, Epstein–Barr nuclear antigen.

EBV is unique among human viruses in that it produces disease by **infecting and transforming B lymphocytes**, via the CD21 molecule on the B-cell surface. Infected B cells multiply like tumour cells, and small numbers may produce free virus which can transform other B lymphocytes. Up to half of the lymphoid cells from the tonsils of EBV-infected patients may be transformed.

Primary EBV infection is stopped by two defences: a T-cell immune response capable of eliminating almost all virus-infected cells, and virus-neutralizing antibodies which prevent the spread of infection from one target cell to another. The characteristic 'atypical lymphocytes' are predominantly CD8+ cytotoxic T lymphocytes, which recognize and destroy EBV-infected B cells (Case 2.1).

The **importance of the immune response** to EBV is illustrated by (i) rare patients with EBV-specific failure of immunity; and (ii) the occurrence of EBV-induced malignant transformation of B cells in patients receiving immunosuppressive therapy (see Case 7.1). For example, the X-linked 'lymphoproliferative syndrome' (Duncan's syndrome) affects males (aged 6 months to > 20 years) who are unable to control EBV infection due to mutation in the gene

CASE 2.1 INFECTIOUS MONONUCLEOSIS

A 20-year-old carpet fitter presented with a 1-week history of a sore throat, stiffness and tenderness of his neck, and extreme malaise. On examination, he was mildly pyrexial with posterior cervical lymphadenopathy, palatal petechiae and pharyngeal inflammation without an exudate. Abdominal examination showed mild splenomegaly. There was no evidence of a skin rash or jaundice.

The clinical diagnosis of infectious mononucleosis ('glandular fever') was confirmed on investigation. His white cell count was 13×10^9/l (NR $4–10 \times 10^9$/l) with over 50% of the lymphocytes showing atypical morphology ('atypical lymphocytosis'). His serum contained IgM antibodies to Epstein–Barr viral capsid antigen (VCA), the most specific test for acute infectious mononucleosis (see Table 2.2). Liver function tests were normal.

He was treated symptomatically and was advised to avoid sporting activity until his splenomegaly had completely resolved, because of the danger of splenic rupture. Many patients show clinical or biochemical evidence of liver involvement and are recommended to abstain from alcohol for at least 6 months.

encoding SAP (SLAM-associated protein). SAP mutations lead to a failure in signal transduction from the 'signalling lymphocyte activation molecule' (SLAM), which is present on the surface of T and B cells. Most patients with this syndrome die, some with lymphoma, some with aplastic anaemia, and others with immunodeficiency.

Some immunosuppressive regimens used in transplantation, such as cyclosporin, antithymocyte globulin or monoclonal anti-T-cell antibodies, are associated with **EBV reactivation**: about 1–10% of certain transplants are complicated by EBV-induced lymphoproliferative disease. Similarly, up to 2% of patients infected with human immunodeficiency virus (HIV) (Chapter 3) develop non-Hodgkin's lymphoma; EBV has been identified in most acquired immune deficiency syndrome (AIDS)-associated lymphomas.

Burkitt's lymphoma is a highly malignant, extranodal tumour of B lymphocytes strongly associated with EBV infection. It is endemic in certain African countries, where it represents approximately 90% of childhood cancers in contrast to 3% in developed countries. The link between EBV and Burkitt's lymphoma was substantiated by the demonstration of the EBV genome and EBV antigens in tumour cells. It is likely that Burkitt's lymphoma is due to EBV-induced lymphoproliferation in individuals rendered susceptible by chronic malaria. EBV infection in this setting leads to chromosomal translocation(s) with consequent activation of the *c-myc* oncogene.

2.3.2 Viruses and the immune response

The clinical spectrum of viral disease is very wide and, because there is such variation, herpes virus infections will be used as a general example (Table 2.3).

Table 2.3 Clinical aspects of herpes virus infections

	Clinical spectrum	Modes of transmission	Site of latency
Herpes simplex virus type 1 (HSV-1)	Acute gingivostomatitis Herpes labialis Keratoconjunctivitis Encephalitis Disseminated infection	• Oral–respiratory secretions • Skin contact	Trigeminal ganglion
Herpes simplex virus type 2 (HSV-2)	Genital herpes Meningitis Disseminated infection	• Sexual • Intrapartum	Sacral ganglion
Varicella zoster virus (VZV)	Herpes zoster Disseminated herpes zoster Congenital varicella	• Oral–respiratory secretions • Skin contact • Congenital	Dorsal root ganglion
Cytomegalovirus (CMV)	Glandular fever-like syndrome Retinitis Pneumonia Hepatitis	• Oral–respiratory secretion • Sexual • Congenital • Intrapartum • Iatrogenic, e.g. blood transfusion, organ transplant	Leucocytes Epithelial cells of parotid salivary gland, cervix, renal tubules
Epstein–Barr virus (EBV)	Infectious mononucleosis Burkitt's lymphoma Nasopharyngeal carcinoma	• Oral–respiratory secretions	B lymphocytes Epithelial cells of nasopharynx
Human herpes virus type 6 (HHV-6)	Exanthem subitum Glandular fever-type syndrome	• Oral–respiratory secretions	? B lymphocytes
Human herpes virus type 7 (HHV-7)	Exanthem subitum	• Oral–respiratory secretions	Unknown
Human herpes virus type 8 (HHV-8)	Kaposi's sarcoma	• ? Sexual	Unknown

The herpes virus group consists of at least 60 viruses, eight of which commonly infect humans (Table 2.3). Two features of **pathogenesis** are common to all human herpes viruses. First, close physical contact must occur between infected and uninfected individuals for transmission of virus and no intermediate host is involved. Exceptions to this rule are blood transfusion and organ transplantation, which are potential routes of transmission for cytomegalovirus (CMV). Second, after a primary infection, herpes viruses will persist in the host throughout life.

To limit virus dissemination and prevent reinfection, the immune response must be able to stop virions entering cells, and to eliminate infected cells to reduce virus shedding. Immunological reactions are thus of two kinds: those directed against the virion and those that act upon the virus-infected cell. In general, immune responses to the virion are predominantly humoral, whilst T-cell-mediated responses act on virus-infected cells. The major humoral mechanism involved is viral neutralization by antibody, but complement-dependent enhancement of viral phagocytosis and complement-mediated lysis of virus also occur.

Viral neutralization prevents attachment of virus to target cell and is the function of IgG antibodies in the extracellular fluid, IgM in the blood and secretory IgA antibodies on mucosal surfaces. *Only antibodies to those viral components responsible for attachment are neutralizing.* The generation of antibodies of the correct specificity is therefore essential for an effective viral vaccine; antibodies to inappropriate antigens not only may fail to protect, but may actually provoke immune complex disease (see section 2.3.5).

Cell-mediated immunity is concerned with virus-infected cells rather than free virus. Virus-immune T lymphocytes recognize viral antigens in association with self major histocompatibility complex (MHC class I) glycoproteins (see Chapter 1). Cytotoxic T (T_C) cells lyse virally modified cells and limit disease by eliminating production of infectious progeny. *T cells are therefore concerned with recovery from virus infections*; containment of the initial infection is mediated by interferons and natural killer cells (Fig. 2.5).

Most viral infections are self-limiting. Recovery from acute viral infections usually produces specific long-term immunity and secondary attacks by the same virus are uncommon.

2.3.3 Direct effects of viruses

The clinical importance of viral infection *depends not only on the number of host cells destroyed but on the function of those cells.* Destruction of relatively few cells with highly specialized function, such as neurotransmission or immunoregulation, can be disabling or life-threatening. In contrast, destruction of larger numbers of less specialized cells, such as epithelial cells, has less drastic results. In order to gain entry into specialized cells, viruses interact with specific receptors on host cells—**viral tropism**. For example, EBV uses the C3d receptor (CD21), HIV uses multiple receptors (CD4, chemokine receptors: CCR5, CXCR-4) and the newly described SARS-Coronavirus (SARS-CoV) uses angiotensin converting enzyme-2 (ACE-2) in order to gain entry into target cells.

Once inside a cell, a virus can kill the cell in several ways. Some viruses, such as poliovirus or adenovirus or their products, can block enzymes needed for cell replication or metabolism, while others may disrupt intracellular structures, such as lysosomes, releasing lethal enzymes. Some viral proteins inserted into the cell membrane can alter its integrity: measles virus, for instance, possesses fusion activity and causes cells to form syncytia.

Some viruses can **alter the specialized function** of a cell without killing it. Usually, such cells belong to the central nervous or endocrine systems. Dementia caused by HIV infection is an example.

Transformation of host cells may occur with certain viruses which are potentially *oncogenic* (Table 2.4). Mostly, these are viruses that establish latency. Cells from Burkitt's lymphoma, for instance, show a characteristic translocation between the long arms of chromosomes 8 and 14, suggesting that the tumour results from the translocation of the

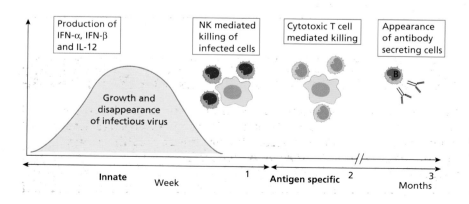

Fig. 2.5 Time sequence of immune response to viral infection.

Table 2.4 Viruses and malignant disease

Malignancy	Virus
Certain T-cell leukaemias	Human T-cell leukaemia virus (HTLV-I)
Carcinoma of cervix	Herpes simplex (type 2)
	Human papillomaviruses
Burkitt's lymphoma	Epstein–Barr virus
Nasopharyngeal carcinoma	Epstein–Barr virus
Skin cancer	Papillomavirus
Hepatocellular carcinoma	Hepatitis B
	Hepatitis C
Kaposi's sarcoma	Human herpes virus 8 (HHV-8)

oncogene, *c-myc*, to an active region of the cellular genome (in this example, the locus for the immunoglobulin heavy chain).

Some viruses can **interfere with the immune response** by suppressing it or infecting cells of the immune system (Table 2.5). The best example of this phenomenon is AIDS (see Chapter 3), caused by HIV types 1 and 2 (HIV-1, HIV-2), which selectively infect and deplete CD4+ T lymphocytes and macrophages. The resulting profound immunosup-pression leads to the development of the severe, disseminated, opportunistic infections and tumours that characterize AIDS.

Measles virus is a less well known but important example. Before treatment for tuberculosis (TB) was available, outbreaks of acute measles infection were associated with the reactivation and dissemination of miliary TB, due to reduced T-cell-mediated immunity.

2.3.4 Viral strategies to evade the immune response

Viruses have evolved ingenious mechanisms for evading or interfering with immune responses. An important viral strategy for evasion is entry into a **latent state**. All human herpes viruses can remain latent (see Table 2.3), undergoing periodic cycles of activation and replication. The viral genome remains within the host cell but no expression of viral antigens occurs. When the equilibrium between virus and host defence is upset, perhaps by other infections, metabolic disturbances, ageing or immunosuppression, the virus may be activated, with subsequent expression of disease.

Herpes zoster is a good example of a disorder caused by a virus which normally lies **latent** in the dorsal root ganglion but gets activated when host immunity is impaired, as in Case 2.2, with prolonged corticosteroid therapy. Frequently, the virus remains latent in other anatomically defined sites

Table 2.5 Examples of viruses infecting cells of the immune system

Cell	Virus	Outcome
B lymphocytes	Epstein–Barr virus	Transformation and polyclonal B-cell activation
T lymphocytes	Measles	Replication in activated T cells
	Human T-cell leukaemia virus I	T-cell lymphoma/leukaemia
	Human immunodeficiency virus 1 and 2	Acquired immune deficiency syndrome
Macrophages	Dengue	
	Lassa	Viral haemorrhagic fevers
	Marburg—Ebola	

CASE 2.2 RECURRENT HERPES ZOSTER

A 72-year-old woman was commenced on oral corticosteroids for giant cell arteritis. Over the next 6 months she had three episodes of a painful, vesicular rash ('shingles') typical of herpes zoster affecting the ophthalmic division of the right trigeminal nerve. Each episode was successfully treated with oral acyclovir, but she experienced considerable post-herpetic neuralgia. A steady improvement in her arteritic symptoms and inflammatory indices allowed a reduction in steroid dosage over a period of 6 months, with no further episodes of zoster.

Table 2.6 Mechanisms of immune evasion by viruses

Mechanism	Example
Non-expression of viral genome	Herpes simplex virus (latent in neurones)
Production of antigenic variants	Influenza, HIV
Inhibition of major histocompatibility complex expression	Adenovirus
Production of inhibitory cytokines	EBV and IL-10

HIV, Human immunodeficiency virus; EBV, Epstein–Barr virus; IL-10, interleukin-10.

(see Table 2.3), for instance, herpes simplex virus in the trigeminal ganglion (producing 'cold sores') and activated by sunlight, stress or intercurrent infection.

Other mechanisms of evading immune responses are given in Table 2.6. Antigenic variation is best illustrated by influenza A, an RNA virus surrounded by a lipid envelope with two inserted proteins—haemagglutinin and neuraminidase—against which most neutralizing antibodies are directed. The virus can evade antibody responses by modifying the structure of these proteins in two ways: antigenic drift and antigenic shift. **Antigenic drift** is minor structural change caused by point mutations altering an antigenic site on haemagglutinin. Such mutations probably account for the 'minor' epidemics of influenza occurring most winters. **Antigenic shift** is a major change in the whole structure of haemagglutinin or neuraminidase, which has caused periodic influenza pandemics this century.

Viral persistence is a feature of certain viral infections. If the provoked immune response does not clear a virus, a low-grade infection with persistent shedding of infectious virus may result. For example, hepatitis C may persist for many months or years with continuous carriage in the liver if treatment is not successful (Chapter 14).

2.3.5 Bystander damage caused by the immune response to viral infection

Although immunological reactions are usually beneficial, they do sometimes initiate or aggravate tissue damage and this may be difficult to distinguish from viral damage. Such mechanisms in viral diseases are less well defined than in bacterial infections.

During recovery from some viral infections, such as infectious mononucleosis or hepatitis B, patients may develop circulating autoantibodies. Viral infections upset tolerance to self-antigens in two ways: (i) viruses, such as EBV, are polyclonal B-cell activators; and (ii) the virus may combine with host antigens to form new antigens (see Chapter 1). Antibodies to these new antigens will recognize healthy host tissue as well as the virus-infected cells. Persistence of a viral infection may eventually cause **autoimmune disease** in susceptible individuals. One example is the development of chronic autoimmune liver disease in some patients following hepatitis B infection (see Chapter 14) or immune complex features such as vasculitis, arthropathy or glomerulonephritis.

Some viruses induce production of **inappropriate antibodies** that facilitate viral damage to the host. Dengue virus, for instance, can infect macrophages efficiently via Fc receptors, and its capacity to enter the target cell is enhanced if it is bound to IgG antibodies. Consequently, a second infection by a different virus serotype may be potentiated by pre-existing antibody.

The best example of **damage mediated by T cells** is lymphocytic choriomeningitis infection of mice. In mice infected in neonatal life, the virus multiplies extensively in many tis-

CASE 2.3 CHRONIC FATIGUE SYNDROME

A 25-year-old woman presented with a 6-month history of extreme lethargy and difficulty in concentration following a flu-like illness. She was unable to work as a physiotherapist and experienced considerable stress as a result of having to give up work. Clinical examination was unremarkable with the exception of globally reduced muscle strength; the rest of the neurological examination was normal. She was assessed by several specialists, who found no explanation for her extreme lethargy. A diagnosis of chronic fatigue syndrome (CFS) of unknown aetiology was made and a programme of graded exercises was recommended. Over the next 2 years she improved steadily, enabling her to resume employment.

sues including the central nervous system, but produces few ill effects. In contrast, inoculation of the virus into the brain of adult mice results in a fatal meningoencephalitis; cerebral damage is limited by pretreating animals with anti-T-cell monoclonal antibodies but worsens if the animals are reconstituted with T cells from immune donors. Cytotoxic T lymphocytes from immune animals lyse those infected brain cells which express virus-coded antigens on their surfaces. Whether or not cell-mediated mechanisms also contribute to the encephalitis sometimes seen in human virus infections is unknown. It has been suggested that liver damage in patients with chronic hepatitis B or C infection results from the lysis of virus-infected hepatocytes by HBV/HCV-specific CD8+ cytotoxic T cells.

2.3.6 Speculative effects of viral infection

The postviral fatigue syndrome, also called the chronic fatigue syndrome (CFS) or **myalgic encephalomyelitis (ME)**, is a somewhat controversial subject. CFS describes severe, prolonged, disabling fatigue, often associated with myalgia, and mood and sleep disturbance. These symptoms seem genuine, and cases have been reported from many countries in the developed world. The condition mainly affects adults between 20 and 50 years old, and women more frequently than men. A preceding infectious illness, such as EBV, CMV, Coxsackie B or HHV-6, is reported by many patients, but there is no convincing evidence causally linking any recognized infectious agent to the condition. Depression is found in about 50% of patients and frequently precedes the physical symptoms.

The diagnosis of CFS is made entirely on clinical grounds in patients presenting with a characteristic symptom complex dominated by fatigue. While detailed laboratory investigation is unhelpful in most patients, it is important to be aware that patients with unrelated disorders, for example hypothyroidism, systemic lupus erythematosus, may occasionally present with severe fatigue.

A variety of immunological alterations have been reported in 10% of patients only and are inconsistent and of uncertain significance. **No treatment**, including intravenous immunoglobulin, has proved reliably effective in the few controlled clinical trials conducted. A programme of graded exercise significantly improves functional capacity and fatigue (Case 2.3). The syndrome appears to be a disease of uncertain aetiology, prolonged duration and considerable morbidity but no mortality.

2.4 Bacterial infection

2.4.1 Normal immune responses to bacterial infections

There are two major categories of bacterial antigens that provoke immune responses: **soluble (diffusible) products** of the cell (e.g. toxins) and **structural antigens** that are part of the bacterial cell (such as LPS). Many bacterial antigens contain lipid in association with cell-wall glycoproteins; the presence of lipid appears to potentiate the immunogenicity of associated antigens.

Most bacterial antigens are **T-cell dependent**, requiring helper T lymphocytes for the initiation of humoral and cell-mediated immunity. However, some bacterial antigens, such as pneumococcal polysaccharide, are relatively **T independent**: these are characterized by their high molecular weight and their multiple, repeating antigenic determinants. In children, adequate antibody responses to these antigens can take 4–6 years to develop. Consequently, younger children are susceptible to invasive disease caused by encapsulated bacterial pathogens.

In the following discussion, streptococci are used as an example, but other bacteria provoke a similar immune response. β-Haemolytic streptococci (especially Group A) most commonly cause localized infection of the upper respiratory tract or skin but they can, and do, infect almost any organ of the body. There are striking differences in the clinical features of streptococcal infection in patients of different

CASE 2.4 ACUTE BACTERIAL TONSILLITIS

A 5-year-old boy presented to his general practitioner with a 36-h history of acute malaise, shivering and vague pains in his legs. For 12 h he had complained of a dry, sore throat and had vomited twice. He was febrile (temperature 40.2 °C) with a tachycardia of 140/min and tender, bilateral, cervical lymphadenopathy. His pharynx, tonsils and buccal mucosa were red and inflamed and his tonsils were studded with white areas of exudate. He was diagnosed as having acute bacterial tonsillitis and treated with phenoxymethyl penicillin for 5 days. A throat swab taken before starting antibiotics grew β-haemolytic streptococci (Group A). After 3 days of treatment, his temperature had returned to normal and he made an uneventful recovery. Haemolytic streptococcal infections illustrate an important point about bacterial infection—namely, that immune defences plus antibiotics cope satisfactorily with most bacterial infections in most people.

CASE 2.5 STREPTOCOCCAL TOXIC SHOCK SYNDROME

A 35-year-old man was admitted to hospital with a 7-day history of high fever, sore throat and a diffuse erythematous rash over the anterior chest wall. Additional findings on examination included hypotension (blood pressure 80/50 mmHg), conjunctival injection and cellulitis of both calves. Over the next 24 h there was increasing pain and swelling of the right calf associated with disappearance of the pedal pulse, necessitating emergency fasciotomies of the anterolateral and posterior compartments of the right leg. At operation, there was marked bulging of muscle in both compartments. Gram

stain of the fluid obtained during fasciotomy showed Gram-positive cocci with an abundant growth of Group A β-haemolytic streptococci on muscle culture. The same organism was also isolated from throat and blood cultures. Exotoxin typing with a gene probe revealed pyrogenic exotoxins A and B.

A diagnosis of streptococcal toxic shock syndrome was made on the basis of the above findings. The patient made a full recovery following treatment with intravenous clindamycin.

ages, which probably reflect differences in **immune status** to this pathogen. The young infant presents with a mild illness of insidious onset, characterized by low-grade fever and nasal discharge. Pharyngeal signs are usually minimal. This picture contrasts sharply with the acute streptococcal tonsillitis seen in older children (Case 2.4) or adults. This more acute and localized response is probably due to previous exposure to the streptococcus and modification of the response by preformed antibodies to streptococcal toxins and enzymes.

Streptococcal antigens include **specific toxins** (streptolysins O and S and pyrogenic exotoxin), which lyse tissue and circulating cells (including leucocytes), **specific enzymes** (such as hyaluronidase and streptokinase), which promote the spread of infections, and **surface components** of the streptococcal cell wall (M protein and hyaluronic acid). All these proteins are immunogenic, but the M protein is the chief virulence factor.

Specific antibodies are slow to appear (4 days) and are unlikely to play a role in limiting acute primary streptococcal infection. *Antistreptolysin O (ASO) and antistreptococcal deoxyribonuclease B (anti-DNase B) are two valuable streptococcal antibody tests for clinical use.* The ASO titre is generally raised after throat infections but not after skin infections: the anti-DNase B titre is a reliable test for both skin and throat infections and therefore useful in the diagnosis of poststreptococcal glomerulonephritis (see Chapter 9).

Some products, such as endotoxin, are powerful **stimulators** of the immune response, leading to polyclonal activation of B lymphocytes. The rise in serum immunoglobulins in some prolonged infections is probably due to this polyclonal stimulation, since *increase in specific antibody forms only a very small proportion of the total immunoglobulin level.*

2.4.2 Bacteria as superantigens

Some streptococcal toxins are potent activators of T cells by virtue of their ability to act as **superantigens**. In contrast to

conventional antigens which are processed intracellularly, superantigens simultaneously activate large numbers of T cells carrying a particular T-cell receptor Vβ gene, by binding directly to MHC class II molecules at a site distinct from the antigen-binding groove (Fig. 2.6). Since there are 50 different Vβ genes in humans, a superantigen will react with $\geq 1:50$ T cells in contrast to a conventional peptide antigen which will react with $1:10^4$ to $1:10^8$ T cells.

Widespread T-cell activation with selective usage of certain T-cell receptor Vβ genes is a feature of superantigen-associated diseases (see Box 2.1). Consequently, these disorders are characterized by marked cytokine release, high fever, hypotension and multisystem involvement (Case 2.5).

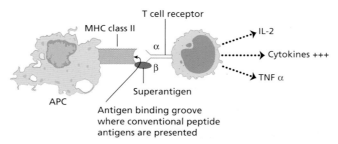

Fig. 2.6 Superantigen-induced T-cell stimulation.

BOX 2.1 SUPERANTIGEN-ASSOCIATED DISEASES

Toxic shock syndrome
- Streptococcal
- Staphylococcal
- Clostridial (Clostridium perfringens)
- Yersinial (Yersinia enterocolitica)

Kawasaki disease
- No organism yet identified (superantigen association based on cytokine profile)

2.4.3 Bacterial evasion of immune defences

Bacteria survive in the host if immune responses kill them at a rate slower than the rate at which they multiply. Complete failure of defences is not needed for infection, only evasion or subversion of the immune response, and bacteria have evolved many mechanisms for achieving this (Table 2.7).

Capsules are important for long-term survival of pathogens; for instance, polysaccharide antigens of Pneumococcus and Meningococcus can inhibit ingestion of bacteria by phagocytes; mucoid secretions prevent activation of the alternate pathway of complement.

Antigenic variation occurs in some bacterial infections. Patients infected by a tick bite experience relapsing fever due to multiplication of Borrelia recurrentis. After a week or so, antibodies destroy the bacteria and the fever subsides. However, **antigenic variants** are formed which reach bacteraemic proportions after 5–7 days, with consequent relapse of the patient. Antibodies to these variants eliminate the bacteria and fever, but further variants are made again. The cycle recurs five to 10 times before the disease finally subsides.

Some bacteria infecting mucous surfaces possess **proteases** that hydrolyse IgA antibody: these include Neisseria gonorrhoeae, N. meningitidis, Haemophilus influenzae and Streptococcus pneumoniae. Others (e.g. some staphylococci) produce enzymes (e.g. catalase) that prevent them being killed inside phagocytic cells.

Bacteria may survive by **sequestration** in non-phagocytic cells where they are not exposed to immune factors or some antibiotics. An example is the chronic carriage of Salmonella typhi in scarred, avascular areas of the gall bladder and urinary tract.

2.4.4 Bystander damage caused by the immune response to bacterial infection

It is often difficult to distinguish between the direct toxic effects of bacterial infection and the damage caused by immune reactions to bacterial antigens. This problem is illustrated by the complications of streptococcal infection (Fig. 2.7).

Rheumatic fever is a systemic illness that occurs about 1–5 weeks after a Group A β-haemolytic streptococcal infection of the upper respiratory tract, although fewer than 1% of untreated infections result in rheumatic fever. After many decades of continuous decline in the incidence of rheumatic fever, there has been a recent resurgence of the condition in the USA. There is evidence of an underlying **genetic susceptibility**. Rheumatic fever clusters in families: 40–60% of patients in the recent USA outbreaks had a family history of the disease. Rheumatic fever is three times more common in monozygotic than dizygotic twins, with a significant association between inheritance of HLA-DR4 in white people and HLA-DR2 in black people with the disease.

Table 2.7 Mechanisms of immune evasion by bacteria

- Capsular polysaccharide—antiphagocytic role
- Mucoid secretions—decreases alternate pathway complement activity
- Antigenic variation—tick-borne relapsing fever due to Borrelia recurrentis
- Proteases—render mucosal IgA ineffective
- Sequestration in non-phagocytic cells—provides shelter from immune response

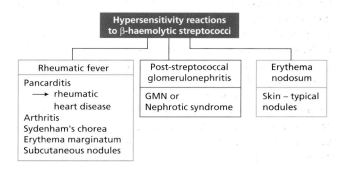

Fig. 2.7 Recognized complications of β-haemolytic streptococcal infection. GMN, Glomerulonephritis.

CASE 2.6 RHEUMATIC HEART DISEASE

A 38-year-old labourer presented with a 3-month history of progressive shortness of breath on effort. Exertion was often associated with central chest pain and irregular palpitations. He had twice woken from sleep with attacks of frightening breathlessness and was unable to lie flat. His general health was good, with no weight loss or anorexia. He had been told that he had suffered from rheumatic fever when he was 9 years old.

On examination, he had the typical physical signs of congestive cardiac failure due to underlying mitral valve stenosis and rheumatic heart disease. There was no evidence of bacterial endocarditis. On treatment with digoxin, diuretics and anticoagulants, his exercise tolerance improved dramatically and cardiac surgery was postponed. Antibiotic cover was provided for any dental or surgical treatment, in order to prevent the development of subacute bacterial endocarditis.

The **pathogenesis of rheumatic fever** has been intensively studied. Streptococcal components or products probably start the tissue damage. Strains of streptococci which are 'rheumatogenic' show certain characteristics (Box 2.2).

However, attention has focused also on the possible *importance of immunological mechanisms in pathogenesis*. Children with rheumatic fever have a high incidence of **antibodies**

BOX 2.2 EVIDENCE FOR THE INVOLVEMENT OF ANTIBODIES IN THE PATHOGENESIS OF RHEUMATIC FEVER

'Rheumatogenic' strains of streptococci:

- are confined to certain M serotypes only
- are heavily encapsulated and form mucoid colonies on culture
- resist phagocytosis by inhibiting alternate complement pathway activation.

'Rheumatogenic' strains of streptococci are cross-reactive between:

- streptococcal Group A carbohydrate and the heart valve glycoprotein
- M protein, cardiac sarcolemma and cardiac myosin
- another cell wall component and human brain
- a cell wall glycoprotein and the glomerular basement membrane
- streptococcal hyaluronidase and human synovium.

---

to extracts of human heart. This suggests that *rheumatic carditis may be caused by antistreptococcal antibodies which cross-react with heart antigens*. Rheumatic fever is not confined to the myocardium (see Fig. 2.7) and lesions are found in heart valves, joints, blood vessels, skin and, in the related condition of chorea, in the central nervous system. It is probable that most of the damage is antibody mediated, since cross-reactivity has been unequivocally demonstrated (Box 2.2).

However, some patients with streptococcal sore throats develop these cross-reacting antibodies without subsequent cardiac disease, while in animals passive transfer of the antibodies alone has no demonstrable effect on the target organ, suggesting that **damage by streptococcal products** is required for antibodies to then be damaging.

The relationship of streptococcal infection to **acute poststreptococcal glomerulonephritis** differs from that in rheumatic fever in two important respects. Glomerulonephritis seems to occur only after infection with one of the few 'nephritogenic' strains, whereas several but not all serotypes of Group A streptococcus are associated with rheumatic fever. Available evidence suggests that poststreptococcal glomerulonephritis is caused by deposition of circulating immune complexes and not by cross-reacting antibodies (see Chapter 9). The two conditions are only rarely associated with each other in epidemics that are caused by a single strain of a known M serotype, suggesting individual host susceptibility.

Many other bacterial and Mycoplasma infections can also trigger a self-damaging immune response (Table 2.8).

Table 2.8 Examples of diseases caused by immune reactions to bacterial antigens

Immune reactions	Diseases
Cross-reacting antigens (type II hypersensitivity)	
Human heart and Group A streptococci	Rheumatic carditis
Human brain and Group A streptococci	Sydenham's chorea
Association of infective antigen with autoantigens (type II hypersensitivity)	
Mycoplasma antigens and erythrocytes	Autoimmune haemolytic anaemia
Immune complex formation (type III hypersensitivity)	
Subacute bacterial endocarditis	Vasculitis, arthritis,
Infected ventriculoatrial shunts	glomerulonephritis
Secondary syphilis	
Gonococcal septicaemia	Vasculitis, arthritis
Meningococcal septicaemia	
Delayed hypersensitivity reactions (type IV hypersensitivity)	
Tuberculosis	Pulmonary cavitation and fibrosis
Leprosy	Peripheral neuropathy

CASE 2.7 TUBERCULOSIS

A 25-year-old Asian man was referred to his local chest clinic with a history of a cough and loss of weight over the preceding 6 months. He had lived in the UK for the past 7 years and a chest X-ray taken immediately prior to entry into the UK was reportedly normal.

On examination, left apical crackles were noted on auscultation of his chest and a chest X-ray revealed left apical shadowing with cavitation. His sputum contained Mycobacterium tuberculosis and a skin test with tuberculin was strongly positive. He was promptly treated with standard antituberculous therapy and made a full recovery. The local public health department was notified, who undertook contact tracing.

This patient presented with postprimary TB, a common form of the disease, which occurs as a result of reactivation of quiescent endogenous primary infection or exogenous reinfection.

2.5 Mycobacterial infection

2.5.1 Mycobacterial infections

Mycobacterium tuberculosis is an *obligate intracellular pathogen* which is responsible for causing 3 million deaths worldwide per year. Only a proportion of infected individuals develop overt disease, underlining the critical role of the host's cellular immune response in successfully containing primary infection (Fig. 2.8). Several risk factors for the development of active disease, including malnutrition, have been identified (Table 2.9). Infection commonly occurs by inhalation, resulting in pulmonary disease; a few patients develop gastrointestinal disease following ingestion of the bacterium. Dissemination of infection beyond the lungs is uncommon in postprimary disease, as in Case 2.7, but bacilli may spread systemically to lymph nodes, the genitourinary tract, spine, joints, meninges and pericardium in immuno-compromised and malnourished individuals.

Two other mycobacterial species are prominent human pathogens. **Mycobacterium leprae** is currently responsible for 5.5 million cases of leprosy worldwide, causing considerable morbidity in the developing world. The severity and extent of disease in leprosy are closely related to the host immune response. Robust cellular immunity leads to localized tuberculoid disease affecting skin and nerve with few bacilli and vigorous granuloma formation. In contrast, patients with poor cellular immunity develop disseminated, bacteraemic disease (see Fig. 2.9). **Mycobacterium avium-intracellulare (MAC)** is an ubiquitous environmental my-cobacterium which is handled satisfactorily by immuno-competent individuals, but causes disseminated disease in patients with advanced HIV infection (CD4 T cell count $< 50/\text{mm}^3$). MAC is estimated to affect 50% of patients with HIV disease and its increasing prominence is a direct result of the HIV epidemic.

2.5.2 Mycobacteria and the normal immune response

Protection against mycobacterial infection is crucially dependent on **intact macrophage and T-cell function**. On entry into the body, mycobacteria are taken up by mononuclear phagocytes and processed prior to presentation to T cells. Several pieces of evidence point to the important role played by CD4 and CD8 T cells and TH1 cytokines in controlling mycobacterial infection (see Box 2.3).

Presentation of mycobacterial antigens to T cells at the site of infection triggers clonal expansion and cytokine release (Fig. 2.8). The pattern of **cytokine release** is an important determinant in controlling infection. A predominant TH1

Table 2.9 Risk factors for the development of tuberculosis

- Impaired cellular immunity
      Human immunodeficiency virus infection
      Immunosuppressive therapy
- Advanced age
- Protein calorie malnutrition
- Alcoholism
- Intravenous drug abuse

BOX 2.3 EVIDENCE THAT T CELLS AND TH1 CYTOKINES ARE CRUCIAL IN PROTECTION AGAINST MYCOBACTERIAL INFECTION

- Patients with HIV infection are particularly prone to M. tuberculosis and M. avium-intracellulare (MAC) infection.
- Patients with interferon (IFN)-γ receptor defects are prone to MAC infection.
- IFN-γ is effective as adjunctive therapy in patients with resistant MAC infection.
- Deletion of the gene for IFN-γ renders mice susceptible to low doses of M. tuberculosis.
- Mice deficient in CD8 T cells, due to deletion of the gene for β₂-microglobulin, are unable to control M. tuberculosis infection.
- Patients treated with biological agents which neutralize TNF (anti-TNF, soluble TNF receptor) have a significant risk of developing tuberculosis.

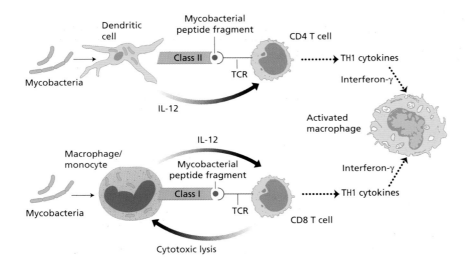

Fig. 2.8 Diagrammatic representation of immune response to mycobacteria resulting in activated macrophages killing intracellular organisms too. TcR, T-cell receptor; IL-12, interleukin-12.

cytokine profile characterized by interferon-γ (IFN-γ), tumour necrosis factor (TNF) and interleukin-2 (IL-2) leads to macrophage activation and granuloma formation, which enables immunocompetent individuals to contain disease.

The pivotal role of IFN-γ in the immune response to mycobacteria has been exploited by the development of IFN-γ assays for the **diagnosis of latent TB**. The production of IFN-γ by a patient's T cells on exposure to the mycobacterial antigen ESAT-6 (Early Secretory Antigenic Target-6) has recently been shown to be a more reliable marker of latent infection with Mycobacterium tuberculosis than conventional skin testing with tuberculin.

2.5.3 Mycobacterial evasion of the immune response

Macrophages fulfil a dual role in the immune response to mycobacteria by acting as **reservoirs of infection** as well as directly killing more bacteria. The balance between these two opposing functions determines the outcome of infection. Disease-causing strains of mycobacteria are particularly adept at evading the host immune response using a variety of strategies (Table 2.10).

Phagocytes engulf M. leprae and M. tuberculosis via complement receptors; from the microbial perspective, this confers a **survival advantage**, since it avoids triggering the oxidative burst and therefore protects bacteria from exposure to damaging oxygen radicals. Once engulfed, disease-causing mycobacterial strains inhibit macrophage activation by the possession of 'inert' lipoarabinomannan, a cell-wall carbohydrate which inhibits release of IFN-γ and TNF. Additional survival strategies adopted by mycobacteria include inhibition of phagolysosome formation, invasion of the cytoplasm of macrophages and shelter within non-professional phagocytes.

2.5.4 Damage caused by the immune response to mycobacteria

A vigorous immune response to mycobacteria may sometimes have undesirable consequences by way of **tissue damage**. This is well illustrated by the immune response in patients with leprosy. The clinical spectrum of disease in leprosy correlates well with the host immune response to M. leprae (Fig. 2.9).

A vigorous cellular immune response characterized by TH1 cytokine release and strong granuloma formation lim-

Table 2.10 Mechanisms of immune evasion by mycobacteria

• Engulfment via complement receptors — avoids triggering respiratory burst
• Inhibition of macrophage activation by lipoarabinomannan
• Inhibition of phagolysosome formation
• Invasion of macrophage cytoplasm — provides protection from killing by phagolysosome
• Invasion of non-professional phagocytes, e.g. Schwann cells by M. leprae

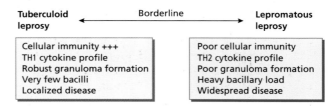

Fig. 2.9 Clinical spectrum of disease in leprosy in relation to immune response.

its spread of M. leprae but produces tissue damage. For example, patients with tuberculoid leprosy develop disabling neuropathies as a direct result of **granulomatous inflammation**, despite having paucibacillary disease. In patients with disease of intermediate severity (borderline tuberculoid, borderline lepromatous), spontaneous improvement in cellular immunity is associated with perineural and skin inflammation, due to entry of T cells secreting IFN-γ. These so-called reversal reactions require prompt treatment with corticosteroids to avert further nerve damage.

Paradoxically, treatment of patients with a heavy bacillary load, as in lepromatous leprosy, may result in **erythema nodosum leprosum (ENL)**, an immune-complex-mediated reaction (type III hypersensitivity) characterized by high fever, glomerulonephritis, rash, iritis and nerve pain. Release of mycobacterial antigens during treatment leads to circulating immune complex formation and systemic deposition. Thalidomide is particularly effective at controlling erythema nodosum leprosum reactions by its anti-TNF effect.

2.6 Fungal infection

2.6.1 Mechanisms of immunity to fungal infections

Fungi cause many diseases, which can be **classified** into superficial, subcutaneous or deep mycoses (Table 2.11). In superficial mycoses, the skin or mucous membranes are the main sites of the attack, while subcutaneous mycoses involve adjacent tissues, such as skin or bone. The term systemic mycosis describes deeper invasion of tissues with involvement of organs such as liver, lung or brain. Fungi causing systemic infections are usually divided into two groups: pathogenic and opportunistic fungi. The term pathogen implies that infection may result from contact with the organism in any individual, *whereas the opportunistic mycoses usually occur only in immunosuppressed hosts*.

Candida infection has been chosen as an example in this discussion, since it is an ubiquitous fungus which frequently causes **superficial infection** in normal hosts. Candida albicans is commonly found in the vagina and in the gastrointestinal tract from the mouth to the anus. The intact skin and mucous membranes present a formidable barrier to the fungus. Although the pH, temperature and skin shedding rate are important, the normal bacterial flora probably play the critical role in preventing fungal colonization and subsequent invasion. Disturbances of gastrointestinal ecology, through the use of antibiotics or via traumatic or hormonal changes, are important predisposing factors in many cases of chronic superficial Candida infection.

A *change in systemic immune responses* is the major factor governing **susceptibility to fungal infection**. Colonization of the susceptible host can occur when the fungus gains access via breaks in the skin or mucosae, via indwelling cannulae (especially if hypertonic solutions of glucose and amino acids are being infused) or via urinary catheters. *Cell-mediated immunity appears to be the most important effector mechanism* in these systemic infections, since disseminated fungal infection is a feature in patients with impaired T cells or neutrophils, although rare in antibody deficiency.

Table 2.11 Some examples of fungal infection in humans

Infection	Clinical presentation
Superficial	
Trichophyton rubrum	Ringworm
	Athlete's foot
Candida albicans	Vulvo-vaginitis, oral thrush
Subcutaneous	
Sporotrichium schenkii	Ulceration, abscess formation
Systemic	
Histoplasma capsulatum	Pulmonary infection
Coccidioides immitis	Acute pneumonitis
Candida albicans	Bronchopulmonary disease, oesophagitis
Cryptococcus neoformans	Meningitis, solid lung lesions
Aspergillus fumigatus	Aspergilloma, cerebral abscess, eye infections
Pneumocystis carinii	Pneumonia

CASE 2.8 ACUTE VULVO-VAGINITIS

A 27-year-old woman presented with a 4-week history of severe irritation and soreness of her vulva. For 2 weeks she had experienced burning pain on micturition but no frequency. In addition, she had a thick, creamy-white vaginal discharge. Her menstrual periods were regular and she was taking the oral contraceptive pill. On examination, her general condition was good. She had marked erythema of her vulva and vaginal mucosa, with white plaques. The appearances were those of acute vulvo-vaginitis. A vaginal swab showed masses of pseudohyphae, with a profuse growth of Candida albicans on culture. She was treated with oral miconazole with rapid symptomatic relief.

2.6.2 Bystander damage caused by immune reactions to fungi

There are several possible **outcomes** of fungal infection. Usually, the specific immune response to the fungus, coupled with topical antifungal drugs, eliminates superficial infection. In contrast, systemic opportunistic fungal infection carries a high mortality rate in the immunosuppressed host, an outcome only partly improved by the use of newer prophylactic and therapeutic antifungal agents.

There is a third possible outcome. If the fungus is not successfully eliminated, or causes persistent reinfection, then the host's immune response to fungal antigen may trigger a **hypersensitivity reaction**. For example, Aspergillus fumigatus infection can present in a disseminated form or as a persistent aspergilloma, in which the fungus grows in pre-existing lung cavities (usually left after successful treatment of pulmonary tuberculosis). Allergic bronchopulmonary aspergillosis can then occur; this happens mainly in atopic patients and is due to **IgE-mediated hypersensitivity** to Aspergillus antigens. Bronchi may be obstructed by fragmented mycelia, and there is an inflammatory reaction in the bronchial wall with eosinophilic infiltration. Clinically, the condition usually presents as recurrent episodes of increased wheezing, coughing, fever and pleuritic pain in an asthmatic (see Chapter 13).

If fungal antigens are inhaled by someone with preformed precipitating antibodies, then **antigen–antibody complexes** may form in the respiratory tract. One example is farmers' lung, a condition resulting from an immune-complex-mediated hypersensitivity response to a fungus (Micropolyspora faeni) present in mouldy hay (see Chapter 13).

2.7 Parasitic infection

2.7.1 Protozoal infection

Protozoa are a diverse group of parasites. In this section, malaria (Case 2.9), leishmaniasis and trypanosomiasis, which globally constitute a huge burden of parasitic disease, are used to illustrate the immunological interactions between host and parasite.

If parasites **elude** the host's immune response and are sufficiently virulent, they kill the host upon whom their own survival depends; yet, if they are too easily destroyed by the immune response, their own survival is jeopardized. *The survival of any parasite therefore represents a balance between induction of immunity in the host and escape from surveillance.*

Parasites may even have induced **mutations** in humans which, due to natural selection, has enabled them to resist the parasite. Plasmodium, the protozoon causing malaria, is an example. The sickle-cell haemoglobin gene confers partial resistance to P. falciparum and limits its multiplication within erythrocytes. Thus, people with the normal haemoglobin genotype (Hb AA) are highly susceptible to falciparum malaria; those with the homozygous sickle-cell genotype (Hb SS) suffer serious and usually lethal sickle-cell anaemia, but those with heterozygous sickle-cell trait (Hb AS) have a survival advantage in endemic malarial areas. A number of other genetic polymorphisms are associated with resistance to malaria, including HLA-B53 and the absence of the red cell Duffy antigen, which is the receptor for P. vivax.

2.7.2 Normal immune responses to protozoa

Patients react to protozoal infection with a spectrum of responses similar to that evoked by other microbes. An early response is **activation of macrophages** and monocytes with release of cytokines, including TNF, IL-1 and IL-6. Their combined actions cause fever, leucocytosis and production of acute-phase reactants such as C-reactive protein. The fever response may itself be a host defence since, for example, certain stages of malarial parasite development are sensitive to elevated temperatures.

CASE 2.9 CEREBRAL MALARIA

A 44-year-old Nigerian man was admitted as an emergency while visiting relatives in England. His symptoms began 4 days after arrival, and over the following 10 days he deteriorated progressively, with vague upper abdominal pain, sweating, rigors and vomiting. In the past, he had been treated twice for malaria but had never taken malarial prophylaxis. On examination he was ill and jaundiced, with a temperature of 39.2 °C. His blood pressure was 90/70 but he showed no signs of visceral perforation. The differential diagnosis included occult gastrointestinal bleeding, septicaemia, hepatitis or recurrence of malaria.

Emergency
(140 g/l) and
was excluded b
a thick blood fil
falciparum. After
was treated with
rapidly deteriorate
a cardiac arrest an
diagnosis was ceret

Although IgM and IgG **antibodies** are made in response to most adult protozoa, these antibodies are not necessarily protective, making it difficult to produce an effective vaccine. Furthermore, some protozoa penetrate and survive within host cells: examples include the malarial parasite, Plasmodium, which invades erythrocytes and hepatocytes, and Leishmania, which survives inside macrophages. Such intracellular protozoa are not accessible to antibodies unless protozoal antigens are also secreted on to the host cell surface.

The role of **cell-mediated immunity** has proved difficult to evaluate in these diseases. In mice, resistance to infection with several intracellular pathogens (mycobacteria, leishmania, salmonella) is controlled by a single gene expressed only in reticuloendothelial cells called the natural-resistance-associated macrophage protein 1 gene (Nramp 1). In addition, sensitized T cells and IFN-γ are important determinants of immunity against protozoa that survive within macrophages, e.g. leishmania. A predominant TH1 cytokine profile (IFN-γ, IL-2, TNF, IL-12) is associated with localized disease in the form of cutaneous leishmaniasis, while disseminated visceral disease occurs in individuals with a TH2 cytokine profile. In such cases, addition of IFN-γ to conventional anti-leishmania treatment hastens recovery.

sion of immune responses

ways in which protozoa can evade or munological attack (Table 2.12): anti-

genic variation, blunting the attack by immune suppression, or hiding in cells where the immune attack is less effective.

Antigenic variation is the most striking example of successful adaptation and is exemplified by sleeping sickness; this is caused by Trypanosoma brucei and spread by the bite of the tsetse fly. After infection, the number of parasites in the blood fluctuates in a cycle of parasitaemia — remission and recrudescence. This is due to destruction of trypanosomes by host antibody, followed by the emergence of parasites expressing different surface antigens (or variant surface glycoproteins — VSGs). Antibodies produced after each wave of parasitaemia are specific for that set of VSGs only. The parasite possesses a number of genes that code for its VSGs and can vary the genes used. The antibodies do not trigger the switch; it occurs spontaneously. By varying the immunodominant antigen, the parasite diverts its host's attack. This type of antigenic variation is known as phenotypic variation and is in contrast to genotypic variation, in which a new strain periodically results in an epidemic, as is the case with influenza virus.

Other protozoa can rapidly change their surface coat to elude the immune response, a process known as **antigenic modulation**. Within minutes of exposure to antibodies, Leishmania parasites can remove ('cap off') their surface antigens, so becoming refractory to the effects of antibodies and complement.

Suppression of the immune response is one of the most obvious adaptive mechanisms for protozoal survival and has been found in all parasitic infections in which it has

Table 2.12 Mechanisms of protozoal survival

Mechanism	Examples of disease
Host variation	
• Genetic factors	Malaria
• Suppression of host immunity	Malaria, leishmaniasis, schistosomiasis
• Active induction of IL-10 producing CD25+ regulatory T cells to prevent parasite clearance	Leishmaniasis
• Inhibition of IL-12 production	Leishmaniasis
• Inhibition of dendritic cell function	Leishmaniasis, trypanosomiasis, malaria
Parasite variation	
• Antigenic variation	Trypanosomiasis, malaria
• Antigenic modulation	Leishmaniasis
• Antigenic disguise	Schistosomiasis
• Premunition	Schistosomiasis
• Resistance to macrophage killing	Leishmaniasis
	Toxoplasmosis
	Trypanosomiasis
• Resistance to complement-mediated lysis	Leishmaniasis
	Trypanosomiasis

been sought. The most striking examples occur in malaria and visceral leishmaniasis. Soluble antigens released by the parasite may inhibit non-specifically the host's immune response by acting directly on lymphocytes or by saturating the reticuloendothelial system. Leishmania and Trypanosoma have stages that are refractory to complement-mediated lysis. Trypanosoma cruzi, for instance, produces molecules that either inhibit the formation or accelerate the decay of C3 convertases, so blocking complement activation on the parasite surface. Leishmania can down-regulate MHC class I expression on parasitized macrophages, reducing the effectiveness of cytotoxic CD8+ T cells.

Some protozoa, including Toxoplasma, Leishmania and Trypanosoma cruzi, not only easily enter but **survive and grow inside macrophages**. Infective Leishmania bind C3 actively and these serve as a molecule for binding the parasite to CR3 receptors on macrophages. Monoclonal antibodies to the CR3 receptor inhibit uptake of the parasite into a safe haven. Toxoplasma has evolved mechanisms that prevent fusion of phagocytic vacuoles (containing the parasite) with lysosomes. Trypanosomes are also resistant to intracellular killing mechanisms in non-activated macrophages.

2.7.4 Helminth infections

Helminths are multicellular (metazoan) parasites that are grouped into three distinct families: nematodes (e.g. Ascaris spp.), trematodes (e.g. Schistosoma spp.) and cestodes (e.g. Taenia spp.). They have complex life cycles with many developmental stages. In the course of a single infection, humans may be repeatedly exposed to larval, adult and egg antigens. For example, free-swimming larval stages (cercariae) of the trematode, S. mansoni, penetrate the skin of humans bathing or swimming in infested water. Following entry, they develop into tissue-stage schistosomula, which migrate via the pulmonary circulation into the liver. In the liver, they trigger a granulomatous inflammatory reaction leading to portal hypertension (as in Case 2.10). Once within the porta-hepatic system, the schistosomula mature into adult worms and take up their final position in small venules draining the intestine, from where they shed eggs into the intestinal lumen.

2.7.5 Normal immunity to helminth infection

The immunological characteristics of helminth infection are increased IgE production, eosinophilia and mastocytosis. These responses are regulated by the TH2 subset of CD4+ T lymphocytes (see Chapter 1). People living in tropical or subtropical countries, where helminth infestation is endemic, have grossly raised serum IgE levels.

Parasite-specific IgE antibodies play an important role in protection, for example to S. mansoni. IgE antibodies react with helminth antigens and lead to the release of pharmacologically active mediators from mast cells, eosinophils and basophils to which the IgE is bound. These mediators cause local accumulation of leucocytes and augment their ability to damage the helminth. They induce local inflammation and act on smooth muscle to aid expulsion of parasites. However, parasite-specific IgE is only a fraction of the massive increase in IgE induced by IL-4 produced by CD4+ TH2 cells (Fig. 2.10). It is possible that the excess polyclonal IgE provoked by helminth infestation may represent a mecha-

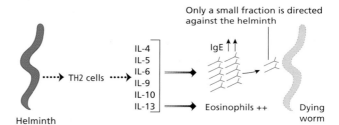

Fig. 2.10 IgE production in helminth infection may be an epiphenomenon.

CASE 2.10 SCHISTOSOMIASIS

A 25-year-old Egyptian student who had lived in England for the past 2 years presented with acute haematemesis. Examination revealed marked hepatosplenomegaly. Oesophageal and gastric varices were identified at emergency upper gastrointestinal endoscopy, thus confirming the presence of portal hypertension. The following disorders were considered in the differential diagnosis as a possible cause of his portal hypertension: alcoholic cirrhosis, chronic active hepatitis, portal and hepatic venous obstruction and schistosomiasis. Alcoholic liver disease was considered unlikely since he was a teetotaller; ultrasound and computed tomography studies of the porta-hepatic circulation excluded vascular obstruction. A liver biopsy was postponed until his deranged clotting was corrected. Schistosomiasis was considered as a possible diagnosis in view of his ethnic background and markedly raised total serum IgE: 2500 kU/l (NR < 130). Examination of stool specimens revealed the characteristic ova of Schistosoma mansoni and high levels of serum antibodies to S. mansoni were subsequently detected by enzyme immunoassay. Endoscopic sclerotherapy was used to sclerose his bleeding varices and he was commenced on Praziquantel, a highly effective antischistosomal drug.

nism to saturate IgE receptors on mast cells, thus rendering them refractory to stimulation by parasite antigens.

Eosinophilia is also characteristic of helminth disease and, like IgE responses, is regulated by CD4+ T cells but is driven by IL-5. Mast cells, degranulated by bound IgE reacting with parasite antigens, release a variety of mediators (see Fig. 1.26). Some parasitic material is even directly attractant to eosinophils. Eosinophils have an effector role in helminth infection: they attach to the parasite surface and degranulate, releasing major basic protein and eosinophil cationic protein, which cause small holes in the tegument of the helminth.

2.7.6 Helminth evasion of immune responses

Antigenic disguise is important in helminth survival. Adult schistosomes 'disguise' their surface antigens (see Table 2.12) by synthesizing host-like antigens, such as α_2-macroglobulin, to mask their own foreignness. Alternatively, they may adsorb host molecules on to their surfaces: red blood cell antigens, immunoglobulins, MHC antigens and complement have all been demonstrated on the outer layer of schistosomes.

Helminth infestation is also associated with **immunosuppression of T- and B-cell responses** through the induction of IL-10. For instance, numerous immune mechanisms are directed against the young schistosomulum as it migrates from the skin to the blood vessels in which it matures. Schistosomes evade such attack by 'disguise', but can also actively protect themselves by releasing peptidases that cleave bound immunoglobulins, and other factors that inhibit either T-cell proliferation, release of IFN-γ or the mast cell signal required for eosinophil activation.

The observation of reduced skin test reactivity to allergens coupled with the inhibition of TH2-associated allergic disease in schistosome-infected children has led to a reappraisal of the '**hygiene hypothesis**' which states that TH2-associated allergic disease would be counteracted by exposure to microorganisms that induce TH1 cells. It is thought that regulatory T cells may play a role in preventing the development of allergic disease in helminth-infested populations who exhibit TH2 immune responses.

The term 'concomitant immunity' or '**premunition**' is used to describe a form of acquired immunity in which the established infection persists but new infection is prevented by immune mechanisms. Schistosomiasis is again the best example: adult schistosome worms can live in the host for many years, often with little or no evidence of any immune response. However, adult schistosomes do stimulate a response that prevents reinfection of the same animal with immature forms of the parasite, called cercaria.

2.7.7 Bystander damage caused by immune reactions to protozoa and helminths

Many of the clinical features of parasite infection result from the host's immune response to parasite antigens. **Immediate (type I) hypersensitivity** reactions, such as urticaria and angioedema, are found in the acute stages of ascariasis, and in many other helminth infections. Rupture of a hydatid cyst during surgical removal may release vast amounts of antigen and trigger anaphylactic shock.

Type II hypersensitivity reactions are caused by antibodies to cell-surface antigens. Parasite antigens which cross-react with host tissue, or host antigens adsorbed on to the parasite surface, may lead to the development of antibodies which recognize self-antigens. Such autoimmunization is an important factor in the immunopathology of Chagas' disease (see Chapter 13).

Circulating immune complexes of parasite antigen and host antibodies cause some of the tissue damage seen in malaria, trypanosomiasis and schistosomiasis. In some cases, chronic deposition of immune complexes may lead to glomerulonephritis (see Chapter 9).

Cell-mediated immunity to parasite antigens can also cause severe tissue damage. For example, in schistosomiasis, portal fibrosis and pulmonary hypertension are probably due to cellular responses to schistosome eggs deposited in the tissues.

FURTHER READING

See website: www.immunologyclinic.com

3.1 Introduction

Once a newborn infant leaves the sterile intrauterine environment, he or she meets many microorganisms and becomes colonized with 'healthy bacteria'. Most microflora are non-pathogenic, so this colonization does not cause symptoms. When exposed to a pathogen which the child has not met before, clinical infection results, expanding the child's immunological memory and producing long-lasting immunity.

In any encounter with a microorganism, the resistance of the host must be balanced against the **virulence** of the microorganism and the size of the inoculums. Infections with certain organisms, for example Pneumocystis carinii, are unknown except in patients with underlying immunodeficiency, and are therefore known as 'opportunistic'. **Host factors** are very variable; they can be inherited or acquired, including environmental, dietary or drug induced. Some infective agents, for example HIV or cytomegalovirus, have potent immunosuppressive effects and can cause serious disease. These causes of secondary immune deficiencies are discussed in this chapter.

Underlying immunodeficiency should be suspected in every patient, *irrespective of age*, who has recurrent, persistent, severe or unusual infections. Defects in immunity can be **classified** into primary disorders, due to an intrinsic defect in the immune system that may be congenital or acquired, or those secondary to a known condition (Fig. 3.1). They may involve adaptive or innate immune mechanisms and maybe be permanent (genetic) or transient (if due to a viral infection). Furthermore, many defects are subtle and defy classification.

The **type of organism** causing the infections may give a clue to the nature of the defect (Fig. 3.2). The speed of the infection is also important. The innate immune system is

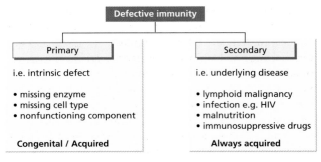

Fig. 3.1 Primary and secondary immune deficiencies.

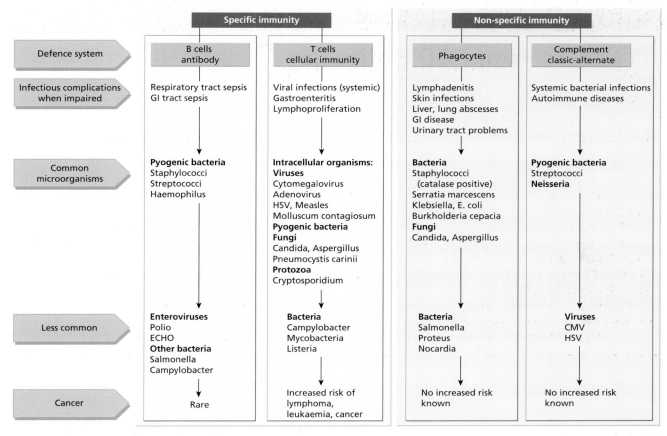

	Specific immunity		Non-specific immunity	
Defence system	B cells antibody	T cells cellular immunity	Phagocytes	Complement classic-alternate
Infectious complications when impaired	Respiratory tract sepsis GI tract sepsis	Viral infections (systemic) Gastroenteritis Lymphoproliferation	Lymphadenitis Skin infections Liver, lung abscesses GI disease Urinary tract problems	Systemic bacterial infections Autoimmune diseases
Common microorganisms	**Pyogenic bacteria** Staphylococci Streptococci Haemophilus	**Intracellular organisms: Viruses** Cytomegalovirus Adenovirus HSV, Measles Molluscum contagiosum **Pyogenic bacteria Fungi** Candida, Aspergillus Pneumocystis carinii **Protozoa** Cryptosporidium	**Bacteria** Staphylococci (catalase positive) Serratia marcescens Klebsiella, E. coli Burkholderia cepacia **Fungi** Candida, Aspergillus	**Pyogenic bacteria** Streptococci **Neisseria**
Less common	**Enteroviruses** Polio ECHO **Other bacteria** Salmonella Campylobacter	**Bacteria** Campylobacter Mycobacteria Listeria	**Bacteria** Salmonella Proteus Nocardia	**Viruses** CMV HSV
Cancer	Rare	Increased risk of lymphoma, leukaemia, cancer	No increased risk known	No increased risk known

Fig. 3.2 Defects in immunity suggested by infections with certain organisms. GI, gastrointestinal; HSV, herpes simplex virus.

the first line of defence and, if this fails, an infection will be acute and severe (even overwhelming). In the main, bacterial infections indicate humoral (antibody and complement) or phagocytic defects and viral or fungal infections suggest T-cell defects.

3.2 Primary antibody deficiencies

3.2.1 Diagnosis of primary antibody deficiencies

The **commonest** forms of primary immune deficiencies are those due to antibody failure and are discussed first. These occur in children and adults and may be congenital or acquired. Congenital antibody deficiencies are rarer than acquired ones; > 90% of patients who fail to produce protective antibodies present after 10 years of age (Table 3.1). It is easier, however, to discuss the various forms of antibody deficiencies in relation to the development of B cells, and so the clinical types are given here in this order too [Case 1 (lack of B cell differentiation) to Case 4 (failure of T cells to help B cells to immunoglobulin class switch)]. Regardless of the precise defect, the outcome is failure of production of protective antibodies.

In **genetic forms** of antibody deficiency, recurrent infections usually begin between 4 months and 2 years of age, because maternally transferred IgG affords some passive protection for the first 3–4 months of life (Fig. 3.3). Some

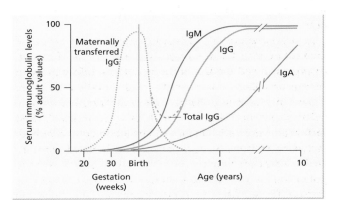

Fig. 3.3 Serum immunoglobulin levels and age. Maternally transferred IgG (···) has mostly disappeared by 6 months. As the neonate synthesizes (—) IgG, the level slowly rises, but a physiological 'trough' of serum IgG is characteristically seen between 3 and 6 months (- - -).

Table 3.1 Major causes of primary antibody deficiencies in children and adults

Age (years)	Children	Adults
< 4	Transient hypogammaglobulinaemia of infancy X-linked agammaglobulinaemia (late diagnosis is unusual but does occur) Hyper-IgM syndromes (diagnosis may be later too)	
4–15	Common variable immunodeficiency disorders Hyper-IgM syndromes Selective IgA deficiency Selective/partial antibody deficiencies	
16–60		Common variable immunodeficiency disorders Selective/partial antibody deficiencies Selective IgA deficiency Antibody deficiency with thymoma

BOX 3.1 CLUES FROM THE HISTORY IN ANTIBODY DEFICIENCY

Recurrent sinus/chest infections are common (see Fig. 3.4)

- History of repeated ENT surgery
- Lobectomy in childhood or adolescence
- Early bronchiectasis

Another system is usually involved

- Skin sepsis (boils, abscesses)
- Gut infections
- Meningitis

Infections are due to common bacteria (Fig. 3.2)

- Streptococcus pneumoniae
- Haemophilus influenzae

Non-infectious features are common

- Autoimmune thyroid disease
- Immune thrombocytopenic purpura
- Arthritis

Fungal and viral infections are uncommon

examination often shows evidence of the consequences of previous severe infections, such as a ruptured tympanic membrane, grommets, bronchiectasis or failure to thrive.

Laboratory investigations are essential to the diagnosis. Measurements of serum immunoglobulin levels will often but not always reveal gross quantitative abnormalities. Complete absence of immunoglobulin, i.e. agammaglobulinaemia, is unusual, and even severely affected patients have very low but detectable IgG and IgM. Defects in antibody synthesis can involve one immunoglobulin isotype alone, such as IgA, or groups of isotypes, often IgA and IgG. The ability of a patient to make antibodies is a better guide to susceptibility to infection than total immunoglobulin levels. *Failure to make specific antibody after immunization is fundamental to the diagnosis.* Tests of specific functional antibodies are shown in Table 3.2. Measurements of IgG subclasses are meaningless unless backed up by test immunizations and detection of specific IgG responses.

Circulating B cells are identified by monoclonal antibodies to **B-cell antigens** (see Chapter 19). In normal blood,

Table 3.2 Tests for functional antibodies

Detection after natural exposure/infection (chicken pox)
Response to prior or test immunization:
- protein (tetanus toxoid, Haemophilus influenzae type b, measles, etc.)
- carbohydrate (bacterial polysaccharide, e.g. pneumococcal, salmonella)

Caution
Live vaccines (e.g. MMR) should never be given to children in whom an immunodeficiency is suspected
Normal children under the age of 2 years do not respond to carbohydrate antigens

forms of primary antibody deficiency are inherited as X-linked or autosomal recessive traits: a history of affected relatives, especially boys, is therefore of diagnostic value, although a negative family history does not exclude an inherited condition or a de novo mutation. Primary immune deficiencies are relatively rare. **A detailed history** (Box 3.1) helps to distinguish them from more common causes of recurrent infection: for example, cystic fibrosis or inhaled foreign bodies are more likely causes of recurrent chest infections in childhood. However, *if tests for cystic fibrosis are done, immunoglobulin measurements should always be performed also.*

Clues from the examination are few: there are rarely any diagnostic physical signs of antibody deficiency, although

these cells comprise about 5–15% of the total lymphocyte population. The absence of mature B cells in an antibody-deficient individual distinguishes X-linked agammaglobulinaemia from other causes of primary antibody deficiency in which B cells are present in low or normal numbers. Mutation analysis is essential to confirm a diagnosis of an inherited condition and enables family members to be tested and counselled. Management with replacement immunoglobulin therapy by a clinical immunologist is important (see below).

3.2.2 Types of primary antibody deficiency
(see Table 3.1 and Box 3.2)

Transient hypogammaglobulinaemia of infancy
Maternal IgG is actively transported across the placenta to the fetal circulation from the fourth month of gestational life, although maximum transfer takes place during the final 2 months (see section 18.4.2). At birth, the infant has a serum IgG at least equal to that of the mother (see Fig. 3.3), but catabolism of maternal IgG outstrips IgG synthesized by the newborn child, resulting in a phase of '**physiological IgG trough**'. However, the normal infant is not unduly susceptible to infection because functioning antibody can be made and some T-cell functions are active (see Chapter 18).

The trough in IgG is more severe if the child is **premature**, as IgG acquired from the mother is reduced (see Case 18.2). Improved neonatal care of babies results in more surviving infants born between 26 and 32 weeks of gestation. These infants are at risk of bacterial infections due to reduction of time for placental transfer, though the incidence of such infections is low in the UK where routine invasive support (e.g. indwelling lines for nutrition, monitoring, etc.) is not used. Low-birth-weight babies in countries where such procedures are common, in whom there is an increased incidence of severe bacterial infections, may benefit from replacement immunoglobulin until they can synthesize their own protective antibodies (see Fig. 3.3).

Transient hypogammaglobulinaemia also occurs when the infant is **slow to synthesize IgG**; as serum levels of

Table 3.3 Prevalence of primary antibody deficiency

Comparison with other diseases	Per 10⁵ population
Rheumatoid arthritis	1000
Insulin dependent diabetes	200
Multiple sclerosis	60
Systemic lupus erythematosus	50
Primary antibody deficiencies	4–6
Scleroderma	1

maternally acquired antibodies continue to fall, the infant may become susceptible to recurrent pyogenic infections for many months, until spontaneous IgG synthesis begins. It is important to distinguish this condition from pathological causes of hypogammaglobulinaemia because the management differs. In most cases, the infant remains well and needs no specific therapy even though immunoglobulin levels remain below the normal range. If infections are severe, then prophylactic antibiotics should prevent further morbidity; these may be needed for 1–2 years or until endogenous IgG synthesis is satisfactory.

X-linked agammaglobulinaemia (Bruton's disease)
Boys with X-linked agammaglobulinaemia (XLA) usually present with **recurrent pyogenic infections** between the ages of 4 months and 2 years (as in Case 3.1). The sites of infection and the organisms involved are similar to other

---

BOX 3.2 TYPES OF PRIMARY ANTIBODY DEFICIENCIES

- Common variable immunodeficiency disorders
- X-linked agammaglobulinaemia
- Hyper IgM syndromes (e.g. CD40 ligand deficiency)
- IgA and IgG subclass deficiencies
- Selective IgA deficiency
- Specific antibody deficiencies
- Transient hypogammaglobulinaemia of infancy

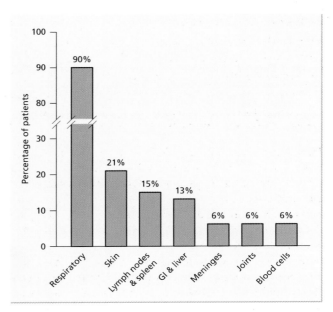

Fig. 3.4 Presenting symptoms in particular organs in patients with primary antibody deficiencies.

CASE 3.1 X-LINKED AGAMMAGLOBULINAEMIA (BRUTON'S DISEASE)

Peter was born after an uneventful pregnancy, weighing 3.1 kg. At 3 months, he developed otitis media; at the ages of 5 months and 11 months, he was admitted to hospital with Haemophilus influenzae pneumonia. These infections responded promptly to appropriate antibiotics on each occasion. He is the fourth child of unrelated parents: his three sisters showed no predisposition to infection.

Examination at the age of 18 months showed a pale, thin child whose height and weight were below the third centile. There were no other abnormal features. He had been fully immunized as an infant (at 2, 3 and 4 months) with tetanus and diphtheria toxoids, acellular pertussis, Haemophilus and Mening. C conjugate vaccines and polio (Salk). In addition, he had received measles, mumps and rubella vaccine at 15 months. All immunizations were uneventful.

Immunological investigations (Table 3.4) into the cause of his recurrent infections showed severe reduction in all three classes of serum immunoglobulins and no specific antibody production. Although there was no family history of agammaglobulinaemia, the lack of mature B lymphocytes in his peripheral blood suggested a failure of B-cell differentiation and strongly supported a diagnosis of infantile X-linked agammaglobulinaemia (Bruton's disease). This was confirmed by detection of a disease-causing mutation in the Btk gene. The antibody deficiency was treated by 2-weekly intravenous infusions of human normal IgG in a dose of 400 mg/kg body weight/month. Over the following 7 years, his health steadily improved, weight and height are now on the 30th centile, and he

Table 3.4 Immunological investigations* in Case 3.1. XLA

Quantitative serum immunoglobulins (g/l):

IgG	0.17	(5.5–10.0)
IgA	Not detected	(0.3–0.8)
IgM	0.07	(0.4–1.8)

Antibody activity

Immunization responses—no detectable IgG antibodies to:
  Tetanus toxoid
  Haemophilus type b polysaccharides
  Polio
  Measles
  Rubella
Isohaemagglutinins (IgM) not detected (blood group A Rh+)

Blood lymphocyte subpopulations (×10⁹/l):

Total lymphocyte count	3.5	(2.5–5.0)
T lymphocytes (CD3)	3.02	(1.5–3.0)
B lymphocytes (CD19)	<0.1	(0.3–1.0)

*Normal range for age 18 months shown in parentheses.

has had only one episode of otitis media in the last 4 years. He is now able to co-operate and is treated with the same dose of replacement immunoglobulin given subcutaneously by his mother at home.

types of antibody deficiency (Figs 3.2 and 3.4), although these young boys are also susceptible to life-threatening enteroviruses.

In almost all patients, **circulating mature B cells are absent** but T cells are normal. There are no plasma cells in the bone marrow, lymph nodes or gastrointestinal tract. Differentiation of pre-B cells into B cells depends on a tyrosine kinase enzyme—known as Bruton's tyrosine kinase (Btk), normally found in developing B cells, though not mature B cells (Fig. 3.5). This enzyme, like the T cell counterpart, Itk, interacts with lipids on the inner cell surface membrane clustered around an antigen receptor and is crucial for maturation. The Btk gene is mutated in XLA patients, resulting in

abnormal enzymes which may be either absent or present but always non-functional.

The diagnosis of XLA rests on the very low serum levels of all isotypes of immunoglobulin, the absence of circulating mature B lymphocytes and a **mutation in the Btk gene**. The identification of the gene allows asymptomatic female carriers to be identified and counselled, and prenatal diagnosis is now feasible. The gene for Btk is located on the long arm of the X chromosome, resulting in X-linked inheritance. Other defects in the B-cell maturation pathway, though still rare, have autosomal recessive inheritance and occur in girls.

Management consists of high levels of **replacement immunoglobulin** for all affected individuals (see section 3.2.5 below), to prevent bronchiectasis (see Fig. 3.6).

Fig. 3.5 An overview of the steps in B-cell maturation. The proteins in red are those in which gene defects have been shown to cause specific failure of B-cell differentiation and therefore primary antibody failure.

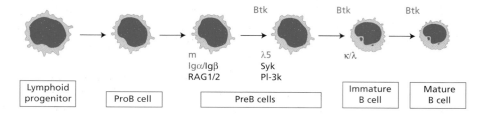

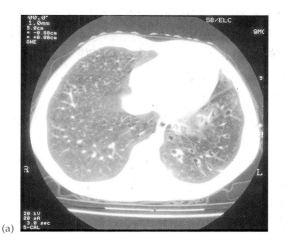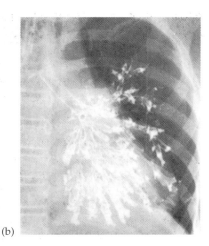

Fig. 3.6 Bronchiectasis— (a) computed tomography scan and (b) bronchogram (no longer performed) show the typical features of damaged terminal bronchioles, leading to structural lung damage. (a)   (b)

Hyper-IgM syndromes

Some children with severe antibody deficiency (including boys with or without affected male relatives) have normal numbers of B cells and normal or raised serum IgM levels at presentation; such syndromes are therefore known as hyper-IgM syndromes as in Case 3.2. In the **X-linked form**, the boys have an additional susceptibility to Pneumocystis carinii infection. Such infection is normally associated with T-cell defects such as HIV or severe combined immune deficiency (see Fig. 3.2). Unlike XLA, this defect is not restricted to B cells, being due to failure of the CD40 ligand accessory molecule on T cells (Fig. 1.26). Normally, this ligand reacts with CD40 on B cells to trigger switching in specific antibody production from IgM to IgG or IgA and the formation of germinal centres. Failure of expression or functional activity of this ligand results in failure of switching and poor organization of the germinal centres (see Fig. 3.7) and is associated with lack of memory B cells, reduced somatic hypermutation and impaired dendritic cell function to prime T cells. The lack of cross-linking of CD40 also results in failure of the B cells to up-regulate CD80 and CD86, important co-stimulatory molecules that interact with CD28 and CTLA-4 on T cells for immune regulation, and defective recognition of tumour cells. This is associated with the development of lymphoid and other malignancies in older patients with this condition. The lack of CD40 ligand in the thymus results in defective purging of autoreactive thymocytes, hence increased susceptibility to autoimmune diseases including neutropenia (as in Case 3.2).

Management of such patients currently consists of replacement immunoglobulin and genetic testing for potential female carriers. **Bone marrow transplantation in childhood** is now considered to be the treatment of choice, since a high proportion of patients develop liver disease or malignancies in later life.

Failure of *any part* of the interaction between CD40 ligand and CD40, or of the other essential components of the pathway (such as the intracellular enzymes involved), results in failure in immunoglobulin switch and germinal centre formation. These **pure B-cell forms of the hyper-IgM syndrome** may have defects in the enzymes responsible for repair of DNA in somatic hypermutation in B cells—such as activation-induced cytidine deaminase (AID). Such patients fail to switch and have a limited antibody repertoire, causing an accumulation of immature B cells in abnormal germinal centres and hence clinically enlarged lymph nodes and spleens.

Common variable immunodeficiency disorders

CVIDs are a heterogeneous group of disorders making up the **commonest form of primary antibody deficiency**, accounting for about 90% of the symptomatic antibody deficiencies.

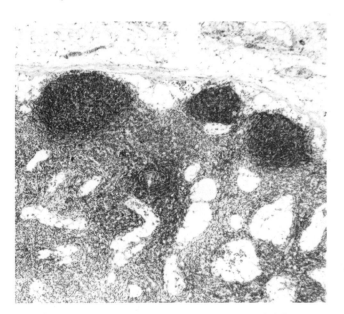

Fig. 3.7 Lymph node from a patient with CD40 ligand deficiency showing impaired germinal centres. (From F. Fachetti with permission.)

CASE 3.2 CD40 LIGAND DEFICIENCY

Michael was seen in OPD at the age of 4 years with a history of painful mouth ulcers, abdominal pain over 7 weeks (associated with going to nursery) but persistent diarrhoea in the last 2 weeks. He had suffered multiple episodes of ear and chest infections, starting with pneumonia at the age of 9 months, when he had been noted to have neutropenia but this had appeared to be transient. He has three healthy sisters. On examination he had multiple oral ulcers, enlarged tonsils, purulent nasal discharge, scarred tympanic membranes, abdominal distension and hepatomegaly.

He was investigated for an early presentation of inflammatory bowel disease, including stool microscopy. In addition, liver function tests and hepatitis serology were done to determine the cause of the enlarged liver, T-lymphocyte enumeration to exclude severe combined immunodeficiency (SCID) and immunoglobulin levels to exclude a CVID. Crytosporidia were found in the stools and liver enzyme levels were raised. Serum IgG and IgA levels were very low but B and T-cell numbers were normal (see Table 3.5). Since C-reactive protein (CRP) and albumin serum levels were normal, an intestinal biopsy was not indicated. A diagnosis of primary antibody deficiency with cryptosporidiosis was made, confirmed by liver biopsy. Abdominal ultrasound showed a diffusely enlarged liver with a dilated common bile duct.

This was most likely to be due to a hyper-IgM syndrome as the serum IgM was raised. Peripheral blood lymphocytes were separated and stimulated in culture; activation markers, including CD40 ligand, were then detected by flow cytometry. CD69 and CD72 were present but there was no CD40 ligand on Michael's T lymphocytes. Mutation analysis confirmed a deletion in the CD40 ligand gene on the X chromosome and a substantive diagnosis of CD40 ligand deficiency was made. He was treated initially with replacement immunoglobulin, co-trimoxazole to prevent Pneumocystis infection and specific antibiotics for Cryptosporidiosis; if this organism can be controlled, bone marrow grafting, with or

without liver transplantation, will be considered. His mother will be tested for carrier status, as will his sisters when they reach the age of consent.

Table 3.5 Immunological investigations in Case 3.2, CD40 ligand deficiency

Serum proteins

Albumin		39 g/l
C-reactive protein		8 mg/l
Immunoglobulins	IgG	0.9 g/l
	IgA	< 0.07 g/l
	IgM	3.2 g/l

There were no detectable IgG antibodies to immunization or exposure antigens

Blood lymphocyte subpopulations (×10⁹/l):

Total lymphocyte count	2.1	(1.5–3.50)
T lymphocytes		
CD3	1.5	(0.9–2.8)
CD4	0.8	(0.6–1.2)
CD8	0.7	(0.4–1.0)
B lymphocytes		
CD19	0.4	(0.2–0.4)
NK lymphocytes		
CD16:CD56	0.2	(0.2–0.4)

Lymphocyte stimulation assays (with phytohaemagglutinin)

	Prestimulation*			Post-stimulation		
	CD69	CD71	CD40 ligand	CD69	CD71	CD40 ligand
Control	3%	5%	< 1%	73%	49%	62%
Patient	1%	2%	< 1%	72%	63%	< 1%

*Percentage of CD3 cells with relevant activation marker on surface.

The several diseases with this type of clinical phenotype will become more distinct over the next several years. Although some patients present in childhood, most (> 90%) are not diagnosed until adulthood (see Cases 3.3 and 16.7). Most patients with a CVID have very **low serum levels of IgG and IgA**, with normal or reduced IgM and normal or low numbers of B cells. About one-third of patients have an abnormality of cell-mediated immunity as well; these variable findings reflect the name of the condition. Affected individuals experience the same range of bacterial and viral infections as other patients with antibody deficiencies (see Figs 3.2 and 3.4).

Currently, most patients lead normal though shortened lives, provided that they receive replacement immunoglobulin therapy (see below). Complications are very varied (see section 3.2.4), probably due to large numbers of disease-

causing and modifying genes, resulting in the different syndromes in this large group of disorders. Affected women have given birth to normal offspring, as in Case 3.3.

Selective or partial antibody deficiencies

So called 'IgG subclass deficiencies' are controversial, since deletion of IgG subclass genes does not necessarily lead to disease. *Investigation of individual patients should be limited to those with significant recurrent bacterial infections.* In such patients, selective deficiencies of one or two of the three protective IgG subclasses (IgG₁, IgG₂ and IgG₃) may be missed, as the total IgG level may appear normal. However, what really matters is the ability to make specific antibodies against infective organisms to prevent recurrent infections. Most significant deficiencies of **IgG subclasses are those associated with IgA deficiency**. IgG subclass measurements are

CASE 3.3 COMMON VARIABLE IMMUNODEFICIENCY DISORDERS (CVID)

A 64-year-old woman developed herpes zoster and lobar pneumonia; over the previous 5 years she had been admitted to hospital with pneumonia on two previous occasions and made a full recovery. There had been no history of recurrent chest infections during childhood. The pathogens isolated were Haemophilus influenza and Streptococcus pneumoniae. At the age of 35, she developed a non-erosive seronegative arthritis. On direct questioning, she gave a history of intermittent diarrhoea since her late teens. These episodes lasted from 2 days to 2 weeks and she passed five to six partly formed stools a day. There was no family history of recurrent infections: she had two sons, aged 10 and 7, both of whom were well. Physical examination was normal, although she was thin.

Investigations showed a haemoglobin of 115 g/l, with normal neutrophil and lymphocyte counts. Immunological studies (Table 3.6) showed very low levels of serum immunoglobulins, and no detectable specific antibodies despite culture-proven Streptococcus pneumoniae and a tetanus toxoid boost 1 year earlier. She had normal numbers of circulating T and B lymphocytes. No infective cause of the intermittent diarrhoea was found; barium enema and colonoscopy were normal.

She was diagnosed as having a common variable immunodeficiency disorder, a diagnosis of exclusion, as no underlying cause was found. She was given fortnightly intravenous infusions of human normal IgG (400 mg/kg body weight/month) for the antibody deficiency.

Table 3.6 Immunological investigations* in Case 3.3, a CVID

Quantitative serum immunoglobulins (g/l):

IgG	3.15	(7.2–19.0)
IgA	0.11	(0.8–5.0)
IgM	0.66	(0.5–2.0)

Antibody activity

Post-immunization IgG to:

Tetanus toxoid	Negative (> 0.85 IU/ml)
Diphtheria toxoid	Negative (> 0.2 IU/ml)
Pneumococcal polysaccharides	Negative (> 80 U/ml)

Blood lymphocyte subpopulations (×10⁹/l):

Total lymphocyte count	1.6	(1.5–3.5)
T lymphocytes		
CD3	1.31	(0.9–2.8)
CD4	0.89	(0.6–1.2)
CD8	0.41	(0.4–1.0)
B lymphocytes		
CD19	0.2	(0.2–0.4)
NK lymphocytes		
CD16: CD56	0.2	(0.2–0.4)

*Normal adult ranges shown in parentheses.

therefore rarely needed, unless there is also a low serum IgA level, the patient suffers from recurrent infections and also fails to make specific antibodies to a group of antigens (see Case 3.4).

Antibodies are produced in different ways to carbohydrate and protein antigens. **Antibodies to polysaccharide capsular antigens** of organisms, such as Streptococcus pneumoniae, Salmonella typhi and Haemophilus influenzae (see Fig. 3.2), are often transient, low affinity and of the IgG_2 subclass. Those to protein antigens, such as **viral coats** and **toxoids**, are usually persistent, high affinity and of the IgG_1 subclass. Failure to produce normal amounts of IgG_1 and IgG_3 may lead to recurrent infections, as in Case 3.4.

Polysaccharide antigens alone do not stimulate immune responses in children under 2 years of age, explaining why severe infections with encapsulated organisms were relatively common in infants until the advent of conjugated polysaccharide:protein vaccines. *Partial antibody deficiencies cannot therefore be diagnosed until children are over 4 years*, to allow for physiological variation (see above in delay maturation).

Selective IgA deficiency

This is the commonest primary defect of specific immunity, with an incidence of 1 : 700 in Europe, Japan and the USA.

It can present at any age, although *most patients are diagnosed by an incidental finding* as young adults. It is characterized by undetectable or very low serum IgA levels with normal concentrations of IgG and IgM and production of normal antibodies to pathogens. So **most individuals are healthy** and do not suffer from recurrent infections.

Nevertheless, selective IgA deficiency **predisposes** the individual to a **variety of disorders** (Fig. 3.8). About one-fifth of people with selective IgA deficiency make antibodies to IgA. A very few of these patients develop adverse reactions after transfusions of blood or plasma, so that measurement of serum IgA is routine in the investigation of transfusion reactions (see section 16.7).

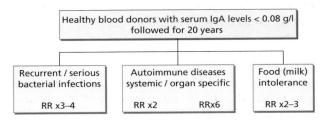

Fig. 3.8 Clinical associations of IgA deficiency. RR, Relative risk.

CASE 3.4 IgA WITH IgG SUBCLASS DEFICIENCIES

A 48-year-old man was admitted for investigation of weight loss associated with intermittent diarrhoea; stool examinations had been unhelpful. He had a history of pneumonia as a child and again as a young man working abroad. At the age of 33 he had developed chronic sinusitis, with persistent headaches. On examination, he was thin but had no signs of malignancy. There was no clubbing, lymphadenopathy or hepatosplenomegaly and his chest was clear on auscultation. Haemoglobin, serum albumin, liver function tests and urine electrophoresis were normal. Immunological tests are shown in Table 3.7. Investigations into the cause of the recurrent diarrhoea revealed Giardia lamblia on jejunal biopsy, even though microscopy was negative. Endoscopic examination of his maxillary sinuses showed considerable inflammation and hypertrophy of the mucosa.

A diagnosis of IgA with IgG subclass deficiencies, with chronic sinusitis and intestinal giardiasis as secondary complications, was made. He was given a course of metronidazole for the giardia infestation and replacement immunoglobulin was started with weekly infusions initially and subsequently 3-weekly at a dose of 0.4 g/kg per month. The sinusitis gradually improved, the diarrhoea did not return and he remained infection free for many years.

Table 3.7 Immunological investigations* in Case 3.4, IgA with IgG subclass deficiency

Serum immunoglobulins (g/l):

IgG	7.6	(6.5–12.0)
IgA	< 0.1	(0.8–5.0)
IgM	1.2	(0.5–2.0)
IgG$_1$	1.1	(3.6–7.3)
IgG$_2$	3.8	(1.4–4.5)
IgG$_3$	0.1	(0.3–1.1)
IgG$_4$	2.6	(0.1–1.0)

Serum and urine electrophoresis—no monoclonal bands

Antibody activity—post immunization

IgG	Tetanus toxoid	Negative	(> 0.85 IU/ml)
	Diphtheria toxoid	Negative	(> 0.2 IU/ml)
	Pneumococcal polysaccharides	Normal	(> 80 U/ml)

Antibody activity—post exposure

IgG	Rubella	Not detectable
	Measles	Not detectable
	Varicella zoster	Not detectable

Blood lymphocyte subpopulations (×10⁹/l):

Total lymphocyte count	2.8	(1.5–3.5)
T lymphocytes		
CD3	2.2	(0.9–2.8)
CD4	1.6	(0.6–1.2)
CD8	0.6	(0.4–1.0)
B lymphocytes		
CD19	0.3	(0.2–0.4)
NK lymphocytes		
CD16:CD56	0.2	(0.2–0.4)

*Normal adult ranges shown in parentheses.

3.2.3 Differential diagnosis

Primary antibody deficiencies are relatively rare causes of recurrent infections and the differential diagnosis is wide. If **infections recur at a single site**, then a local cause is likely. For example, cases of recurrent meningitis are usually caused by a passage communicating the ear or sinuses with cerebrospinal fluid, while recurrent pneumonia may be due to structural lung damage or aspiration of a foreign body.

Secondary causes of immunoglobulin deficiency (see section 3.5) *are far more common* than primary defects. Many textbooks provide long lists of causes. From the practical viewpoint, however, this is not a particularly helpful approach. For example, although the nephrotic syndrome is relatively common in childhood (compared with primary antibody deficiency) and certainly causes low serum IgG levels, recurrent infections are rarely a significant problem, since **antibody production** is normal.

It should be remembered that patients with primary antibody deficiency can present at any age and a search for an underlying cause for antibody deficiency should always be made in patients with recurrent/severe/persistent/unusual infections (as in Cases 3.1–3.4).

3.2.4 Complications of antibody deficiencies

Patients with all forms of primary antibody deficiency suffer from a wide range of bacterial infections (Fig. 3.2). Chronic sepsis of the upper and lower **respiratory tracts** can lead to chronic otitis media, deafness, sinusitis, bronchiectasis, pulmonary fibrosis and ultimately cor pulmonale.

Mild **gastrointestinal disease** occurs in up to two-thirds of patients with antibody deficiencies, and in about 20% it warrants further investigations. Diarrhoea, with or without malabsorption, is most frequently caused by infestation with Giardia lamblia, bacterial overgrowth of the small intestine, or persistent infection with cryptosporidium (in those with hyper-IgM syndromes), salmonella, campylobacter, rotavirus or enteroviruses. Chronic cholangitis may be due to ascending bacterial infection of the biliary tract; some cases progress to hepatic cirrhosis.

Virus infection of the central nervous system is rare, but patients with X-linked agammaglobulinaemia or a CVID are susceptible to **chronic echovirus infection**. This can result in severe, persistent meningoencephalitis, sometimes with an associated dermatomyositis-like syndrome. Death often follows, despite high doses of immunoglobulin therapy. **Urea-plasma** may cause genitourinary infections.

Arthropathy complicates about 12% of cases of antibody deficiency, usually the CVID group. Septic arthritis is uncommon. Of the remainder, some patients develop a chronic arthritis of large joints and some a monoarticular arthritis, but without circulating rheumatoid factor. It is still not uncommon for patients with antibody defects to be initially misdiagnosed as having Still's disease or rheumatoid arthritis.

Autoimmune phenomena are common, with 15% of CVID patients presenting with or developing autoimmune haemolytic anaemia or immune thrombocytopenia. Autoimmune thyroid disease affects > 10% and a pernicious-anaemia-like syndrome is also fairly common, but differs from classic pernicious anaemia in that autoantibodies to parietal cells and intrinsic factor are usually absent and the atrophic gastritis involves the entire stomach without antral sparing. Autoimmune enteropathy may be gluten-sensitive (as in coeliac disease) or more commonly resistant to gluten withdrawal.

In some patients with CVID, hyperplasia of gut-associated lymphoid tissue occurs. This nodular lymphoid hyperplasia is benign. Thirty percent of CVID patients have an **enlarged spleen**, causing diagnostic confusion with lymphoma (see section 6.4). Further, as yet unexplained, late complications are those of non-mycobacterial granulomata, usually outside lymphoid tissue, and lymphoid infiltration of the lung, known as interstitial lymphoid pneumonitis.

Patients with immunodeficiency involving humoral and/or cell-mediated immunity have a 10- to 100-fold increase in incidence of **malignant disease**. Most tumours are of lymphoid in origin, although carcinoma of the stomach may follow atrophic gastritis.

3.2.5 Management of antibody deficiencies

Early diagnosis is essential if further infections are to be prevented and the incidence of complications reduced.

Immunoglobulin replacement therapy is mandatory for children and adults with persistently defective antibody production. Preparations are available for intravenous or subcutaneous use; the choice depends on the severity of failure of antibody production, pre-existing complications

and venous access as well as convenience and patient choice. Most patients require 400–600 mg of immunoglobulin/kg per month to prevent further infections and reduce complications, especially those of chronic lung or gut disease. Intravenous immunoglobulin (IVIG) is usually given at 2- or 3-weekly intervals, the dose and timing being adjusted *to provide maximum reduction in infections for each patient*. Serum immunoglobulin levels are monitored and, once a steady state is reached (usually after about 6 months), trough (pre-infusion) levels are maintained at a level that keeps the patient infection free. Adverse reactions are uncommon with modern, highly purified IVIG preparations. This makes IVIG safe for self-infusion by the patient at home, provided they are trained and registered on a recognized programme.

The **dose per month** of replacement immunoglobulin by the subcutaneous route is equivalent to that given intravenously; most patients receive twice-weekly infusions of 30–60 ml of a 15% solution, given into several sites simultaneously. A syringe driver usually controls infusion rates and each site infusion takes about 30 min. Serum levels equivalent to those with IVIG are achieved. Adverse reactions are most unusual, enabling this route to be used at home also.

Immunoglobulin is derived from a plasma pool of 6000–10 000 donor units, in order to give the widest possible range of protective antibodies. Transmitted viruses are, therefore, of great concern. Cold ethanol precipitation, the initial process involved in the manufacture of both intravenous and subcutaneous preparations, has been shown to kill retroviruses (such as human immunodeficiency virus) and probably kills many other viruses transmitted in blood or blood products (see Chapter 16). **Screenings** of donor units and **viral inactivation** steps have reduced the risks of hepatitis. However, in the past there were cases of transmission of hepatitis C (see Case 16.7) and all patients must have **regular monitoring** including liver function tests.

General management measures include the early recognition and diagnosis of new infections or complications. Coexistent problems may be mistakenly attributed to the complications of antibody deficiency, e.g. an inhaled foreign body may be overlooked in a child with fresh chest symptoms. Antibody-deficient patients respond promptly to appropriate antibiotics but it is best to give a course of 10–14 days' therapy.

3.3 Combined primary T- and B-cell immunodeficiencies

3.3.1 Types of defects

Depressed T-cell immunity is usually accompanied by variable abnormalities of B-cell function, reflecting the T–B-cell cooperation needed for antibody synthesis to most antigens. Most defects of specific immunity, other than antibody deficiencies, are therefore **combined immune deficiencies** of the

CASE 3.5 SEVERE COMBINED IMMUNODEFICIENCY

David was born at full term after a normal pregnancy; his parents were first cousins. He was not given Bacille Calmette–Guérin (BCG) at birth. He was well until 2 months, when he became 'chesty' and needed antibiotics. Routine immunizations were postponed until he had recovered, but he then developed 'antibiotic-related' diarrhoea, which did not settle after the antibiotics were stopped. After 3 months a further chest infection occurred, his weight fell from the 25th centile to below the third. He was admitted for investigation for failure to thrive and was found to have a silent atypical pneumonia on initial chest X-ray.

On examination, he was a thin, scrawny infant on the 25th centile for length. There were no rashes or lymphadenopathy, but his liver was palpable just below the right costal margin. He had slight tachycardia and tachypnoea; bronchoscopy to obtain a sample for microbiological tests revealed Pneumocystis carinii on staining of the fluid. Investigations (Table 3.8) showed a marked deficiency of T cells with normal numbers of B cells but no immunoglobulin production. He had a T⁻B⁺NK⁻ form of SCID. He was treated with high dose co-trimoxazole for the Pneumocystis and referred promptly to a specialist unit for bone marrow transplantation, where he was put in isolation and given immunoglobulin therapy to prevent further infections. The diagnosis was investigated further by mutation analysis, starting with the commonest form of this type of SCID, X-linked common γ chain cytokine receptor deficiency, which was positive.

Table 3.8 Immunological investigations* in Case 3.5, severe combined immune deficiency

Full blood count

Haemoglobin	108 g/l
Neutrophil count	3.5×10^9/l
Lymphocyte count	0.5×10^9/l (4–15)

Microbiology results

Blood	Negative for HIV by PCR
Urine	Negative for cytomegalovirus
Nasopharyngeal swab	Rhinovirus
Stool	Echovirus-22
Sputum	Negative for bacterial culture
Lavage fluid	Pneumocystis: PCR +ve and staining

Immunological results

IgG	0.9 g/l
IgA	< 0.1 g/l
IgM	0.1g/l

Lymphocytes

CD3⁺/CD4⁺	0.09×10^9/l
CD3⁺/CD8⁺	0.04×10^9/l
CD19⁺	0.23×10^9/l
CD3⁻/CD16⁺56⁺	0.07×10^9/l
CD4⁺/CD25⁺	0.08×10^9/l
CD3⁺/HLA-DR⁺	0.11×10^9/l

Lymphocyte stimulation assays

	SI†		CD69‡	
	Patient	Control	Patient	Control
Phorbol ester and ionophore	6	300	< 1%	49%
Phytohaemagglutinin	4	385	< 1%	29%
Mab to CD3	3	165	1%	17%

Mab, monoclonal antibody

*Normal range for 3 months shown in parentheses (see Fig. 3.9).
†Stimulation index.
‡Percentage of CD3⁺ cells expressing CD69 after 6 hours.

adaptive system. These severe deficiencies (Case 3.5) usually present within the first few months of life (see Box 3.3).

Those infants in whom there is complete failure of both T- and B-lymphocyte function have **severe combined immune deficiency (SCID)**. Several variants are recognized (Table 3.9), depending on the presence or absence of T, B and NK cells, even though the cells may not function normally. These infants present in the first few weeks of life with chronic or persistent infection and failure to thrive. The condition should be suspected in any sick infant with infection, who should be checked for a low lymphocyte count (Box 3.3 and Fig. 3.9). Bone marrow transplantation (see section 8.5)

has proved successful in repairing many types of immune defect. Some types of SCID, e.g. cytokine receptor common γ chain deficiency, are prototypes for gene therapy, but only if a suitable bone marrow donor is not available.

The **variety of different forms of SCID** (Table 3.9) reflects the complexity of the cell surface receptors and the corresponding intracellular signalling enzymes. Recognition of these immune deficiencies in patients has contributed substantially to the further understanding of immune physiology.

Some combined immune deficiencies affect other systems as well as the immune system (Table 3.10). The severity, and

Table 3.9 Examples of some well-described severe combined immunodeficiencies (SCID) defined by the numbers of T, B and natural killer (NK) cells present in the blood. This list is not intended to be exhaustive but gives examples of several mechanisms by which SCID can occur

Condition	Pathogenesis	Inheritance
T– B– NK– SCID		
Reticular dysgenesis	No stem cells	Autosomal recessive
Adenosine deaminase (ADA)	Defective ADA genes lead to toxic metabolites in T, B and NK cells	Autosomal recessive
T– B– NK+ SCID		
RAG1/2 defect	RAG1/2 enzymes snip DNA for VDJ rearrangement for TCR and BCR—partial defect known as Omen's syndrome	Autosomal recessive
Artemis deficiency	Failure to repair DNA after RAG1/2 snips	Autosomal recessive
T– B+ NK– SCID		
X linked	Absent IL receptors for range of cytokines due to lack of common γ chain	X linked
Jak 3 kinase deficiency	No Jak 3 kinase to follow signal via IL-R binding	Autosomal recessive
T– B+ NK+ SCID		
IL-7 receptor deficiency	No IL-7α chains lead to failure of T cells differentiation	Autosomal recessive
CD3δ chain defect	Defective CD3 molecules, as CD3δ essential for assembly	Autosomal recessive
CD3 activation failure	Defective signal transduction, e.g. ZAP-70 deficiency	Autosomal recessive
T+ B+ NK+ MHC failure		
MHC class I deficiency ('bare lymphocyte syndrome')	Failure to express MHC class I due to defect in TAP-2 transcription	Autosomal recessive
MHC class II deficiency	Defect in transcription of MHC class II proteins	Autosomal recessive

IL, Interleukin; RAG, recombination activation genes; TAP, transporter associated with antigen processing; ZAP-70, an intracellular tyrosine kinase.

BOX 3.3 CLUES IN SEVERE COMBINED IMMUNE DEFICIENCY

- Present in first few weeks/months of life
- Infections are often viral or fungal rather than bacterial
- Chronic diarrhoea is common and often labelled as 'gastro-enteritis'
- Respiratory infections and oral thrush are common
- Failure to thrive in absence of obvious infections should be investigated
- Lymphopenia is present in almost all affected infants and is often overlooked (Fig. 3.7)

---

therefore the **clinical significance**, of the immune defect vary from patient to patient. The Di George anomaly is an example: this consists of a group of developmental abnormalities resulting in distinctive clinical features (Table 3.10), and now known to be due to defects on chromosomes 22 q11 or 10. The immune defect is usually mild.

3.3.2 Management of defects in cellular immunity

Early recognition and *differentiation from paediatric HIV are essential*. Prevention of defects is obviously better than cure

and genetic counselling is important. Where a molecular or biochemical defect has been defined, recognition of heterozygote carriers and prenatal diagnosis become possible by amniocentesis.

The management of patients with severe defects in cell-mediated immunity, including SCIDs, involves not only appropriate **antimicrobial therapy** but prophylactic measures also. To **avoid potentially infecting** situations, infants are nursed in positive pressure areas. Immunization with *live vaccines and conventional blood transfusions must be avoided* in patients with proven or suspected T-cell defects: live vaccines can lead to disseminated infection and blood transfusion may result in graft-versus-host disease (GVHD) (see section 8.5.3 and Case 8.4) unless irradiated blood is used.

Grafting of viable immunocompetent cells offers the only hope of permanent restoration of immune responsiveness. Bone marrow transplantation (see Chapter 8) is the treatment of choice for all forms of SCID; intrauterine infusion of bone marrow has also been shown to be feasible. Replacement of missing factors is a logical approach for enzymes and cytokines, but is temporary and fails to produce a permanent cure. For example, adenosine deaminase (ADA) replacement is successful in the short term, provided a chemically modified enzyme with a prolonged in vivo life is used, but early bone marrow transplantation is preferable.

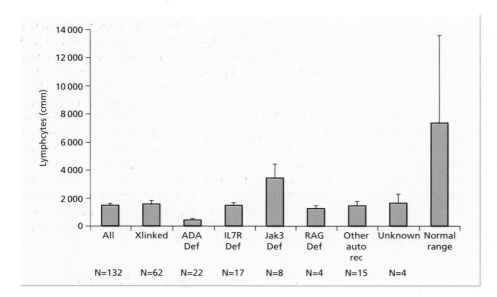

Fig. 3.9 Absolute lymphocyte count (mean ± SD) in 132 infants with severe combined immune deficiency. Buckley R. Molecular defects in human severe combined immunodeficiency and approaches to immune reconstitution. Ann Rev Immunol 2004; 625–55 (with permission).

Table 3.10 Some primary combined immune deficiencies with other non-immunological features, to show the wide range of these associated defects

Condition	Distinctive clinical features
DiGeorge anomaly	1 Hypoparathyroidism, convulsions, tetany 2 Cardiovascular defects 3 Abnormal facies 4 Recurrent or severe infections are rare
Chronic mucocutaneous candidiasis	1 Candida albicans infections of mucous membrane/nails/skin 2 Associated endocrine abnormalities—hypoparathyroidism, Addison's disease, etc. 3 Recurrent bacterial infections
Purine nucleoside phosphorylase	1 Recurrent infections, bacterial, fungal and viral 2 Neurological disorders (60%) 3 Autoimmune diseases 4 Failure to thrive
Ataxia telangiectasias	1 Cerebellar ataxia with progressive neurological deterioration and radiation sensitivity 2 Oculocutaneous telangiectasia 3 Recurrent viral infections 4 Gonadal dysgenesis 5 Chromosomal abnormalities 6 Malignant disease
Wiskott–Aldrich syndrome	1 Thrombocytopenia 2 Bleeding due to small platelets 3 Eczema 4 Recurrent bacterial infections 5 Malignant disease

Gene mapping of many of the defects involved in SCID has led to the relevant genes being cloned. Successful **transfection of genes** into benign retroviral vectors has shown that gene therapy is now practical. However, there is a risk of leukaemia if the vector inserts next to a regulator gene and a few cases have been reported in children who have been treated in this way. New vectors, or inbuilt auto-destruction of the vector, may resolve this problem. Until now, gene

Table 3.11 Prerequisites for gene therapy in humans

1 Absence of reasonable present therapy
2 Determination of precise genetic defect in patient requiring therapy (i.e. no complex gene regulation)
3 Cloning of normal gene for the missing product
4 Identification of target cell which will replicate and mature
5 Transfer of normal gene efficiently to appropriate target cell
6 Synthesis of gene product by that cell
7 Assurance that the transfected gene has no deleterious effects or oncogenic potential

therapy has been reserved for those in whom bone marrow transplantation is unlikely to be successful, but the increasing success of stem cell transplantation now provides viable therapy for many patients. There are a number of prerequisites before gene transfer becomes routine in any human system (Table 3.11), but work in the primary immune deficiencies has led the way. Common γ chain deficiency, leucocyte adhesion deficiency and chronic granulomatous disease show promising results.

3.4 Primary defects in non-specific immunity

The clinical significance of defects in non-specific immunity has been appreciated for many years; patients with low neutrophil counts have been known to be at risk of over-

whelming infection. Furthermore, since **innate immunity** is responsible for host defence very early in infection and adaptive humoral immunity requires non-specific dendritic cells to **initiate antigen-specific responses**, the role of innate immunity is gaining new importance (see Chapter 1). These two systems work in tandem to provide efficient protection against infection. The best known example is the opsonization of microorganisms, i.e. coating (opsonized) with IgG antibodies and complement; these pathogens are then readily bound, ingested and destroyed by phagocytic cells, such as neutrophils. This interdependence partly explains some similarities between the infectious complications experienced by patients with defects of antibody or complement synthesis and those with neutrophil or macrophage/monocyte dysfunction (see Fig. 3.2).

3.4.1 Defects in monocytes and dendritic cells

The major role of the macrophage is to ingest opsonized bacteria and to kill them intracellularly by fusing phagosomes with lysosomes—intracellular structures containing digestive enzymes (see section 1.3.3). Activation occurs non-specifically via large numbers of germline surface glycoprotein receptors—**pattern recognition receptors (PRRs)**—that are distinct from the phagocytic receptors. These recognize conserved ligands on the surfaces of the pathogens, known as pathogen-associated molecular patterns (PAMPs) (Fig. 1.4). Macrophage PRRs are not specific for individual or-

CASE 3.6 IRAK-4 DEFICIENCY

A 9-year-old girl was admitted with meningitis due to Shigella; previously she had been in hospital with septic arthritis due to Streptococcus pneumoniae as well as several deep-seated abscesses with Staphylococci or Strep. pyogenes. On each occasion, full blood counts were normal, including lymphocyte and neutrophil counts. Curiously, her CRP had also been low despite severe infections, never higher than 35 mg/l. Other screening tests such as liver function tests, functional complement (CH_{50} and AP_{50}) were normal, as were serum immunoglobulin levels and antibody production (see Table 3.12). The only abnormality was failure to reduce dihydrorhodamine on stimulation with lipopolysaccharide in vitro, the significance of which was unknown at the time. Years later, when more was known about the innate immune system, peripheral blood mononuclear cells were isolated from her blood and tested in vitro for IL-6 production following stimulation with a variety of agents including lipopolysaccharide; poor production of IL-6 was seen. It was thought that she might have a defect in the NF-κB pathway; on sequencing of her IRAK-4 gene, this was found to be the case.

Table 3.12 Immunological investigations in case 3.6, IRAK-4 deficiency

Investigation	Patient	Normal ranges
Dihydrorhodamine reduction test:		
Medium only	2%	8.7 ± 7.3%
Phorbol myristate acid	99%	99.2 ± 0.9%
Lipopolysaccharide	7%	> 60%
Serum immunoglobulin concentrations:		
IgG	16.7	6.0–13.0 g/l
IgA	1.1	0.8–3.0 g/l
IgM	1.9	0.4–2.5 g/l
IgE	400	< 125 kU/l
Post-immunization IgG antibodies to:		
Tetanus	0.06	> 0.01 IU/ml
Diphtheria	0.18	> 0.01 IU/ml
23 valency Pneumovax	> 100	> 50 IU/ml
Haemophilus influenzae type b	1.36	> 1 µg/ml

ganisms, unlike T-cell receptors and B-cell receptors but are communal; they do not undergo gene rearrangement. Macrophages use these to distinguish non-self from self-molecules. Like the adaptive system, defects in the genes for these receptors can lead to absent or non-functional proteins, resulting in excessive or persistent infections, i.e. immune deficiency disorders.

One family of non-phagocytic receptors, known as **Toll-like receptors (TLRs)**, is implicated in such immune deficiencies (see Fig. 1.2). In the same way as patients with adaptive immune deficiencies suffer from a range of bacterial or viral infections, so in TLR deficiencies patients have a range of pathogens, including intracellular mycobacteria and salmonellae and extracellular streptococci and staphylococci. Many more TLR deficiencies will be found. Already there are similar patients who lack the enzymes in the pathways (as Case 3.6) which signal activation of the cell to switch on killing mechanisms, drawing a parallel with common γ chain SCID, in which the clinical disease resulting from absence of the enzyme JAK3 resembles that of missing the surface receptor, common γ chain.

Monocytes and dendritic cells respond to microorganisms very early in infection, to produce cytokines that stimulate the antigen-specific system to produce activated T cells and antibodies. They also trigger **acute-phase responses** to provide additional mechanisms for the limitation of spread of pathogens. Defects in any of the immune receptor signalling pathways lead to increased susceptibility to infection. These include abnormalities in cytokine receptors for cell activation (IL15R/IL17R and IL1R/TLRs), as well as some intracellular receptors (such as NOD) that lead to the common pathway for gene transcription. Since this transcription factor, NF-kappa B, regulates the expression of numerous genes controlling the immune and stress responses, inflammatory reactions, cell adhesion, and protection against apoptosis, defects result in severe infections due to a wide range of organisms. IL-1 receptor-associated kinase (IRAK)-4 deficiency (Case 3.6) is specifically associated with defects affecting the responses to TLRs and IL-1 receptors (IL1Rs), essential for both the innate and adaptive immune systems. TLRs sense various microbial products and initiate the immune response by leading to the production of key inflammatory cytokines, IL-1 and IL-18, which then amplify the response. IL-1 receptors are responsible for acute-phase responses. Known protein defects in NF-κB activation so far include NEMO, IκB and IRAK-4 (see Box 1.1) and these are now known to result in primary immune defects in man and mice. As in the adaptive immune system, defects in either receptors or in the intracellular enzymes of this innate pathway can result in significant immune deficiency (see Table 3.13).

3.4.2 Defects in neutrophil function

The major role of the neutrophil is to ingest, kill and digest invading microorganisms, particularly bacteria and fungi. Failure to fulfill this role leads to infection. Defects in neutrophil function can be quantitative—neutropenia—or qualitative—neutrophil dysfunction. However, irrespective of the basic cause, clinical features are similar and certain generalizations are possible.

The circulating neutrophil count normally exceeds $1.5 \times 10^9/l$. While mild degrees of **neutropenia** are usually asymptomatic, moderate to severe reductions in numbers are associated with a progressive increase in the risk and severity of infections (Fig. 16.7). Episodes of infection are

Table 3.13 Some parallels between adaptive and innate immune systems: examples of missing immune components leading to immune deficiencies

	Adaptive system	Innate system		
Type of component	**Lymphocytes**	**Dendritic cells**	**Neutrophils**	**Macrophages**
Differentiation defect leading to low numbers	XLA for B cells Di George for T cells	Unknown at present	Neutropenia	Unknown at present
Receptors	Cytokine receptor common γ chain	Toll like receptor 2	Leucocyte adhesion molecules	IL-12/IFN-γ receptors
Signalling pathway/ activation defects	JAK 3–tyrosine kinase	IRAK-4 NEMO		
Effector function defects	Perforin defect in CD8 deficiency		Chronic granulomatous disease – cytochromes for oxidative burst	Chediak–Higashi—failure of fusion of lysosomes

CASE 3.7 CHRONIC GRANULOMATOUS DISEASE

Mark was born by Caesarean section and weighed 3.1 kg. He is the sixth child of unrelated white parents. At the age of 4 weeks, he developed an axillary abscess which healed spontaneously, followed by a staphylococcal abscess of the chest wall, requiring surgical incision and a course of flucloxacillin. He had a total white-cell count of $45 \times 10^9/l$, of which 90% were neutrophils.

At the ages of 3 and 7 months, he was readmitted to hospital with large staphylococcal abscesses, first on his face and then on his right buttock; both abscesses were treated by surgical incision and systemic antibiotics for 10 days. By the age of 2 years, he had been admitted to hospital five times with staphylococcal abscesses. The family history was remarkable: three elder brothers had died of infections at ages ranging from 7 months to 3 years, but his parents and two sisters were healthy.

On examination, he was pale and persistently pyrexial. His height and weight were below the third centile. He had bilateral axillary and inguinal lymphadenopathy with marked hepato-splenomegaly.

Laboratory tests showed mild anaemia (Hb 104 g/l) with marked polymorphonuclear leucocytosis. His immunological investigations are summarized in Table 3.14. There was gross polyclonal elevation of all immunoglobulin classes, particularly IgG and IgA. His neutrophils moved and phagocytosed Staphylococcus aureus normally; however, they showed impaired intracellular killing of staphylococci. Further tests on this boy showed that his polymorphs failed to consume oxygen or to produce hydrogen peroxide during phagocytosis. These findings, and the probable X-linked nature of the condition, are diagnostic of chronic granulomatous disease (CGD).

Table 3.14 Immunological tests* in Case 3.7, chronic granulomatous disease

Quantitative serum immunoglobulins (g/l):		
IgG	17.8	(5.5–10.0)
IgA	4.8	(0.3–0.8)
IgM	2.0	(0.4–1.8)
Antibody activity		
IgG antibodies: post immunization		
Tetanus toxoid	89	(> 1.0 IU/ml)
Diphtheria toxoid	3.0	(> 0.6 IU/ml)
Nitroblue tetrazolium (NBT) test†		
Unstimulated	2	(normal < 10)
Stimulated	4	(normal > 30)
Neutrophil mobility‡		
In medium alone	18	(17 μm)
In presence of chemoattractant	129	(148 μm)

*Normal range for age (or value for healthy control studied in parallel) is shown in parentheses.
†Percentage of neutrophils showing reduction of NBT before and after stimulation with endotoxin (see Chapter 19).
‡Distance moved (in μm) by test (and healthy control) neutrophils (see Chapter 19).

Now aged 7 years, Mark continues to have periodic abscesses despite long-term co-trimoxazole. Since most antibiotics fail to penetrate cells effectively, treatment of acute infections is continued for at least 8 weeks. He has not had a major infection necessitating therapy with IFN-γ but is on a prophylactic antifungal agent. He will be considered for bone marrow transplantation if a matched donor can be found.

likely to be life threatening when the neutrophil count falls below $0.5 \times 10^9/l$.

Neutropenia is more common than neutrophil dysfunction and *secondary causes of neutropenia are more common than primary ones* (Fig. 3.10); for example, neutropenia is a frequent side-effect of chemotherapy for malignant disease. Primary neutropenia is rare; congenital forms range in severity and, if severe, are often fatal. Treatment with recombinant human granulocyte–colony-stimulating factor (G-CSF) stimulates myeloid stem cells, although long-term complications include vasculitis. **Neutrophil function** can be conveniently subdivided into stages: mobilization from bone marrow or spleen, chemotaxis to a site of infection, phagocytosis of pathogen, fusion with lysosome to release enzymes to kill organism (see Fig. 19.17). Qualitative defects in these functional steps result in typical infections and some unexplained accompanying features (Table 3.15).

When intracellular killing mechanisms fail, ingested bacteria may survive and proliferate in an intracellular environment free from the effects of antibodies and most antibiotics.

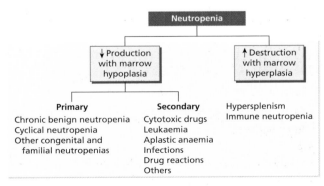

Fig. 3.10 Some causes of neutropenia. Secondary causes are far more common than primary ones.

Table 3.15 Features of some primary defects of neutrophil function resulting in recurrent infections

Condition	Distinctive clinical features	Functional defect	Inheritance
Leucocyte adhesion deficiency	1 Delayed separation of umbilical cord 2 Skin infections and gingivitis 3 Deep abscesses, peritonitis, osteomyelitis	Fail to adhere to endothelial cells and so to traverse into tissues to ingest and kill bacteria	Autosomal recessive
Chediak–Higashi syndrome	1 Giant lysosomal granules in secretory cells 2 Partial oculocutaneous albinism	Abnormal chemotaxis, so fail to reach bacteria, and reduced microbicidal activity as lysosomes fail to fuse with phagosomes	Autosomal recessive
Hyper-IgE: recurrent infection syndrome	1 Coarse facial features 2 Mucocutaneous candidiasis 3 Huge level of serum IgE 4 Lung abscesses and pneumatocoeles 5 Abnormal calcium metabolism	?Abnormal chemotaxis	Familial and non-familial cases
Chronic granulomatous disease	1 Abscesses with catalase positive organisms 2 Granuloma formation	↓Oxidative metabolism and fail to kill Staph. and fungi	X-linked or autosomal recessive

One of the most severe types of neutrophil defect occurs in **chronic granulomatous disease (CGD)**. CGD is a group of disorders resulting from a failure to produce high concentrations of highly toxic reactive oxygen species during the 'respiratory burst' that accompanies activation of phagocytes. Although it was originally thought that these toxic oxygen species were directly bactericidal, it is now known that mice deficient in neutrophil-granule proteases, but normal in respect of superoxide production, are unable to resist staphylococcal and Candida infections. It is the proteases, released by the efflux of potassium ions that follows superoxide production, which is primarily responsible for the destruction of the bacteria.

The classic type of CGD is inherited as an X-linked recessive disorder, and typically presents in males in the first 2 months of life as in Case 3.7, although the diagnosis may not be made until young adulthood (see Box 3.4). The usual **complications** include regional lymphadenopathy, hepatosplenomegaly, hepatic abscesses and osteomyelitis.

Affected organs show multiple abscesses caused by Staphylococcus aureus, Gram-negative bacilli or fungi and non-caseating, giant cell granulomas.

The simplest **screening test** for CGD is the nitroblue tetrazolium test (see section 19.10), which depends on the ability of polymorphs to generate superoxide radicals during phagocytosis. Sensitive assays enable diagnosis of the carrier state in X-linked CGD and prenatal diagnosis on cells obtained by fetal blood sampling — the dihydrorhodamine reduction test (section 19.10). X-linked CGD is caused by the lack of one specific cytochrome involved in the 'respiratory burst'. Female carriers have half the normal amount of this cytochrome and their white cells have about half the normal capacity for generating oxygen radicals.

Treatment of CGD relies on prophylactic antibiotics (usually co-trimoxazole) and antifungal agents when required. Studies with the cytokine IFN-γ have shown some reduction in the numbers of infections without apparently improving the killing capacity of neutrophils. Allogeneic bone marrow transplantation from an HLA-matched related donor offers the only long-term hope of cure for patients with CGD. This procedure has a significant mortality rate of about 10%, and it should be reserved for patients with debilitating or life-threatening complications. Gene therapy is also an option.

3.4.3. Defects of effector functions of macrophages

As in SCID, there are also cytokine receptor defects on the surface of macrophages that result in primary immune deficiencies. All species of Mycobacteria enter these cell types to reproduce, but this is normally controlled by the intracellular production of IL-12, which in turn activates T cells

---

BOX 3.4 CLUES FROM THE HISTORY IN CHRONIC GRANULOMATOUS DISEASE

Infections are recurrent and prolonged

Clinical features may be minimal despite severe infection

Infections are:
- poorly responsive to antibiotics
- commonly staphylococcal
- involve skin and mucous membranes
- complicated by suppurative lymphadenopathy

CASE 3.8 IL-12 RECEPTOR DEFICIENCY

A 3-year-old girl, Sophia, born to consanguineous parents, came to OPD with a newly enlarged and persistent single lymph node in the supraclavicular region. Her parents were extremely anxious about leukaemia, although the child was well and a full blood count done in advance was normal. She had not been exposed to Mycobacteria tuberculosis, nor had she received BCG. She had had a few episodes of otitis media after an upper respiratory tract infection but no infections elsewhere. Biopsy of the lymph node was performed under general anaesthetic; histology showed a granuloma and the presence of a few acid-fast bacilli; an atypical (environmental) mycobacterium was grown on culture.

In order to be sure that this was not due to HIV disease, the child was tested after parental consent was given; the result was negative. Analysis of T, B and NK cells was normal, excluding a late presentation of SCID or another combined defect. IFN-γ and IL-12 production by monocytes and T cells were shown to be normal by Elispot. Markedly reduced expression of IL-12 receptors on the surface of activated T cells was found and a diagnosis of complete IL-12 receptor deficiency was confirmed on mutation analysis. She has three healthy older siblings who were found to be heterozygous for the defect, as were her parents.

to produce IFN-γ. Not surprisingly, **absence of either these cytokines or their receptors** results in susceptibility to both Mycobacterium tuberculosis and atypical (less pathogenic) forms of mycobacteria (see Case 3.8).

Structural defects can result in failure of intracellular killing mechanisms in macrophages, though these are very rare indeed. The severe immune deficiency of Chediak–Higashi syndrome is an example, in which the relationship of the

mild accompanying defects of partial albinism and defective platelets with the failure to fuse lysosomes and thus kill pathogens remains unexplained (see Tables 3.13 and 3.15).

3.4.4. Complement deficiency

Impaired complement activity is usually secondary to those diseases in which complement is consumed via the classical

CASE 3.9 ISOLATED DEFICIENCY OF COMPLEMENT COMPONENT

A 26-year-old West Indian man presented with a 24-h history of occipital headache and vomiting. He was pyrexial (temperature 38.3 °C), confused, irritable and had marked neck stiffness with a positive Kernig's sign. There was no other history of serious infections. His immediate family were healthy.

Lumbar puncture produced turbid cerebrospinal fluid (CSF) with a protein concentration of 4.5 g/l (NR 0.1–0.4), glucose content of < 0.1 mmol/l (NR 2.5–4.0) and a leucocyte count of 8000/mm³ (97% neutrophils). Neisseria meningitidis was cultured from the CSF. The patient was treated with intravenous penicillin and oral chloramphenicol and made a rapid recovery over the following 2 weeks.

A search was made for an underlying cause of his meningitis. X-rays of the skull and sinuses showed no abnormal communication with the CSF. The possibility of an underlying immune defect was then considered and the results of immunological tests are shown in Table 3.16. Antibody production to a variety of bacterial and viral antigens was normal. However, total classical pathway haemolytic complement activity (CH₅₀) and alternate pathway (AP₅₀) were consistently undetectable in his serum during convalescence, indicating a complete functional absence of one or more complement components of the terminal lytic pathway. Eventually, he was shown to have an isolated deficiency of C6, with normal levels of all other components. Half normal levels of C6 were found in the sera of his parents and in three of his four siblings: the other sibling had a normal level.

Table 3.16 Immunological investigations* in Case 3.9, complement deficiency

Quantitative serum immunoglobulins (g/l):
IgG	15.0	(7.2–19.0)
IgA	3.2	(0.8–5.0)
IgM	1.2	(0.5–2.0)

Antibody activity
Normal titres of antibodies to tetanus toxoid, diphtheria toxoid and pneumococci
Detectable antibodies to herpes simplex, measles, influenza A and adenovirus
Complement activity
CH₅₀	No detectable activity
AP₅₀	No detectable activity

*Normal ranges shown in parentheses.

Unlike immunoglobulin deficiency, long-term replacement of missing complement components is not feasible at present because their half-lives are so short (< 1 day). Nasopharyngeal carriage of Neisseria meningitidis by the patient and his close contacts can be eradicated by antibiotics but at the risk of inducing resistant strains. Prophylactic penicillin is used in those patients with symptomatic complement deficiencies.

or alternate pathways. A common example is systemic lupus erythematosus (SLE) (see section 10.7), in which consumption of the early classical pathway complement components C1, C4 and C2 impairs the ability of complement to solubilize immune complexes, the degree of impairment correlating with disease activity.

In humans, **inherited deficiencies of complement** components are associated with characteristic clinical syndromes (Fig. 3.11). Many patients with C1q, C4 or C2 deficiency have presented with a lupus-like syndrome of malar flush, arthralgia, glomerulonephritis, fever or chronic vasculitis and, in the case of C1q deficiency, with recurrent pyogenic infections. Antinuclear and anti-dsDNA antibodies (see section 10.7) may be absent. Deficiency of any of these early classical pathway components probably compromises the ability of the host to eliminate immune complexes. Such a defect can be demonstrated by failure to detect haemolytic activity in the classical complement pathway, whilst the alternate pathway is normal.

Patients with **C3 deficiency**, occurring as a primary or secondary defect, for example following deficiencies of C3b inhibitors, i.e. factor I or factor H (see Chapter 1), have an increased susceptibility to recurrent bacterial infections. Affected individuals typically present with life-threatening infections such as pneumonia, septicaemia and meningitis, illustrating the important role of C3 in defence against infection (see Chapter 1). Tests of both haemolytic pathways are abnormal.

There is a striking association between **deficiencies of C5, C6, C7, C8 or properdin** and recurrent neisserial infection. Most patients present with recurrent gonococcal infection, particularly septicaemia or arthritis, or recurrent meningococcal meningitis, as in Case 3.9. However, patients should be tested after only one episode of meningitis as many years may elapse between attacks.

C1 inhibitor deficiency is the commonest inherited deficiency of the complement system and causes hereditary angioedema (see section 11.5.1).

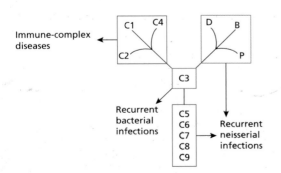

Fig. 3.11 Inherited complement deficiencies: characteristic clinical syndromes are associated with deficiencies of certain groups of components.

3.5 Secondary immunodeficiency

3.5.1 Secondary causes of immunodeficiency

Secondary causes of immunodeficiency are far more common than primary causes. Levels of immune components, as in any system, represent the **net balance** of failure of synthesis or apoptosis of producing cells vs. consumption, catabolism or loss. Low levels reflect either depressed production or accelerated consumption (Fig. 3.12).

Protein loss severe enough to cause low antibody levels and hypoproteinaemia occurs mainly via the kidney (the nephrotic syndrome) or through the gut (protein-losing enteropathy). The primary diagnosis of nephrotic syndrome usually presents little difficulty; renal loss of immunoglobulin is at least partially selective, so that IgA and IgM levels are maintained despite the fall in serum IgG and albumin. Recurrent infections are rarely a significant problem as specific antibody synthesis is intact. Protein can also be lost from the gut in a variety of active inflammatory diseases such as Crohn's disease, ulcerative colitis or coeliac disease. In intestinal lymphangiectasia, the dilated lymphatics leak lymphocytes as well as proteins.

Impaired synthesis is exemplified by malnutrition. Severe protein deficiency causes profound changes in many organs, including the immune system. Malnourished people show an increased incidence of infectious disease but the association is complex, since low-grade infection itself may cause malnourishment. Impaired specific antibody production following immunization, and defects in cell-mediated immunity, phagocyte function and complement activity are associated with **extreme poor nutrition**. These reverse after adequate protein and caloric supplementation of the diet.

Patients with **lymphoproliferative diseases** are very prone to infection (see Case 6.2). Untreated chronic lymphocytic leukaemia is often associated with antibody failure and recurrent chest infections, which tend to become more severe as the disease progresses. Non-Hodgkin's lymphoma may be associated with defects of both humoral and cell-mediated immunity. Hodgkin's disease is usually associated with marked impairment of cell-mediated immunity, especially following chemotherapy.

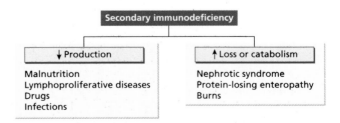

Fig. 3.12 Common causes of secondary immunodeficiency.

The infection risk in patients with multiple myeloma is five- to 10-fold higher than in age-matched controls. Initially, the plasma-cell tumour mass is treated aggressively with chemotherapy (section 6.6). Even before treatment, there is considerable suppression of polyclonal (non-paraprotein) antibody production and chemotherapy results in added suppression of T cells and phagocytic cells. The resultant infections reflect combined B- and T-cell deficiencies and thus may be bacterial, viral or fungal. During remission (plateau phase) the incidence and range of infections decrease; infections at this stage are mainly bacterial, reflecting the domi-nant polyclonal humoral immune suppression associated with myeloma itself.

The frequency of opportunistic infections in patients with disseminated non-lymphoid malignancies suggests a significant underlying immune defect, although it is difficult to distinguish between the immunosuppressive effects of the disease and those of the treatment. **Immunosuppressive drugs** affect lymphocyte and neutrophil activity, although low antibody levels are unusual. Patients on drugs to prevent organ transplant rejection also develop unusual opportunistic infections (see section 3.5.8). Another iatrogenic form of secondary immune deficiency is that associated with splenectomy (see also Case 7.5). Every year there are deaths from sudden, overwhelming infection due to Streptococcus pneumoniae in patients who have been **splenectomized**, often years before. The overall risk of death from infection following splenectomy is 1–2% over 15 years. All such patients should receive immunization with pneumococcal conjugate vaccine (see section 7.7) as well as prophylactic penicillin.

In a number of infections, the **microorganism paradoxically suppresses** rather than stimulates the immune system (see section 2.3). Severe, though transient, impairment of cell-mediated immunity has been noted in many viral illnesses, particularly cytomegalovirus, measles, rubella, infectious mononucleosis and viral hepatitis, and in some bacterial infections, such as tuberculosis, brucellosis, leprosy

---

BOX 3.5 IMPORTANT POINTS EMPHASIZED BY HIV CASES

- Not all patients with HIV present with recognizably HIV-related symptoms or signs

- A careful 'high-risk' history is important but not always helpful

- If there is a possibility of HIV infection, an HIV antibody test should always be done, after appropriate counselling

- If there is still a strong clinical suspicion, PCR testing should be done

- Absolute compliance with therapy is essential to prevent disease progression

---

CASE 3.10 ACQUIRED IMMUNE DEFICIENCY SYNDROME: KAPOSI'S SARCOMA

A 45-year-old man presented with a skin 'rash' of 2 months' duration. This had started as a single, small spot on his trunk, followed by widespread crops of similar lesions; they were painless and did not itch. He had no other symptoms; in particular, no cough, chest symptoms, fever, weight loss or lymphadenopathy. He was homosexual, with one regular sexual partner over the preceding 2 years, though he participated in casual, unprotected sexual intercourse whilst on holiday (Box 3.5). He had never used intravenous drugs.

He was apyrexial, with bilateral axillary and inguinal lymphadenopathy. About 20 purplish-red nodules were present on his trunk, face and palate as well as at the anal margin. His nose showed similar discoloration and swelling. White, wart-like projections of 'hairy leucoplakia' were present on the sides of his tongue.

Investigations showed a normal haemoglobin, a normal white-cell count (4.9×10^9/l) and normal absolute lymphocyte count (1.8×10^9/l). After counselling, blood was sent for an HIV antibody test; this was positive by enzyme-linked immunosorbent assay (ELISA) and confirmed by Western blotting (see Chapter 19). A second test was also positive. Immunological studies (Table 3.17) showed a raised serum IgA and analysis of lymphocyte subpopulations showed absolute depletion of CD4+ cells.

Biopsy of one of his skin lesions showed the typical histological features of Kaposi's sarcoma, so the clinical diagnosis was that of the acquired immune deficiency syndrome, caused by HIV-1.

He was started initially, in 1994, on combination therapy and prophylactic co-trimoxazole and undertook regular monitoring. He remains well more than 12 years later, now on HAART.

Table 3.17 Immunological investigations* in Case 3.10, HIV infection

Quantitative serum immunoglobulins (g/l):		
IgG	16.00	(8.0–18.0)
IgA	7.90	(0.9–4.5)
IgM	1.65	(0.6–2.8)
Peripheral blood lymphocytes ($\times 10^9$/l):		
Total lymphocyte count	1.8	(1.5–3.5)
T lymphocytes (CD3)	1.51	(0.9–2.8)
CD4+	0.20	(0.6–1.2)
CD8+	1.26	(0.4–1.0)
B lymphocytes (CD19)	0.14	(0.2–0.4)

*Normal ranges shown in parentheses.

and syphilis; however, the most florid example is infection with HIV (Cases 3.10 and 3.11).

3.5.2 Acquired immune deficiency syndrome

Acquired immune deficiency syndrome (AIDS) is the final stage in the progression of infectious disease caused by HIV. According to a **United Nations report**, more than 5 million people worldwide contracted the AIDS virus in 2004 alone, bringing the total number of those infected to 50 million. About 70% of patients are in sub-Saharan Africa.

HIV produces a **spectrum of disorders** from a transient, acute glandular fever-like illness to life-threatening tumours and opportunistic infections. HIV also causes dementia, autoimmune disorders and atrophy of particular organs (e.g. brain).

Seventy per cent of the global spread of HIV infection is thought to be by **heterosexual transmission**. In contrast to the USA and Europe, the African male-to-female ratio of cases is almost 1 : 1, with severe implications for the numbers of infants born to HIV-positive mothers. The prognosis was dismal prior to antiviral therapy, but new therapeutic regimens have changed the outlook for HIV-infected individuals in the West and politicians are now finding ways to bring these expensive therapies to patients in developing countries too.

3.5.3 Transmission of human immunodeficiency virus infection

HIV has been isolated from semen, cervical secretions, lymphocytes, cell-free plasma, cerebrospinal fluid, tears, saliva, urine and breast milk. Not all these fluids transmit infection, since the concentration of virus varies considerably: semen, blood, breast milk and cervical secretions have been proved to be infectious.

Transmission occurs mainly through sexual intercourse, heterosexual or homosexual, but also through blood and blood products. Sharing of contaminated needles and syringes by intravenous drug abusers and by therapeutic procedures in areas of the world where re-use of contaminated equipment occurs, resulting in HIV transmission. There

---

CASE 3.11 ACQUIRED IMMUNE DEFICIENCY SYNDROME: PERSISTENT GENERALIZED LYMPHADENOPATHY

A 29-year-old man had a history of fatigue, night sweats, diarrhoea and axillary lymphadenopathy for 6 months. Fine-needle lymph-node biopsy suggested a reactive cause rather than malignancy. At a follow-up visit 2 months later he was found to have palpable, non-tender cervical and inguinal nodes and considerable weight loss (8.5 kg) associated with the colitis. Further investigations were done to exclude a lymphoma. Computed tomography scan of his chest and abdomen showed no lymph-node enlargement and no organomegaly (Box 3.5).

Immunological investigations are shown in Table 3.18. Full blood counts were normal, as was the CRP level. In view of these findings, he was asked about previous blood transfusions (none) and high-risk activity for HIV infection (three heterosexual partners), counselled and tested for HIV antibody. He was HIV-antibody positive. A clinical diagnosis of AIDS was made, on the basis of a positive HIV antibody test and weight loss of more than 10% in 12 months.

Viral load measurement showed 46×10^3 copies of HIV-RNA per millilitre and he was positive for cytomegalovirus infection by PCR. In view of the low CD4 count he was started on prophylactic co-trimoxozole and combination therapy. CMV colitis was treated with Ganciclovir. He was initially reviewed at 4-weekly intervals and monitored with regular viral load measurements, but became a poor attender and there was some doubt about compliance with therapy. Four years later he complained of headaches, vomiting, a dry cough, sweats and profound breathlessness on minimal exertion. A chest X-ray showed bilateral lower-lobe shadowing and subsequently bronchial washings were positive for Pneumocystis carinii; rapid deterioration occurred and he died of respiratory failure.

At post-mortem examination, cytomegalovirus and Mycobacterium avium-intracellulare were also isolated from the lungs. A particular surprise was the presence of localized, unsuspected central nervous system lymphoma.

Table 3.18 Immunological investigations* in Case 3.11, HIV infection

Serum immunoglobulins (g/l):		
IgG	20.2	(8.0–18.0)
IgA	2.1	(0.9–4.5)
IgM	0.9	(0.6–2.8)
Electrophoresis—hypergammaglobulinaemia		
β_2-microglobulin	3.8 mg/l	(< 3.5)
Lymphocyte subpopulations ($\times 10^9/l$):		
Total lymphocyte count	2.80	(1.5–3.5)
T lymphocytes		
CD3+	2.35	(0.9–2.8)
CD4+	0.23	(0.6–1.2)
CD8+	2.04	(0.4–1.0)
B lymphocytes		
CD19+	0.36	(0.2–0.4)

*Normal adult ranges shown in parentheses.

should be no new HIV seroconversions in blood product recipients in developed countries, since all blood is now screened and blood products treated to inactivate any possible virus. **Vertical transmission** from mother to child in utero or at delivery is the dominant route of infection of children, although fewer than 20% of children born to HIV-positive mothers become infected. Since maternal antibody to HIV crosses the placenta, *a positive test in an infant does not indicate infection.* Vertical transfer of HIV may also occur after birth through breast milk (see section 18.4.3). Neonatal diagnosis depends on detection of nucleic acid [by polymerase chain reaction (PCR)] or viral antigen (by ELISA) and the mother must be tested also. In a previously undiagnosed family it is essential to test both parents; the mother for vertical trans-

mission and father in case mother is infected but as yet HIV antibody negative (see below).

Cases of **seroconversion** among healthcare workers are still reported after needlestick injuries but there is no evidence, despite many studies, that the virus is spread by mosquitoes, bed bugs, swimming pools, or by sharing eating utensils or toilets with an infected person.

3.5.4 The clinical spectrum of human immunodeficiency virus infection

HIV produces a spectrum of disorders (Fig. 3.13). A transient, acute glandular fever-like illness occurs in patients but this usually goes unsuspected. Like other viral illnesses, this

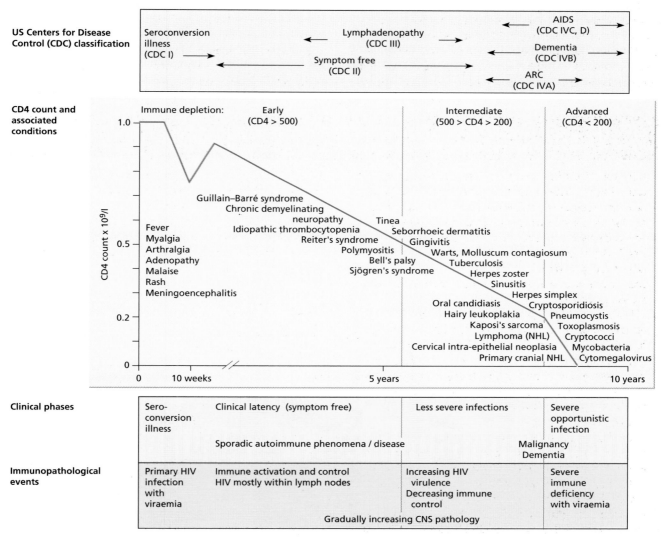

Fig. 3.13 Chronology of HIV-induced disease correlated with time since infection. CD4+ T-cell depletion, immunopathology and CDC classification. ARC, AIDS-related complex; CD4, CD4+ T lymphocytes; CNS, central nervous system; NHL, non-Hodgkin's lymphoma. (Redrawn, with permission, from Stewart, 1997.)

is accompanied by the findings of atypical lymphocytes and an increased number of CD8$^+$ T cells in the blood, followed by seroconversion; the time interval between infection and the production of antibodies to HIV (the '**window period**') may be as long as 6 months.

Most HIV-seropositive individuals then remain symptom-free for up to 10 years; development of AIDS depends on the contribution of many **cofactors** such as genetic background (those with HLA-B57 or HLA-B27 have a better prognosis), repeated stimulation by foreign antigens (multiple co-infections speed the rate of progression) or pregnancy. Almost all patients developed recurring opportunistic infections in the early stages before antiviral therapy. Some individuals develop asymptomatic persistent generalized lymphadenopathy (Case 3.11), whilst others suffered from autoimmune diseases (Fig. 3.13). The most important **prognostic factor** for progression to AIDS is the concentration of HIV-RNA in the blood — viral load — at diagnosis.

The major clinical manifestations of AIDS are **tumours** and **opportunistic infections**. Kaposi's sarcoma (due to HHV8) is the commonest tumour (Case 3.10), but non-Hodgkin's lymphoma (due to EBV) of B-cell phenotype and often within the central nervous system, and squamous carcinoma of the mouth or anorectum are also frequent. The many opportunistic infections affect virtually all systems of the body; however, the commonest organs involved are the lung, gut and central nervous system (Fig. 3.13).

HIV is **neurotrophic** as well as lymphotrophic: acute aseptic meningitis, encephalopathy, myelopathy and neuropathy have been reported around the time of seroconversion, while chronic meningitis, lymphoma, encephalopathy and dementia may occur later. Up to 70% of AIDS patients suffer from HIV-related dementia, which is probably a direct effect of HIV.

Most patients in the USA and Europe present with Pneumocystis carinii pneumonia, other opportunistic infections or Kaposi's sarcoma. The **presentation** in African patients is different: in Africans, AIDS is characterized primarily by a diarrhoea–wasting syndrome ('slim disease'), Kaposi's sarcoma and opportunistic infections such as tuberculosis, cryptococcosis or cryptosporidiosis.

Infants with HIV infection (< 20% of those born to infected mothers) present at around 6 months, whilst cases associated with neonatal blood transfusion present later, at 12–15 months of age. These children fail to thrive and nearly all have oral candidiasis and recurrent bacterial infections. Chronic interstitial pneumonitis is characteristic. In the late stage, typical opportunistic infections may occur but Kaposi's sarcoma and other tumours are rare.

Once AIDS has developed, the **prognosis** is dismal if untreated. Prior to antiviral therapy, survival was about 9–12 months for patients with Pneumocystis carinii pneumonia, 6–12 months for other opportunistic infections, and 20–30 months for Kaposi's sarcoma. The survival time for patients treated with new therapies will depend on previous treatment (due to viral resistance to the drug), size of the viral load, HLA type of patient and, of course, the virulence and genetic mutation rate of the virus. Rare resistance to HIV in those exposed repeatedly is associated with genetic variants of CCR5, a chemokine receptor used for entry of the virus (see below).

3.5.5 Immunopathogenesis of acquired immune deficiency syndrome

AIDS is a pandemic form of immunodeficiency, caused by several different variants of HIV retroviruses. **Retroviruses** belong to the lentivirus group, so called for the slow development of the disease. They are RNA viruses that possess a unique enzyme, reverse transcriptase, to synthesize virus-specific double-stranded DNA from the viral RNA genome (Fig. 3.14). The new DNA is integrated into the genome of the infected cell and may remain latent in these cells. Once reactivated, the DNA is used as a template for the RNA required for virus production. Viral release takes place at the cell surface by budding; the envelope of the virus is formed from the host cell membrane, modified by the insertion of viral glycoproteins.

HIV enters susceptible cells either through binding of viral envelope glycoprotein (gp120) to specific receptors on the cell surface or by fusion between the viral lipid envelope and the target cell membrane. The variant of HIV determines the **major route of entry**. Lymphotrophic variants use the CD4 molecule itself, with CXCR4 as a cofactor. Cells, such as macrophages and dendritic cells, with low levels of surface CD4 are infected via the chemokine receptor, CCR5. Other cells, such as glial cells of the central nervous system and epithelial cells in the gut and uterine cervix, have differ-

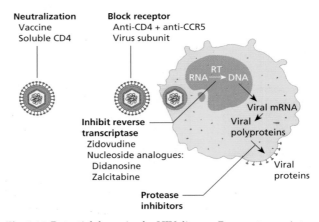

Fig. 3.14 Potential therapies for HIV disease. Reverse transcriptase can be inhibited not only by nucleoside analogues but also by nucleotide analogues and by non-nucleoside substances.

ent receptors for HIV and are also susceptible. At mucosal surfaces, where contact with HIV usually occurs, infection occurs predominantly either in the mucosal cells themselves or in intra-epithelial dendritic cells; these cell types can then pass the virus to CD4 cells by fusion of the viral lipid envelope and the target cell membrane, bypassing any neutralizing antibodies which may be present.

Since HIV **replicates** at a rate of 10^9–10^{10} new virions per day, resulting in as many as 10^8 new mutants per day, the immune response has an enormous task to limit HIV. In addition, the fast replication results in intrinsically unstable B cell binding epitopes. Production of high-affinity antibodies for neutralization does not keep up with the mutations. Cytotoxic T cells are less susceptible since, depending on the HLA type, they bind to more stable epitopes.

HIV-associated disease is characterized by major defects in immunity, following the elimination of CD4 cells. When normal CD4 T lymphocytes are stimulated by antigen, they respond by release of lymphokines, including IL-2, interferons and B-cell growth factors (see Chapter 1): these regulate growth, maturation and activation of cytotoxic T cells (antiviral), macrophages (anti-intracellular bacteria, protozoa and fungi) and natural killer cells (involved in tumour surveillance). The most **striking effects of HIV** are therefore on T-lymphocyte-mediated responses. As with other viruses which affect the immune system, autoimmunity and malignancies (both lymphoid and non-lymphoid) reflect loss of immune regulation due to HIV.

3.5.6 Diagnosis of human immunodeficiency virus infection

Primary HIV infection in adults provokes antibodies to the virus envelope and core proteins that are the principal evidence for HIV infection, provided infection with HIV is > 6 months prior to testing. These antibodies are directed typically at the envelope glycoproteins (gp120 and gp41) and are detectable throughout most of the life of the infected host. As in other viral infections, **anti-HIV antibodies** only provide indirect evidence of past infection. Absence of antibody, as in the 'window period', does not exclude the presence of the virus, which can be detected by PCR amplification (see Chapter 19).

The hallmark of **disease progression**, in addition to development of new symptoms, is an inexorable fall in the absolute number of CD4$^+$ T cells. As in other virus infections, there may be a rise in the number of CD8$^+$ suppressor/cytotoxic cells within a few weeks of infection but, subsequently, seropositive asymptomatic individuals may have normal numbers of circulating lymphocyte subsets until disease progression begins. Lymph node biopsies show many enlarged follicles, often infiltrated by CD8 lymphocytes, with depletion of CD4 cells, and destruction of the normal network structure.

Later, **polyclonal B-cell activation** results in a rise of serum immunoglobulin concentrations in 80–90% of patients with AIDS.

3.5.7 Therapeutic options in acquired immune deficiency syndrome

Management of the disease involves **early recognition of opportunistic infections**. Responses to new antigens are impaired as a result of dysfunction of CD4$^+$ dendritic cells. Even in patients with widespread opportunistic infections there may be no detectable antibody response. Consequently, *conventional serological diagnosis of intercurrent infections is unreliable* in those with AIDS; PCR is essential. In infants, the failure of antigen presentation and the subsequent humoral immune defect result in repeated bacterial infections. Immunization with pathogen-specific vaccines, including live vaccines such as MMR and BCG, have been shown to be safe in all but the most immune suppressed children and are usually recommended in order to give as much protection as possible.

Knowledge of the way in which HIV gains access into cells and its method of replication has led to exploration of **potential therapies** (Fig. 3.14). Attempts to provide antibodies to block binding of receptors on the viral envelope have so far proved fruitless. To be protective, antiviral antibody must also be neutralizing, although, even so, prevention of cell-to-cell spread by syncytium formation is very difficult. Once long-lived memory T cells are infected, patients are difficult to treat; additionally, macrophages and dendritic cells act as **reservoirs of infection** as well as a means of spread to the brain.

Inhibition of viral replication is achieved by inhibiting activity of reverse transcriptase (RT), as this is a unique retroviral enzyme with no mammalian counterpart. Zidovudine is an analogue of thymidine that yields inactive proviral DNA. Patients who received zidovudine had significantly improved survival over matched patients given placebo in blinded trials. This is not, however, a cure and significant bone marrow toxicity, coupled with viral resistance, limit its long-term usefulness. Other agents have been developed (see Fig. 3.14). Less toxic nucleoside analogues enable lower doses of zidovudine to be used in combination regimens: these have slowed progression significantly in patients with less advanced disease. A major advance was the advent of protease inhibitors, which **prevent the assembly of new infectious viruses**. The efficacy of this type of treatment has been demonstrated even in advanced cases. However, resistance to protease inhibitors, as well to some nucleoside analogues, appears after only a few days. By contrast, **resistance**

to zidovudine takes months to develop as it requires three or four mutations in the viral reverse transcriptase, whereas a single mutation can confer resistance to the protease inhibitors and other reverse transcriptase inhibitors. The advent of enfuvirtide, a **fusion inhibitor** that bars the entry of the virus by preventing viral fusion via envelope gp41 with the membrane of cell, showed improved efficacy.

Combinations of drugs (Box 3.6) and early treatment are therefore important and reduce the viraemia quickly; monitoring with quantitative measurements of viral load enable tailoring of the dose, resulting in improved compliance and therefore efficacy of drug therapy. Within weeks of starting treatment, the viral load drops below the limit of detection and CD4 count rises in the blood, due to mobilization of new CD4 cells from lymphoid tissues, prevention of reinfection

---

BOX 3.6 HIGHLY ACTIVE ANTI-RETROVIRAL THERAPY, KNOWN AS HAART

This regime is the combination of drugs:

- Nucleoside analogues, i.e. reverse transcriptase inhibitors—prevent transcription of viral RNA into cDNA copy, so blocking viral replication
- Non-nucleoside reverse transcriptase inhibitors—also inhibit reverse transcriptase
- Protease inhibitors— prevent the cleavage of viral proproteins to prevent formation of structural viral proteins and viral enzymes

Also in trials—prevention of viral entry to CD4 cells:

- CD4:Ig fusion products binding to gp120
- Block CCC5R entry
- Improved fusion inhibitors to prevent syncytium formation between viral envelope and cell membrane
- Prevention of viral incorporation into genome by inhibition of the HIV integrase

---

of these new T cells provided compliance with HAART is complete.

Monitoring for therapeutic purposes routinely involves regular viral load measurements and frequent measurements of absolute numbers of CD4+ T cells, with serum β_2-microglobulin levels. Prophylaxis against pneumocystis infection is started when the circulating CD4 count falls below 0.2×10^9/l. Prophylactic antibiotics and antiviral agents have reduced the risk of opportunistic infections, although these now occur later in the disease rather than being prevented totally. The high rate of replication allows the accumulation of numerous variants of HIV over time and many of these are resistant to antiviral therapy. Considerable mortality from HIV remains.

The response of CD8+ lymphocytes early in infection and the finding that some individuals have mounted a brisk cytotoxic T-cell response leading to apparent clearance of HIV have encouraged **potential vaccine therapy**. Traditional vaccines, using killed or attenuated organisms (see section 7.7) are unlikely to be of value, since the fragile nature of the HIV envelope makes it a poor immunogen and the high mutation rate pose difficulties of selecting a stable, common epitope to provoke useful immune responses. Since mutation of an attenuated HIV back to its virulent state would be catastrophic, safety concerns are paramount and these exclude live virus vaccines. The use of recombinant DNA technology has generated a number of novel approaches to vaccine development (discussed in Chapter 7), all of which are being explored actively in the search for a candidate 'AIDS vaccine'. However, success is elusive. The most effective *controls for HIV diseases continue to be education and prevention.*

3.5.8 Infections in the immunosuppressed host

People who are medically immunosuppressed are also **predisposed to infection** (see Cases 7.2 and 8.2). Such immu-

---

CASE 3.12 LISTERIA MONOCYTOGENES MENINGITIS AFTER IMMUNOSUPPRESSION FOR SLE

A 24-year-old woman presented with a 3-week history of tiredness, a facial rash and progressive swelling of her ankles. There was no past medical or family history of note. On examination, she was pale and pyrexial (temperature 38.2 °C) with a 'butterfly' rash on her face. There was gross oedema to the level of her sacrum and blood pressure was 180/100. Urinalysis showed haematuria (2+) and proteinuria (3+). The clinical diagnosis was nephrotic syndrome, probably due to systemic lupus erythematosus. This was supported by laboratory results: her haemoglobin was 91 g/l with a white-cell count of 3.2×10^9/l and an erythrocyte sedimentation rate (ESR) of 110 mm/h. CRP was normal. Her antinuclear antibody was strongly positive (titre > 1/10 000) and she had serum

antibodies to dsDNA (98% binding; normal < 25%). There was marked complement consumption: C3 was 0.36 g/l (NR 0.8–1.4) and C4 0.08 g/l (NR 0.2–0.4). Her serum albumin was 27 g/l, with proteinuria of 7.5 g per day.

The renal lupus (see section 9.6) was treated aggressively with high-dose methylprednisolone, azathioprine and thrice-weekly plasma exchange. However, 4 weeks later, she suddenly became unusually agitated and disorientated, with mild neck stiffness. CSF showed a raised protein concentration of 0.85 g/l (NR 0.1–0.4) with 10^4 polymorphs/mm³. Cultures of blood and CSF grew Listeria monocytogenes. The meningitis was treated with Ampicillin and her mental state rapidly returned to normal.

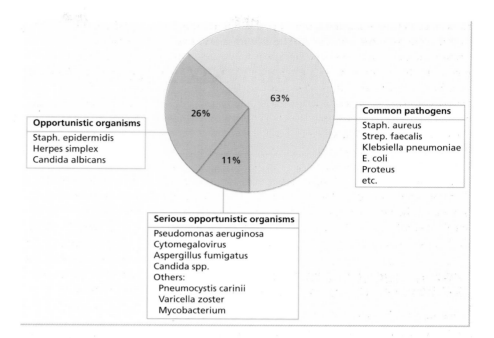

Fig. 3.15 Organisms causing infections in patients on immunosuppressive treatment.

nocompromised patients are at risk from two sources: they can be infected by common pathogens that invade even the immunologically healthy, or by truly 'opportunistic' agents, i.e. those organisms that inflict damage on weakened hosts (Fig. 3.15, see Cases 7.2 and 8.2). Opportunistic agents account for only one-third of infections but are responsible for most infective deaths.

This highlights two fundamental points about infections in the compromised host: first, most infections are due to common pathogens—these are usually readily identified and controlled by appropriate therapy; second, difficult problems are those caused by opportunistic organisms because these are often elusive or impossible to isolate and they may not respond to available drugs. In practical terms, therefore, the clinician needs to know **when to suspect opportunistic infections**.

Several studies have documented diagnostically helpful **patterns of infection** in the immunosuppressed host. The best-studied patients are those who have undergone renal transplantation (see Fig. 8.9). The major causes of infection in the first month are bacteria related to surgical wounds, indwelling cannulae or postoperative lung infections. After 1–4 months of therapeutic immunosuppression, cytomega-

lovirus infection dominates a picture that includes various fungal, viral and protozoal infections. Infections occurring beyond 4 months are due either to chronic viral infections, occasional opportunistic infections or infections normally present in the community.

The **major portal of entry of opportunistic** organisms is the oropharynx, so the lung is the commonest site of infection in the compromised host. The clinical picture is nonspecific: fever, dyspnoea and an unproductive cough with widespread pulmonary infiltrates on chest X-ray. Unfortunately, sputum, blood cultures and serology are of little help in identifying the organism; more invasive methods such as bronchoalveolar lavage, transbronchial biopsy or open lung biopsy are frequently needed. The importance of early diagnosis and treatment (where feasible) is emphasized by the grim results: the overall mortality usually exceeds 50%. However septicaemia, meningitis and gastrointestinal infections with local spread to the liver are not uncommon (see Case 3.12).

FURTHER READING

See website: www.immunologyclinic.com

CHAPTER 4

Anaphylaxis and Allergy

4.1 Introduction

Allergic diseases are common: about 20–30% of the population experience some form of allergy and this imposes a substantial physical and economic burden on the individual and society. Some patients have an occasional mild allergic reaction, some suffer life-long debilitating disease, while, more rarely, some react with severe or fatal anaphylactic shock. The prevalence of allergic diseases is increasing: in the USA, UK and many European countries, the prevalence of asthma diagnosed in children has risen at a rate of about 5% per year. Multiple factors contribute to the overall risk of developing allergy (Box 4.1), but the decline in family size

BOX 4.1 RISK FACTORS FOR ALLERGIC DISEASES

- Atopy
- Age—commoner in children than adults
- Gender—commoner in boys than girls
- Family size— less common in large families
- Reduced microbial burden in developed countries (hygiene hypothesis)
- Smoking—active and passive
- High levels of antigen exposure
- Dietary factors—poor intrauterine nutrition

and a reduced microbial burden during childhood in Westernized societies—the hygiene hypothesis—may partly account for the rising prevalence.

Allergic reactions to antigens that enter the systemic circulation, through an insect sting or intravenous administration of an antibiotic, can produce life-threatening anaphylactic reactions. More commonly, antigens are inhaled or ingested, usually triggering more local reactions in the upper or lower respiratory tracts (rhinitis or asthma) or in the mouth or upper gastrointestinal tract. However, some ingested (peanut) or inhaled (latex particles) antigens can cause severe systemic reactions.

Unfortunately, the term allergy is often used loosely to describe any intolerance of environmental factors irrespective of any objective evidence of immunological reactivity to an identified antigen.

In this chapter, we cover not only conditions in which immunological reactivity to key antigens is well defined, but also those which often present to an allergy clinic because of a popular public perception that they are allergic in origin.

4.2 Immediate (type I) hypersensitivity

Unfortunately, the recognition of antigen by antibodies and cellular receptors can cause incidental tissue damage. Such reactions are often called hypersensitivity reactions (section 1.6) and the term allergy is often used synonymously with immediate (type I) hypersensitivity. In this situation, antigen-

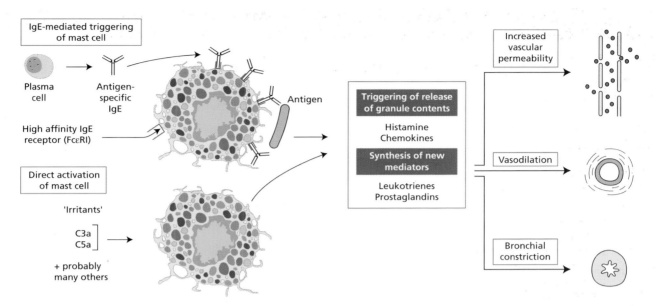

Fig. 4.1 Mast cell triggering and the results of mediator release.

specific IgE plays a key role. IgE is only a trace component of normal serum immunoglobulins but is the major class of antibody involved in 'arming' mast cells and basophils. IgE is bound via its Fc regions to the high-affinity FcεRI receptor on mast cells (Fig. 4.1). The reaction of antigen with surface-bound IgE causes cross-linking of receptors, an influx of calcium ions into the cell and explosive degranulation of the cell with release of preformed mediators (Fig. 4.1): these include histamine, heparin, lyososomal enzymes and proteases, and several chemoattractant cytokines (chemokines) such as interleukin-8 (IL-8) and RANTES (Table 1.6). Other mediators are newly generated and derived from the metabolism of arachidonic acid via two enzyme pathways; one leads to production of prostaglandins and thromboxane, the other to formation of leukotrienes. Histamine is a dominant mediator in the upper airways and leukotrienes are a significant contributor to lower airways disease.

Type I hypersensitivity reactions are rapid; for example, if the antigen is injected into the skin (a skin-prick test), **immediate hypersensitivity** can be seen within 5–10 min as a 'weal-and-flare' response. Reactions to insect venom or drugs cause immediate and systemic symptoms via this mechanism. However, IgE-mediated reactions are more commonly directed against antigens which enter at epithelial surfaces — inhaled or ingested antigens — and allergic reactions occur in the upper and lower airways or the gastrointestinal tract. Within the upper airways, this is associated with nasal itch, sneeze and rhinorrhoea, which are neurally mediated, as well as nasal obstruction, which is vascular in origin. In the lower airways, mediator release is associated with bronchoconstriction and mucus hypersecretion, giving rise to symptoms of wheeze, breathlessness, chest tightness

and cough. Where allergen exposure is persistent, there is also tissue accumulation of neutrophils and eosinophils. Release of mediators from eosinophils and from activated epithelial cells contributes to symptoms (see section 4.6.2).

Exposure of allergic patients to antigen challenge may trigger both 'immediate' and 'late' phases of bronchoconstriction. This **late-phase response** (LPR) starts 4–6 h after exposure and can last 24 h. The LPR is characterized by accumulation of activated inflammatory cells, including eosinophils and T lymphocytes. Two mechanisms have been suggested: in one, the LPR is primarily an IgE- and mast cell-dependent reaction; in the other, it is mainly mediated by IL-4 released by CD4[+] T lymphocytes. These mechanisms are not mutually exclusive.

Not all rapid clinical features resulting from mast cell degranulation necessarily involve IgE-mediated sensitivity. Direct activation of mast cells will result in release of histamine or other mediators having similar effects (see Fig. 4.1). Aspirin, tartrazine and preservatives which cause asthma or urticaria in sensitive patients probably do so by directly triggering basophils or mast cells. Substances which directly activate complement (with the production of C3a and C5a) also cause immediate reactions because these anaphylatoxins release histamine from mast cells.

4.3 Atopy

Allergic diseases tend to run in families. **Atopy** defines a state of disordered immunity in which TH2 lymphocytes drive an inherited tendency for hyperproduction of IgE antibodies to common environmental allergens. About 80% of atopic individuals have a family history of 'allergy', compared with only 20% of the normal population. However, this trait is not absolute as there is only 50% concordance in monozygotic twins.

The susceptibility to atopic disorders is under genetic control, but the evidence suggests that there are many genes with moderate effects (Table 4.1) rather than one or two major genes. Total serum IgE levels, production of antigen-specific IgE and bronchial hyperreactivity are all under some degree of **genetic control**. Genes on chromosome 5 (the IL-4 gene cluster) are implicated in the regulation of IgE production and genes on chromosome 11q to the atopic phenotype. Inheritance of the HLA-DR3 haplotype is linked to the development of allergy to rye grass.

Although genetic susceptibility to allergic disease is clearly important, environmental risk factors must play a significant role (see Box 4.1). The epidemiological observation that allergic sensitization is less common in children with older siblings and in those with early exposure to animals or brought up on farms has given rise to the 'hygiene hypothesis', which argues that children growing up in affluent societies are exposed to lower levels of bacterial or parasite antigens, which in turn causes their T lymphocytes to polarize towards a TH2 rather than a TH1 cytokine profile, so posing a greater risk of allergic disease.

4.4 Anaphylaxis

4.4.1 Anaphylaxis

Systemic anaphylaxis is the most dramatic example of an immediate hypersensitivity reaction. Clinically, the term refers to the sudden, generalized cardiovascular collapse or bronchospasm (Table 4.2) that occurs when a patient reacts to a substance to which he or she is exquisitely sensitive (Box 4.2). Generalized degranulation of IgE-sensitized mast

Table 4.1 Candidate genes implicated in development of atopy, asthma and atopic dermatitis

Chromosome	Candidate gene
5q	TH2 cytokine cluster (IL-3, IL-4, IL-5, IL-13 and GM-CSF)
11q	High-affinity IgE receptor β-subunit
16q	IL-4 receptor α-subunit
17q	RANTES
3q	CD80/CD86
20p	ADAM 33 metalloproteinase

Listed in order of likely significance but this may change.

Table 4.2 Clinical features of anaphylaxis

Organ	Feature
Cardiovascular system	Cardiovascular collapse
Respiratory system	Bronchospasm
	Laryngeal oedema
Skin	Erythema
	Angioedema
	Urticaria
Gastrointestinal system	Vomiting
	Diarrhoea

CASE 4.1 WASP VENOM ANAPHYLAXIS

A 69-year-old woman was fit and well until one August when she was stung on the back of her right hand by a wasp. She had previously been stung on several occasions, the last time 2 weeks earlier. Within 5 min, she felt faint, followed shortly by a pounding sensation in her head and tightness of her chest. She collapsed and lost consciousness and, according to her husband, became grey and made gasping sounds. After 2–3 min, she regained awareness but lost consciousness immediately when her husband and a friend tried misguidedly to help her to her feet. Fortunately, a doctor neighbour arrived in time to prevent her being propped up in a chair: he laid her flat, administered intramuscular epinephrine (adrenaline) and intravenous antihistamines and ordered a paramedic ambulance. She had recovered fully by the next day.

Her total serum IgE was 147 IU/ml (NR < 120 IU/ml). Her antigen-specific IgE antibody level to wasp venom was 21 U/ml [ra-dioallergosorbent test (RAST) class 4], but that to bee venom was 0.3 U/ml (RAST class 0). The patient was a candidate for specific allergen injection immunotherapy (hyposensitization) for her wasp venom anaphylaxis. The slight but definite risk of desensitization was explained and balanced against the major risk of anaphylaxis should she be stung again. The first injection consisted of 0.1 ml of 0.0001 μg/ml of wasp venom vaccine given subcutaneously. No reaction occurred. Over the next 12 weeks, gradually increasing doses were given without adverse effects. Over this period, she tolerated injections of 100 μg venom. She then continued on a maintenance regimen of 100 μg of venom per month for 3 years.

At the age of 76 years, she was stung by a wasp which had come into her bathroom. She remained calm, lay down and experienced no significant systemic reaction.

BOX 4.2 THE MOST COMMON CAUSES OF ANAPHYLAXIS

- Bee and wasp stings (Case 4.1)
- Foods (Case 4.8)
- Latex rubber (Case 4.2)
- Drugs

cells or basophils follows antigen exposure and previous sensitization is therefore required. While anaphylaxis is uncommon, it is extremely dangerous, as it is so unexpected, and can be fatal.

When the antigen is introduced systemically, as in a wasp sting or intravenous antibiotic, *cardiovascular collapse is the predominant clinical feature*. When the antigen is absorbed through the skin or mucosa, as in latex rubber anaphylaxis, the reaction develops more slowly (see Case 4.2). Allergy to latex rubber is increasingly common: several high-risk groups are recognized and latex allergy may cross-react with certain foods (Table 4.3). Foods which are absorbed via the oral mucosa seem especially likely to trigger angioedema of the lips, tongue and larynx. In some cases, hypotension and collapse may occur if certain foods are eaten immediately prior to exercise — food-related, exercise-induced anaphylaxis.

Anaphylaxis can also occur in those **allergic to drugs**, such as penicillin. Penicillin allergy is commonly self-reported, but true anaphylactic reactions are much rarer, with a rate of 25 per 100 000 treated patients. The risk of a severe reaction is greater following parenteral than oral penicillin, and over

six times more likely in a patient with previous reactions to penicillin. However, most serious reactions occur in patients with no previous history of penicillin allergy. Skin-prick testing using major and minor penicilloyl determinants is of limited value, since up to 90% of skin-test-positive patients subsequently tolerate penicillin. On the other hand, a negative skin-prick test usually indicates patients who are not at risk or in whom reactions will be mild.

The only **laboratory test** that is useful at the time of an apparent anaphylactic reaction is blood mast cell tryptase. This is an indicator of mast cell degranulation, but an elevated level identifies neither the mechanism of mast cell activation nor its cause. Antigen-specific IgE (RAST) tests are helpful to confirm the nature of the insect venom prior to desensitization but skin testing is more useful for latex rubber.

As in Cases 4.1 and 4.2, intramuscular epinephrine (adrenaline) is the most important drug in **treating anaphylaxis** and is nearly always effective. It should be followed by parenteral administration of hydrocortisone and chlorpheniramine. Epinephrine (adrenaline) by inhalation is much less effective. A note of caution: a detailed history is vital in distinguishing anaphylaxis from idiopathic angioedema and urticaria (section 4.8.1), with which it is often confused. While injection of epinephrine can be lifesaving in anaphylaxis, it can be harmful, even fatal, in elderly arteriosclerotic patients with urticaria and angioedema.

Long-term management requires detailed advice on avoidance to prevent further attacks. Preloaded epinephrine (adrenaline) syringes are readily available and effective, but patients must receive training on when and how to use them. Wearing a medical alert bracelet alerts paramedic staff and doctors to the possible cause of collapse. **Hyposensitization, or specific allergen immunotherapy**, is over 90% effective in patients with bee or wasp venom anaphylaxis provided recommended guidelines are followed (Box 4.3). Venom immunotherapy leads to a marked change in cytokine secre-

Table 4.3 Key features of latex rubber allergy

High-risk groups
- Patients with spina bifida or multiple urological procedures (10–50% risk)
- Healthcare workers (5–10% risk)
    Operating theatre staff
    Females
    Atopics
- Rubber industry workers (5–10% risk)

High-risk latex products
- Surgical latex gloves
- Latex rubber gloves for home use
- Balloons
- Catheters and enema tubes
- Condoms
- Teats and dummies (pacifiers)

Cross-reactivity with food allergies
- Kiwi fruit, banana, avocado, melon, chestnut

BOX 4.3 RECOMMENDED GUIDELINES FOR SPECIFIC ALLERGEN IMMUNOTHERAPY (HYPOSENSITIZATION)

- Only high-quality standardized allergen extracts should be used
- Administered in hospitals or specialized clinics only
- Medical staff should have appropriate training and experience in immunotherapy
- Epinephrine (adrenaline) should always be immediately available
- Ensure ready access to resuscitative facilities with attendant staff trained in resuscitative techniques
- Patients should be kept under close supervision for 60 min after each injection

CASE 4.2 LATEX-INDUCED ANAPHYLAXIS

A 38-year-old woman was referred for investigation following an anaphylactic reaction whilst visiting a relative in hospital. She gave a 5-year history of recurrent conjunctival oedema and rhinitis when blowing up balloons for her children's birthday parties. In the year prior to admission, three successive visits to her dentist triggered marked angioedema of her face on the side opposite to that requiring dental treatment. The swellings took 48 h to subside.

On the day of admission, she visited a critically ill relative in hospital. The patient was being reverse barrier nursed and visitors were required to wear gown and gloves. About 20 min after putting on the gloves her face and eyes became swollen, she felt wheezy and developed a pounding heart beat and light-headedness. Her tongue started to swell and she was taken to the Emergency Department where she was given intramuscular epinephrine (adrenaline) and intravenous hydrocortisone. She recovered rapidly but was kept under observation overnight.

She had no history of atopy or other allergies. Ten years earlier she had undergone a series of operations for ureteric reflux and in the preceding 2 years had received colposcopic laser treatment for cervical intra-epithelial neoplasia (CIN-III).

Skin-prick testing to a crude latex extract produced a very strong reaction and her antigen-specific IgE antibody level to latex was significantly elevated at 57 U/ml (RAST class 5).

The diagnosis was that of latex-induced anaphylaxis. She was advised to avoid contact with all materials containing latex, and warned that she could react to certain foods (see Table 4.3). It was suggested that she wears a medical alert bracelet, in case she required future emergency surgery, and carry a self-injectable form of epinephrine. The diagnosis has important implications for any further dental, surgical or anaesthetic procedures. Hospitals should have written procedures for latex-free surgery for planned and emergency operations.

---

tion, with a switch from the proallergic TH2 cytokine profile to a TH1 response (see Chapter 7).

4.4.2 Anaphylactoid reactions

Anaphylaxis should be distinguished from **anaphylactoid (i.e. anaphylaxis-like) reactions**. These are not mediated by IgE antibodies. Similar pharmacological mediators (such as histamine) are responsible for the clinical features but the stimulus for their release differs. Substances inducing anaphylactoid reactions do so by a direct action on mast cells or by alternate pathway complement activation (see Fig. 4.1). Since this is not immunologically specific, *the person does not need to have been previously sensitized to the substance*. Collapse following intravenous injections of radio-opaque organic iodines in radiology or intravenous

induction agents for anaesthesia may fall into this category. Non-steroidal anti-inflammatory drugs (NSAIDs) divert arachidonic acid metabolism towards production of leukotrienes, which are potent inducers of allergic-type reactions via their interactions with specific receptors on target tissues.

The **emergency treatment** of an anaphylactoid reaction is the same as that of anaphylaxis, but the distinction is important in ensuring the appropriateness and interpretation of investigations and in long-term management of the clinical problem (Case 4.3). In anaphylactoid reactions, skin-prick tests and measurements of antigen-specific IgE are of no value: the only test available is in vivo challenge. Management requires avoidance of the offending agent, since specific allergen immunotherapy is of no benefit in non-IgE-mediated reactions.

CASE 4.3 DRUG-INDUCED REACTION

A 77-year-old woman was referred from the Accident and Emergency Department, having been admitted overnight because of sudden onset of massive angioedema of her tongue associated with laryngeal stridor. She was treated with intravenous hydrocortisone only. This was her fifth such episode: an anaphylactoid attack 2 months earlier was severe enough for her to be intubated and ventilated on the Intensive Care Unit.

She had no history of previous allergy and no family history of atopy. A drug history revealed that, in addition to oral prednisolone prescribed in the Accident and Emergency Department, she was taking oral furosemide and captopril. Captopril is an angiotensin-converting enzyme (ACE) inhibitor and this group of drugs is known to cause severe episodes of angioedema. Captopril was discontinued and her mild hypertension was managed with alternative medication. The attacks have not recurred.

CASE 4.4 SEASONAL ALLERGIC CONJUNCTIVITIS

A 7-year-old boy developed itchy eyes and swollen lids after playing tennis in the garden. Because his mother had hay fever, the boy's symptoms were also presumed to be an allergy to grass pollen. After several episodes of increasing severity, medical help was sought. He was skin tested; a weal-and-flare reaction appeared 5–15 min after prick testing with extracts of grass pollens, cat fur and house dust mite. The speed and nature of the reaction con-

firmed immediate (type I) hypersensitivity to these antigens, and he was told to try to avoid exposure to high concentrations of grasses in the pollen season. He developed similar reactions the following summer, particularly in June and July; they were sometimes accompanied by sneezing and rhinorrhoea. He was therefore started on prophylactic eye drops containing sodium cromoglycate, which helped control his seasonal allergic conjunctivitis.

4.5 Allergic conjunctivitis

4.5.1 Seasonal (hay fever) and perennial (vernal) conjunctivitis

Seasonal conjunctivitis is common and mainly affects children and young adults. This is a mild, bilateral disease characterized by itching, redness and excessive tear production (Fig. 4.2). It is usually associated with the nasal symptoms of hay fever and follows the same seasonal variation. Antigen-specific IgE is involved; this has been demonstrated by passive transfer of specific antigen hypersensitivity to a 'volunteer' by serum. The IgE is attached to conjunctival mast cells but its site of production is uncertain, and excess free IgE is not necessarily found in the tears. Although pollen-specific IgE is responsible for hay-fever conjunctivitis, affected individuals often react to additional antigens when skin-tested (as in Case 4.4) (since this is one of the 'atopic' diseases), without necessarily developing clinical reactions on exposure. Treatment includes pollen avoidance where possible, sodium cromoglycate eye drops to reduce mast cell sensitivity and topical or systemic antihistamines to block the effects of mediators released from mast cells.

A more severe form of conjunctivitis, persisting throughout the year (with exacerbations in the spring), is known as **vernal conjunctivitis**. It is a self-limiting condition of young

people (usually lasting 3–5 years) and is characterized by red eyes, photophobia, itching and a mucous discharge. The diagnostic feature is the formation of giant papillae (known as cobblestones) on the upper tarsal conjunctiva. These are due to oedema and hypertrophy of underlying tissue, which contains IgA- and IgE-secreting plasma cells, mast cells and eosinophils. Vernal conjunctivitis is often associated with atopic diseases (eczema and asthma) and most patients have high serum IgE levels, with IgE detectable in their tears. Vernal conjunctivitis probably represents immediate and late-phase reactions. When the conjunctiva over the limbus (corneal–scleral junction) is affected, it is called **limbal vernal conjunctivitis**. Severe diseases may provoke outgrowth of epithelium, even extending over the corneal surface. Although rare, this can lead to corneal damage, permanent scarring and blindness.

Immediate (type I) reactions in the eye can be caused by a variety of other antigens, the commonest being topical agents such as antibiotics or contact lens solutions. In severe cases a cobblestone appearance of the upper tarsal conjunctiva is seen. The development of papillae is not unique to atopy-associated diseases; they are occasionally seen in contact dermatoconjunctivitis (a type IV reaction) and contact lens-associated conjunctivitis (an autoimmune reaction to conjunctival antigens adherent to contact lenses) (see Chapter 12). Decisions to treat with anti-inflammatory drugs or steroids should be made in conjunction with an ophthalmologist.

4.6 Respiratory allergy

4.6.1 Allergic rhinitis

Allergic rhinitis may be seasonal or perennial (Fig. 4.3). In the USA, it is the sixth most prevalent chronic disease, outranking heart disease. **Seasonal allergic rhinitis** is often referred to as hay fever and its prevalence is rising. Patients **present** with rhinorrhoea, sneezing and nasal obstruction following antigen exposure. Those with chronic symptoms develop sinusitis, serous otitis media and conjunctivitis, and lose their senses of taste and smell. Many

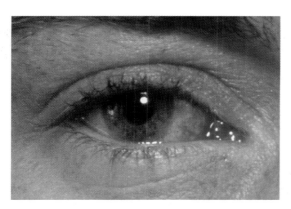

Fig. 4.2 Acute conjunctivitis.

CASE 4.5 PERENNIAL ALLERGIC RHINITIS

A 29-year-old doctor developed intense itching of her eyes and nose and a tickling sensation in her ears and palate, followed by sneezing and rhinorrhoea. These symptoms developed within 15 min of visiting an elderly patient who kept four cats. The symptoms settled down over the next 2 h but started to recur whenever home visits were made to houses where cats were present. Symptoms occurred even though the cats were excluded from the interview room. Each episode took slightly longer to resolve and some were accompanied by a dry cough.

The doctor had suffered from asthma in childhood and her non-atopic parents had a cat. During her years in medical school and in hospital posts, she had no respiratory symptoms. The move into general practice and exposure to cat dander had triggered perennial allergic rhinitis. On investigation, she had strongly positive skin tests to cat dander, house dust mite and grass pollen. She started prophylactic use of a nasal spray and eye drops containing sodium cromoglycate, with abolition of most of her symptoms. Sometimes, she also needed to use a local antihistamine spray to relieve breakthrough attacks of rhinitis. The value of hyposensitization (antigen-specific immunotherapy) to cat dander was discussed because occupational exposure was unavoidable, but not undertaken while her symptoms continued to be controllable. It remains a therapeutic option.

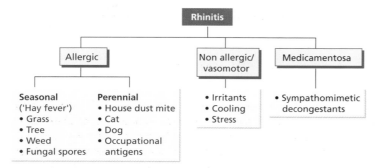

Fig. 4.3 Causes of rhinitis.

patients also have asthma and, as with asthma, there is an increased susceptibility to irritating fumes, cold or emotional stress. The antigens which cause this condition are usually 'large' and mainly deposited in the nose (Fig. 4.4). However, many particles (10–40 μm diameter), such as grass pollens, release soluble antigenic material whilst lodged in the nasal mucus. When the causative antigen is present all the year round, for instance house dust mite or animal dander, the patient may suffer **perennial allergic rhinitis**. Such patients are often misdiagnosed as having a 'permanent cold'.

A careful history is essential if the causative antigen is to be found. Positive **skin tests** help to distinguish allergic rhinitis from non-allergic rhinitis. RAST tests are useful only occasionally, if skin tests are conflicting or contraindicated.

Histopathologically, the nose shows mucosal swelling, with excessive production of nasal fluid containing basophils and eosinophils. The **pathogenesis** is similar to asthma, with mediators of inflammation liberated from mast cells. IgE mechanisms are involved and IgE, IgG and IgA can be detected in nasal secretions. In a few patients with severe chronic hay fever or perennial rhinitis, mucosal hyperplasia

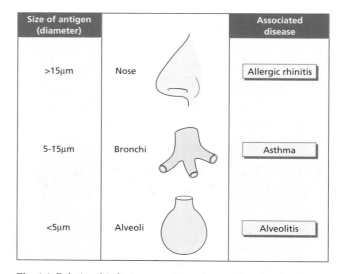

Fig. 4.4 Relationship between antigen size and the site of major symptomatology.

may result in the formation of polyps, but only a few cases of nasal polyps are due to an allergic cause.

The differential diagnosis of allergic rhinitis is **vasomotor or irritant, non-allergic rhinitis**. This is a non-seasonal condition in which there is no itching, few eosinophils in the nasal fluid and a normal level of serum IgE. In contrast to allergic rhinitis, it responds poorly to nasal disodium cromoglycate. Chronic non-allergic rhinitis is probably the nasal equivalent of idiopathic asthma.

Topical sodium cromoglycate and intranasal corticosteroids are effective prophylactic **treatment** for most patients with allergic rhinitis. Prolonged use of nasal decongestants leads to rebound rhinitis when treatment is stopped — **rhinitis medicamentosa**. Local or oral antihistamines may be needed for relief of troublesome symptoms. In patients with severe symptoms which are not controlled by anti-allergic medication, **hyposensitization (antigen-specific immunotherapy)** to grass pollen or cat dander can be effective. Selection of patients is critical and immunotherapy should be carried out by experienced specialists in departments with full resuscitative facilities because of the danger of anaphylaxis (see Box 4.3).

4.6.2 Asthma

Asthma is a syndrome with three cardinal features:
- generalized but reversible airways obstruction;
- bronchial hyper-responsiveness; and
- airways inflammation.

It arises as a result of complex interactions between multiple genes and environmental factors (Fig. 4.5) and cannot be explained solely on the basis of IgE-mediated triggering of mast cells. Although not all cases are allergic in origin (Table 4.4), most cases occur in patients who also show immediate hypersensitivity to defined environmental allergens, as in Case 4.6. It is a common condition, affecting 5–10% of the population in the UK. The prevalence and severity of asthma are rising. Despite medical awareness about the dangers of asthma, and an effective range of therapies, *many asthmatics die each year during a severe attack*, although deaths are now less common following decreased use of high-dose formulations of relatively unselective β-agonist drugs.

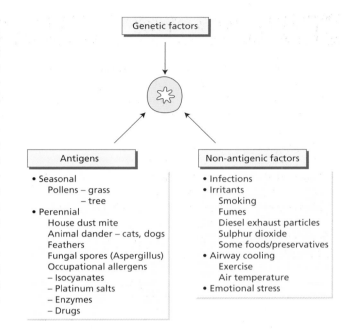

Fig. 4.5 Some precipitating factors in asthma.

Asthma is **familial** and many genetic loci predispose to the disease (Table 4.1). Asthma is less common in less affluent populations and those who grow up in large families, possibly because transmission of viral or bacterial infections from older siblings leads to preferential stimulation of TH1 lymphocytes over TH2 lymphocytes, so reducing allergic sensitization.

The **pathogenesis** of asthma can be subdivided into inflammatory and remodelling components. Dendritic cells in the airways play a vital role in the inflammatory component. These professional antigen-presenting cells direct T-lymphocyte development down the TH2 pathway through the interaction between CD28 on T cells and B7 on dendritic cells (see Fig. 1.14) and their secretion of cytokines (especially IL-1 and IL-12). Sensitized T cells are identified readily in bronchial biopsies and bronchoalveolar lavage fluid from asthmatic individuals, and allergen-specific, TH2-like

CASE 4.6 ALLERGIC ASTHMA

A 15-year-old girl presented with a prolonged wheezing attack which had come on suddenly 36 h earlier. She had experienced several episodes of 'wheezy bronchitis' as a child and eczema as an infant. She was a non-smoker. Her father suffered from hay fever but there was no family history of asthma. On examination, she was tired and unwell, with a rapid respiratory rate and tachycardia (140/min). There were bilateral expiratory wheezes on chest auscultation. Investigations showed a normal haemoglobin but a raised white cell count (14 × 10⁹/l). Her sputum contained many eosinophils. A chest X-ray was normal but lung function tests showed reversible airways obstruction. Skin tests showed an immediate reaction to six common antigens. The clinical diagnosis was asthma and the family history and skin tests suggested this was allergic asthma. She continues to have periodic attacks of asthma, although they are controlled, in part, by prophylactic inhaled steroids and β₂-adrenergic stimulants (salbutamol) as needed.

Table 4.4 Features of asthma

	Allergic	Idiopathic	Others
Proportion of total asthmatics	60%	30%	10%
Age of onset	Childhood	> 40 years	Variable
Other atopic diseases	Common	Unusual	Unusual
Family history	Yes	No	No
Causes	Seasonal	None known	Aspergillus
	Perennial		Carcinoid
	Occupational		Carcinoma, aspirin
			Churg–Strauss syndrome
Prognosis	Often persists into adult life (30%)	Many become chronic	Variable
	Deaths rare	Deaths do occur	

clones have been produced which preferentially release IL-3, IL-4, IL-5, IL-13, tumour necrosis factor-α (TNF-α) and granulocyte–macrophage colony-stimulating factor (GM-CSF) (Fig. 4.6). IL-3, IL-5 and GM-CSF influence eosinophil development, maturation, activation and survival, while IL-4, IL-5, IL-13 and TNF-α are important in the up-regulation of a leucocyte–endothelial cell adhesion molecule, called VCAM-1 (see Chapter 1), that enables neutrophils, monocytes and eosinophils to adhere to vascular endothelium prior to migration into the tissues.

IL-4 and IL-13 produced by these TH2 cells promote B lymphocytes to switch to IgE synthesis; effective signalling also requires the engagement of a second set of co-stimula-tory molecules, CD40 on B cells and CD40 ligand on T cells (see Fig. 1.16).

When the asthmatic patient is exposed to the relevant antigen, **immunological recognition** can occur via both the T-cell receptor and IgE bound to mast cells (Fig. 4.6). The frequency of antigen exposure determines whether the response is acute reversible airways obstruction alone or a chronic allergic response with bronchial hyper-responsiveness. In the case of single antigen exposure, the symptoms are due to the release of preformed and newly generated mediators released by mast cells, as described in section 4.2. Epithelial cells of the airways, when inflamed and activated, also generate IL-8 and RANTES and recruit further eosinophilic infiltration (Box 4.4; Fig. 4.7).

Acute inflammation usually resolves as repair processes restore normal structure and function. In chronic asthma, this process is disturbed and leads to remodelling, which is reflected in the **pathological changes** (Fig. 4.7). Epithelial damage and loss of barrier function expose deeper airway structures. Inflammatory and structural cells produce growth factors and profibrinogenic cytokines that lead to angiogenesis, proliferation of smooth muscle, basement membrane thickening, a cellular infiltrate of eosinophils (see Box 4.4) and mononuclear cells, and fibrosis.

The **diagnosis** of asthma is a clinical one but may not always be obvious. Any sputum should be examined for cells

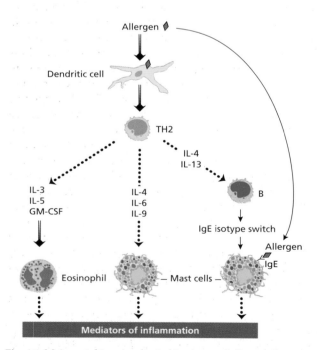

Fig. 4.6 Major cytokines implicated in airways inflammation.

BOX 4.4 CAUSES OF EOSINOPHILIC INFILTRATION IN CHRONIC ALLERGEN EXPOSURE (FIG. 4.5)

- Up-regulation of VCAM-1 enabling eosinophil recruitment
- Maturation and increased survival mediated by IL-3, IL-5 and GM-CSF
- Selective eosinophil migration induced by IL-8 and RANTES (Table 1.6)

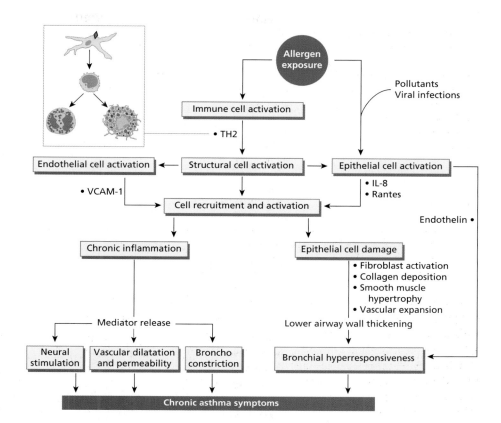

Fig. 4.7 The development of airways inflammation and bronchial hyper-responsiveness in chronic asthma.

and pathogens because many attacks are precipitated by infection. Sputum or blood eosinophilia may be present. Lung function tests show a reduced forced expiratory volume (FEV_1), reversible with bronchodilators — this is the *essential diagnostic test*.

Laboratory tests, such as the total serum IgE level, are unhelpful in distinguishing patients with allergic asthma from those with idiopathic asthma. Twenty percent of children with 'wheezy bronchitis' eventually develop asthma; these children have high IgE levels, but this is not sufficiently predictive to be of clinical diagnostic value. There is no evidence that the routine use of RASTs to identify antigens suspected of causing inhalant allergy adds anything to a careful history and the judicious use of skin tests.

Bronchial challenge is an important test of occupational asthma. It not only proves the reversibility of the airways obstruction, but also indicates which inhaled antigens will trigger the asthma. Bronchial challenge often results in immediate bronchoconstriction (within 10 min) and a late-phase reaction. Such challenge has definite risks and is performed only in specialized centres.

Avoidance of precipitating factors (see Fig. 4.5) is important in patients with asthma caused by indoor allergens such as mites, cats and dogs, but these allergens have different aerodynamic characteristics. Mite allergens are present as large particles in bedding and soft furnishings, but only become airborne after vigorous disturbance and settle quickly. In contrast, cat and dog allergens are small particles which, following disturbance, remain airborne for long periods. Dust mite-allergic patients experience predominantly low-grade exposure overnight in bed. In contrast, cat or dog-allergic patients develop symptoms within minutes of exposure due to inhalation of large amounts of easily respirable allergens. Even after permanent removal of a cat or dog from the home, it may take 6–12 months before the huge concentrations of allergens in the home drop to normal. The value of mattress covers to reduce exposure to house dust mite is controversial: while allergen exposure may fall, there is an inconsistent effect on symptoms or respiratory function.

Treatment, although usually effective, is largely palliative because there is no way to correct permanently the fundamental genetic predisposition. Most asthma treatment guidelines recommend a stepwise approach to drug treatment. Bronchodilators (β_2-adrenoceptor agonists) are good for relieving bronchospasm but do not inhibit other mechanisms that produce airways hyper-responsiveness. Steroids down-regulate proinflammatory cytokine production, especially those released by TH2 cells and activated epithelial cells. The use of potent, topically active, inhaled steroids has reduced the need for systemic steroids other than to control a severe attack, or in a few patients with severe, chronic asthma. Leukotriene receptor antagonists have recently been shown to be effective as add-on treatment in asthmatics whose disease is poorly controlled by standard therapy. Ciclosporin is also of benefit in severe, intractable, chronic asthma, illustrating the importance of T cells in pathogenesis. There are several new therapeutic approaches in asthma. Clinical trials of a recombinant humanized monoclonal antibody to IgE—called omaluzimab or Rhu-Mab-E25—have shown a dramatic fall in free serum IgE and clinical benefit in some patients with a reduction in the therapeutic dose of inhaled steroids.

4.7 Food allergy and intolerance

Food 'allergy' undoubtedly exists, but extravagant claims that a wide array of symptoms are due to allergies to foods has confused the subject. One cause of confusion lies in poor definition of terms. Several **categories of adverse reactions to foods**—immunological, biochemical (enzyme deficiency) and psychological (food fads and aversion)—can lead to gastrointestinal, respiratory, skin and even neurological symptoms. An adverse reaction cannot be considered immunological until there is proof of an immune-mediated mechanism. The term **food intolerance** should be used to

---

CASE 4.7 ORAL ALLERGY SYNDROME

A 40-year-old man knew he had longstanding 'hay fever', although his symptoms were worse in March and April each year rather than in summer months. For the previous 4 years he had noticed that eating certain fruits, particularly apples, pears and peaches, produced tingling, burning and swelling of his lips and gums. These symptoms occurred within seconds of starting to eat these fruits and lasted about 30 min, but were never associated with vomiting, urticaria, bronchospasm or circulatory collapse. He found that he could eat cooked or preserved apples without any reactions. He was worried that these reactions heralded an increasing potential to develop anaphylaxis to fruit.

He was skin-prick tested to a variety of allergens: he showed strongly positive reactivity to tree pollen and peach but a negative

reaction to the commercial apple solution. However, when the skin test lancet was first pricked into a fresh apple and then into the patient's skin—so-called 'prick-prick' testing—a strongly positive immediate reaction developed.

He has the oral allergy syndrome. This occurs in patients allergic to birch tree pollen because of allergic cross-reactivity between pollen and certain fruits. The allergens are heat-labile and destroyed by cooking, so patients can tolerate cooked fruit or jams. Skin-prick testing with commercial fruit extracts is often negative, as the relevant proteins are destroyed during extraction, but sensitivity to fresh fruit can be demonstrated by 'prick-prick' testing as here. The oral allergy syndrome does not normally progress to cause systemic anaphylaxis.

CASE 4.8 NUT ALLERGY

A 15-year-old schoolgirl was admitted to hospital as an emergency whilst on holiday. Her parents believed her to be allergic to nuts. At the age of 5 years, she vomited about 1 min after eating a bar of chocolate containing nuts. Three years later, she developed marked angioedema of her face, lips and tongue, followed by tightness of her throat and vomiting: this occurred 2–3 min after friends of her brother decided to test her allergic status by pushing peanuts into her mouth and holding her jaws shut! Less severe attacks had followed inadvertent ingestion of hazelnuts and almonds. As a consequence, she avoided peanuts and tree nuts wherever possible.

The emergency admission occurred following a single lick of a vanilla ice cream. Within seconds, she developed angioedema of her lips and tongue, difficulty in breathing, and felt light-headed. Following an emergency call, she was injected with intramuscular adrenaline and intravenous hydrocortisone by the paramedical service, and admitted to hospital overnight. She made a rapid and

uneventful recovery. Her parents later recalled that one ice-cream scoop was used by the vendor to dispense all flavours: the customer immediately before the patient had been served a nut-flavoured ice cream.

On investigation, she had a grade 6 RAST (see Chapter 19) to peanut with significant but lesser (grade 2) reactivity to hazelnut, almonds and brazil nuts. She was also atopic, with strongly positive RASTs to grass pollen (grade 4) and cat dander (grade 3).

The management of her nut allergy comprised advice on strict avoidance of peanuts and tree nuts, with particular attention to 'hidden' nuts in food. She was advised to wear a medical alert bracelet as a warning to emergency personnel of a possible cause of sudden collapse, and to carry with her at all times a self-injectable form of epinephrine (adrenaline). There is no place for hyposensitization in peanut-allergic patients.

Table 4.5 Adverse reactions to foods

	Reproducible reaction on challenge		
	Open challenge	Blind challenge	Immune mediated
Food fad	–	–	–
Psychological aversion	+	–	–
Food intolerance (mechanism unknown)	+	+	?
Food allergy (immune mechanism)	+	+	+
Food idiosyncrasy	+	+	–

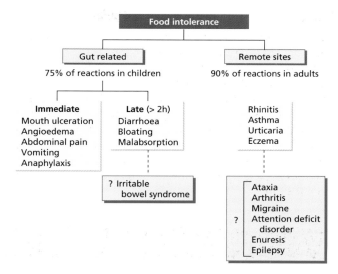

Fig. 4.8 Putative clinical spectrum of food intolerance.

describe all abnormal but reproducible reactions to food when the causative mechanism is unknown (Table 4.5). **Food allergic disease** should be used when the abnormal reaction is proved to be immunologically mediated. If the mechanism involved is non-immunological, the adverse response is best called **food idiosyncrasy**, e.g. a patient with biliary tract disease who cannot tolerate fatty meals is not 'allergic' to fat. The public perception of their illnesses being caused by food is over 10 times greater than the proven prevalence of food intolerance.

4.7.1 Food allergy and intolerance

Food intolerance is a relatively common problem in childhood, especially in the first year of life. Nearly three-quarters present with immediate gastrointestinal symptoms (Fig. 4.8). However, some clinical syndromes of food intolerance in children are more common than others (Table 4.6)

and food intolerance must be considered to be a rare or unproven cause of certain symptoms that occur at sites remote from gut, such as attention deficit disorders, arthritis or enuresis. Those children who have apparently benefited from dietary manipulation in some reports have been from highly selected groups. In food intolerance proven by blind challenge, a single food (most commonly cow's milk) is responsible in just under half of the cases.

Allergy to peanuts is becoming more common (Box 4.5) and most patients are atopic. A minute quantity of peanut antigen can cause a life-threatening reaction, as in Case 4.8. Avoidance is thus vital, but difficult to achieve, because nuts are ubiquitous and often 'hidden' in inadequately labelled foods.

Most reports of proven food intolerance in adults incriminate nuts, milk, eggs, fish, wheat and chocolate. Some children and adults report itching and swelling of the mouth,

Table 4.6 Clinical syndromes of food intolerance in children

Common	Occasionally important	Unusual	Rare
Acute angioedema/ urticaria in infants under 1 year	Atopic eczema in infants under 1 year	Atopic eczema in children over 1 year	Asthma
Perioral erythema		Chronic urticaria	
Atopic infants with gastrointestinal symptoms		Loose stools	
		Migraine	
Infantile colitis			

BOX 4.5 KEY POINTS ABOUT PEANUT ALLERGY

- Peanuts are legumes, botanically distinct from nuts
- Peanut allergy is accompanied by increased risk of allergy to tree nuts
- Commonest cause of fatal or near-fatal food-related anaphylaxis in USA and UK
- Affects 1% of children but is seven times more common in siblings of patients with peanut allergy
- Life-long problem, starting in early childhood (< 7 years)
- Most patients do not 'outgrow' peanut allergy
- T-cell clones from patients produce high levels of IL-4 and low levels of interferon-γ—consistent with a TH2-like profile
- Hyposensitization is not available

tongue and soft palate after eating fresh fruit, typically apples, pears, cherries, plums and peaches—the oral allergy syndrome (see Case 4.7).

There are many **mechanisms of adverse reactions to food** other than immunological ones. These include irritant, toxic, pharmacological or metabolic effects of foods, enzyme deficiencies, or even the release of substances produced by fermentation of food residues in the bowel. For instance, some foods contain pharmacologically active substances (such as tyramine or phenylethylamine) that may act directly on blood vessels in sensitive subjects to produce symptoms such as migraine.

However, traces of drugs or antibiotics (e.g. penicillin in the milk of penicillin-treated cows), foods rich in natural salicylates (e.g. fruits and vegetables), food additives (e.g. monosodium glutamate), colouring agents (e.g. tartrazine) or preservatives (e.g. benzoic acid) can also cause symptoms in susceptible people by mechanisms which are ill understood, but are probably due to direct effects on mast cells and not to an immunological mechanism. Salicylates, for instance, inhibit synthesis of prostaglandins and cause release of mast cell mediators.

4.7.2 Diagnosis of food allergy and intolerance

The diagnosis depends on a careful clinical history and thorough examination to exclude other, perhaps more likely, causes of the patient's symptoms such as a food fad or an anxiety state. *Elimination and challenge diets form the basis of the diagnosis of food allergic disease.* A food challenge must be carefully monitored and conducted under double-blind conditions.

No **laboratory test** is diagnostic. Immediate-hypersensitivity skin tests and antigen-specific IgE antibodies (RAST) only identify some antigens, even where there is a strongly positive history. Only one-third of patients with a clear history of egg, fish or nut intolerance give positive skin reactions and RAST results and most of those with milk intolerance do not. A negative blood test for IgE antibodies is not proof of lack of food allergic disease; conversely, a RAST result may be positive in a patient who is perfectly able to tolerate the food in question. Testing the blood or skin of a

CASE 4.9 IS THIS FOOD ALLERGY?

A 38-year-old woman presented with a 2-year history of abdominal bloating, cramping abdominal pains and loose stools. Attacks occurred every 7–10 days but lasted only 2–3 h. One attack occurred about 8 h after a meal of pasta in a local restaurant and led her to believe her symptoms were food-related. She initially eliminated wheat-based products from her diet and then, because the attacks continued, dairy products as well. She was referred to a gastroenterologist and investigated extensively: gastroduodenal endoscopy, duodenal biopsy, barium meal, colonoscopy and pancreatic function tests were all normal.

She continued to believe her symptoms were food related: vague muscular pains, headaches, poor concentration and fatigue were attributed to other foods which were also eliminated from her diet. She was referred to an allergy clinic for further assessment.

Physical examination showed an undernourished woman with no other abnormal findings. As this was a second opinion, a wide range of tests were done. Her haemoglobin and erythrocyte sedimentation rate were normal. Her serum immunoglobulins were normal and her serum IgE was only 8 IU/ml. She had no detectable antibodies to tissue transglutaminase, endomysium or gliadin (see Chapter 19). While waiting for her outpatient appointment, she had responded to an advertisement in a health food shop and undergone electrodermal or 'Vega' testing. The report listed 24 foods to which she was allergic, many of which she had felt able to tolerate previously. Her diet had become increasingly restricted: expert dietetic assessment showed her diet to be nutritionally unsound, with deficient intake of protein, fat, fat-soluble vitamins and trace elements. The diagnosis was that of psychological food aversion and irritable bowel syndrome. She was reluctant to accept this diagnosis and asked her GP for referral to another specialist.

patient clearly does not always reflect what is happening at the level of the gut mucosa.

Other tests are at best misleading, at worst dangerous. A diagnostic procedure used by 'clinical ecologists' is symptom provocation by intradermal or sublingual extracts of test substances. When evaluated under double-blind conditions, this method lacked validity: the high frequency of positive responses to the extracts appeared to be due to suggestion and chance. Other methods, such as hair analysis, are more a matter of gullibility and faith than evidence-based medicine. A double-blind, randomized trial of electrodermal ('Vega') testing found that this method could not distinguish between atopic and non-atopic people. A study of five commercial 'allergy' testing clinics in the UK, conducted by the Consumers' Association, found that these clinics did not reliably identify food allergies in patients known to have them; they gave different results for paired samples from the same patient; and they often gave dubious and risky dietary advice. Be warned!

Recognition of the offending food and its elimination from the diet is the cornerstone of treatment. Some patients know that a certain food, such as peanuts, regularly produces their symptoms; this food can be avoided — a simple **elimination diet**. Certain foods are eliminated empirically because they are frequently implicated in that form of food 'allergy', e.g. milk and eggs in infant atopic eczema. Rare patients who seem intolerant of a wide range of foods may need a very restricted diet — a 'few-food' or 'oligoantigenic' diet. Dietary exclusion has many risks: nutritional deficiency, expense, disruption of lifestyle and psychological consequences. If symptoms are improved, then foods can be reintroduced one at a time. This is a diagnostic procedure, but care is essential, as anaphylaxis can occur on reintroduction. The lack of objective tests causes some parents to insist that their children suffer from food 'allergy' despite any clinical evidence and to put them on nutritionally deficient diets, a situation that has been called 'induced or fabricated illness', previously known as 'Munchausen's syndrome by proxy'.

4.8 Skin disease and allergy

4.8.1 Urticaria and angioedema

Urticaria is a physical sign, not a disease. Urticaria refers to transient episodes of demarcated, oedematous, erythema-

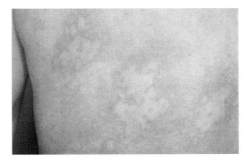

Fig. 4.9 Typical urticaria.

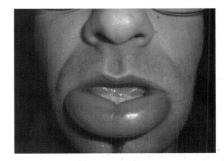

Fig. 4.10 Angioedema.

CASE 4.10 CHRONIC URTICARIA AND ANGIOEDEMA

A 25-year-old joiner presented with a 12-month history of an intensely itchy 'nettle rash' on his chest and back (see Fig. 4.9). The lesions appeared suddenly and lasted from 6 to 12 h, to be replaced by new lesions at other sites. The lesions varied in size from a few millimetres to several centimetres. Attacks occurred two to three times each week. In addition, he had experienced four episodes of sudden swelling of lips that took 48 h to subside. He said he looked as though he had been punched (see Fig. 4.10). He was unaware of any triggering factors and there was no personal or family history of atopy. His general health was excellent and he was not taking any medications. On examination, the lesions consisted of raised, red, irregular patches, some with white centres, and were typically urticarial. General examination was entirely normal.

Laboratory investigations showed a normal haemoglobin and white cell count, with no eosinophilia. His complement C4 and C1 inhibitor levels were normal, excluding hereditary angioedema (see Case 11.5).

Since certain food additives may trigger urticaria and angioedema, he was challenged with tartrazine (a colouring substance) and sodium benzoate (a food preservative) by mouth; neither substance induced a new crop of lesions. The urticaria was fairly well controlled by a long-acting antihistamine (levocetirizine) but he was reluctant to take these tablets on a long-term basis. Three years later, his urticarial lesions are still present, although less severe; their cause is unknown.

tous, pruritic lesions with a raised edge. It has such a distinctive appearance that clinical diagnosis is usually easy; the difficult task is finding the cause, since laboratory tests are frequently unhelpful. Urticaria results from sudden, localized accumulation of fluid in the dermis. Angioedema is a similar process occurring in the deep dermis, subcutaneous tissues or mucous membranes. Urticaria and angioedema commonly coexist.

Any sudden increase in local vascular permeability in the dermis will cause urticaria. A variety of **mechanisms** may be responsible (Fig. 4.11); some are immune but many are not. Mast cells in the dermis are an important source of these vasoactive mediators.

Spontaneous urticaria can be classified into acute and chronic (Box 4.6). **Acute urticaria** is short-lived, although the cause is identified in only 50% of cases. Episodes caused by an IgE-mediated reaction to extrinsic antigens, such as food, are usually obvious from the history and can be confirmed by skin-prick testing. Attacks can also be related to drug ingestion (Fig. 4.11) or to acute viral infections.

Chronic urticaria is conventionally defined as the occurrence of widespread urticarial weals on a daily or almost daily basis for at least 6 weeks. It affects over one in 200 of the population and can be very disabling. The term 'chronic idi-

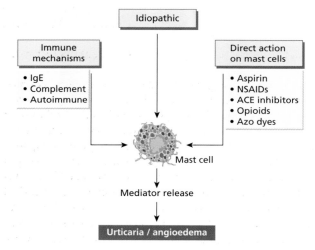

Fig. 4.11 Mechanisms of urticaria production.

BOX 4.6 CLASSIFICATION OF URTICARIA

- Spontaneous urticaria
  - Acute
  - Chronic
- Physical urticarias
- Contact urticaria
- Urticarial vasculitis

BOX 4.7 CLINICAL IDENTIFICATION OF URTICARIAL VASCULITIS

- The weals are usually tender and painful rather than itchy
- They generally last longer than 24 h
- They fade to leave purpura or bruising
- They are often accompanied by systemic features such as fever and arthralgia

opathic urticaria' is used when physical urticarias and urticarial vasculitis have been excluded. Chronic idiopathic and physical urticarias commonly coexist in the same patient.

In patients with **physical urticarias**, itching and weals are provoked by physical stimuli such as scratching the skin (dermographism), rapid cooling (cold urticaria), sun exposure (solar urticaria), water (aquagenic urticaria) or exercise, heat or emotion (cholinergic urticaria).

Urticarial vasculitis (Boxes 4.6 and 4.7) is regarded as an immune-complex disease with histological evidence of vasculitis on skin biopsy. The diagnosis is important because patients may have underlying disease, such as systemic lupus erythematosus (SLE), and the treatment differs.

By definition, no cause can be found for **chronic idiopathic urticaria**. However, up to 30% of patients have circulating IgG autoantibodies which bind to the high-affinity IgE receptor ($Fc_{\varepsilon}RI$) on mast cells and basophils and trigger mediator release. Chronic urticaria can be triggered by food additives, namely azo-dyes and preservatives, or by a variety of drugs, including aspirin, other NSAIDs, ACE inhibitors and opioids (Fig. 4.11). IgE antibodies to these drugs are not involved.

Treatment of chronic urticaria is empirical. Avoidance of triggering factors is an obvious step. Elimination of Helicobacter pylori infection has been associated with remission of chronic urticaria. Long-acting antihistamines are the mainstay of treatment: they reduce itch and decrease the frequency and duration of weals. Care must be taken using mizolastine, which has weak potential to prolong the QT interval, in patients with liver disease or in combination with cytochrome P450 inhibitors, which include azole antifungals and macrolide antibiotics, to avoid potential cardiac arrhythmias. Systemic steroids are not indicated in chronic urticaria because of the high doses required, the development of intolerance and the problems of steroid toxicity. For patients with severe autoimmune disease, high-dose intravenous immunoglobulin or ciclosporin therapy may be effective. Despite treatment, about 20% of patients still have chronic urticaria 10 years following presentation.

4.8.2 Atopic eczema

Atopic eczema is a common, chronic, severely pruritic, ecze-

CASE 4.11 ATOPIC ECZEMA

Sam was born at full term, after a normal pregnancy, and weighed 3.4 kg. He was breast-fed. At the age of 4 weeks, he was admitted with a 2-day history of screaming attacks, loose motions and rectal bleeding. He was treated conservatively, but 3 days after discharge his symptoms recurred, together with patches of eczema on his arms and trunk. On detailed questioning, it transpired that a health visitor had told Sam's mother that her breast milk was of 'poor quality' and had advised her to 'top up' each feed with cow's milk. His mother had been following this advice from the time Sam was 2 weeks old. When investigated at the age of 6 weeks, strongly positive IgE-specific antibodies to cow's milk were present on RAST testing (see Chapter 19). His mother returned to exclusive breast-feeding and excluded dairy products from her own diet, to eliminate any possibility that cow's milk antigens might be excreted in her breast milk. Within 2–3 days, the screaming attacks stopped.

At the age of 10 months he was referred back to hospital with extensive atopic eczema. It had recurred behind his knees at the age of 7 months, when solids were first introduced into his diet, and steadily worsened. The areas affected were the popliteal and antecubital fossae, arms and abdomen. He scratched the eczematous lesions, especially at night, with the result that his and the family's sleep was badly disturbed. Sam had a strong family history of atopic disease; his mother and maternal grandmother both suffered from asthma. On examination, his height and weight were around the 50th centile. He was covered in extensive eczema, involving 60% of the total skin area.

Laboratory investigations showed a normal haemoglobin (123 g/l) with a raised white cell count (16.0×10^9/l): the differential count showed relative (9%) and absolute (650/mm^3) eosinophilia. His total serum IgE level was markedly raised at 4600 IU/ml (NR for age < 50 IU/ml) with strongly positive RASTs (see Chapter 19) to grass pollen, cat epithelium, dog dander, house dust mite, cow's milk, wheat and peas. Skin-prick testing was not considered in the presence of such widespread eczema. Samples of dust from his home showed very high levels of house dust mite in the carpet and on several toys.

He was treated with antihistamines at night and liberal applications of an emollient cream to his skin lesions. Environmental control of antigen exposure was also attempted: the mite count was lowered by changing carpets, and covering the mattress, pillows and duvet with covers impermeable to mite allergens, and the cat was found a new home. Sam was put on a diet free of cow's milk, wheat, oats, peas, beans, nuts, food preservatives and food colourings. Over the following 3 months, there was only partial improvement in the severity of his eczema.

---

matous skin disease, usually occurring in individuals with a hereditary predisposition to all atopic disorders, and frequently in association with a high serum IgE level.

The **prevalence** of atopic eczema is increasing. It affects about 10–20% of children worldwide and some 2% of adults. Over half of children present during the first year of life. In infants, the dermatitis often appears on the face first, followed by the flexural aspects of the arms and legs. In older children and adults, the flexures are frequently involved, with thickening, lichenification and scaling of the epidermis, which tends to crack and weep. Spontaneous resolution occurs in many patients; about half clear by the age of 7 and 90% by their late teens but, in the remainder, eczema persists into adult life.

The commonest **complication** is superadded bacterial infection, but some children may develop ocular complications, such as cataracts, psychological problems or side-effects from prolonged treatment (particularly with corticosteroids). Although atopic children handle most viruses normally, *superadded infection with herpes simplex virus is life-threatening*.

The **diagnosis** of atopic eczema is based on the clinical features, usually with a personal or family history of atopy. There are no pathognomonic clinical or laboratory findings, and although a raised IgE and multiple positive prick tests and RASTs are commonly found, they are unhelpful in management.

There is a strong **genetic** predisposition to atopic eczema. The concordance rate is up to 85% in monozygotic twins compared with 30% in dizygotic twins. Familial aggregation analysis shows a stronger clustering of atopic eczema between siblings than between siblings and parents, suggesting that **environmental factors** are also important. Allergen exposure in atopic eczema is often via the skin. House dust mite is one provoking factor and reduction in the house dust mite allergen load in the home may result in significant clinical improvement. The role of food intolerance is controversial: controlled studies of dietary manipulation in children suggest that it is an uncommon trigger, particularly in older children (see Table 4.6). Staphylococcus aureus colonization and infection is found in over 90% of patients with atopic eczema. Staphylococcus aureus may exacerbate skin inflammation by acting as a superantigen (see section 2.4.2), activating macrophages and T cells, particularly T cells expressing the skin homing receptor, cutaneous lymphoid antigen (section 11.1).

The most obvious **immunological abnormality** is a raised serum IgE level in about 90% of patients. The highest levels are found in patients with both eczema and asthma. Since IgE production is under T-cell control, the abnormal regulation of IgE production reflects defective T-cell function (Box 4.8). Evidence suggests that activation of the TH2 subset of CD4$^+$ lymphocytes leads to the release of cytokines important in the **pathogenesis** of atopic eczema. TH2 cells produce IL-4, IL-5, IL-6 and IL-13 but not interferon (IFN)-γ. IL-4 and IL-13 act as IgE isotype-specific switch factors and induce the expression of VCAM-1 (see Chapter 1), an adhesion molecule involved in the migration of mononuclear cells into sites of allergic tissue inflammation. T lymphocytes migrating into the skin are highly enriched for cutaneous lymphoid antigen-expressing memory TH2 cells, implying the selective migration of these cells. Once the 'itch–scratch' cycle is triggered, mechanical stimulation of the keratinocytes further releases cytokines to sustain the inflammatory process.

BOX 4.8 EVIDENCE THAT ATOPIC ECZEMA IS LINKED TO ABNORMAL T-CELL FUNCTION

Clinical evidence

- Increased susceptibility to skin infections normally controlled by T cells

  Disseminated vaccinia (eczema vaccinatum)

  Herpes simplex (eczema herpeticum) or Kaposi's varicelliform eruption

  Viral warts

  Dermatophyte fungal infection

- Temporary improvement during measles infection (?TH1 cell response with interferon-γ production)

- Occurrence of eczema in primary immunodeficiency diseases, e.g. Wiskott–Aldrich syndrome; hyper-IgE recurrent infection syndrome

- Response to T cell immunomodulatory therapy

Laboratory evidence

- Disappearance of eczema in children with Wiskott–Aldrich syndrome following bone marrow transplantation

- Decreased CD8$^+$ T-cell number and function

- Decreased number of interferon-γ-secreting TH1 cells

- Expansion of IL-4-, IL-5- and IL-13-secreting TH2 cells in the skin and peripheral blood

- Chronic macrophage activation with increased secretion of GM-CSF, PGE$_2$ and IL-10

Animal evidence

- Absence of T cells prevents eczema in mouse model

IL, Interleukin; GM-CSF, granulocyte–macrophage colony-stimulating factor; PGE$_2$, prostaglandin E$_2$.

Current **management** of atopic eczema is directed at the reduction of cutaneous inflammation and the elimination of exacerbating factors including allergens, infection and irritants. Bland emollients provide some symptomatic relief of itching and help to repair and rehydrate the skin. Topical corticosteroids suppress inflammation and also help to reduce itching; they are the most successful agents currently available to treat eczema. Long-term use of potent steroids may lead to atrophy of the dermis and epidermis and may even be accompanied by significant systemic absorption if they are applied in excess. Systemic steroids are rarely justified, but may sometimes be used in short bursts to control otherwise intractable eczema, or in an attempt to 'reset' the 'itch–scratch' cycle. There is limited and conflicting evidence that the use of bed covers impermeable to mite allergens and other measures to reduce the allergen load is associated with clinical improvement in randomized controlled trials.

A number of **therapeutic approaches** are now directed at modulating signal transduction in TH2 lymphocytes. Ciclosporin A has proved safe and effective as a short-term treatment for severe, refractory atopic eczema. Controlled trials have shown topical calcineurin inhibitors (section 7.2), such as tacrolimus or pimecrolimus, to be effective in controlling moderate to severe atopic eczema without the atrophic side-effects of topical steroids. Randomized controlled trials of IFN-γ therapy have demonstrated reduction in clinical severity scores and reduction in eosinophil counts, but IFN-γ therapy is limited by side-effects (section 7.3.2). Ultraviolet phototherapy may be beneficial in severe and resistant atopic eczema, but carries the risk of premature skin ageing and cutaneous malignancy. When used as monotherapy, mycophenolate mofetil clears skin lesions, but not all patients benefit and those who do usually take 4-8 weeks to respond.

4.8.3 Contact dermatitis

Contact dermatitis is an inflammatory skin disease caused by T-cell-mediated (type IV) hypersensitivity to external agents which come into contact with the skin rather than an IgE (type I) hypersensitivity. It is an important cause of occupational skin disease. Contact dermatitis is quite distinct from atopic dermatitis, both clinically and in immunopathogenesis, and is discussed fully in section 11.4.

FURTHER READING

See website: www.immunologyclinic.com

5 Autoimmunity

5.1 Definition of autoimmunity and autoimmune disease

Autoimmunity is an immune response against a self-antigen or antigens. Autoimmune disease is tissue damage or disturbed physiological function due to an autoimmune response. This distinction is important, as autoimmune responses can occur without disease (Case 5.1) or in diseases caused by other mechanisms (such as infection). Proof that autoimmunity causes a particular disease requires a number of criteria to be met, as in Koch's postulates for microorganisms in infectious diseases (Table 5.1). The best **evidence** for autoimmunity in human disease comes from active transfer of IgG across the placenta in the last trimester of pregnancy, which may lead to the development of transient autoimmune disease in the fetus and neonate (Table 5.2 and Case 5.2). In contrast, there are diseases which are reliably associated with autoimmune responses but where the relationship between autoimmunity and disease is unclear. For example, the chronic liver disease primary biliary cirrhosis (section 14.8.2) is strongly associated with autoantibodies directed against mitochondria (and more specifically against a single isoform of the mitochondrial enzyme pyruvate dehydrogenase), but it seems unlikely that these antibodies play any role in liver dam*age. Caution is therefore required in making the assumption that autoimmune responses necessarily imply autoimmune disease.*

CASE 5.1 IS THIS RHEUMATOID ARTHRITIS?

A 43-year-old woman presented to her general practitioner (GP) with sudden onset of acute back pain while gardening, followed by more sustained but less severe pain over the next 2 weeks. The GP felt that this was mechanical back pain but performed some 'screening investigations' which included an erythrocyte sedimentation rate (ESR) of 4 mm in the first hour (normal < 10) and a positive test for rheumatoid factor at a titre of 1 in 256. She was then referred to her local rheumatology department with a possible diagnosis of rheumatoid arthritis. This caused the patient considerable anxiety as her aunt had had severe rheumatoid arthritis,

leading to a very high level of disability. When she was seen in the rheumatology clinic 3 months later she still had minor back pain, but this was overshadowed by her anxiety. She had no other musculoskeletal symptoms and examination was normal apart from mild restriction of the lumbar spine. The rheumatologist agreed with the initial diagnosis of mechanical back pain and explained that around 5% of healthy normal people have a positive test for rheumatoid factor. Testing for rheumatoid factor is useful only in patients with a clinical picture consistent with rheumatoid arthritis, where it is an important prognostic indicator.

Table 5.1 Criteria that must be fulfilled to confirm that a particular autoimmune response causes a corresponding autoimmune disease

Criterion	Comment
1 Autoantibodies or autoreactive T cells with specificity for the affected organ are found reliably in the disease	This criterion is met in most endocrine autoimmune diseases. It is more difficult to fulfil where the target antigen (if any) is unknown as in rheumatoid arthritis. Autoantibodies are much easier to detect than autoreactive T cells but autoantibodies can also be detected in some normal subjects
2 Autoantibodies and/or T cells are found at the site of tissue damage	True for some endocrine diseases, SLE and some forms of glomerulonephritis
3 The levels of autoantibody or T-cell response reflect disease activity	Demonstrable only in acute systemic autoimmune diseases with rapidly progressive tissue damage such as some subjects with SLE, systemic vasculitis or antiglomerular basement membrane disease
4 Reduction of the autoimmune response leads to improvement	Benefits of immunosuppression are seen in many disorders, but most immunosuppressive treatments are non-specific and anti-inflammatory
5 Transfer of antibody or T cells to a second host leads to development of autoimmune disease in the recipient	Easily demonstrated in animal models. In humans by transplacental transfer of autoreactive IgG antibodies during the last third of pregnancy (see Case 5.2) and by development of autoimmune disease in the recipient of bone marrow transplants when the donor has an autoimmune disease
6 Immunization with autoantigen and consequent induction of an autoimmune response causes disease	Many self-proteins induce an autoimmune response in animals when injected with an appropriate adjuvant. Harder to demonstrate in humans, but rabies immunization once involved use of infected (but non-infective) mammalian brain tissue, which could induce autoimmune encephalomyelitis

SLE, Systemic lupus erythematosus.

Table 5.2 IgG antibody-mediated diseases capable of placental transfer

Maternal autoantibody to	Disease induced in neonate
Thyroid-stimulating hormone	Neonatal Graves' disease
Epidermal basement membrane cell adhesion molecules	Neonatal pemphigoid
Red blood cells	Haemolytic anaemia
Platelets	Thrombocytopenia
Acetylcholine receptor	Neonatal myasthenia gravis
Ro and La	Neonatal cutaneous lupus and congenital complete heart block

5.2 Patterns of autoimmune disease

Autoimmune diseases can affect any organ in the body, although certain systems seem particularly susceptible (e.g. endocrine glands). Autoimmune diseases have been conventionally classified into (i) organ-specific and (ii) non-organ-specific disorders.

5.2.1 Organ-specific autoimmune disease

Organ-specific autoimmune disorders (Cases 5.2 and 5.3) affect usually a **single organ** and the autoimmune response is directed against multiple antigens within that organ. Most of the common organ-specific disorders affect one or another endocrine gland. The antigenic targets may be molecules expressed on the surface of living cells (particularly hormone receptors) or intracellular molecules, particularly intracellular enzymes (Table 5.3). The reasons for the restricted pattern of affected organs and target antigens are unclear.

5.2.2 Non-organ-specific autoimmune disease

Non-organ-specific disorders affect **multiple organs** and

CASE 5.2 MYASTHENIA GRAVIS AND NEONATAL MYASTHENIA GRAVIS

A 21-year-old woman was referred to a neurology clinic with a 1-month history of double vision, difficulty swallowing and weakness in her upper arms. These symptoms were mild or absent in the morning and tended to worsen through the day. When she was seen towards the end of an afternoon neurology clinic she was found to have a bilateral ptosis and disconjugate eye movements that could not be ascribed to any individual cranial nerve lesion. Her upper limb power was initially normal but deteriorated with repeated testing. An intravenous injection of edrophonium, a short-acting cholinesterase inhibitor, completely abolished the neurological signs but her eye movements deteriorated again 30 min after the injection. A clinical diagnosis was made of myasthenia gravis. Subsequent blood testing showed the presence of a high level of antibodies against the acetylcholine receptor.

She was treated with oral cholinesterase inhibitors with some improvement. However, 1 month later she deteriorated and corticosteroids were introduced with no improvement. A computed tomography scan of her thorax showed no evidence of a thymoma but she was nevertheless referred to a thoracic surgeon for thymectomy, as this can sometimes induce remission in myasthenia even in the absence of a thymoma. A small thymic remnant was removed

and she recovered uneventfully and was able to withdraw from all medication without deterioration in her symptoms. Acetylcholine receptor antibody levels fell but remained detectable. One year later, she became pregnant and after an uneventful 41-week pregnancy she delivered a 4-kg male infant. There were immediate concerns about the baby, who failed to make adequate respiratory efforts and who appeared limp and hypotonic. The baby was intubated and ventilated on the neonatal intensive care unit. In the light of the mother's history, a provisional diagnosis of neonatal myasthenia gravis was made, although care was taken to exclude other causes of neonatal respiratory insufficiency such as maternal analgesia with pethidine, hypoglycaemia and sepsis. A cranial ultrasound showed no evidence of bleeding or other pathology. Subsequent testing of a blood sample taken from the umbilical cord showed low levels of acetylcholine receptor antibody. The baby needed ventilation and feeding via a nasogastric tube for 3 days, at which time the ventilation was successfully withdrawn. There were some initial feeding problems due to difficulty sucking and swallowing, but these resolved over the next 48 h. The child's subsequent development has been entirely normal. The mother also remains well.

CASE 5.3 FUNGAL INFECTIONS, FITS AND HYPOCALCAEMIA

A 14-year-old boy presented to a dermatologist with sore, cracked hypertrophic lips, chronic paronychia (tender, swollen nail beds with dystrophic nails) and curious horn-like lesions in the scalp. The dermatologist made a clinical diagnosis of chronic mucocutaneous candidiasis, and subsequently cultured the yeast Candida albicans from the boy's mouth and a dermatophyte fungus from the lesions on the scalp. The dermatologist noted a history of epilepsy starting at the age of 5. Subsequent investigation demonstrated profound hypocalcaemia with corrected serum calcium of 1.1 mm/l (normal 2.2–2.6) with undetectable levels of parathyroid hormone. His 4-year-old sister had also recently developed epilepsy and was

also found to be severely hypocalcaemic. No assay for antibodies against endocrine parathyroid tissue was available, but the classical clinical picture allowed a confident diagnosis of autoimmune hypoparathyroidism as a feature of APECED (Autoimmune Polyendocrinopathy, Candidiasis and Ectodermal Dysplasia). The patient subsequently developed fatigue and vomiting and a short synacthen test revealed evidence of adrenal cortical failure. The presence of antibodies to adrenal cortex suggested this was caused by autoimmune adrenalitis. As yet there is no evidence of diabetes mellitus.

are usually associated with autoimmune responses against self-molecules that are widely distributed through the body, and particularly with intracellular molecules involved in transcription and translation of the genetic code (Table 5.3). Many of these non-organ-specific disorders fall within the group of multisystem disorders labelled as 'connective tissue diseases'; this is a misleading term since the 'connective tissues' are neither abnormal nor specifically damaged, but the term is in very widespread use.

5.3 Who gets autoimmune disease?

The burden of autoimmune diseases is considerable in western society. Around 3% of the population have an autoimmune disease. Many of the major chronic disabling diseases affecting people of working age are usually considered to have an autoimmune basis. These include multiple sclerosis (MS), rheumatoid arthritis and insulin-dependent diabetes mellitus. Autoimmune diseases are rare in childhood and

Table 5.3 Some examples of self-antigens and associated diseases. More information can be found in the appropriate organ-based chapters. In general, tissue-specific antigens are associated with organ-specific diseases and those antigens found in all cells are associated with systemic disease

Self antigen	Disease
Hormone receptors	
TSH receptor	Hyper- or hypothyroidism
Insulin receptor	Hyper- or hypoglycaemia
Neurotransmitter receptor	
Acetylcholine receptor	Myasthenia gravis
Cell adhesion molecules	
Epidermal cell adhesion molecules	Blistering skin diseases
Plasma proteins	
Factor VIII	Acquired haemophilia
β_2-glycoprotein I and other anticoagulant proteins	Antiphospholipid syndrome
Other cell-surface antigens	
Red blood cells (multiple antigens)	Haemolytic anaemia
Platelets	Thrombocytopenic purpura
Intracellular enzymes	
Thyroid peroxidase	Hypothyroidism
Steroid 21-hydroxylase (adrenal cortex)	Adrenocortical failure (Addison's disease)
Glutamate decarboxylase (β-cells of pancreatic islets)	Autoimmune diabetes
Lysosomal enzymes (phagocytic cells)	Systemic vasculitis
Mitochondrial enzymes (particularly pyruvate dehydrogenase)	Primary biliary cirrhosis
Intracellular molecules involved in transcription and translation	
Double-stranded DNA	SLE
Histones	SLE
Topoisomerase I	Diffuse scleroderma
Amino-acyl t-RNA synthases	Polymyositis
Centromere proteins	Limited scleroderma

TSH, Thyroid-stimulating hormone; SLE, systemic lupus erythematosus.

the peak years of onset lie between puberty and retirement age, the major exception being the childhood-onset form of diabetes mellitus.

There are striking sex differences in the risk of developing an autoimmune disease. Almost all are **more common in women**, and for some autoimmune diseases the risk may be increased eight times in females. There are, however, notable exceptions, such as ankylosing spondylitis.

The prevalence of autoimmunity tends to be higher in northern latitudes and is probably higher in westernized, industrialized societies, and seems to increase progressively as this pattern of social and economic organization develops. It is unclear whether this geographic and socioeconomic variation in autoimmunity reflects differential exposure to pathogens, variations in nutrition or other factors.

Autoimmune diseases also show evidence of **clustering within families** (Case 5.3, Table 5.4). These genetic factors are discussed in more detail below in section 5.6.1.

5.4 What prevents autoimmunity?

Autoimmune responses are very similar to immune responses to non-self antigens. Both sorts of response are driven by antigen, involve the same immune cell types and produce tissue damage by the same effector mechanisms. The development of autoimmunity, however, implies a failure of the normal regulatory mechanisms. These regulatory mechanisms are discussed first so that reasons for their breakdown can be examined.

5.4.1 Autoimmunity and self-tolerance

Strong protective mechanisms exist to prevent the development of autoimmune disease. As outlined in Chapter 1, the immune system has the ability to generate a vast diversity of different T-cell antigen receptors and immunoglobulin molecules by differential genetic recombination. This proc-

Table 5.4 Single gene defects that provide an insight into autoimmune diseases

Gene defect or experimental genetic manipulation	Autoimmune disease seen as consequence of gene defect	Implications for autoimmunity
Deficiency of early classical complement pathway components, C1q, C2, C4. Rare human disease and knockout mouse	Systemic lupus erythematosus	Early classical complement pathway important in immune-complex clearance and disposal of intracellular debris; thus limits presentation of self-antigens
Chronic granulomatous disease (defect in NADPH oxidase enzyme complex). Rare human disease	Discoid lupus erythematosus	Phagocytes scavenge and destroy cell debris
Fas (CD95) deficiency. (Binding of cell surface Fas triggers apoptosis.) Rare human disease and inbred strain of mouse	Mice: lupus-like disorder Humans: lymphoproliferation and red cell/platelet autoimmunity	Apoptosis deletes potentially autoreactive lymphocytes, particularly B cells
Bcl-2 deficiency in knockout mice (Bcl-2 is intracellular molecule which inhibits apoptosis)	Lupus-like disorder	As above
Over-expression of tumour necrosis factor (TNF)-α in TNF-α transgenic mice	Destructive joint disease resembling rheumatoid arthritis	Key role of TNF in joint inflammation
Over-expression of human HLA-B27 in transgenic mice	Multisystem disease with some similarity to ankylosing spondylitis (AS): development critically dependent upon bowel flora	Direct link between this HLA molecule and pattern of inflammation found in AS. Implicates infection as trigger
Absence of CTLA-4, (T-cell molecule involved in negative second signal) CTLA-4 knockout mice	Lupus-like disorder with lymphoproliferation	Negative second signal is important in switching off autoreactive cells
Absence of transforming growth factor (TGF)-β (a cytokine with potent inhibitory effects on T cells) TGF-β knockout mouse	Florid multisystem autoimmune disorder	Negative regulation of T cells is important in limiting autoimmunity
Abnormal or absent expression of transcription factor, AIRE. Human disease or knockout mouse	Autoimmunity in multiple endocrine organs	AIRE controls expression of self-molecules (such as insulin) in the thymus. Thus influences thymic tolerance

ess produces many antigen-specific receptors capable of binding to self-molecules. To avoid autoimmune disease, the T and B cells bearing these self-reactive molecules must be either eliminated or down-regulated. Because T cells (in particular CD4+ T cells) have a central role in controlling nearly all immune responses, the process of T-cell tolerance is of greater importance in avoidance of autoimmunity than B-cell tolerance, since most self-reacting B cells will not be able to produce autoantibodies unless they receive appropriate T-cell help.

5.4.2 Thymic tolerance

T-cell development in the thymus plays a major role in eliminating T cells capable of recognizing peptides from self-proteins (Fig. 5.1). By a process called positive selection, cells survive by binding to major histocompatibility complex (MHC) molecules. This binding induces a signal which stops the cell from dying. T-cell receptors which fail to bind in any way to self-MHC molecules in the thymus die through apoptosis. T cells which survive this process will bind, with a variety of affinities, to the MHC molecules and self-peptide complexes present in the thymus. Those T cells which bind with low affinity are allowed to survive and have the potential to bind to MHC plus a foreign peptide with high affinity and so initiate protective immune responses at a later time. However, T cells which bind to MHC plus self-peptides with high affinity in the thymus have clear potential for self-recognition elsewhere in the body with consequent induction of autoimmunity. These cells are therefore eliminated on the basis of their high-affinity binding. This elimination of self-reactive cells is known as **negative selection**.

This process of **thymic education** is only partially successful as autoreactive T cells can be detected in healthy persons. The most important reason for failure of thymic tolerance is that many self-peptides are not expressed at sufficient level

CORTEX

MEDULLA

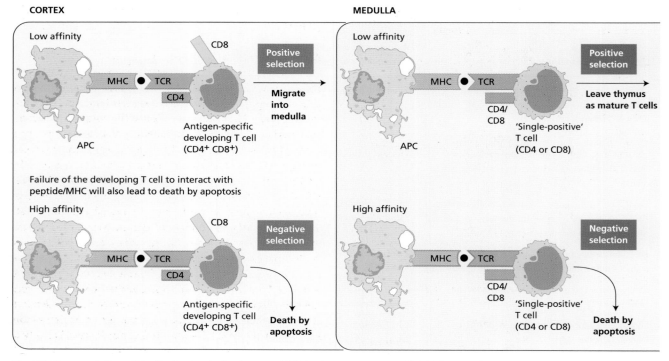

Fig. 5.1 Representation of T-cell selection in the thymus. APC, Antigen-presenting cell; MHC, major histocompatibility complex; TcR, T-cell receptor; ●, self-peptide.

in the thymus to induce negative selection. Most peptides found bound to MHC molecules in the thymus are from either ubiquitous intracellular or membrane-bound proteins or proteins present in the extracellular fluid, although some antigens that have been conventionally considered to be tissue specific are expressed in the thymus (such as insulin). This means that thymic tolerance is induced to some, but not all, tissue-specific proteins (errors in this process may underlie one well defined genetic cause of autoimmunity—Table 5.4 and section 5.6.1). It is not surprising therefore that T cells responsive to tissue-specific proteins [for example, cartilage collagens or some central nervous system (CNS) antigens] can be detected in healthy people under certain laboratory conditions. A second level of control exists over these potentially autoreactive cells: this further level is known as peripheral tolerance.

5.4.3 Peripheral tolerance

There are several mechanisms by which peripheral tolerance is maintained. These are outlined below.

Ignorance

A form of peripheral tolerance exists to some self-antigens because the antigen is effectively invisible to the immune system. This is known as immunological ignorance (Fig. 5.2). Immunological ignorance can occur because the antigen is

sequestered in an avascular organ such as the intact vitreous humour of the eye, although when limited amounts of antigen do escape from these sites active peripheral tolerance develops by mechanisms discussed below. More importantly, immunological ignorance occurs because CD4+ T cells (which are required to initiate most immune responses via their helper function) will only recognize antigens presented in association with MHC class II molecules. The very limited distribution of these molecules, on professional antigen-presenting cells such as dendritic cells, means that most organ-specific molecules will not be presented at levels high enough to induce T-cell activation.

Separation of autoreactive T cells and autoantigens
Self-antigens and lymphocytes are also kept separate by the restricted routes of **lymphocyte circulation** which limit naive lymphocytes to secondary lymphoid tissue and the blood (Fig. 5.3). To prevent large amounts of self-antigen from gaining access to antigen-presenting cells, debris from self-tissue breakdown needs to be cleared rapidly and destroyed. This is achieved by cell death through **apoptosis**, preventing widespread spilling of cell contents, plus a variety of scavenger mechanisms clearing up cell debris. These include the complement system, certain acute-phase proteins (such as serum amyloid P and C-reactive protein) and a number of receptors found upon phagocytes. Defects of complement or phagocytes are associated with the devel-

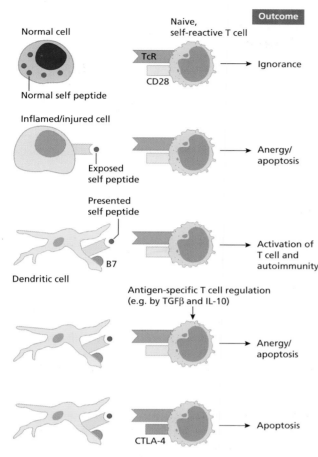

Fig. 5.2 How peripheral tolerance is maintained.

(Labels in figure:)

Normal cell
Normal self peptide

Naive, self-reactive T cell
Outcome
TcR
CD28
→ Ignorance

Inflamed/injured cell
Exposed self peptide
→ Anergy/apoptosis

Presented self peptide
Dendritic cell
B7
→ Activation of T cell and autoimmunity

Antigen-specific T cell regulation (e.g. by TGFβ and IL-10)
→ Anergy/apoptosis

CTLA-4
→ Apoptosis

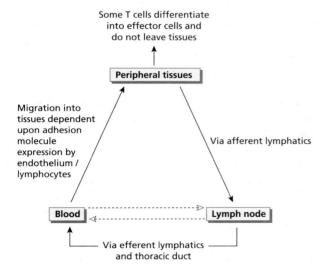

Fig. 5.3 Diagrammatic representation of the different recirculation pathways taken by naive T cells (dotted line) and T cells that have been previously exposed to antigen (solid line).

(Labels in figure:)

Some T cells differentiate into effector cells and do not leave tissues

Peripheral tissues

Migration into tissues dependent upon adhesion molecule expression by endothelium / lymphocytes

Via afferent lymphatics

Blood

Lymph node

Via efferent lymphatics and thoracic duct

opment of autoimmunity against intracellular molecules (Table 5.4).

Anergy and costimulation

More active mechanisms of peripheral tolerance also operate (see Fig. 5.2). These involve either deletion of self-reactive cells by apoptosis or induction of a state of unresponsiveness called **anergy**. Naive CD4+ T cells need two signals to become activated and initiate an immune response: an antigen-specific signal through the T-cell antigen receptor and a second, non-specific co-stimulatory signal, usually signalled by **CD28** (on the T cell) binding to one of the **B7 family (CD80 or CD86)** on the stimulator (see Chapter 1). If the T cell receives both signals, then it will become activated and proliferate and produce cytokines. If **no co-stimulatory molecules are engaged**, then stimulation through the T-cell receptor alone leads to longstanding unresponsiveness or death of the T cell by apoptosis. The expression of these co-stimulatory molecules is tightly controlled. Constitutive expression is confined to specialized antigen-presenting cells such as dendritic cells; given their distribution and patterns of recirculation, interaction between CD4 cells and dendritic cells is likely to happen only in secondary lymphoid tissues such as lymph nodes. The restricted expression of co-stimulatory molecules means that, even if a T cell recognizes a tissue-specific peptide/MHC molecule complex (e.g. an antigen derived from a pancreatic islet cell), then anergy rather than activation is likely to follow, as no antigen-presenting cell (and therefore co-stimulatory signal) will be available in healthy tissue. Expression of co-stimulatory molecules can be induced upon other cells by a variety of stimuli, usually in association with inflammation or cell damage. However, because of the restricted pattern of lymphocyte recirculation, only previously activated cells will gain access to these peripheral sites and these peripheral co-stimulatory molecules are more likely to sustain than initiate an autoimmune response.

The pattern of stimulation through the T-cell antigen receptor may also be important in determining whether a cell becomes activated or anergic: continuous low-level stimulation of a small number of T-cell antigen receptors (as might occur with a self-antigen) would tend to produce anergy, while strong and rapidly increasing stimulation (as would tend to happen in infection) would favour activation.

Activated T cells can also express cell-surface molecules similar in structure to co-stimulatory molecules, but which exert a negative effect upon T-cell activation, in particular **CTLA-4**, which has a similar structure to CD28 and binds to the same ligands. Binding of CD80 or CD86 to CTLA-4 induces anergy or death by apoptosis, in a negative counterpart to co-stimulation that may be important in terminating an immune response (see Fig. 1.1.6). The importance of apoptotic death of autoreactive lymphocytes in preventing autoimmune disease is emphasized by the development of autoimmunity in patients with genetic defects in the control of apoptosis (see Table 5.4).

Regulation and suppression

Other mechanisms for peripheral tolerance include active suppression of self-reactive T cells by inhibitory populations of T cells which recognize the same antigen: so-called **suppressor or regulatory T cells**. The existence of suppressor T cells has generated a great deal of debate over many years: antigen-specific suppression has always been relatively easy to demonstrate in animals, but it proved difficult to isolate a discrete population of cells with suppressor function. It is now clearer how some forms of T-cell suppression operate. Many regulatory T cells have a distinctive $CD4^+$ $CD25^+$ phenotype. The best-defined mechanism for suppression involves cytokines produced by antigen stimulation, which either inhibit or alter the activation of nearby T cells. For example, this can occur by a TH2 response specifically inhibiting a TH1 response with IL-10 or through T-cell production of the potent immunosuppressive cytokine transforming growth factor (TGF)-β (see Fig. 5.2). TGF-β-producing T cells are sometimes called TH3 cells.

5.4.4 B-cell tolerance

B-cell tolerance is less complete than T-cell tolerance since no equivalent of the thymus exists in B-cell development. B-cell tolerance operates at a peripheral rather than central level: the production of self-reactive antibodies is limited mainly by the lack of T-cell help for self-antigens. New B cells are being produced continuously from bone marrow precursors and many of these are autoreactive. The process of somatic hypermutation of immunoglobulin genes in mature B cells in the germinal centres of lymph nodes also has the potential for the generation of autoantibodies. If newly developed or recently hypermutated B cells bind the appropriate antigen in the absence of T-cell help, then the B cell will undergo apoptosis or anergy. Thus, there are some similarities between T- and B-cell activation and tolerance, in that two signals are required for activation and the presence of an antigen-specific signal alone leads to death or anergy. As with T cells, low-level chronic stimulation via the antigen receptor favours anergy and rapidly increasing stimulation favours activation.

5.5 How does tolerance break down?

Overcoming peripheral tolerance

A complete understanding of the breakdown of tolerance is currently not possible; many separate mechanisms may be involved. Overcoming T-cell peripheral tolerance seems likely to be the major hurdle and this may involve reversal of active mechanisms or overcoming protective processes. Situations in which transient breakdown of tolerance and autoimmunity can occur include infections and other non-specific tissue damage. Autoimmune disease is also easy to induce in experimental animals, usually by combining immunization with a self-protein together with a powerful non-specific immune stimulant (or **adjuvant**). Sustained production of autoantibodies occurs in some people without disease, particularly the close relatives of patients with autoimmune disease and with advancing age. Reversal of anergy can occur on exposure to certain cytokines, particularly IL-2. Development or worsening of autoimmune disease has been seen following IL-2 treatment for malignancy.

CASE 5.4 LYMPHOCYTE-DEPLETING MONOCLONAL ANTIBODY TREATMENT FOR MULTIPLE SCLEROSIS AND GRAVES' DISEASE

A 38-year-old woman with progressive MS underwent treatment with the monoclonal antibody Campath-1H (alemtuzumab) as part of a clinical trial. The treatment did not seem to slow the progress of her neurological disease, although she developed no new lesions on magnetic resonance imaging scanning of her brain over an 18-month period of follow-up. About 2 years after treatment with Campath-1H she developed a fine tremor, 5 kg weight loss and heat intolerance. Examination revealed a tachycardia and mild exopthalmos. The clinical impression of thyrotoxicosis was confirmed by thyroid-stimulating hormone (TSH) suppressed at < 0.03 mU/l (normal range 0.4–4 mU/ml) and free T4 elevated at 76 pmol/l (normal range 5–20). A radioisotope scan of the thyroid showed diffusely increased uptake and antibodies stimulatory to the TSH receptor were found in the patient's blood; a diagnosis of Graves' disease or autoimmune hyperthyroidism was made.

Campath-1H targets the CD52 antigen, which is expressed on both T and B cells. Treatment with Campath-1H produces prolonged suppression of peripheral blood lymphocyte numbers. Clinical trials suggest that this form of treatment may slow clinical and radiological progression of MS. However, around 25% of patients treated for MS with Campath-1H subsequently develop Graves' disease. The mechanisms underlying this unusual adverse reaction are unclear, but the most plausible explanation is that in genetically susceptible individuals, Campath-1H depletes an inhibitory or suppressor T-cell population which would otherwise prevent the development of antithyroid autoimmunity.

Reversal of suppression has been demonstrated in animal models as, in mice and rats, suppressor T cells seem to be unusually sensitive to cytotoxic drugs such as cyclophosphamide. Selective inhibition of T-cell suppression has been harder to demonstrate in humans, although occasionally paradoxical development of autoimmune disease can been seen in patients receiving immunosuppression. For example, some patients receiving the anti-T-cell monoclonal antibody, Campath-1H, for the treatment of MS subsequently develop autoimmune hyperthyroidism (Case 5.4). The potential importance of suppression in preventing autoimmunity is seen in animal models, where loss of immunosuppressive cytokines leads to widespread autoimmunity (see Table 5.4).

Overcoming peripheral tolerance might result from inappropriate access of self-antigens to antigen-presenting cells, inappropriate local expression of co-stimulatory molecules or by alterations in the ways in which self-molecules are presented to the immune system (Fig. 5.4). All of these are more likely to happen when inflammation or tissue damage is present, induced either by local infection or physical factors. Local inflammation increases traffic of self-antigens to regional lymph nodes (and hence to antigen-presenting cells) and also induces expression of MHC molecules and, under certain circumstances, co-stimulatory molecules. The increased activity of proteolytic enzymes in inflammatory sites can also cause both intra- and extracellular proteins to be broken down, leading to high concentrations of peptides

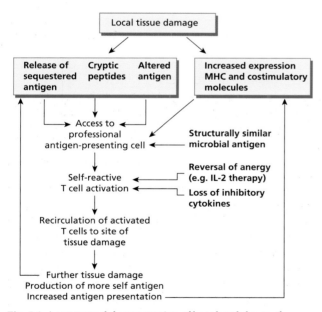

Fig. 5.4 A conceptual demonstration of how breakdown of tolerance leads to autoimmune disease and spreading of responses to epitopes.

(not present at significant levels in normal thymus) being presented to responsive T cells (see Fig. 5.1). These may include novel peptides known as **cryptic epitopes**. The structures of self-peptides may also be altered by viruses, free radicals or ionizing radiation, thus bypassing previously established tolerance. For antigens that are sequestered from the immune system, sufficient antigen may be released by tissue damage to initiate an immune response.

Molecular mimicry

Structural similarity between self-proteins and those from microorganisms may also trigger an autoimmune response. A self-peptide in low concentration and with no access to appropriate antigen-presenting cells may cross-react with a structurally similar microbial peptide. In systemic infection, this cross-reactivity will cause expansion of the responsive T-cell population, which may then recognize the self-peptide if local conditions (such as tissue damage) allow presentation of that peptide and access of the T cell to the tissue. This process is known as **molecular mimicry** (Case 5.5 and Table 5.5).

Once tolerance has broken down to a particular peptide, the resulting process of inflammation may allow presentation of further peptides. The immune response broadens and local tissue damage accelerates. This domino-like process is known as epitope spreading (see Fig. 5.4). This is best demonstrated in experimental models where immunization with a single peptide from a protein found in myelinated nerve sheaths (known as myelin basic protein or MBP) can lead to widespread inflammation in the CNS with an immune response against many peptides found in both MBP and other CNS proteins.

The requirements for co-stimulation for T-cell activation vary with the differentiation of the T cell: T cells not previously exposed to antigen (naive T cells) require co-stimulation via CD28 in order to take part in an immune response. However, previously activated T cells can be induced to proliferate and produce cytokines by a much wider variety of co-stimulatory signals, triggered through adhesion molecules expressed in increased amounts upon these cells. This means that previously activated autoreactive cells will not only recirculate more freely to inflamed tissues (because of their increased expression of adhesion molecules), but will also be much easier to activate once they arrive in the tissue containing the appropriate self-peptide/MHC complex. *This implies that once the barrier of tolerance is broken down, autoimmune responses may be relatively easy to sustain.*

It is therefore clear how a state of local inflammation, particularly in the presence of a pathogen that has some structural similarity to a self-antigen present at the site of inflammation, could potentially induce a **self-sustaining au-**

CASE 5.5 GUILLAIN–BARRÉ SYNDROME

A 23-year-old man developed flu-like symptoms, severe diarrhoea and abdominal pain 4 days after attending a dinner party at which he had eaten a chicken casserole. Three other people who had attended the same party developed gastrointestinal symptoms. These symptoms settled within a few days. Stool cultures taken from all four individuals grew Campylobacter jejuni. About 10 days after the onset of diarrhoea, he developed diffuse aching around his shoulders and buttocks and pins and needles in his hands and feet. Over the next week the sensory changes worsened and spread to involve his arms and legs. His limbs became progressively weaker and 8 days after the onset of neurological symptoms he could not hold a cup or stand unaided.

He was admitted to hospital and found to have severe symmetrical distal limb weakness and 'glove and stocking' sensory loss to the elbows and knees. Nerve conduction studies showed evidence of a mixed motor and sensory neuropathy and examination of his cerebrospinal fluid (CSF) showed a very high total protein level at 4 g/l but without any increase in the number of cells in the CSF. High titres of IgM and IgG antibodies to Campylobacter jejuni were found in his peripheral blood. A diagnosis was made of the Guillain–Barré syndrome (acute inflammatory polyneuropathy) probably triggered by Campylobacter jejuni infection.

He was treated with high-dose intravenous immunoglobulin but his condition deteriorated with respiratory muscle weakness and he required mechanical ventilation. His condition slowly improved and he was able to breathe spontaneously after 2 weeks. His strength and sensory symptoms slowly improved with vigorous physiotherapy, but 1 year after the initial illness he still had significant weakness in his hands and feet.

toreactive pathogenic process (see Fig. 5.4). What is equally clear, however, is that while transient autoimmune responses occur commonly after infection or other forms of tissue damage, the development of sustained immunity is relatively rare. Our knowledge of the factors curtailing autoimmune responses is poor, but is important for understanding both pathogenesis and treatment of autoimmune disease. It seems likely that minor genetic or acquired defects in the normal control mechanisms may combine to allow failure of the switching off process.

5.6 What triggers autoimmunity?

As with most complex chronic illnesses, interactions between genetic and environmental factors are critically important in the causation of autoimmune disease, although it is simpler to deal with these factors separately.

5.6.1 Genetic factors

The use of twin and family studies has confirmed a genetic contribution in all autoimmune diseases studied (Table 5.6). *Multiple autoimmune diseases may cluster within the same family* (see Case 5.3) and subclinical autoimmunity is more common among family members than overt disease. The genetic contribution to autoimmune disease almost always involves multiple genes. There are, however, a number of single gene defects in both humans and laboratory animals which can lead to autoimmunity (see Table 5.4). Rarely, endocrine autoimmunity affecting multiple organs is inherited in an autosomal dominant fashion. In some of these families this is caused by mutations in a gene on chromosome 21 known as **AIRE (AutoImmune REgulator)**. Affected subjects in families expressing an abnormal AIRE gene also have chronic mucocutaneous candidiasis and skin/tooth changes; this

Table 5.5 Molecular mimicry: microbial antigens and self-antigens potentially involved in this process

Microbial antigen	Self-antigen with similar structure	Disease in which consequent molecular mimicry may play a role*
Group A streptococcal M protein	Antigen found in cardiac muscle	Rheumatic fever
Bacterial heat shock proteins	Self-heat shock proteins	Links suggested with several autoimmune diseases but nil proven
Coxsackie B4 nuclear protein	Pancreatic islet cell glutamate decarboxylase	Insulin-dependent diabetes mellitus
Campylobacter jejuni glycoproteins	Myelin-associated gangliosides and glycolipids	Guillain–Barré syndrome

*In general, it has been much easier to demonstrate structural similarity between microbial and self-antigens than to prove that this similarity plays any role in disease pathogenesis.

Table 5.6 The genetic contribution to autoimmune disease — increased risk in the brothers and sisters of those with an autoimmune disease (adapted from Vyse TJ, Todd JA. Review: genetic analysis of autoimmune disease. Cell 1996; 85:311–8)

	Frequency of the disease in the population (prevalence) (%)	Frequency of the disease in individuals with an affected sibling (%)	Increase in risk with an affected sibling*	Frequency of the disease in individuals with an affected identical twin (%)	Increase in risk with an affected identical twin compared with a non-twin sibling†	Increase in risk with an affected identical twin compared with the general population
Rheumatoid arthritis	1	8	8×	30	3.5×	30×
Insulin-dependent diabetes mellitus	0.4	6	15×	34	5.7×	85.5×
Ankylosing spondylitis	0.13	7	54×	50	7.1×	383×
Multiple sclerosis	0.1	2	20×	26	13×	260×
Systemic lupus erythematosus	0.1	2	20×	24	12×	240×

*Increased risk in a sibling may reflect both genetic and environmental factors.

†The additional increase in risk in identical (monozygotic) twins gives an additional measure of the genetic component in these diseases. Even though the risks of disease are massively increased in identical twins, the diseases still affect only a minority of those with an affected twin, emphasizing that environmental factors have some role to play.

syndrome is known as **APECED** (Autoimmune Polyendocrinopathy Candidiasis Ectodermal Dysplasia — see Chapter 15.10). The AIRE gene is expressed in the thymus, where it is believed to control the transcription of genes for non-thymic self-proteins, and hence influence the central tolerance to these proteins. In addition to these autoimmune polyendocrine syndromes, there are a number of other single gene defects where some understanding exists of the mechanism of autoimmunity. Some of these single gene defects involve defects in apoptosis or the breakdown of self-anergy and are compatible with the mechanisms for peripheral tolerance and its breakdown discussed above (see Table 5.4). These disorders give useful insights into ways in which multiple minor genetic differences (each in themselves incapable of producing autoimmunity) and environmental factors could interact to allow autoimmune disease to develop.

Many of the strongest and best characterized associations between genes and autoimmunity involve different variants or alleles of the MHC, as might be expected from the central role of the products of many of these genes in T-cell function, and the involvement of other MHC genes in control of immunity and inflammation (e.g. the genes encoding the tumour necrosis factors). The biology of the MHC is discussed in Chapter 1. The understanding of the relationship between MHC variants and autoimmunity has progressed from rather crude association studies to more precise relationships being identified between disease and particular molecular motifs within certain MHC alleles (Table 5.7). Associations between HLA and disease were initially described in terms of one or another HLA allele. Further genetic studies and increased understanding of the molecular genetics of the MHC/HLA system have led to a more precise relationship being defined between HLA type and disease. For some diseases the association can be pinpointed to the possession of one or more amino acids at a particular location in the HLA molecule. Alleles without these particular amino acids at

Table 5.7 Possible mechanistic associations between some common autoimmune diseases and certain HLA alleles

Disease	HLA association	Molecular specificity	Relationship to pathogenesis
Rheumatoid arthritis	DR4 + DR1	Sequence of five amino acids lying in the peptide-binding groove of HLA-DR	Unclear ?Influences binding of antigenic peptide to MHC
Insulin-dependent diabetes mellitus	DR3 + DR4	Single amino acid at position 57 in the β chain of HLA-DQ	As above
Organ-specific autoimmune disease: Type 1 diabetes, Addison's disease, pernicious anaemia	DR1*03 (in association with A1 B8 DR3 DQ2 haplotype)	Unknown but this haplotype is associated with promotor polymorphism in TNF-α gene	Unclear but this haplotype is associated with high levels of TNF and vigorous antibody responses

this site are not associated with disease. Despite this description of the association at the molecular level, the relationship to disease pathogenesis remains unclear in most cases. Some of the most significant insights have been gained from analysis of strains of laboratory animals that spontaneously develop autoimmunity, e.g. the non-obese diabetic (NOD) mouse. A hierarchy of genes is involved in the development of autoimmunity: MHC genes are the most important but 12–14 other genes also participate, their functions ranging from control of the immune response to factors affecting the functioning of the relevant target organ (in this case the islets of Langerhans).

5.6.2 Environmental factors

Environmental factors identified as possible triggers in autoimmunity include hormones, infection, therapeutic drugs and miscellaneous other agents such as ultraviolet radiation.

Hormones

One of the most striking epidemiological observations regarding autoimmune diseases is that **females are far more likely to be affected than males**. While this is obviously a genetic factor, hormonal factors appear to play a major role in the increased prevalence in females, and since these can be externally manipulated, they are perhaps best considered with other environmental factors. Most autoimmune diseases have their peak age of onset within the reproductive years and much experimental and some clinical evidence exists to implicate oestrogens as triggering factors. Removal of the ovaries inhibits the onset of spontaneous autoimmunity in animal models [particularly models of systemic lupus erythematosus (SLE)] and administration of oestrogen accelerates the onset of disease. The mechanism underlying this relationship is unclear, but evidence suggests that oestrogens can stimulate certain types of immune response. The pituitary hormone prolactin also has immunostimulatory actions, particularly on T cells. Prolactin levels surge immediately after pregnancy and this may be linked with the tendency of some autoimmune diseases, particularly rheumatoid arthritis, to present at this time.

Infection

The relationship between infection and autoimmunity is clearest in the situation of molecular mimicry discussed above (see Table 5.5), but other possible links exist. Infection of a target organ may play a key role in local **up-regulation of co-stimulatory molecules** and also in inducing altered patterns of antigen breakdown and presentation, thus leading to autoimmunity without molecular mimicry. Attempts have been made repeatedly in some 'autoimmune' diseases,

particularly rheumatoid arthritis and MS, to look for hidden infection, but so far without success.

Infection may also exert a completely different influence upon autoimmune disease. As noted in section 5.3, autoimmune diseases tend to be less common in parts of the world that carry a high burden of parasitic diseases and other infections. Intriguingly, in some animal models of autoimmunity (e.g. the NOD mouse) the development of disease can be dramatically inhibited by keeping the animals in a laboratory environment with a high prevalence of infection. Keeping the same animals in germ-free conditions promotes the development of autoimmunity. The mechanisms behind non-specific protection from autoimmunity by infection (and possibly other environmental factors) are unclear.

Drugs

Many drugs are associated with the development of idiosyncratic side-effects which may have an autoimmune component in their pathogenesis. Drugs may induce a variety of pathological immune responses and it is important to distinguish between an immunological response to the drug, either in its native form or complexed with a host molecule, and a true autoimmune process induced by the drug. The former mechanism of **drug hypersensitivity** is usually reversible on drug withdrawal, whereas the second process may progress independently of drug treatment and require some form of immunosuppressive treatment (Table 5.8). This distinction is comparable to that between autoimmune syndromes triggered by infection and those syndromes with autoimmune features caused by persistent infection. The boundaries between drug hypersensitivity and autoimmunity may be blurred, in that some syndromes may respond eventually to drug withdrawal but still continue for a variable period in the apparent absence of the drug (Case 5.6).

The mechanisms underlying drug-induced autoimmunity are poorly understood but may involve mechanisms comparable to molecular mimicry, whereby the drug or a drug–self-molecule complex have a structural similarity to self and hence allow bypass of peripheral tolerance. Some drugs (e.g. penicillamine) have the ability to bind directly to the peptide-containing groove in MHC molecules, and hence have a very direct capacity to induce abnormal T-cell responses. *Drug-mediated autoimmunity (and drug hypersensitivity in general) affects only a small proportion of those treated.* This differential susceptibility is probably largely genetically determined. Genetic variation within the MHC would potentially influence recognition of drug–self-complexes by T cells, or may directly influence drug binding to the MHC. For example, HLA-DR2 is associated with penicillamine-induced myasthenia gravis, whereas DR3 is associated with nephritis. Genetic variation in drug metabolism is also important, the best characterized example being the relationship between drug-induced SLE and the rate of acetylation

Table 5.8 Syndromes of probable autoimmune aetiology triggered by therapeutic drugs. NB: many of these drugs such as D-Penicillamine and Hydralazine are now only rarely used therapeutically, in part due to the risk of this type of reaction

Syndrome	Drug
Chronic active hepatitis	Halothane (*general anaesthetic*)
Haemolytic anaemia	Methyl-dopa (*antihypertensive*)
Antiglomerular basement membrane	D-penicillamine (*rheumatoid arthritis*)
Myasthenia gravis	D-penicillamine
Pemphigus	D-penicillamine
Systemic lupus erythematosus	Hydralazine (*antihypertensive*)
	Procainamide (*antiarrhythmic*)
	D-penicillamine
	Minocycline (*antibiotic given for acne*)
Glomerulonephritis	D-penicillamine
Scleroderma-like syndrome	Tryptophan (*antidepressant*)

of the triggering drug: slow acetylators are prone to SLE. It seems likely that this partial defect in metabolism may allow the formation of immunogenic conjugates between drug and self-molecules.

Drugs may also have intrinsic adjuvant or immunomodulatory effects which disturb normal tolerance mechanisms, for example, thyroid autoimmunity can be seen following interferon-α treatment.

Other physical agents

Exposure to ultraviolet radiation (usually in the form of sunlight) is a well-defined trigger for skin inflammation and sometimes systemic involvement in SLE. It is most likely that this acts merely to cause flares in a pre-existing autoimmune response, rather than being a true aetiological factor. Ultraviolet radiation could cause worsening of SLE by a number of mechanisms. Ultraviolet radiation can cause free-radical-mediated structural modification to self-antigens, thus enhancing their immunogenicity. More subtly, it can also lead to apoptotic death of cells within the skin. This process is associated with cell-surface expression of lupus autoantigens which are associated with photosensitivity (known as Ro and La) usually only found within cells. Surface Ro and La are then able to bind appropriate autoantibodies and trigger tissue damage.

Other forms of physical damage may alter the immunogenicity of self-antigens, particularly damage to self-molecules by oxygen free radicals produced as part of the inflammatory process.

A variety of other triggers have been suggested to trigger autoimmune disease, including psychological stress and dietary factors. The importance of these factors is unclear.

5.7 Mechanisms of tissue damage

Tissue damage in autoimmune disease is mediated by antibody (types II and III hypersensitivity) or by CD4+ T-cell activation of macrophages or cytotoxic T cells (type IV hypersensitivity) (Tables 5.3 and 5.9). Although many autoim-

CASE 5.6 MINOCYCLINE-INDUCED SYSTEMIC LUPUS ERYTHEMATOSUS

A previously healthy 23-year-old woman was referred to a rheumatology clinic with a 4-month history of pain and swelling in the small joints of her hands associated with a blotchy rash over the bridge of her nose and over her knuckles. Examination revealed mild symmetrical synovitis in the hands and red scaly patches over her knuckles and face consistent with a photosensitive rash. Her blood pressure was normal and dipstick testing of her urine showed no blood or protein. Investigations showed a normal full blood count, urea and creatinine. Her erythrocyte sedimentation rate was significantly elevated at 43 mm/h. Antinuclear antibodies were present at a titre of 1/1000 with a homogeneous pattern. Antibodies to double-stranded DNA and extractable nuclear antigens were absent. A diagnosis of mild SLE was made and she was treated with non-steroidal anti-inflammatory drugs and hydroxychloroquine. She was also given advice on protection from ultraviolet light.

Her symptoms failed to improve over the next 6 months and treatment with low-dose corticosteroids was considered. However, she refused to consider steroid treatment as she had read about side-effects and was concerned that this drug would cause her previously troublesome acne to return. At this point it transpired that she had been receiving treatment with daily low doses of the antibiotic minocycline for the last 4 years because of previously severe acne. She had not mentioned this previously as she had been taking this form of treatment for so long that she did not feel it could be relevant to her more recent problems. The minocycline was discontinued and the clinical and laboratory features of SLE disappeared over the next 6 months, confirming the revised diagnosis of minocycline-induced SLE. Her acne remained in remission with no treatment.

Table 5.9 Mechanisms of hypersensitivity which predominate in autoimmune diseases*

Type II hypersensitivity†
Type IIA
  Idiopathic thrombocytopenic purpura
  Autoimmune haemolytic anaemia
  Myasthenia gravis
  Antiglomerular basement membrane disease
Type IIB
  Graves' disease
  Insulin receptor antibody syndrome
  Myasthenia gravis

Type III hypersensitivity
Systemic lupus erythematosus
Mixed cryoglobulinaemia
Some forms of vasculitis (e.g. rheumatoid vasculitis)

Type IV hypersensitivity
Insulin-dependent diabetes mellitus
Hashimoto's thyroiditis
Rheumatoid arthritis
Multiple sclerosis

*Different aspects of the same disease (e.g. rheumatoid disease) can have different pathogenic mechanisms.
†Type II sensitivity has been subdivided as to whether antibody induces cell damage (IIa) or receptor stimulation or blockade (IIb). In some diseases both mechanisms occur.

The importance of this phenomenon to autoimmune disease is unclear.

Many of the serious and irreversible consequences of autoimmune disease are caused by deposition of extracellular matrix proteins in the affected organ. This process of fibrosis leads to impairment of function in, for example, the lungs (pulmonary fibrosis), liver (cirrhosis), skin (systemic sclerosis) and kidney (interstitial and glomerular fibrosis). No effective treatments exist for the treatment of established fibrosis. Historically, an assumption has been made that fibrotic changes are a consequence of previous chronic inflammation and that treatment with anti-inflammatory and immunosuppressive drugs has the potential to ameliorate the fibrotic process. However, there is now evidence that some forms of tissue injury can lead to fibrosis without any significant intervening inflammation. This would explain the lack of response to conventional immunosuppression in systemic sclerosis and idiopathic pulmonary fibrosis. Fibrosis may be mediated by fibrocytes, circulating cells of haematopoietic origin, which migrate into sites of tissue injury, proliferate and produce extracellular matrix proteins. Future strategies for limiting tissue damage due to fibrosis are likely to focus on manipulating fibrocyte function, perhaps using inhibitors of fibrogenic cytokines (such as antibodies to TGF-β) or interfering with the chemokine gradients that attract fibrocytes into sites of tissue damage.

5.8 Treatment of autoimmune disease

The treatment of autoimmunity is currently unsatisfactory. The two principal strategies are either to suppress the immune response or to replace the function of the damaged organ (Fig. 5.5).

Replacement of function is the usual mode of treatment in endocrinological autoimmune diseases, which usually present with irreversible failure of the affected organ. Replacement of function is a satisfactory treatment for some forms of endocrine failure, such as hypothyroidism, in which the physiological output of the missing hormone is fairly constant. However, when the requirements for the deficient hormone vary considerably over time, the failure of replacement therapy to match physiological changes in hormone output can lead to major metabolic problems, such as the long-term treatment of insulin-dependent diabetes mellitus. Suppression of the autoimmune response before tissue damage is irreversible is a more attractive option, but the detection of preclinical endocrine autoimmunity presents a major challenge.

In many autoimmune diseases, such as SLE, rheumatoid arthritis and autoimmune kidney disease, immunosuppression may be the only means of preventing severe disability or death. As discussed in Chapter 7, however, all currently

mune diseases involve a predominance of one or another form of hypersensitivity, there is often considerable overlap between antibody and T-cell-mediated damage. Immune-complex disease (type III hypersensitivity) is discussed further in Chapter 1.

In addition to organ damage mediated by the usual mechanisms of hypersensitivity, autoantibodies can also cause disease by binding to the functional sites of self-antigens such as hormone receptors, neurotransmitter receptors and plasma proteins. These autoantibodies either mimic or block the action of the endogenous ligand for the self-protein, and thus cause *abnormalities in function without necessarily causing inflammation or tissue damage*. This phenomenon is best characterized in endocrine autoimmunity, where autoantibodies can mimic or block the action of hormones such as thyroid-stimulating hormone and hence induce over- or underactivity of the thyroid (see Table 5.9).

Antibody-mediated damage in autoimmunity is usually considered to occur only when the autoantibody recognizes an antigen that is either free in the extracellular fluid or expressed upon the cell surface. However, there is some in vitro evidence that some autoantibodies against intracellular antigens can enter living cells and perturb their function.

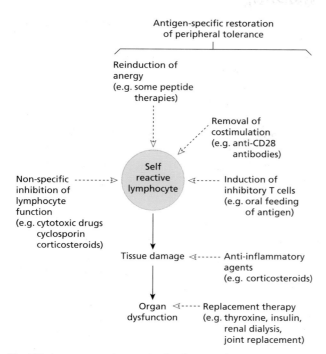

Fig. 5.5 A summary of strategies for therapy of autoimmune disease. Antigenic-specific modulation of tolerance remains experimental.

used modes of immunosuppression are limited by their lack of specificity and other toxic side-effects.

Numerous potential strategies have been developed for selective suppression of the autoimmune response, many of which have shown clear benefit in animal models. Many of these approaches to treatment are now being evaluated in clinical trials. These strategies are discussed further in Chapter 7.

FURTHER READING

See website: www.immunologyclinic.com

6 Lymphoproliferative Disorders

6.1 Introduction

The cells involved in immune responses (Fig. 1.1) may undergo malignant proliferation, giving rise to leukaemias, lymphomas or myeloma. In contrast, 'benign' (or 'reactive') proliferation is a normal response to infection or inflammation.

Leukaemia is defined as a malignant proliferation of those bone marrow cells whose mature forms are normally found in blood or bone marrow. The **circulating malignant cells** often infiltrate other organs and may present as lymphadenopathy, bone marrow infiltration or meningeal lesions. Complications therefore include bone marrow failure, bleeding, infection and meningeal irritation.

Tumours of **non-recirculating lymphoid cells** constitute the lymphomas. Overspill of malignant cells from a lymphoid organ results in a 'leukaemic' state and may be confused with a leukaemia of circulating cell origin. Metastases of these malignant cells may cause organ failure in liver, brain, bone marrow or lungs. Since there is considerable physiological recirculation of B and T lymphocytes (see Fig. 1.31) through solid lymphoid organs, the distinction between leukaemia and lymphoma is not always clear-cut.

Classifications of leukaemias, lymphomas and plasma cell dyscrasias are based on the normal physiological pathways. It is important to distinguish different types of lymphoid malignancies in order (i) to provide a reliable diagnosis and prognosis for a given patient, and hence (ii) to choose the most effective form of therapy.

Each leukaemia or lymphoma is thought to arise from a single cell, which undergoes **malignant transformation** to uncontrolled division. These malignancies are therefore monoclonal and all the malignant cells express the same cellular antigens, i.e. phenotype, and have the same activated genes, i.e. genotype. The immunological techniques that can be used to identify the phenotype of the malignant cell, and thus to distinguish and classify these lymphoid malignancies, are shown in Table 6.1. These techniques are discussed fully in Chapter 19.

6.2 Biology of malignant transformation

The precise stimulus for malignant transformation is still not clear and is beyond the scope of this book. Examples of general principles that are applicable to leucocytes are given here as an introduction, but readers are referred to the Further reading section for more details. The majority of tumours in man arise spontaneously; though a small group of tumours may be inherited, most cancers involve **gene mutations** that accumulate in cells of susceptible individuals (Fig. 6.1). Such mutations arise in genes responsible for cell proliferation, apoptosis or DNA repair. Viruses known to be involved in causing lymphoid tumours include the Epstein–Barr virus (EBV) in Burkitt's lymphoma and the retrovirus human T-cell leukaemia virus I (HTLV-I) in adult T-cell leukaemia/lymphoma. In neither case does infection cause the tumour directly, since only 1% or less of infected individuals in endemic areas develop the malignancy. **Cofactors**

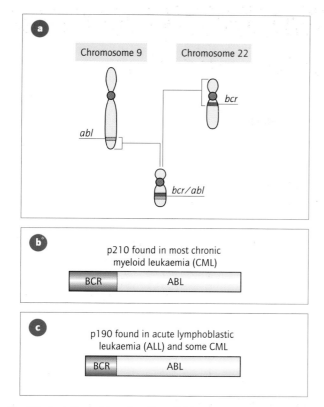

Fig. 6.1 A malignant translocation: Abl is an oncogene on chromosome 9. Bcr is a similar oncogene on chromosome 22. When these two are joined by translocation between the two chromosomes, activation of the fused gene produces a new tyrosine kinase, which enables uncontrolled proliferation of the cells. This translocation is visualized as the Philadelphia chromosome in almost all patients with chronic myeloid leukaemia and some with acute lymphoblastic leukaemia. Reproduced from *Medicine*, 2nd edn, eds Axford and O'Callaghan, with permission.

are needed, which may include other genetic abnormalities, such as DNA repair gene defects as in ataxia telangiectasia, or environmental factors, such as radiation.

Cellular proto-oncogenes (see Box 6.1) are **potential malignancy genes** within the DNA of cells and are involved with cell division and differentiation (by production of growth factors). When activated to oncogenes, they become deregulated by mutation and result in malignancy. An example of a translocation resulting in a new cell proliferation enzyme is given in Fig. 6.1. **Tumour suppressor genes** are responsible for restriction of cell proliferation and induction of DNA repair and apoptosis if such repair is not successful. In this way, they control B-cell proliferation in lymph node follicles. For example, the Bcl-6 protein is necessary for the survival of B cells in the lymph node follicles, where many B cells normally undergo cell degeneration by apoptosis

Table 6.1 Techniques used to identify lymphoid malignancies*

1 Morphology — how the cell and its nucleus look by light (and electron) microscopy
2 Special cytochemical stains — to identify characteristic enzymes, carbohydrates or lipids
3 Immunophenotyping—use of monoclonal antibodies (MAbs) to identify myeloid/lymphocytic origin by surface and intracellular antigens using flow cytometry
4 Precise identification of type of leukaemia by determining particular stage of differentiation by flow cytometry
5 Cytogenetic analysis — to identify characteristic abnormal translocations and deletions on chromosomes by visualization and banding
6 Gene rearrangement studies — to identify or confirm monoclonality, especially in T-cell tumours

*Not all these techniques are needed for every diagnosis of lymphoid malignancy.

BOX 6.1 INTEGRATION OF DNA CAN RESULT IN MALIGNANCY IF:

- Activation of a positive regulator gene, if the DNA is inserted next to a promoter gene, e.g. 'insertional mutagenesis'
- Inactivation of a negative gene if the DNA is inserted next to an apoptosis or apoptosis promoter gene, e.g. 'insertional mutagenesis of apoptosis'
- Activation of a growth factor production gene if the DNA is inserted next to a growth factor gene, resulting in unregulated cell division
- Inactivation of a DNA repair gene if the DNA is inserted next to a DNA repair gene or promoter gene
- Inactivation of a differentiation gene if the DNA is inserted next to a differentiation gene or promoter gene
- Recombination between host cell genes and viral DNA can result in host genes becoming replicating and therefore oncogenic
- Silent 'proto-oncogenes' (c-onc genes),
  - incorporated into mammalian cells eons ago,
  - are inherited in a Mendelian fashion,
  - and normally used for growth factor receptors or signal transducers
  - these can be activated by mutagenesis
- Loss of function if tumour suppression gene inactivated

to control an immune response. Bcl-6 protein is normally present in secondary follicles in a stimulated lymph node. In contrast, activation of the Bcl-2 oncogene by chromosomal

CASE 6.1 ACUTE LEUKAEMIA (COMMON TYPE)

A 7-year-old boy presented with malaise and lethargy of 6 months' duration. He had become inattentive at school, anorexic and had lost 3 kg in weight. On examination he was thin, anxious and clinically anaemic. There was mild, bilateral, cervical lymphadenopathy and moderate splenomegaly.

On investigation, his haemoglobin (80 g/l) and platelet count (66 × 10^9/l) were low, but the white-cell count was high (25 × 10^9/l). The blood film showed that most leucocytes were blasts; the red cells were normochromic and normocytic. Bone marrow examination showed an overgrowth of primitive white cells with diminished numbers of normal erythroid and myeloid precursors. Acute leukaemia was diagnosed.

The circulating blast cells were typed by immunological methods: they did not react with monoclonal antibodies to human T-cell precursor antigens (CD2, CD7), but they were positive for major histocompatibility complex class II (DR), common acute lymphoblastic leukaemia (CD10) and B-cell precursor (CD19) antigens, and contained the enzyme terminal deoxynucleotidyl transferase (Tdt) (Table 6.2). The phenotype of the blasts was that of acute leukaemia of early precursor B cells (see Fig. 6.2), and the prognosis in this child is relatively good.

Table 6.2 Immunophenotyping in Case 6.1

Lymphocyte marker

Tdt	CD19	CD10	CIg	SIg	CD3	CD2	Diagnosis
+	+	–	–	–	–	–	Null ALL
+	+	+	–	–	–	–	Early pre-B-cell (Common)
+	+	+	+	–	–	–	Pre-B ALL
–	+	–	±	+	–	–	B-ALL
+	–	–	–	–	+	–	Pre-T ALL
+	–	–	–	–	+	+	T-ALL
+	+	+	–	–	–	–	Case 6.1

CD antigens are defined by monoclonal antibodies (see Chapters 1 and 19). ALL, Acute lymphoblastic leukaemia; CIg, cytoplasmic immunoglobulin; SIg, surface immunoglobulin; Tdt, terminal deoxynucleotidyl transferase.

translocation results in exaggerated survival and division of B cells to form a follicular lymphoma. The Bcl-2 gene has been implicated in about 80% of follicular lymphomas but is unlikely to be the only factor, or even the only oncogene, involved in the pathogenesis.

6.3 Leukaemia

6.3.1 Acute leukaemia

Acute leukaemias may be of lymphoid, myeloid, monocytic or myelomonocytic origin (Fig. 6.2) and the cells may retain some of their original characteristics; however, many are sufficiently undifferentiated that they bear little resemblance to the cells of origin. Leukaemias of non-lymphoid origin are not discussed in this chapter but are added to Figure 6.2 for clarification.

Acute lymphoblastic leukaemia (ALL) is largely a disease of children and young people; it is less common over the age of 20 years (Fig. 6.3). Patients with ALL often **present** with anaemia, bleeding or infection. Many (70%) have palpable lymphadenopathy and a small proportion (10%) have a mediastinal mass apparent on chest X-ray. Over 80% of patients are thrombocytopenic and in some this is severe and results in petechiae. Many (60%) have a low haemoglobin

below 80 g/l. The blood white cell count varies enormously at presentation but exceeds 25 × 10^9/l in only about a third. However, most of these cells are malignant blasts and so easy to see on a blood film; there is considerable suppression of mature leucocytes, sometimes resulting in bacterial infections. The **diagnosis** is confirmed by performing a bone marrow examination and finding that > 25% of cells are lymphoblasts as in Case 6.1.

ALL is a fatal condition if untreated, but aggressive chemotherapy and radiotherapy eliminate the clone of malignant cells and prevent the **complications** of the disease (see Box 6.2). These include anaemia and thrombocytopenia, resulting in bleeding due to marrow infiltration. Concentrated red cells are given to correct anaemia and platelet concentrates to prevent and treat bleeding. Infection is a common complication of ALL and preventive measures, such as prophylactic antifungal and antiviral agents, are important. It may be difficult to distinguish if symptoms are due to an infection or leukaemic infiltration, an important distinction as their **management** is radically different.

The **immunophenotype** of the malignant cell indicates the stage of development at which the malignancy occurred. The markers commonly used to determine the developmental origin of cells in ALL (Fig. 6.4) include the myelomonocytic markers, CD13 and CD117, CD3 and CD7 to determine

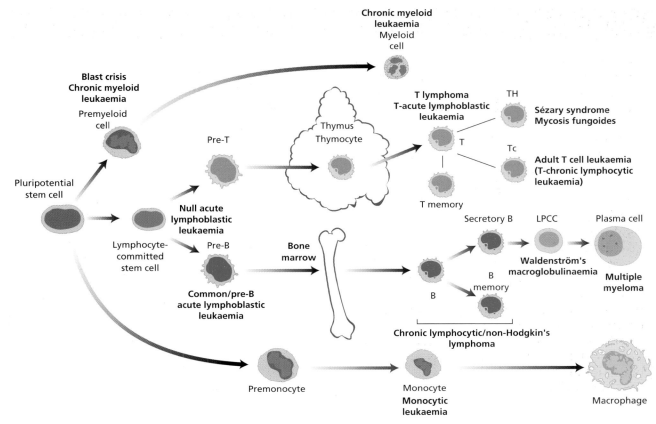

Fig. 6.2 Malignant counterparts at each step in the leucocyte differentiation pathway. LPCC, Lymphoplasma cytoid cell; T, T cell; TH, T helper cell; T_C, T cytotoxic cell; B, B cell.

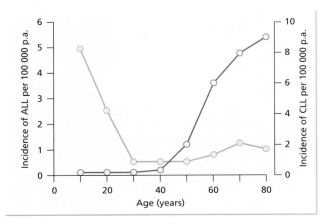

Fig. 6.3 Decade of onset in acute lymphoblastic leukaemia (ALL) (○) and chronic lymphocytic leukaemia (CLL) (○).

BOX 6.2 OBJECTIVES OF TREATMENT IN ALL

1 To induce remission of the disease

2 To eradicate all leukaemic cells and their precursors

3 To replace the bone marrow with autologous stem cells purged of any potentially malignant cells

4 To prevent infiltration of the meninges and other tissues

T lymphoid origin and CD10 and CD79a to detect B-cell stages (see Tables 6.2 and 6.3). Although 80–90% of acute leukaemias can be correctly classified by a combination of morphology and special cytochemical stains, this differentiation can be improved to 98% by immunophenotyping. Precise classification is most important as the management, in terms of drugs used and the use of prophylactic cerebral irradiation, as well as the prognosis of ALL, differs from the non-lymphoid acute leukaemias. Cytogenetic and gene re-arrangement studies are not helpful at present.

Various factors have been used as **prognostic** criteria in ALL, particularly the concentration of circulating blast cells and age at diagnosis. Children under 2 years old or over 15

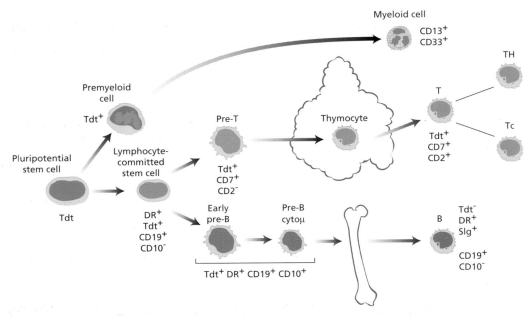

Fig. 6.4 Markers of various forms of acute lymphoblastic leukaemia (ALL). See Fig. 6.2 for abbreviations.

Table 6.3 Panel of antibodies for the diagnosis of acute leukaemias

	B lymphoid	T lymphoid	Myeloid	Non-lineage-restricted
First line	CD19, CD10 (early B cells), CD79a (BCR), CD22	CD3, CD2	CD117 (stem cell growth factor receptor), CD13 Anti-myeloperoxidase	Tdt
Second line	Surface Ig κ:λ Cytoplasmic Ig CD138	CD7	CD33, CD41, CD42, CD61	CD45

From Bain *et al.* 2002.

years and those with a high blast cell count at presentation (> 50×10^9/l) do less well. Patients with mature B cell ALL also have a poor outlook. **High-dose chemotherapy** is used to induce remission followed by **bone marrow transplantation**. Graft-versus-host disease (GvHD) is another common complication after bone marrow transplantation, though some GvHD is helpful for the anti-leukaemic effect. Around 80% of patients are now cured. Controlled clinical trials continue to improve therapeutic regimens. An example is Imatinib; this drug inhibits the constitutively active fusion product arising from the Philadelphia (Ph) chromosome of chronic myelogenous leukemia (CML) and c-kit (CD117).

There are **complications** associated with therapy, both with induction chemotherapy and bone marrow transplantation (Table 6.4). The incidence of profound neutropenia (as a result of intensive therapy) is reduced by the use of granulocyte colony-stimulating factor (G-CSF) and that of late bacterial infections by prophylactic antibiotics and immunization. An additional risk of irradiation-induced damage to the lungs, combined with T-cell defects due to immunosuppression, may result in viral pneumonia (see Chapter 8). **Long-term complications of survivors** have now become significant and prevention of these is paramount; for example, by giving cardiotoxic chemotherapy slowly rather than as a bolus to protect non-reparable cardiac tissue.

Table 6.4 Complications of acute lymphoblastic leukaemia (ALL) associated with disease or induction chemotherapy and bone marrow transplantation

Due to disease	Due to treatment
Early	
Anaemia—bone marrow suppression or hypersplenism	
Infection—neutropenia due to bone marrow suppression	Infection—poor neutrophil function as a result of chemotherapy —neutropenia as result of chemotherapy
Bleeding—low platelets	Low platelets as result of chemotherapy
	Graft-versus-host disease following bone marrow transplantation
Late	
Leukaemic infiltrates, e.g. meninges testis	TBI—lung fibrosis, cataracts, precocious puberty, thyroid tumours
	Poor growth
	Intellectual impairment—cranial irradiation
	Cardiac dysfunction

TBI, Total body irradiation.

CASE 6.2 CHRONIC LYMPHOCYTIC LEUKAEMIA

A 62-year-old man presented with increasing shortness of breath on exercise and loss of weight. He had suffered five chest infections during the previous winter, despite being a non-smoker. On examination, there was moderate, bilateral cervical lymphadenopathy and left inguinal lymph node enlargement. The spleen and liver were enlarged 5 cm below the costal margins. There was no bone tenderness and there were no lesions in the skin. On investigation, his haemoglobin (132 g/l) and platelet count (251×10^9/l) were normal but his white cell count was increased to 150×10^9/l; the film showed that 98% of these were small lymphocytes.

The features on the blood film were suggestive of chronic lymphocytic leukaemia and immunophenotyping confirmed this diagnosis (Table 6.5). Ninety percent of the cells were B cells (CD 19[+]); they all expressed surface immunoglobulin (μ, δ and κ chains), major histocompatibility complex class II antigens (DR) and CD5. The serum immunoglobulins were low: IgG 2.2 g/l (NR 7.2–19.0 g/l); IgA 0.6 g/l (NR 0.8–5.0 g/l) and IgM 0.4 g/l (NR 0.5–2.0 g/l). There was no monoclonal immunoglobulin in the serum or the urine.

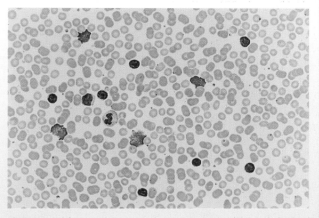

Fig. 6.5 CLL blood film. Reproduced from *Medicine*, 2nd edn, eds Axford and O'Callaghan, with permission.

Table 6.5 Immunophenotyping in Case 6.2

| | Lymphocyte markers* | | | | | | | | | |
| | Surface membrane immunoglobulin (SIg) | | | | | | | | | |
Case	κ	λ	μ	γ	α	CD3	CD19	CD5	CD11c	Diagnosis
Normal/reactive lymphocytosis	7	4	6	3	2	75	12	2	0	Normal/reactive lymphocytosis
Case 6.2	90	0	90	0	0	10	90	90	0	Chronic lymphocytic leukaemia
Differential diagnosis	1	1	2	0	0	92	2	0	0	Sézary syndrome
	60	2	60	1	0	10	60	0	60	Hairy cell leukaemia

*Results expressed as percentage of peripheral blood lymphocytes positive for marker.

6.3.2 Chronic lymphocytic leukaemia

Chronic lymphocytic leukaemia (CLL) is a relatively common disease of elderly patients (20 per 10^5 prevalence in those > 60 years old). It is uncommon in people under 50 years of age (see Fig. 6.3), and usually runs a relatively benign course, although speed of progression varies enormously. Excessive numbers of small lymphocytes are found in the peripheral blood (Fig. 6.5); in over 90% of cases of CLL, the neoplastic cells are B-cells (Fig. 6.6). They have the **characteristic cell surface markers** of immature, circulating B cells (Tables 6.5 and 6.6). The cells represent a malignant proliferation of a *single clone of B cell* and are therefore 'monoclonal'. The lymphocytes are *not* sufficiently mature to secrete monoclonal immunoglobulin (detectable as a band on serum electrophoresis), *nor* is there sufficient intracellular immunoglobulin to be detectable by immunofluorescence.

Estimation of the number of cells with surface κ or λ light chains is helpful in **distinguishing a reactive** from a malignant lymphocytosis (see Table 6.5). In a reactive state, such as a viral infection, the lymphocytes are derived from many different clones (i.e. polyclonal) and the ratio of cells with κ or λ light chains on their surfaces is therefore normal, i.e. 3 : 2. In a monoclonal B-cell proliferation, this ratio is changed in favour of the malignant clone, so *all the cells express the same light-chain type.*

Although most of the elderly patients with CLL usually have a relatively benign illness and survive for over 8–10 years, the **prognosis is variable**. Treatment is not always necessary. The aim of **treatment** is to control symptoms. Those due to hypersplenism (such as anaemia, thrombocytopenia and neutropenia) may be improved by steroids, splenic irradiation or mild cytotoxic therapy such as chlorambucil. Some untreated CLL patients have severe recurrent bacterial infections; such patients often have low serum immunoglobulin levels and reduced production of protective antibodies (as in Case 6.2). Immunoglobulin replacement therapy should be considered as this will prevent serious bacterial infections. Treatment of CLL with cytotoxic or immunosuppressive drugs also makes patients more susceptible to infections, particularly by viruses such as herpes zoster and herpes simplex, as well as bacteria. Late complications (such as haemolytic anaemia or thrombocytopenia) or progressive disease may need more aggressive chemotherapy such as Fludarabine (an adenosine deaminase inhibitor) or Rituximab (a therapeutic monoclonal antibody to the B cell marker, CD20).

6.3.3 Differential diagnosis of chronic lymphoid leukaemias

Sézary syndrome is part of a spectrum of T-cell malignancies that often involve the skin. The skin is infiltrated with the large, cleaved, mononuclear cells diagnostic of the condition. Immunological markers on peripheral blood have shown these cells to be T helper cell (CD4+) in origin (see Tables 6.5 and 6.6). Many patients die within 8 years from a frank lymphoma after a period of remission.

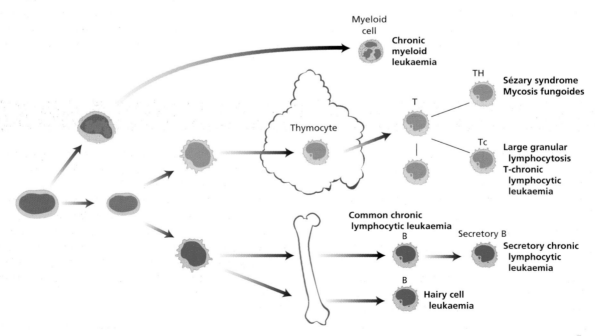

Fig. 6.6 Origins of various forms of chronic leukaemia. See Fig. 6.1 for abbreviations.

Table 6.6 Panel of markers for the diagnosis of chronic leukaemias/lymphoid malignancies of mature cells

	B cell	T cell	B and T cell
First line	CD19, CD33, CD23, CD79b (BCR-β chain) FMC7, surface Ig κ;λ	CD2	CD5
Second line to determine particular disorders			

Hairy cell leukaemia	Early B-cell disorders	Sézary syndrome and other T-cell disorders	Mantle cell lymphoma
CD11c, CD103, HC2	Cytoplasmic Ig, CD79a (BCR-α chain), CD138	CD3, CD7, CD4, CD8	Cyclin D

Other T-cell malignancies include **adult T-cell leukaemia/lymphoma** (ATL), which occurs in clusters, particularly in Japan and the Caribbean, where the associated retrovirus (HTLV-I) is endemic. ATL is an aggressive systemic disorder, often with skin and neurological involvement.

Hairy cell leukaemia is a rare condition of middle aged males, which although termed a 'leukaemia', is not necessarily associated with a high white cell count at presentation. Pancytopenia, leading to an increased risk of infection, is commoner. Two-thirds of the patients have splenomegaly. The abnormal cells are often diagnosed as 'atypical lymphocytes' on the blood film, but close inspection and the use of enzymatic and immunological markers confirm the diagnosis (see Tables 6.5 and 6.6). The 'hairy cell' is a late-stage B cell with characteristic reactions with monoclonal antibodies to B-cell-restricted antigens, as well as the integrin CD11c. Interferon (IFN) and Claribine induce remission in nearly all patients, with 75% achieving complete remission for >5 years. Deoxycoformycin prevents the detoxifica-

tion of T- and B-cell metabolites and causes a mild form of severe combined immune deficiency (SCID) as in adenine deaminase (ADA) deficiency (see Chapter 3). Splenectomy is reserved for those who develop pancytopenia or splenic infarction.

6.4 Lymphomas

The term 'lymphoma' implies a malignant proliferation of **non-recirculating lymph node cells**. Traditionally, there have been two distinct types: Hodgkin's disease and non-Hodgkin's lymphoma (NHL). The different courses of these diseases suggested that these were separate entities, though *both are now known to be of lymphoid origin*. Patients may **present** with painless lymphadenopathy, unexplained fever, night sweats, weight loss, itching or increased/severe infections with opportunistic pathogens such as herpes simplex virus (severe cold sores) or varicella zoster virus (shingles, see Fig. 6.7).

CASE 6.3 HODGKIN'S DISEASE

A 23-year-old man presented with malaise, night sweats, loss of weight and intermittent fever dating from a flu-like illness 3 months previously. On examination, he had bilateral, cervical and axillary lymphadenopathy; the glands were 2–5 cm in diameter, firm, rubbery, discrete and fairly mobile. His liver and spleen were not enlarged. Investigation showed that his haemoglobin was low (113 g/l) and the white cell count was normal (4.2×10^9/l) but his erythrocyte sedimentation rate (ESR) was 78 mm/h; the blood film did not show any abnormal cells. No enlargement of the hilar glands was seen on chest X-ray. A cervical lymph node was removed for histology. The gross architecture of the node was de-

stroyed; the tissue consisted of histiocytes, eosinophils, lymphocytes and giant cells known as Reed–Sternberg cells. These large binucleate cells are characteristic of Hodgkin's disease. A bone marrow examination was normal and computed tomography (CT) showed no involvement of other lymph nodes. This patient had stage 2 Hodgkin's disease, because, although only lymphoid tissue above the diaphragm was involved, his ESR was above 40 mm/h. In view of his symptoms, the suffix 'B' was added to the stage, suggesting a poorer prognosis associated with systemic symptoms, and he was given cytotoxic therapy.

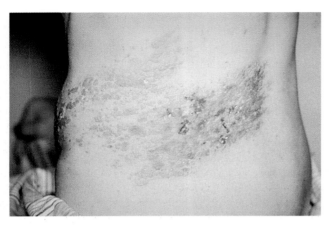

Fig. 6.7 Zoster infection. Reproduced from *Medicine*, 2nd edn, eds Axford and O'Callaghan, with permission.

6.4.1 Hodgkin's disease

The presence of characteristic binucleate Reed–Sternberg cells and their variant (mononuclear Hodgkin cell) is **diagnostic** of Hodgkin's disease (Case 6.3). These cells have B-cell markers on their surface, suggesting that they are malignant B cells, although how or why they gain their particular morphology remains unknown.

Presentation is bimodal, with the larger peak in young adulthood and a smaller peak in the 60s. Painless lymphadenopathy, especially in the neck region, is a common feature.

Therapy depends on the Rye stage of the disease, which is determined by CT scanning of related groups of lymph nodes, since malignant cells spread via lymphatics in Hodgkin's disease. Those with only local disease (stages 1A and 2A) are treated with radiotherapy. The **15-year survival figures** for this group are good, with 70–90% of the patients deemed 'cured'. Patients with constitutional symptoms (known as 'B' symptoms—those without are staged as 'A') or a raised ESR indicative of widespread disease, and those with stage 3

or 4 disease are treated with aggressive chemotherapy; most (80%) remit and remain disease free for at least 5 years; over half of them are still disease-free at 15 years.

Hodgkin's disease is associated with marked depression of cell-mediated immunity and patients are prone to bacterial, fungal and viral infections (see Chapter 3), both prior to and during therapy. Long-term **complications** include second tumours associated with the chemotherapy and thyroid failure after irradiation to the neck

6.4.2 Non-Hodgkin's lymphoma

The **incidence** of this type of lymphoid tumour is increasing at a rate of 4–5% p.a., as immunosuppressive therapy is more widely used. For example, there is a 13–15-fold risk of Hodgkin's disease or lymphoma after alkylating agents are used to treat rheumatoid arthritis. Increased ascertainment also contributes due to early diagnosis, by use of CT scanning and immunophenotyping of biopsy material from bone marrow and any affected tissues (Case 6.4).

Patients **present** with a variety of symptoms, many similar to those in Hodgkin's disease, i.e. weight loss, unexplained fever, night sweats and lymphadenopathy (Fig. 6.8), as well as evidence of bone marrow suppression, i.e. anaemia, bruising due to thrombocytopenia, or lymphoid infiltration of other organs such as liver, skin, brain or lungs.

As with other lymphoid malignancies, the **aetiology** is unknown, although oncogenes, activated by **translocation** during proliferation in **response to a viral infection**, is a likely mechanism at present (Fig. 6.9). An example is the EBV-provoked lymphoma seen in transplanted patients receiving aggressive anti-rejection therapy, i.e. cyclosporin or anti-CD3 monoclonal antibodies (see Case 7.1). Reduction in immunosuppression is associated with tumour regression, indicating a role for T cells in controlling this type of proliferation. Thus, there may be three phases in the development of the tumour (Fig. 6.9); an early reversible stage with

---

CASE 6.4 NON-HODGKIN'S LYMPHOMA

A 59-year-old man presented with a gradually increasing lump in his right groin of 6 months' duration, which he thought was a 'hernia'. This was a large inguinal lymph node. He had suffered repeated urethritis in the past. He had no other symptoms, but was found on examination to have splenomegaly (7 cm below the costal margin) without hepatomegaly.

On investigation, his haemoglobin was low (118 g/l) but his white cell count and differential were normal. His ESR was 58 mm/h and the lactate dehydrogenase level was also high. His serum immunoglobulins were all reduced: his IgG was 5.2 g/l (NR

7.2–19.0 g/l); IgA 0.3 g/l (NR 0.8–5.0 g/l); and IgM 0.3 g/l (NR 0.5–2.0 g/l). Serum electrophoresis showed no monoclonal bands. The lymph node was excised; light microscopy showed irregular follicles with mixtures of small and large cells throughout but no organized germinal centres. Reactive follicular hyperplasia was a possibility but immunophenotyping of tissue sections showed monoclonality, with strong cellular staining of the cells in the multiple follicles with anti-IgG and anti-κ antisera. Normal interfollicular T-cell staining was present. This patient had a follicular type of NHL.

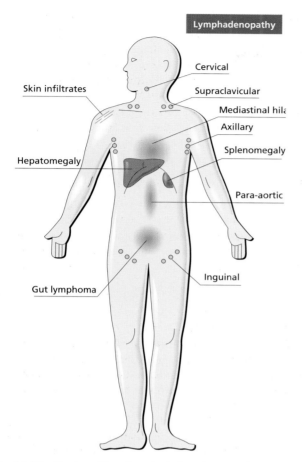

Lymphadenopathy

- Skin infiltrates
- Cervical
- Supraclavicular
- Mediastinal hila
- Axillary
- Hepatomegaly
- Splenomegaly
- Para-aortic
- Inguinal
- Gut lymphoma

Fig. 6.8 Distribution of lymph nodes in lymphoma. Reproduced from *Medicine*, 2nd edn, eds Axford and O'Callaghan, with permission.

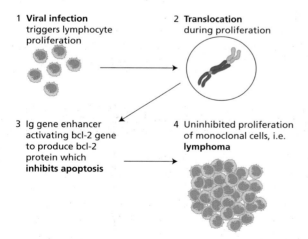

1 **Viral infection** triggers lymphocyte proliferation

2 **Translocation** during proliferation

3 Ig gene enhancer activating bcl-2 gene to produce bcl-2 protein which **inhibits apoptosis**

4 Uninhibited proliferation of monoclonal cells, i.e. **lymphoma**

Fig. 6.9 Immunopathogenesis in lymphoma.

polyclonal proliferation, a later reversible phase associated with oligoclonality and an irreversible, late phase when progression, probably associated with translocation of genetic material, is inevitable. Most patients present only when the tumour is in the final stage.

The **diagnosis** of NHL *depends on a lymph node biopsy*. The area of the lymph node from which the malignant cells arise does not necessarily indicate the cell of origin but is helpful, given the caveat that predominantly B-cell germinal centres and follicular areas do contain T lymphocytes and the paracortex (T-cell area) has some B cells. Precise cell lineage is achieved by staining tissue sections with labelled monoclonal antibodies (MAbs) to different surface antigens. The panel of MAbs is designed to confirm that the abnormal cells are lymphoid (leucocyte common antigen, CD45), their lineage (T or B) and their monoclonality. **Monoclonality of B-cell lymphomas** is easily confirmed with antisera to κ and λ light chains (as in Case 6.4). T-cell lymphomas require T-cell receptor (*TCR*) gene rearrangement studies to prove monoclonality, though an excess of apoptotic proteins, such as Bcl-2, is also a useful marker of lack of proliferative control, i.e. malignancy.

Assessing the **extent of disease** is helpful, although truly localized disease is uncommon. CT and abdominal ultrasound are accurate ways of assessing intra-abdominal involvement. Bone marrow examination is probably the most important investigation in NHL, as marrow involvement is associated with a poor prognosis.

Complications of NHL include autoimmune haemolytic anaemia and thrombocytopenia. Low serum immunoglobulin levels, often resulting in recurrent bacterial infections, are seen in about half the patients.

The natural history of NHL is enormously variable. The aim of a **classification in pathology** is to break up a heterogeneous group of diseases in order to provide the most effective form of treatment. There have been several classifications of NHL, largely based on morphology that failed to distinguish between the different origins of the malignant cells. To be useful, a classification must take into account the grade of malignancy and distinguish between aggressive and indolent tumours—general principles are outlined in Box 6.3. The Revised European American Lymphoma

---

BOX 6.3 DIFFERENT TYPES OF B-CELL LYMPHOMA

Most NHLs are of B-cell lineage

Malignancies of immature B cells include CLL and small lymphoid cell lymphomas

Tumours of antigen-stimulated B cells may be follicular or large cell lymphomas

More mature B cells give rise to more malignant lymphomas

Exceptions are well-differentiated tumours of lymphoplasmacytoid cells in Waldenström's macroglobulinaemia

(REAL) classification does this and has been shown to have **prognostic** value.

Treatment is determined by immunohistological findings, the bulk and site of the disease, and the patient's age and clinical history. Nearly all patients with low-grade malignancies have widespread disease at diagnosis, indicating that chemotherapy is required, as for those with high-grade disease. The rationale behind treatment needs to take into account the widespread involvement and susceptibility of cells turning over slowly. Combination chemotherapy, with Rituximab (anti-CD20 monoclonal antibody) to wipe out all B cells, is used increasingly. Antifungal and antiviral prophylaxis, for the inevitable immune suppression and the transient antibody deficiency resulting from Rituximab,

have improved survival. High-dose ablative therapy is combined with rescue of bone marrow function with autologous (self) bone marrow transplantation. Bone marrow, taken before chemotherapy, must be purged of lymphoma cells (see Chapter 8) and checked for residual malignant cells before it is returned to the patient. The *bcl-2* oncogene in residual malignant cells is amplified by the polymerase chain reaction (Chapter 19); this makes detection sufficiently sensitive to be sure that the marrow is 'clean' for autologous transplantation. Such treatment is successful, with a 90% disease-free survival at 8 years for those whose returning marrow has been completely purged.

The overall prognosis for patients with NHL has improved by the use of combined chemotherapy, though long-term survival remains uncertain. There is also a risk of a second malignancy after treatment is finished.

6.5 Plasma cell dyscrasias

6.5.1 Multiple myeloma

Multiple myeloma is defined as a malignant proliferation of plasma cells (see Fig. 6.2), probably provoked by excess production of interleukin (IL)-6. Theses cells overproduce their specific monoclone of immunoglobulin molecules which are detected in serum or urine or both (Figs 6.10 and 19.4). Patients **commonly present** with recurrent infections (associated with the immunosuppressive effect of the malignancy), renal failure (due to hypercalcaemia or deposition of the paraprotein in the kidney), pathological fractures or bone pain of acute onset (due to osteolytic lesions or osteoporosis) (see Fig. 6.11), or anaemia (due to marrow infiltration) (see Fig. 6.12). Myeloma may also be a rare cause of peripheral neuropathy, pancreatic dysfunction or the hyperviscosity

Table 6.7 Comparison of clinical features of multiple myeloma and Waldenström's macroglobulinaemia

	Multiple myeloma	Waldenström's macroglobulinaemia
Lytic bone lesions	+++	
Bone pain	+++	
Pathological fractures	++	
Anaemia	+++	++
Recurrent infection	++	
Hypercalcaemia	++	
Renal failure	++	
Thrombocytopenia	+	
Leucopenia	+	
Neuropathy	+	+
Lymphadenopathy	+	+++
Hepatosplenomegaly	+	+++
Hyperviscosity	+	+++

CASE 6.5 MULTIPLE MYELOMA

A 66-year-old man presented with sharp, constant, low back pain, dating from a fall from a ladder 6 weeks earlier. On direct questioning, he did admit to vague malaise for over 6 months. On examination, he was in considerable pain but otherwise seemed fairly fit. He was mildly anaemic but had no lymphadenopathy and no fever. There were no signs of bruising, no finger clubbing, no hepatosplenomegaly and no abdominal masses. On investigation, his haemoglobin was low (102 g/l) but his white cell count was normal (6.2 × 10⁹/l). He had a normal differential white cell count and a normal platelet count but his ESR was 98 mm/h. Total serum proteins were raised at 98 g/l (NR 65–75 g/l) but his serum albumin, creatinine and urea were normal. He had a raised serum calcium level (3.2 mmol/l) but a normal alkaline phosphatase. Serum protein electrophoresis revealed a monoclonal band in the

γ region, with considerable immunosuppression of the rest of this region (see Fig. 6.10). The band was typed by immunofixation and shown to be IgG of κ type. Quantification of serum immunoglobulins showed a raised IgG of 67 g/l (NR 7.2–19.0 g/l), a low IgA of 0.3 g/l (NR 0.8–5.0 g/l), and a low IgM of 0.2 g/l (NR 0.5–2.0 g/l). Electrophoretic examination of concentrated urine showed a monoclonal band in the β region, which was composed of free κ light chains. X-rays of his back showed a small, punched-out lesion in the second lumbar vertebra but a subsequent skeletal survey did not show any other bone lesions.

Bone marrow examination showed an increased number of atypical plasma cells; these constituted 45% of the nucleated cells found on the film (see Table 6.8). This man showed the features required for a diagnosis of multiple myeloma (see Box 6.4).

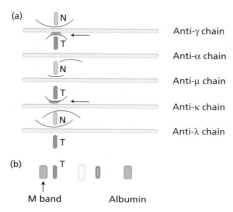

(a) N

Anti-γ chain

T

Anti-α chain

N

Anti-μ chain

T

Anti-κ chain

N

Anti-λ chain

T

(b) T

↑
M band   Albumin

Fig. 6.10 Serum and urine electrophoresis from a patient with multiple myeloma. T, test; N, normal control.

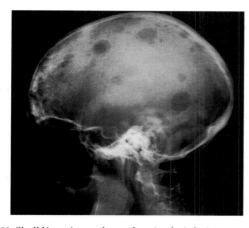

Fig. 6.11 Skull X-ray in myeloma showing lytic lesions. Reproduced from *Medicine*, 2nd edn, eds Axford and O'Callaghan, with permission.

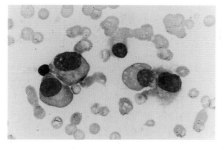

Fig. 6.12 Bone marrow in myeloma showing an excess of plasma cells. Reproduced from *Medicine*, 2nd edn, eds Axford and O'Callaghan, with permission.

syndrome (Table 6.7). It is a relatively common malignancy among the elderly (prevalence of 3 per 10^5 population) but is very rare below the age of 40 years.

The **diagnostic criteria** (used in Case 6.5) are shown in Box 6.4. The finding of a paraprotein in the serum is not di-

---

BOX 6.4 CRITERIA* REQUIRED FOR A DIAGNOSIS OF MULTIPLE MYELOMA

1 Paraprotein in serum and/or urine

2 Increased numbers of abnormal plasma cells in the bone marrow (over 20%) or proven monoclonality of plasma cells (over 12% with one light-chain type)

3 Osteolytic lesions in bones

*Two of the three criteria are essential for diagnosis.

---

agnostic of multiple myeloma; serum paraproteins are also found in some benign conditions (see section 6.5.2). The paraproteins found in the sera of patients with myeloma are usually IgG, IgA or free monoclonal light chains; IgM myelomas are rare and large amounts of IgM monoclonal protein nearly always indicate the more benign disease, Waldenström's macroglobulinaemia (see below).

Free monoclonal light chains indicate a lymphoid malignancy if found in the urine. They are known as Bence-Jones proteins. They may be associated with a serum paraprotein and, if so, then the **urinary light chains** are, of course, the same type. Only proteins of small molecular size are filtered by the normal renal glomerulus, so light chains (mol. wt 22 kDa) can be excreted, but whole immunoglobulin molecules (mol. wt of IgG 150 kDa; mol. wt of IgM 800 kDa) are too large unless there is glomerular damage. When a normal plasma cell makes immunoglobulin, it always produces an excess of the particular light chains compared with heavy chains. This normal polyclonal excess is excreted in the urine and rapidly metabolized by the renal tubules. Since all plasma cells synthesize both heavy and light chains, the free light-chain excess in normal individuals is polyclonal and can be detected only in highly concentrated (× 500) urine.

It is important to realize that *light chains are not detected by routine chemical/dipstick methods* for detecting protein in the urine. Free light chains are detected only by immunofixation (see Fig. 19.5), using specific antisera (see Chapter 19). In patients who have significant glomerular damage, leakage of all serum proteins into the urine may occur, including the serum paraprotein.

The bone marrow in myeloma usually shows abnormal **plasma cells in excess of 15%** (Fig. 6.12). This figure can be reached in some reactive conditions and is not, by itself, diagnostic, but if in doubt, immunohistology of the marrow will confirm the monoclonal nature of the cells (Table 6.8).

The X-ray appearance of a myeloma deposit is typically described as a 'punched-out' lesion (Fig. 6.11). This is often found in the skull, although any part of the skeleton can be involved and myeloma may present with pathological or osteoporotic fractures. Plasma cells release IL-6, which acts as an **osteoclast-activating factor** that may be responsible for the lytic lesions and the associated generalized osteoporosis.

Table 6.8 Interpretation of representative bone marrow studies

Plasma cells in marrow (%)*	Plasma cells with intracytoplasmic immunoglobulin (%)					Laboratory interpretation	Likely clinical diagnosis
	κ	λ	γ	α	μ		
5	3	2	2	1	2	Normal	Normal
12	7	5	6	1	5	Reactive hyperplasia	Infection
12	13	1	2	1	11	Monoclonal proliferation of IgM — κ type	Waldenström's macroglobulinaemia (early stage)
72	2	70	1	70	1	Monoclonal proliferation of IgA — λ type	Myeloma
45	43	2	45	1	1	Monoclonal proliferation of IgG — κ type	Myeloma Case 6.5

* As percentage of nucleated cells.

The **suppression of** polyclonal immunoglobulin production and failure to produce antibodies, demonstrated by a poor response to immunization, are associated with recurrent infections.

Light-chain myeloma is particularly associated with **renal tubular damage** (see Case 9.11). In myeloma, where there is excessive production of free light chains, the tubules become dilated and plugged with eosinophilic, homogeneous casts. If this material is not removed by diuresis, the tubular cells eventually atrophy or even undergo frank necrosis. Forced diuresis of patients who present with a raised serum creatinine improves their early survival. A longer-term complication of myeloma is light-chain-associated amyloid (compare with Case 9.9).

If untreated, myeloma is rapidly progressive and patients die within a year. Estimates of the tumour cell mass in myeloma have been made by measuring the rates of synthesis and catabolism of monoclonal proteins. These, together with β_2-microglobulin and C-reactive protein levels (see Chapters 1 and 19), have proved useful in **predicting survival** in individual patients. The overall prognosis depends on the presence of complications, such as anaemia, renal failure, hypercalcaemia or immunosuppression (see Table 6.7).

Standard therapy for the last three decades, in Europe, has been based on melphalan and prednisone, but **intensive regimens** followed by autologous peripheral stem cells or bone marrow transplantation have improved the prognosis of myeloma, with complete remission rates improving from 5 to 40% and overall survival extended to greater than 5 years. Current trials to reduce toxicity of such regimens, with erythropoietin (to treat the anaemia) and biphosphonates (to prevent osteoporosis and possibly bone metastases) and experimental treatments with anti-IL-6 receptor monoclonal antibodies or multiple drug resistance modulating therapies continue. G-CSF is used to increase the number of circulating CD34+ stem cells in the blood before harvesting to store for **subsequent transplantation**; following high-dose chemotherapy and autologous transplantation, these stem cells re-colonize the marrow. However, multiple myeloma remains a fatal disease, possibly due to premalignant CD34+ stem cells themselves.

The search for curative therapies includes the possibility of using cytotoxic T lymphocytes with specificity for the malignant plasma cells idiotypic marker or tumour-associated antigens (such as Mucin 1), as well as IFN-α therapy. Whether such therapies would eradicate the clonal precursor B cells remains to be seen.

6.5.2 Benign paraproteinaemia (monoclonal gammopathy of unknown significance)

Benign monoclonal gammopathy is **defined as** the presence of a monoclonal protein in a person showing no manifestations of malignant disease (see Case 6.6). About 25% of all patients with paraproteins have benign monoclonal gammopathy, also known as MGUS (Box 6.5). Benign paraproteinaemia is very uncommon under 50 years, but occurs in 1% in those of 50 years, 3% of persons over 70 and 8% of people over 85 years. **Long-term follow-up** has shown that

---

BOX 6.5 UNDERLYING CONDITIONS TO CONSIDER IN PATIENTS FOUND TO HAVE A PARAPROTEIN

- Myeloma
- Waldenström's macroglobulinaemia
- Non-Hodgkin's lymphoma
- Plasmacytoma
- Chronic lymphocytic leukaemia.
- Infection in an immunosuppressed patient
- Benign paraprotein, i.e. monoclonal gammopathy of uncertain significance (MGUS)

CASE 6.6 BENIGN PARAPROTEINAEMIA

A 49-year-old woman presented with a 6-month history of vague aches and pains in her chest. On examination, she was overweight but had no abnormal physical signs.

Her haemoglobin was 136 g/l with a white cell count of 6.7×10^9/l and a normal differential. Her ESR was 34 mm/h. Tests of thyroid function were normal. However, protein electrophoresis showed a small paraprotein band in the γ region; this band was an IgG of λ type. Her serum IgG was raised at 20.1 g/l (NR 7.2–19.0 g/l), with an IgA of 1.9 g/l (NR 0.8–5.0 g/l) and an IgM of 3.0 g/l (NR 0.5–2.0 g/l). Electrophoresis of concentrated urine

showed no proteinuria. The paraprotein measured 10 g/l by densitometry (Chapter 19). A bone marrow examination showed only 12% plasma cells. Together with the absence of osteolytic lesions, the absence of monoclonal free light chains in the urine and normal serum IgA and IgM levels, these findings supported a diagnosis of benign monoclonal gammopathy, also known as a monoclonal gammopathy of unknown significance (MGUS). This woman has been followed at 6-monthly intervals for 3 years with no change in the paraprotein level, and the urine remains free of monoclonal light chains. She will continue to be seen at yearly intervals.

a quarter of patients with a benign band develop multiple myeloma, amyloidosis, macroglobulinaemia or a similar malignant lymphoproliferative disorder (Fig. 6.13). All pa-

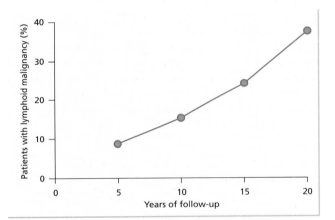

Fig. 6.13 Development of lymphoid malignancy after monoclonal gammopathy of unknown significance diagnosis. (Data from Kyle, 2002.)

tients should be investigated for multiple myeloma if they develop symptoms, if the paraprotein level increases with time or if the features described in Tables 6.7 and 6.9 are present. There are no precise findings at diagnosis that reliably distinguish patients who will remain stable from those in whom a malignant condition will develop, though the finding of an intermediate group between frank myeloma and benign gammopathy (Table 6.9) indicates that there will be markers of incipient malignancy. Until these are determined, all patients must have serial measurements of the serum M protein at yearly intervals; the median interval from recognition of the paraprotein to diagnosis of multiple myeloma is over 8 years, but can range from 2 to > 20 years.

6.5.3 Waldenström's macroglobulinaemia

The clinical **presentation** of Waldenström's macroglobulinaemia is variable. It tends to present after the age of 50 years and, in most patients, follows a relatively benign course.

Unlike myeloma (see Table 6.7), **symptoms** of Waldenström's macroglobulinaemia are usually directly attribut-

CASE 6.7 WALDENSTRÖMS MACROGLOBULINAEMIA

A 76-year-old woman presented with a 6-month history of weakness, malaise, exertional dyspnoea and abdominal discomfort. In the previous month she had experienced epistaxes and headaches but did not have visual disturbances, weight loss, bone pain or recurrent infections. On examination she was pale, with moderate axillary and cervical lymphadenopathy. Her liver and spleen were enlarged.

On investigation, she had an ESR of 112 mm/h and a haemoglobin of 108 g/l. Her white cell count and differential were normal. The total serum protein was increased to 130 g/l. Protein electrophoresis and immunofixation showed a dense paraprotein in the γ region which proved to be an IgM of κ type. Quantification

of the serum immunoglobulins showed normal IgG (9.4 g/l) and IgA levels (1.1 g/l), but her IgM was markedly raised at 64.5 g/l (NR 0.5–2.0 g/l). By densitometry (Chapter 19), the paraprotein measured 63 g/l. Electrophoresis of concentrated urine showed no free monoclonal light chains and there were no bone lesions on X-rays of her chest and skull. Her serum viscosity, relative to water, was 4.7 (NR 1.4–1.8). A bone marrow examination showed a pleomorphic cellular infiltrate composed of a mixture of small lymphocytes, plasma cells and cells of an intermediate appearance, called lymphoplasmacytoid cells. These are features of Waldenström's macroglobulinaemia.

Table 6.9 Comparison of monoclonal gammopathy of unknown significance (MGUS), smouldering myeloma and multiple myeloma

	MGUS	Smouldering myeloma	Multiple myeloma
Age at onset	Elderly	Elderly	Elderly
Symptoms	None	None	Almost invariable
Concentration of paraprotein	< 25 g/l	> 25 g/l	> 25 g/l
Change in paraprotein with time	None	↑	↑↑
Bone marrow findings (plasma cells as % nucleated cells)	< 15%	15–20%	> 20%
Free monoclonal light chains in urine	None	Minimal	Almost invariable
Lytic bone lesions	None	None	Present
Immunosuppression of other immunoglobulins in serum	None	None	Usually present
Haemoglobin, calcium, etc.	Normal	Usually normal	Often abnormal
Treatment	None	Wait for symptoms	Urgent

able to the effects of the monoclonal IgM (see Case 6.7). IgM is a large molecule (mol. wt 800 kDa) confined entirely to the intravascular pool. Increased IgM concentrations (particularly in excess of 40 g/l) cause a marked rise in serum viscosity. Although there is considerable variation in the level of viscosity that induces symptoms, these are unusual if the relative serum viscosity (see Chapter 19) is below 3.8. The symptoms of **hyperviscosity** include headaches, confusion, dizziness, and changes in visual acuity or, in some cases, sudden deafness. Nose bleeds and bruising may also occur. Examination of the optic fundi may reveal dilated vessels, haemorrhages, exudates, intravascular rouleaux formation or papilloedema.

Vigorous plasmapheresis can reduce the serum IgM level quite quickly and, once the viscosity has been lowered, maintenance **plasmapheresis** will keep the patient asymptomatic. However, plasmapheresis does not affect the disease itself; **chemotherapy** is needed to control the monoclonal proliferation.

The **prognosis** of macroglobulinaemia is quite good. The mean survival is 4–5 years, but many patients live for 10 years or more following diagnosis. Complications are due to hyperviscosity or cryoglobulinaemia (see section 11.6.3); infections are uncommon. A small proportion of patients have a rapidly progressive disease; symptoms resemble those of NHL, are usually followed by the appearance of circulating lymphoplasmacytoid cells and patients die fairly rapidly.

6.5.4 Other plasma cell dyscrasias

Almost all malignant plasma cells produce an excess of monoclonal light chains, resulting in a high risk of light chain associated **amyloid** (see section 9.7.3). This type of amyloid is associated with frank myeloma or is 'idiopathic' if the malignant clone is not detected.

A few plasma cell tumours produce incomplete heavy chains without associated light chains. The commonest example is α-**chain disease** in which most patients present with severe diarrhoea, intestinal malabsorption, weight loss, abdominal pain and finger clubbing. Incomplete α chains infiltrate the intestinal mucosa; thus, α-heavy-chain disease is also called immunoproliferative small-intestinal disease. It seems to develop in two stages: an early pre-malignant infiltrative phase followed by progression to an immunoblastic lymphoma. Although no specific dietary agent or enteric pathogen has been implicated, complete remissions have been achieved by oral antibiotics in the early phase, implying that B-cell proliferation stops if the putative antigen is eliminated. This disease is similar to the Maltomas—malignancies of lymphoid follicles in the gut (section 14.4)—which also respond to elimination of causative micro-organisms such as Helicobacter pylori.

FURTHER READING

See website: www.immunologyclinic.com

7 Immune Manipulation

7.1 Introduction

Although the immune system usually responds appropriately to foreign antigens, there are patients whose disease is caused by immune responses which are excessive or defective. The aim of clinical immunology is to correct these abnormalities. Two major approaches are possible: immunosuppression or immunopotentiation. An overactive, self-damaging immune system requires some degree of **immunosuppression**; this is the mainstay of the management of organ transplantation and certain life-threatening autoimmune diseases. With the major exceptions of immunization and bone marrow transplantation (BMT), **immunopotentiation** to improve a naive or defective immune system is still in its infancy, although gene therapy has exciting potential. Some methods of immune manipulation produce definite clinical benefit by mechanisms which are poorly understood, e.g. therapy with intravenous immunoglobulins (IVIG) and monoclonal antibodies: they can suppress, potentiate or modify immune responses depending on their specificity and the clinical circumstances.

7.2 Immunosuppression

7.2.1 Drugs

There are several groups of immunosuppressive drugs (Fig. 7.1). Their effects on the immune system are divided into *short-lived changes on cell traffic and more persistent effects on individual cell functions*. Their anti-inflammatory properties are separate from those on the immune system. In general, azathioprine and cyclophosphamide act on the maturation of cells, while steroids and fungal derivatives inhibit the functions of mature cells.

Corticosteroids have long been known to alter immune responses. A single dose of corticosteroids causes changes in cell traffic within 2 h of administration; the result is a transient lymphopenia, which peaks at 4 h but is no longer apparent after 24 h. Lymphopenia occurs because blood lymphocytes are sequestered in the bone marrow; helper T cells are predominantly affected (Table 7.1).

The influence of steroids on cell function varies according to species, dose and timing. *The major effect in humans is on 'resting' macrophages* (Table 7.1); activated macrophages are

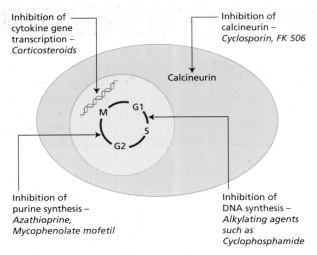

Inhibition of cytokine gene transcription – *Corticosteroids*

Inhibition of calcineurin – *Cyclosporin, FK 506*

Calcineurin

M G1

S

G2

Inhibition of purine synthesis – *Azathioprine, Mycophenolate mofetil*

Inhibition of DNA synthesis – *Alkylating agents such as Cyclophosphamide*

Fig. 7.1 Schematic depiction of the main intracellular sites of action of the major groups of immunosuppressive drugs (blue line depicts the outer cell membrane and the grey line the nuclear membrane and the stages of nuclear cycle in division. DNA is represented in red).

not sensitive to corticosteroids. **Reduced antigen handling by macrophages** probably accounts for the poor primary antibody response seen following corticosteroid administration. The secondary antibody response is not affected, as memory cells are resistant to the effects of corticosteroids. At higher doses of steroids, inhibition of interleukin (IL)-2 production by helper T cells becomes increasingly important.

In humans, corticosteroids are used for two main purposes: the prevention or reversal of graft rejection and the treatment of autoimmune and malignant diseases. In transplantation (see Chapter 8) their anti-inflammatory action and reduction of macrophage activity results in a reduction of cellular infiltration. *Steroids alone are ineffective in preventing rejection in the early phase*, although high doses do reverse acute rejection. Corticosteroids have a wide range of side-effects (Fig. 7.2). They are known to **increase the patient's susceptibility to infections** of all kinds. Failure to export neutrophils into the tissues (Table 7.1) and reduced macrophage function is most relevant to this increased risk. Side-effects are related to the duration of treatment as well as the dose. By giving larger doses for shorter periods, it is often possible to reduce unwanted side-effects while conserving immunosuppression. Side-effects can also be reduced by alternate-day therapy, or by giving steroids with other immunosuppressive drugs as steroid-sparing agents.

The development of **thiopurines** in the 1950s provided another important immunosuppressive drug, namely **azathioprine**. It is inactive until metabolized by the liver and takes a few weeks to be effective. The metabolites can affect all dividing cells by inhibition of DNA synthesis. Azathioprine affects several aspects of immune function (Table 7.2), which accounts for its bone marrow toxicity. Most patients on long-term therapy eventually show granulocytopenia and thrombocytopenia. Homozygous deficiency of **thiopurine methyl transferase (TPMT)**, a key enzyme responsible for metabolizing azathioprine, is associated with life-threatening marrow aplasia. It is important to do weekly leucocyte and platelet counts in order to detect these side-effects. Azathioprine is widely used in two main clinical situations: (i) prevention of rejection after organ transplantation; (ii) treatment of systemic autoimmune disease.

Table 7.1 Actions of corticosteroids on the human immune system

	Effect	Mechanism
1 Cell traffic	↑ Neutrophils in blood	Released from bone marrow but not exported into tissues
	↓ Monocytes in blood	
	↓ Lymphocytes, especially CD4 T cells	Apoptosis of CD4 T cells and TH1, TH2, T_C sequestered in bone marrow
2 Cell function	Macrophages	Membrane stabilization
	↓ Antigen handling	↓ maturation of monocytes to macrophages
	↓ Cytokine (IL-1, IL-6, TNF-α) production	
	↓ Chemotaxis	
	↓ Bactericidal activity	
	↓ T-cell activation	Inhibition of cytokine gene transcription (IL-1, IL-2, IL-3, IL-4, IL-6, IFN-γ)
	↓ Endothelial cell function	↓ Expression of adhesion molecules
	↓ Natural killer cell function	↓ Nitric oxide synthase activity
3 Effects on inflammation	↓ Prostaglandin synthesis	Inhibition of phospholipase A_2 and cyclooxygenase enzymes

TH, Helper T cells; T_C, cytotoxic T cells; IL, interleukin; TNF-α, tumour necrosis factor-α; IFN-γ, interferon-γ.

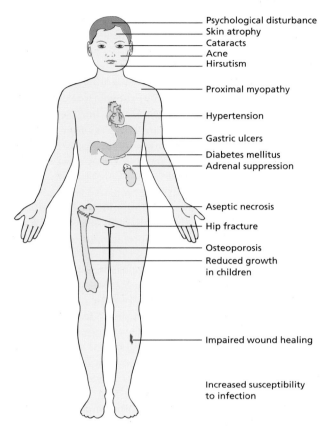

Fig. 7.2 Side-effects of long-term treatment with corticosteroids.

Table 7.2 Actions of thiopurines on the human immune system

1 Cell traffic
Acute	↓Lymphocytes, especially NK and T cells	
	↓Monocytes	
Chronic	↓Granulocytes	due to bone marrow
	↓Platelets	suppression

2 Cell function (effects are seen only in long-term experiments)
   Do not usually alter antibody responses at normal doses;
   can do so at higher doses
3 Effects on inflammation
       ↓Inflammatory infiltrate correlates with
       ↓ monocytes in blood

Mycophenolate mofetil is a new purine inhibitor which inhibits inosine monophosphate dehydrogenase (IMP), a key enzyme in the de novo synthesis of purines by activated T and B lymphocytes. It is an excellent substitute for azathioprine treatment failure or marrow toxicity and is now a well-established component of maintenance immunosuppressive regimens following organ transplantation. **Alkylating agents** interfere with DNA duplication at the premitotic phase and are most effective in rapidly dividing cells. Tissues vary in their ability to repair DNA after alkylation, which accounts for their differing sensitivities to this group of drugs. *They have little anti-inflammatory activity* and so are often given with steroids. **Cyclophosphamide**, like azathioprine, requires metabolism by the liver to form its active metabolites. When cyclophosphamide is given with, or immediately after, an antigen there is **reduced antibody production** and **impaired delayed-type hypersensitivity**. The precise mechanism of action is unknown. At low doses, $CD8^+$ cells show a short-lived fall in number. As the dose is increased, numbers of $CD4^+$ cells fall progressively (Case 7.1). After stopping cyclophosphamide, recovery takes weeks or months. Prolonged high doses are associated with bladder cancer. Clinically, cyclophosphamide is particularly useful in aggressive autoimmune diseases (such as Wegener's granulomatosis or vasculitis associated with systemic lupus erythematosus), and in conditioning bone marrow transplant recipients (see Chapter 8). Another alkylating agent, chlorambucil, is widely used for treating low-grade B-cell neoplasms, such as chronic lymphocytic leukaemia and non-Hodgkin's lymphoma. It appears to act on B cells directly. Chlorambucil is given either intermittently or in low dosage, because persistently high doses are associated with subsequent development of leukaemia.

Cyclosporin is a naturally occurring fungal metabolite. It has no effect on lymphocyte traffic but suppresses both humoral and cell-mediated immunity. Cyclosporin becomes active only when complexed to its intracellular receptor (cyclophilin) and inhibits early, calcium-dependent events, particularly the activation of several cytokine genes (Fig. 7.3). The major effect is **inhibition of IL-2 production** and thus $CD4^+$ cell-dependent proliferative responses. Natural killer (NK) cell activity is also affected, because of its dependence on IL-2 production. Cyclosporin causes a striking **prolongation of graft survival** and virtually all trans-

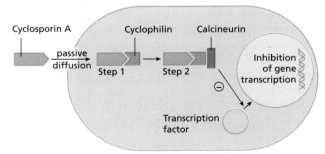

Fig. 7.3 Mechanism of immunosuppressive action of cyclosporin. In step 2 the CyA–Cyp complex binds to and inhibits calcineurin, a key enzyme responsible for translocation of transcription factors from the cytoplasm to the nucleus. Interruption of this event prevents gene transcription for interleukins IL-2, IL-3, IL-4, IL-5 and IFN-γ.

plantation protocols now include cyclosporin, usually in association with prednisolone and azathioprine (see Chapter 8). In animals, short-term administration of cyclosporin has resulted in prolonged graft survival even after the drug was withdrawn; this is not the case in humans where long-term cyclosporin is necessary. Cyclosporin is partially successful both in preventing and reversing acute graft-versus-host disease following BMT.

Cyclosporin is also used in a range of **autoimmune diseases mediated by helper T cells**. Its effectiveness has been established in controlled trials in psoriasis, uveitis and severe rheumatoid arthritis (RA). Several features are common to these reports (Box 7.1).

The timing and dose of cyclosporin must be balanced against the risk of toxicity including **nephrotoxicity** and **hepatotoxicity**. Other side-effects include gingival hyperplasia, tremor, hirsutism and striking changes in facial appearances in children. One of the most worrying side-effects of cyclosporin is **lymphoma induction** due to an increased susceptibility to the oncogenic effects of the Epstein–Barr virus (EBV). There is a disproportionately high prevalence of malignancy (1–10% of transplants), mainly non-Hodgkin's lymphoma or Kaposi's sarcoma, occurring within 2–3 years of transplantation, particularly in those treated concurrently

with anti-CD3 antibody or anti-lymphocyte globulin. This risk of malignancy is not a contraindication to its use in transplantation.

In contrast to immunocompetent individuals who are able to contain EBV as a chronic latent infection, patients with defective cellular immunity are unable to do so and are at risk of developing B-cell lymphoma, as in Case 7.2. EBV-induced lymphoma in transplant patients often regresses on withdrawal or reduction of immunosuppressive medication, but this has to be balanced with the attendant risk of inducing graft rejection.

The success of cyclosporin has stimulated the search for other novel immunosuppressive drugs. **FK506 (tacrolimus)** is derived from a soil fungus. Although its structure is quite different from that of cyclosporin and it binds to a different intracellular protein, it has a similar mode of action but is 10–100 times more potent. Like cyclosporin, it inhibits IL-2, IL-3, IL-4 and interferon (IFN)-γ secretion, so preventing early activation of CD4$^+$ T lymphocytes. Tacrolimus is currently used as an alternative to cyclosporin for primary immunosuppression in liver and kidney allograft recipients; tacrolimus is also of benefit in the treatment of allograft rejection unresponsive to conventional immunosuppressive regimens. Side-effects resemble those of cyclosporin, but the incidence of nephrotoxicity is greater.

Rapamycin (sirolimus) is yet another immunosuppressive drug of fungal origin, which in combination with cyclosporin and steroids is successful in preventing renal transplant rejection. It is structurally similar to FK506 but has a different immunosuppressive effect: sirolimus does not inhibit calcineurin and consequently cytokine gene transcription is unimpaired. However, it inhibits T-cell proliferation induced by IL-2 and IL-4.

BOX 7.1 FEATURES OF CYCLOSPORIN THERAPY

- Cyclosporin has a quick effect (within 2–12 weeks)
- Relapse occurs when the drug is stopped
- The clinical course of the disease is unaffected
- High doses are nephrotoxic and cause hypertension

CASE 7.1 PNEUMOCYSTIS PNEUMONIA COMPLICATING IMMUNOSUPPRESSIVE THERAPY

A 35-year-old man with Wegener's granulomatosis (WG) was admitted to hospital with a 2-week history of fever and shortness of breath. The diagnosis of WG had been made 18 months earlier when he presented with haemoptysis and glomerulonephritis. Disease remission was achieved with aggressive immunosuppressive therapy using a combination of pulse methylprednisolone and cyclophosphamide, enabling him to be maintained on his current tapering dose of steroids and azathioprine. The results of investigations on his current hospital admission were as follows:

- Chest X-ray: diffuse bilateral shadowing
- Serum C-reactive protein (CRP): 80 mg/l (NR < 10)
- Antineutrophil cytoplasmic antibody directed against proteinase 3: weakly positive at a titre of 1 : 40 (> 1 : 640 at disease diagnosis)

- Serum creatinine: 102 µmol/l (NR 50–140)
- Urea: 4.5 mmol/l (NR 2.5–7.1)
- Urine microscopy: clear.

The differential diagnosis was between active WG and infection complicating immunosuppressive therapy. It was crucial to distinguish between infection and active vasculitis in this situation, since an increase in immunosuppressive therapy in the face of sepsis could be potentially fatal. Further investigations, including bronchoalveolar lavage, revealed the presence of Pneumocystis carinii, a recognized lung pathogen in patients on long-term immunosuppressive therapy. He made a full clinical and radiological recovery following 2 weeks of co-trimoxazole therapy and was discharged home on his usual dose of maintenance immunosuppression.

CASE 7.2 EPSTEIN–BARR VIRUS-INDUCED LYMPHOMA IN A TRANSPLANT RECIPIENT

A 65-year-old insulin-dependent diabetic man underwent cadaveric renal transplantation for end-stage renal failure. The immediate post-operative course was complicated by acute rejection, which was successfully reversed by anti-thymocyte globulin. He was discharged from hospital 2 weeks later on insulin, prednisolone, azathioprine and cyclosporin (to prevent transplant rejection), co-trimoxazole (to prevent Pneumocystis infection), erythropoi-etin and ranitidine. Five months later, he developed progressive dyspnoea, fever and fatigue. Clinical examination revealed bilateral lung crackles and hepatosplenomegaly. Bilateral diffuse interstitial shadowing was noted on chest X-ray. The differential diagnosis is summarized in Table 7.3. His haemoglobin was 84 g/l and he was severely leucopenic at $1.0 \times 10^9/l$. Blood cultures were sterile and a bone marrow biopsy showed normal myeloid and erythroid matura-tion with no acid-fast bacilli or fungi evident on special stains. A transbronchial biopsy showed no histological abnormality; special stains for acid-fast bacilli, Pneumocystis and cytomegalovirus were negative. Open lung biopsy showed fibrinous pneumonia with obstructive bronchiolitis associated with a dense cellular infiltrate

of highly atypical lymphoid cells containing pleomorphic nuclei. The lymphoid cells expressed B-cell markers (CD20, CD79) and stained positively for a number of EBV gene products (EBV nuclear antigens, EBV latent membrane proteins).

The lung biopsy results were diagnostic of a B-cell lymphoma secondary to EBV. Following the diagnosis, his immunosuppressive medication was stopped but the patient died 2 weeks later from progressive respiratory failure.

Table 7.3 Differential diagnosis of fever and lung shadows in a renal transplant recipient

- Bacterial pneumonia (unlikely at 5 months post-transplant)
- Reactivation of tuberculosis
- Fungal infection (Aspergillus, Pneumocystis)
- Viral infection (cytomegalovirus)
- Epstein–Barr-virus-induced lymphoproliferative disease

Despite their undoubted efficacy, immunosuppressive drug therapy is inherently unsatisfactory in view of the adverse effects discussed earlier, illustrated in Cases 7.1 and 7.2. As a result, there is much interest in the develop-ment of more effective and less toxic immunosuppressive agents. One such method of maximizing local therapeutic immunosuppression without systemic adverse effects is the development of **topical immunosuppressive agents**. Tacrolimus and a related agent, pimecrolimus, are effective in ointment form in the treatment of moderate to severe eczema unresponsive to conventional therapy (see Chap-ter 11).

7.2.2 Antibodies as immunosuppressive agents

Antibodies can be used to suppress the immune response.

Prevention of sensitization by removal of antigen is illus-trated by the use of antibodies to the rhesus D blood group antigen. Haemolytic disease of the newborn due to rhesus incompatibility between the mother (rhesus D negative) and a rhesus D-positive fetus (see Chapter 18) is prevented by the administration of anti-D antibodies to 'at-risk' mothers immediately after delivery. These antibodies destroy any rhesus-positive fetal red cells, thus preventing sensitization of the mother's immune system.

A wide array of monoclonal antibodies have been de-veloped with the aim of **interrupting interaction between antigen-presenting cells, T cells and B cells** (Fig. 7.4 and Table 7.4).

A major concern of using rodent monoclonal antibodies is the potential for triggering reactions after repeated usage, with loss of efficacy due to antibodies to the species part of the therapeutic antibody. Production of human monoclonal antibodies, by transforming B cells with EBV or fusing anti-body-producing cells with human cell lines, may overcome

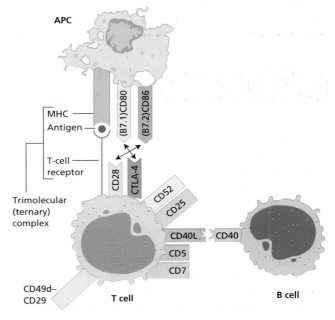

Fig. 7.4 Targets for monoclonal antibodies as immunosuppressive agents.

Table 7.4 Antibodies as immunosuppressive agents

Antibody	Targets	Clinical use	Comments	Adverse effects
Anti-lymphocyte globulin	T and B lymphocytes	Treatment of graft rejection	Polyclonal antiserum prepared by immunizing rabbits/horses with human lymphoid cells	Serum sickness Increased malignancy
Anti-CD52 (CAMPATH-1H)	Lymphocytes and monocytes	T-cell depletion of bone marrow grafts to prevent GVH; CLL, RA	In RA, marked prolonged CD4 lymphopenia	
Anti-CD3	All mature T cells	Treatment of renal and cardiac graft rejection	Induces cytokine release leading to fever, rigors, meningism and hypotension	Incidence of malignancy among recipients increased
Anti-CD4	Mainly helper T cells	Clinical trials in rheumatoid arthritis (RA)	Original murine anti-CD4 immunogenic in humans; non-depleting chimeric and humanized versions undergoing trials	Marked circulatory CD4 lymphopenia lasting months with some preparations
Anti-TNF (Infliximab)	TNF	RA, Crohn's disease resistant to conventional immunosuppression	Chimeric antibody Benefit confirmed in double-blind placebo-controlled trials	Tuberculosis Histoplasmosis
CTLA4-Ig	T cells	Encouraging results in murine lupus	Fusion protein composed of extracellular portion of CTLA-4 and Fc portion of mouse IgG	Not known
Anti-CD40 L	Activated T cells	Encouraging results in murine lupus	Caution required in humans in view of immunodeficiency associated with lack of CD40L	Human trials abandoned due to thrombosis in recipients
Anti-CD20 (Rituximab)	B cells	B-cell lymphoma	Of proven benefit in lymphoma; increasing interest in autoimmune diseases	Transient modest fall in serum immunoglobulins
Anti-CD49d-CD29 (anti-α4-integrins, Natalizumab)	α4-integrins	Crohn's disease, multiple sclerosis	Beneficial in randomized placebo-controlled trials. Value of natalizumab relative to other treatments for MS and Crohn's is not known	JC virus-related progressive multifocal leucoencephalopathy. Peripheral monocytosis, lymphocytosis and eosinophilia due to interruption of α4-integrin-mediated homing

CTLA4-Ig, cytotoxic T-lymphocyte antigen 4; GVH, graft versus host disease; TNF, tumour necrosis factor.

this problem. An alternative approach has been to '**humanize**' mouse monoclonal antibodies genetically by transposing their antigen-binding sites (hypervariable regions) onto a human antibody framework (Fig. 7.5); this retains the full range of effector properties of human Fc regions while minimizing the immunogenicity of the mouse component (see Case 7.3).

The use of **anti-tumour necrosis factor antibodies** (anti-TNF) as a therapeutic agent is an excellent example of targeted immunotherapy (Case 7.3). The success of TNF blockade in RA underlines the pivotal proinflammatory role of TNF in this disease (Chapter 10). TNF blockade can be achieved by either the use of a chimeric anti-TNF antibody (infliximab, adalimumab) or a soluble TNF receptor (etanercept).

In clinical practice, therapeutic TNF inhibition is associated with a range of infective complications, in particular a significant risk of reactivation of Mycobacterium tuberculosis. In contrast to tuberculosis (TB) in the immunocompe-

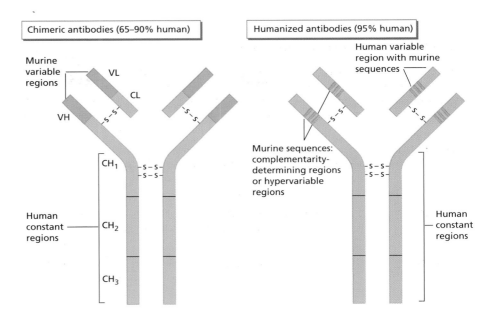

Fig. 7.5 Schematic depiction of humanized and chimeric antibodies.

tent, characteristics of TB in the setting of anti-TNF therapy include a preponderance of extrapulmonary disease and poor granuloma formation on histology. The risk of TB associated with TNF blockade in humans is mirrored by the predisposition of TNF knock-out mice to disseminated TB. It is interesting to note that an increased risk of serious infections was not noted during clinical trials of anti-TNF but soon became apparent with widespread clinical use, thus highlighting the importance of rigorous surveillance of new drugs.

7.2.3 Plasmapheresis and plasma exchange

Plasmapheresis involves taking blood, separating off the plasma and returning the red cell-enriched fraction to the patient. In contrast, **plasma exchange** involves the withdrawal of blood, removal of plasma and the return to the patient of the red cell-enriched fraction plus donor plasma. In plasmapheresis, improvement may be due to the removal of mediators of tissue damage, whereas in plasma exchange it may be due to the replacement of deficient factors or to the immunomodulating effects of human immunoglobulins (section 7.4). Therapeutic plasmapheresis is used as an adjunct in many diseases in which immunological mechanisms are proven or suspected, but clear benefit has been shown in only a few of these diseases (Table 7.5). It is useful in the emergency treatment of hyperviscosity (see Chapter 6), but long-term treatment also requires correction of the underlying disorder.

7.2.4 Total lymphoid irradiation

Total lymphoid irradiation (TLI) produces long-term suppression of helper T-lymphocyte function. Remission of autoimmune disease has been induced in various animal models. TLI has also been used in humans and produces partial (about 25%) palliation in patients with intractable RA or severe lupus nephritis. Serious side-effects, such as neu-

---

CASE 7.3 SEVERE RHEUMATOID ARTHRITIS TREATED WITH ANTI-TUMOUR NECROSIS FACTOR-α ANTIBODIES

A 55-year-old woman with active RA, previously unresponsive to multiple disease-modifying agents, was treated with a humanized mouse monoclonal antibody to TNF-α (anti-TNF-α) as part of a clinical trial. Following her first infusion of anti-TNF-α a significant reduction (60–70%) in clinical indices of inflammation (number of swollen and tender joints, duration of morning stiffness and pain score) and serum CRP was noted within 3 days. Unexpectedly, clinical and laboratory improvement was sustained for 12 weeks following the first infusion.

Table 7.5 Effects of plasmapheresis in various diseases

System	Examples of diseases	Benefit/indications
Renal	Goodpasture's syndrome	Treatment of choice in severe disease
	Rapidly progressive glomerulonephritis	
	Systemic lupus erythematosus	Only if desperate
Neurological disease	Myasthenia gravis	Yes — in severe disease only
	Guillain–Barré syndrome	Yes—as efficacious as intravenous immunoglobulin
Haematological disease	Isoimmunization in pregnancy	Yes
	Thrombotic thrombocytopenic purpura	No — only if plasma replacement therapy is given
Lymphoproliferative disorders	Waldenström's macroglobulinaemia	
	Myeloma	Yes — for hyperviscosity
	Cold agglutinin disease	
	Cryoglobulinaemia	

tropenia, thrombocytopenia, pericarditis and pleurisy, limit the potential use of TLI to severe cases.

7.2.5 Ultraviolet light

The known value of psoralen and ultraviolet A (PUVA) treatment in psoriasis has led investigators to assess the use of psoralens in autoimmune diseases. **Extracorporeal photochemotherapy (photopheresis)** is a form of immunotherapy in which peripheral blood lymphocytes treated with the photosensitizing compound 8-methoxypsoralen are exposed to ultraviolet A irradiation and reinfused into the patient. Psoralens, once photoactivated, bind covalently to target molecules and interrupt function. In autoimmune disorders, expanded populations of disease-provoking T cells should be affected more than the multitude of smaller clones of normal T cells. Studies in experimental animal models show that this approach leads to profound suppression of pathogenic T-cell clones. In humans, photopheresis is of palliative benefit for patients with advanced forms of cutaneous T-cell lymphoma and improves survival. Photopheresis has also been reported to be of benefit in the treatment of patients with pemphigus vulgaris and systemic sclerosis.

7.3 Immune potentiation

The best-established form of immune potentiation is **immunization** and this is discussed in section 7.7. Other ways of manipulating the immune response have been tried increasingly in recent years, with variable success. There are three other groups of potentiating agents: thymic hormones, cytokine therapies and gene replacement.

The most specific form of restoration of immune function is to replace a missing enzyme, cytokine or the gene coding for a receptor by gene therapy.

7.3.1 Hormones

Thymic hormones are produced by the thymic epithelium and bind to lymphoid cells via specific receptors. Several have been isolated and purified, including thymopoietin (TP5) and thymosin. There is no evidence of beneficial effect in humans and their use in cellular immunodeficiency has long been overtaken by BMT.

7.3.2 Cytokine therapy

Interferons are antiviral glycoproteins produced in response to virus infections which have wide-ranging immunomodulatory and anti-tumour effects (Table 7.6). There are three families of human interferon: alpha (α), beta (β) and gamma (γ). Interferons bind to cell-surface receptors and trigger secondary intracellular changes which inhibit viral replication. As a group, interferons have attracted much interest as immunotherapeutic agents. Genetically engineered, recombinant IFN-α, -β and -γ are available, but **IFN-α** is the best studied. Response rates to IFN-α therapy vary in different malignancies. In hairy cell leukaemia, cutaneous T-cell lymphoma and metastatic renal cell carcinoma, IFN-α has an important role in management of otherwise poorly responsive malignancies.

IFN-α is the treatment of choice for **hepatitis B and C** (Table 7.7). Given systemically, IFN-α produces significant clearing of hepatitis B in chronic carriers infected during adolescence or adult life, but has no effect on those infected

Table 7.6 Anti-tumour and immunomodulatory properties of interferons

Anti-tumour effects	Immunomodulatory effects
1 Direct antiproliferative effect on certain tumour cells 2 Increased tumour cell antigenicity • Enhanced MHC expression • Enhanced expression of receptors for TNF • Stimulation of NK cell activity	1 Macrophage activation 2 Induction of MHC antigens 3 Stimulation of NK cell activity 4 Activation of cytotoxic T cells

TNF, Tumour necrosis factor; MHC, major histocompatibility complex; NK cells, natural killer cells.

Table 7.7 Antiviral activity of interferon-α (IFN-α)

Local application
   Genital warts
   Herpes keratoconjunctivitis
   Laryngeal papillomatosis
Systemic administration
   Hepatitis B and hepatitis C infections
   Limited effect on human immunodeficiency virus
   Kaposi's sarcoma in AIDS

at birth (see Chapter 14). It also induces marked biochemical and histological improvement in some patients with chronic hepatitis C (see Chapter 14). Although IFN-α has **toxic effects**, these are usually tolerable. Most commonly, it produces flu-like symptoms, fever, malaise, anorexia and mental confusion. More serious problems are reversible bone marrow suppression, proteinuria, liver dysfunction and cardiotoxicity. There have also been reported exacerbations of autoimmune disease, including thyroiditis. Some patients make low-titre antibodies to IFN-α whilst on treatment, but have not developed clinical problems as a result.

IFN-β (interferon β-1b, interferon β-1a) has been shown, in randomized trials, to reduce the frequency of attacks in patients with relapsing–remitting multiple sclerosis (MS) (see Chapter 17). IFN-β-1a also slowed progression of disability, but it is unclear whether this will prove to be a sustained effect. Despite these results, the precise therapeutic role of IFN-β in MS remains controversial. The exact mechanism of action of IFN-β in MS is also unclear but may be related to inhibition of expression of HLA-DR on glial cells.

IFN-γ is a potent activator of macrophages and is most impressive in conditions in which defective macrophage function occurs, for instance lepromatous leprosy, leishmaniasis and chronic granulomatous disease (CGD). In CGD (Chapter 3), IFN-γ increases phagocyte bactericidal activity but only some patients show enhanced superoxide production, implying that IFN-γ works by several mechanisms. Following the results of an international double-blind study, IFN-γ is currently used in selected patients with CGD in whom prophylactic co-trimoxazole is inadequate to prevent infection.

IL-2 is produced by stimulated CD4$^+$ T cells (see Chapter 1). IL-2 acting on recently synthesized IL-2 receptors (CD25 antigen) induces clonal expansion of IL-2-positive T and B cells and stimulates activity of NK cells. IL-2 is used in immunodeficiency syndromes where IL-2 production is defective, such as human immunodeficiency virus (HIV) infection, and in malignant diseases or infections where weak immune responses are amplified by IL-2 (Fig. 7.6). In patients with HIV infection and baseline CD4 counts above 200 cells/mm^3, intermittent IL-2 infusions have been shown in controlled trials to produce substantial and sustained increases in the CD4 count. Genetically engineered, recombinant IL-2 is currently used in the treatment of metastatic renal cell carcinoma and malignant melanoma.

Treatment is limited by the **toxicity of IL-2**: common side-effects are flu-like malaise, mild bone marrow suppression and abnormal liver function. The most serious side-effect is the vascular leak syndrome: IL-2 infusion provokes massive release of IL-1, IFN-γ and TNF, all mediators of vascular permeability, with consequent marked hypotension, fluid retention, pulmonary oedema and neuropsychiatric symptoms.

Granulocyte colony-stimulating factor (G-CSF) and **granulocyte/macrophage colony-stimulating factor (GM-CSF)** are cytokines readily synthesized by recombinant DNA technology. They have not only a powerful stimulating effect on production of granulocytes (G-CSF) and monocytes/macrophages (GM-CSF) but also enhance the function of mature granulocytes and monocytes. When infused into patients, G-CSFs shorten the period of severe neutropenia

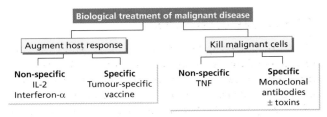

Fig. 7.6 Biological treatment of malignant disease. IL-2, Interleukin-2; TNF, tumour necrosis factor.

Table 7.8 Potential clinical applications of recombinant haematopoietic colony-stimulating factors

Use	Examples
1 Reduce duration/degree of myelosuppression following chemotherapy	Small-cell lung cancer Carcinoma of bladder Carcinoma of breast Metastatic melanoma
2 Augment haematological reconstitution following bone marrow transplantation	Non-Hodgkin's lymphoma SCID
3 Facilitate harvesting of bone marrow stem cells	Prior to autologous bone marrow transplant
4 Treatment of leukaemia with cytotoxic drugs or toxins	Acute myeloid leukaemia
5 Treatment of other neutropenic states	Aplastic anaemia Cyclical/congenital neutropenias Myelodysplastic syndromes AIDS
6 Improve host defence against potential infection	Burns

caused by radiotherapy or cytotoxic drugs, in which infections are the major cause of morbidity and mortality. The myeloprotective effect of these factors has allowed oncologists to boost the doses of cytotoxics used, with a consequent improvement in the chance of cure, without apparently increasing the morbidity of treatment.

Growth factors have **other uses** (Table 7.8). Haematopoietic malignancies and some solid tumours, like the cells from which they arise, can express growth factor receptors. Treatment with growth factors could result in accelerated growth and therefore increased sensitivity to cell cycle-dependent cytotoxic drugs. Such receptors could also be used as targets for receptor-specific antagonists or toxins. The main concern is that these growth factors may promote the growth of malignant cells and so provoke clonal disorders, such as myeloid leukaemia. Bone pain is a common side-effect, as is a vascular leak syndrome similar to that seen with IL-2 therapy.

7.3.3 Gene therapy

Since the demonstration that genes could be successfully transferred into humans in 1990, gene therapy has become established as an alternative strategy to BMT in carefully selected individuals (Box 7.2).

Building on promising results in severe combined immunodeficiency (SCID) due to adenosine deaminase deficiency, gene therapy has recently been extended to X-linked SCID associated with mutations in the common γ-chain cytokine receptor and chronic granulomatous disease. Using a retroviral vector (Fig. 7.7), several children with this form of

---

BOX 7.2 REQUIREMENTS FOR SUCCESSFUL GENE THERAPY

- A single genetic abnormality being responsible for the defect
- The normal gene being identified, cloned and inserted into a suitable vector (retroviruses, adenoviruses, plasmid–liposomal complexes)
- Cells with the inserted gene proliferating normally when reintroduced into the host to replace the defective cell population
- The gene product being detectable, to allow evaluation of the outcome

---

SCID are currently in remission with durable restitution, to date, of T and B cell function. Delight at the apparent success of gene therapy has recently been dampened by the development of T-cell leukaemia several years after engraftment due to **insertional mutagenesis** affecting the LMO2 oncogene, a possibility that had been feared. New vectors may overcome this.

The potential for somatic gene therapy is enormous, but this form of treatment must be shown to be ethically acceptable. Cloning of non-reproductive cells is permitted under strict regulatory approval in the UK purely for the purposes of therapeutic research. Recipients face the **risk** of vector-induced inflammation (as seen with adenoviral vectors), overwhelming viral infection by the vector (not seen yet) and the possibility, with retroviral vectors, of insertional mutagenesis, though inclusion of inactivation genes may prevent this.

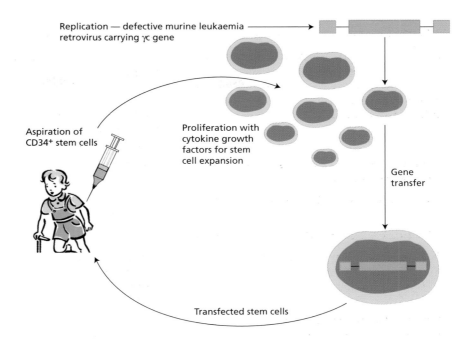

Fig. 7.7 Gene therapy for severe combined immunodeficiency (SCID) associated with mutations in the common γ-chain gene.

In addition to correcting single gene disorders, gene therapy is **potentially useful** in delivering therapeutic anti-inflammatory proteins to specific locations, a strategy that would be useful in inflammatory disorders such as cystic fibrosis.

7.4 Immunomodulation by intravenous immunoglobulin

Immunoglobulin replacement is *essential* for patients with primary antibody deficiency (section 3.2.8) and of proven value in several forms of secondary hypogammaglobulinae-mia, particularly infants with HIV infection and patients with lymphoproliferative malignancy. The serendipitous observation that IVIG raised the platelet count in two hypogam-maglobulinaemic children with idiopathic thrombocytopenia inspired a new approach to the therapy of **autoimmune disease**. The beneficial effect of IVIG must be established by controlled trials against placebo or conventional treatment and has been demonstrated in relatively few disorders (Table 7.9). More frequently, benefit has been claimed from open trials or anecdotal reports. In autoimmune diseases, IVIG is given usually at a daily dose of 1 g/kg body weight for 2 days, repeated every 4–8 weeks if necessary.

In acute idiopathic thrombocytopenia, the rise in platelet count occurs within hours of infusion but is often only

---

CASE 7.4 KAWASAKI'S DISEASE TREATED WITH INTRAVENOUS IMMUNOGLOBULIN

A 2-year-old boy was admitted to hospital with a 7-day history of high fever, lymphadenopathy, conjunctivitis and an erythematous exfoliative rash affecting his trunk and extremities. On the basis of the characteristic clinical picture, a clinical diagnosis of Kawasaki's disease (also known as acute mucocutaneous lymph node syndrome), an acute vasculitic disorder of infants affecting small and medium-sized blood vessels, was made. Other infective causes of a similar clinical presentation were excluded on the basis of negative blood and urine cultures. The results of initial investigations were as follows:

- Hb 110 g/l (NR 120–150)

- White cell count 14×10^9 (NR 4–11)
- Platelets 550×10^9 (NR 250–400)
- C-reactive protein 80 mg/l (NR < 10)

Since untreated or delayed treatment of Kawasaki's disease is associated with the development of coronary artery aneurysms, urgent treatment with high-dose IVIG (total dose 2 g/kg) was given in conjunction with anti-inflammatory doses of aspirin. This led to rapid resolution of fever and normalization of CRP (within 48 h). While IVIG is undoubtedly effective in Kawasaki's disease, the mechanism of action is unclear. For maximum benefit, treatment should be administered within 10 days of onset of fever.

Table 7.9 Intravenous immunoglobulin (IVIG) as an immunomodulatory therapeutic agent

Efficacy proven in randomized controlled trials (RCT)
- Immune thrombocytopenia
- Guillain–Barré syndrome
- Chronic inflammatory demyelinating polyneuropathy
- Kawasaki's disease
- Dermatomyositis
- Lambert–Eaton myasthenic syndrome
- Multifocal motor neuropathy

Ineffective in RCT
- Postviral fatigue (chronic fatigue syndrome)
- Rheumatoid arthritis
- Juvenile rheumatoid arthritis

Encouraging results in open trials/small numbers of patients
- Systemic vasculitis
- Steroid-dependent asthma
- Anti-factor VIII antibody-induced coagulopathy
- Myasthenia gravis in crisis
- Intractable epilepsy

transient; in other diseases, the effect of IVIG is long lasting. These differing patterns of response imply that different **mechanisms** operate. One mechanism of particular interest in autoimmune disease is the role of FcRn, the MHC class-I related Fc receptor for IgG (also binds albumin) which protects IgG from lysosomal degradation. Blockade of FcRn by high-dose exogenous IgG is likely to result in accelerated catabolism of endogenous pathogenic IgG with consequent clinical improvement (Fig. 7.8). In addition to monomeric

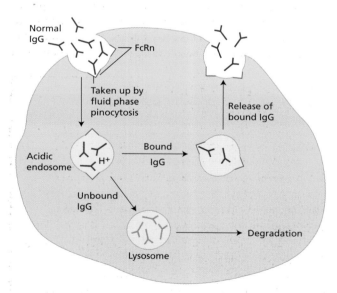

Fig. 7.8 Schematic representation of the role of the endothelial FcRn receptor in IgG homeostasis.

IgG, IVIG contains several other immunologically active constituents including antibodies to cytokines, anti-idiotypic antibodies, soluble CD4, soluble CD8 and HLA molecules which may contribute to its immunomodulatory effects at high doses.

7.5 Other uses of monoclonal antibodies

Monoclonal antibodies have great potential in diagnosis and treatment (Box 7.3).

Monoclonal antibodies have promise as **anti-tumour agents** (Box 7.3). Specific targeting and killing of tumour cells can be achieved by linking the monoclonal antibody to a cytotoxic drug (e.g. methotrexate or vincristine), a toxin (e.g. ricin) or a radioisotope (e.g. iodine-131 or yttrium-90), but any cross-reactions of the antibody with normal tissues will prove toxic. The demonstration of cytotoxicity of a monoclonal antibody in vitro has not always been paralleled by effectiveness in vivo.

Radiolabelled antibodies have been used for **immunolocalization** of tumour deposits, staging of malignant disease and determining the whole body distribution of amyloid deposits (Chapter 9). The monoclonal antibody is conjugated to a γ-emitting isotope (such as indium-111 or technetium-99), injected intravenously and the body scanned with a γ-camera to detect the label in presumed tumour-bearing sites. Intravenous injection results in substantial uptake in the reticuloendothelial system. Timing of scanning, the use of Fab fragments of antibody and computed tomographic techniques help to reduce background interference and improve specificity. The concern of using mouse monoclonal antibodies applies as much to diagnosis as it does to treatment (section 7.2.2.).

Autologous bone marrow grafting requires removal of bone marrow from the patient prior to supralethal therapy. Graft-versus-host disease is avoided, but, if tumour cells have already metastasized to bone marrow, they are returned to the patient in a viable form. Various methods have been developed for **purging bone marrow** of tumour cells. Monoclonal antibodies can kill targeted cells by subsequent addition of complement; however, tumour cells of low antigen density may escape cytolysis, and some tumours are relatively resistant to complement-mediated lysis. An alter-

---

BOX 7.3 OTHER CLINICAL USES OF MONOCLONAL ANTIBODIES
(in addition to Table 7.4)

- Direct action of monoclonal antibodies on tumour cells
- Diagnostic immunolocalization of tumours
- Removal—'purging'—of malignant cells from bone marrow in autologous marrow transplantation

native approach has been to link the antibody to toxins such as ricin or abrin. Cells can also be physically trapped, using monoclonal antibodies attached to magnetic beads, and removed with cobalt magnets.

7.6 Psychological factors

The concept that immune responses can be influenced by **psychological factors** is not new. *Stress undoubtedly affects immunity*, possibly via corticosteroid production or synthesis of other hormones and peptides, such as β-endorphin, by the central nervous system. Lymphocyte responses to mitogen stimulation in vitro are depressed after bereavement, and similarly impaired responses (lymphopenia, reduced NK cell activity and reduced IFN-γ production) have been noted in medical students during examinations! While the link between psychological factors and the immune system is unclear, it would be unwise to ignore the relationship and its potential for influencing treatment.

7.7 Immunization against infection

Prevention of infectious diseases depends on controlling (or eliminating) the source of infection, breaking the chain of transmission and increasing the resistance of individuals. In developed countries, the major factors in the virtual elimination of certain infectious diseases have been the supply of clean water and an increased resistance to infection resulting from better nutrition and improved personal hygiene. In recent years, however, immunization has been one of the most effective measures in controlling infectious diseases. With the emergence of 'new' pandemic infections, such as hepatitis C, AIDS and severe acute respiratory syndrome, novel approaches are needed to generate safe, cheap and effective vaccines.

7.7.1 Theoretical basis of immunization

There are two methods of achieving immunity: active and passive immunization. These may be naturally acquired or artificially induced (Fig. 7.9).

Active immunity is acquired when exposure to an immunogenic stimulus triggers an immune response by the host. The best type of active immunization follows **natural infection**, which may be clinical or subclinical: with many diseases, this gives lifelong protection at little or no cost to the individual or to the community. **Artificial active immunization** involves the deliberate administration of an immunogen in the form of a vaccine. Vaccines may be live organisms, killed organisms or their modified toxins. An ideal vaccine should mimic the immunological stimulus associated with natural infection, have no side-effects, be readily available, cheap, stable and easily administered, and produce long-lasting immunity. This latter property is dependent on it fulfilling certain immunological requirements (see Box 7.4). No current vaccine is ideal; each has its problems, but those encountered with live vaccines are generally related to their safety, while those of killed vaccines relate mainly to effectiveness (Table 7.10).

Live vaccines are selected so that they infect, replicate and immunize in a way which duplicates natural infection without causing significant illness. Examples include bacillus Calmette–Guérin (BCG) for TB, and poliomyelitis (Sabin), measles, mumps and rubella virus vaccines. Live vaccines must not contain fully virulent organisms. The organisms are therefore **attenuated**, so that their virulence is decreased without removing their ability to stimulate an immune response. The final vaccine represents a balance (see Table 7.10) between diminished pathogenicity and retained immunoreactivity. Even attenuated vaccines may induce disease in the immunocompromised host; an example is paralytic poliomyelitis after oral polio vaccination of hypogammaglobulinaemic individuals. **Killed vaccines** consist either of suspensions of killed organisms (e.g. typhoid, cholera and whole pertussis) or of products or fractions of the microorganisms (acellular pertussis). These include toxoids, prepared from the toxins of diphtheria or tetanus, and

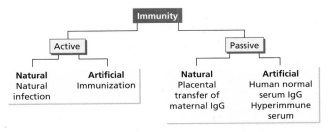

Fig. 7.9 Classification of immunity.

BOX 7.4 IMMUNOLOGICAL REQUIREMENTS OF A VACCINE

(After Ada G. *Lancet* 1990; 335:523–6)

1 Activation of antigen-presenting cells to initiate antigen processing and production of cytokines

2 Activation of both T and B cells to give a high yield of memory cells

3 Generation of T cells to several epitopes to overcome:

   (a) antigenic variation of pathogens

   (b) genetic variability in the host's immune response due to MHC polymorphism

4 Persistence of antigen on follicular dendritic cells in lymphoid tissue where memory B cells are recruited. Live attenuated vaccines fulfil these criteria par excellence

Table 7.10 Relative advantages and disadvantages of vaccines

	Live vaccines	Killed vaccines
Advantages	1 Single, small dose	1 Safe
	2 Given by natural route	2 Stable, therefore the potential of single batch of vaccine is known (i.e.
	3 Invokes local and systemic immunity	safety and efficacy)
	4 Resembles natural infection	
Disadvantages	1 Contaminating virus ?oncogenic	1 Multiple doses and boosters required
	2 Reversion to virulence	2 Given by injection — unnatural route
	3 Inactivation by climatic changes	3 High antigen concentration needed
	4 Disease in immunocompromised host	4 Variable efficiency

subunits of viruses (split vaccines), which are immunogenic but not infectious (e.g. hepatitis B surface antigen).

The *poor immunogenicity of pure polysaccharide vaccines*, particularly in infancy, has led to the development of **protein–polysaccharide conjugate** vaccines. Unlike pure polysaccharides, conjugate vaccines elicit sustained antibody responses and induce B- and T-cell memory. Examples of conjugate vaccines include those against Haemophilus influenzae type B (Hib), Neisseria meningitidis group C and certain serotypes of Streptococcus pneumoniae. The success of conjugate vaccines is exemplified by the dramatic reduction in the incidence of invasive Hib disease following the inclusion of Hib conjugate vaccine in the routine immunization schedule for infants (Fig. 7.10).

In general, killed vaccines are less successful than live vaccines; when a live vaccine is used, the replicating agent provides an immunogenic stimulus over many days (see Box 7.4). To produce the equivalent stimulus with inactivated vaccine would require a vast dose of antigen, with the risk of producing severe reactions. This problem is partly overcome by combining the vaccine with an adjuvant, a substance that enhances the immune response to the antigen (see below).

7.7.2 Adjuvants

Many purified or synthetic antigenic determinants show poor immunogenicity. *Adjuvants enhance the immune response to another antigen given simultaneously.* Thus, combinations of antigenic subunits and appropriate immunostimulatory compounds may provide a safe and effective vaccine. The best known adjuvant is **Freund's complete adjuvant**, which has been used for many years to stimulate specific antibody production in animals. It contains mycobacteria, oil and a detergent. *Unfortunately, it cannot be used in humans because it induces granulomatous reactions in the spleen, liver and skin.* The active component of mycobacterial membranes is **muramyl dipeptide (MDP)**, an adjuvant that seems free of toxic

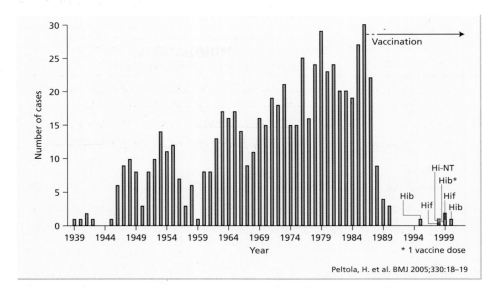

Fig. 7.10 Effect of introduction of Haemophilus influenzae type B (Hib) conjugate vaccine on the incidence of Hib meningitis in Helsinki. Hif, H. influenzae type f; Hi-NT, non-typeable H. influenzae. (Reproduced with permission Peltola *et al.* Incidence of Haemophilus influenzae type B meningitis during 18 years of vaccine use: observational study using routine hospital data. BMJ 2005; 330:18–19.)

side-effects and has now been synthesized. Its major action is dendritic cell and macrophage stimulation, with enhancement of T- and B-cell functions.

In humans, the most widely used adjuvants are **aluminium compounds (alums)**. These form a precipitate with protein antigens and result in slow release of the antigen. Alums are present in vaccines such as tetanus toxoid and diphtheria toxoid. **Biodegradable polymers** can be used as delayed-release capsules, dissolving weeks after injection to release a booster dose of antigen.

7.7.3 Routine immunization

Immunization of **children** is one of the most cost-effective activities in healthcare. Table 7.11 shows the schedule currently recommended in the UK, but recommendations for most other developed countries are similar.

Rubella vaccine is given to females to avoid the potentially disastrous effects of rubella on the fetus during early pregnancy. When maternal rubella occurs in the first 3 months of pregnancy, the risk of congenital infection is about 80%. At present, the vaccine is offered to all children and to all unimmunized girls aged from 10 to 14 years, plus any seronegative women with an occupational risk of acquiring rubella (e.g. nurses). Immunized women must be warned against becoming pregnant for 8–12 weeks after vaccination because the vaccine virus can also infect the fetus.

The risk of TB is now so low in some areas of the UK that authorities question the health benefit in giving **BCG** unless there is a special indication. This policy may be reconsidered in view of the increase in TB in countries where the prevalence of HIV infection is high.

Every vaccine can produce unwanted **side-effects** in some people. The *risk of these reactions must be weighed against the consequences of natural infection*. A historical example is whooping cough. The acceptance rate of whooping cough immunization in the UK fell from 80% in 1974 to 31% in 1978 following widespread adverse publicity about the possible risks of severe nervous system reactions. Whooping cough is a highly infectious and serious disease. Over 110 000 cases of whooping cough were notified in the UK between 1977 and 1979, an incidence many times higher than that before the adverse publicity; in this time, 26 children died and a similar number suffered brain damage. In contrast, the risk of serious nervous system damage attributable to the full course of pertussis immunization is about 1 : 100 000 children. About 750 000 children died from pertussis in developing countries and it would be a tragedy if **preventable deaths** on such a scale were to continue because confidence in a vaccine had been undermined unjustifiably. Immunization uptake may also fall if the public perceives scientific controversy, as evidenced by the drop in use of the MMR vaccine. In reality, there is overwhelming scientific evidence in support of MMR, but this message has been obscured by unbalanced media coverage. The benefits of immunization for a child (and for society) clearly outweigh the risks, provided that there are no contraindications to immunization (Table 7.12).

Patients with hyposplenism or those who have undergone **splenectomy** are at risk from overwhelming pneumococcal infection (Case 7.5). This is because splenic B lymphocytes are important in the production of protective antibody (IgG_2) against pneumococcal cell wall and other carbohydrate antigens. Pneumococcal vaccine contains polysaccharide antigens of the 23 most common serotypes encountered in Europe. Immunization offers some protection (about 60% efficacy) in these patients and should therefore be performed before elective splenectomy and in all patients with known functional hyposplenism. In the UK, immunization is also offered to patients with lymphoma, chronic renal failure,

Table 7.11 Current recommended immunization schedule for the UK

Age	Vaccine and timing
2 months	Diphtheria/tetanus/pertussis + polio vaccine + Haemophilus influenzae type b-conjugate vaccine (Hib) (first dose) + Pneumococcal conjugate vaccine (Pneu) (first dose)
3 months	Diphtheria/tetanus/pertussis + polio vaccine + Hib (second dose) + Men C (first dose)
4 months	Diphtheria/tetanus/pertussis + polio vaccine + Hib (third dose) + Pneu (second dose)
12 months	Hib (foruth dose) + Men C (second dose)
13 months	Measles/mumps/rubella (MMR) + Pneu (third dose)
4–5 years (school entry)	Diphtheria/tetanus + polio
10–14 years (if tuberculin-negative)	Bacillus Calmette–Guérin (BCG)
10–14 years (girls only)	Rubella
15–18 years (school-leaving)	Tetanus + polio vaccine booster

Table 7.12 General contraindications to immunization

Absolute contraindications
- Acute systemic febrile illness
- Any severe, local or generalized or neurological reaction to a previous dose of vaccine, particularly pertussis

Special consideration needed
- A documented history of cerebral damage in the neonatal period, convulsions or idiopathic epilepsy
- Children whose parents or siblings have a history of idiopathic epilepsy
- Children with evolving neurological disease
- Immunosuppressed patients—primary or secondary
- Pregnancy
- Egg allergy—since some vaccines are prepared in chicken eggs

HIV infection, and to those undergoing transplantation; in the USA, the recommendations are more liberal. Children under 2 years old respond poorly to this carbohydrate vaccine but mount adequate antibody responses to the new pneumococcal conjugate vaccine.

Despite new methods for producing vaccines (section 7.7.6), there are many infections for which no vaccines are available at present, for instance HIV, EBV, leprosy and malaria.

7.7.4 Immunization for travellers

Many diseases acquired by travellers are not preventable by vaccination. Cases of malaria continue to increase, particularly among travellers to West Africa. Travellers should be advised of mosquito bite prevention methods, such as nets and repellents, and the use of chemoprophylaxis. Travellers should also be **informed and educated** on food and water consumption, personal hygiene and the high risks of sexually transmitted diseases, particularly HIV infection.

Although no vaccine is 100% effective, vaccine-preventable diseases affect significant numbers of UK travellers each year. A very high proportion of typhoid and paratyphoid cases in the UK are acquired abroad, mainly in South Asia.

Typhoid vaccine should be considered for any UK resident travelling to endemic areas, as should inactivated **hepatitis A** vaccine, which is safe and immunogenic in 86% of recipients.

7.7.5 Passive immunization

At-risk patients exposed to certain infections can be given some degree of passive protection using human normal immunoglobulin or human-specific immunoglobulin. Passive immunity is short-lived because these IgG antibodies are slowly catabolized (half-life 3–4 weeks). **Human normal immunoglobulin**, in the form of intravenous or subcutaneous immunoglobulin, is essential treatment for patients with primary antibody deficiency (section 3.2.8), but can also be used as short-term prophylaxis against measles in immunosuppressed children, and to provide immediate short-lived protection against hepatitis A in non-immunized individuals. **Human-specific immunoglobulins** are in short supply and given only when certain criteria are fulfilled. Varicella zoster hyperimmune immunoglobulin may be indicated in children and adults with acute leukaemia or on immunosuppressive treatment who have been exposed to chickenpox, because varicella can be severe and fatal in such hosts. *Immunoglobulin preparations meant for intramuscular use should never be injected intravenously, as anaphylactic reactions can result.*

Monoclonal antibodies allow more specific protection against infection, but the results to date in humans have been disappointing. Randomized trials of antibodies against endotoxin and TNF have shown no benefit in patients with sepsis. Indeed, in a study of septic shock, blockade of TNF-α actually increased mortality. Although TNF-α is a mediator of sepsis, it has an important role in the generation of a protective immune response. It is possible that blocking TNF-α in this situation proved deleterious because of interference with the host's immune response.

7.7.6 Developing new vaccines

Many traditional vaccines are not ideal, and new approaches to vaccines are needed for infectious diseases of high viru-

---

CASE 7.5 FATAL PNEUMOCOCCAL SEPSIS 8 YEARS FOLLOWING SPLENECTOMY

A 35-year-old man felt non-specifically unwell for 24 h before being found collapsed at home. Despite intensive attempts at resuscitation by ambulance staff he was pronounced dead on arrival in hospital. Post-mortem examination revealed acute bacterial pneumonia and meningitis due to Streptococcus pneumoniae. His previous medical history was unremarkable except for a ruptured

spleen following a road traffic accident, necessitating emergency splenectomy, 8 years previously. It transpired that immunization with 'Pneumovax' (23 valent pneumococcal polysaccharide) had been overlooked at the time and the patient's compliance with subsequent antibiotic prophylaxis had been erratic.

lence, such as hepatitis C, AIDS or SARS. Rapid advances in immunology and recombinant DNA technology (see Chapter 19) have provided fresh impetus for production of chemically uniform and safe vaccines.

Polypeptide vaccines are made by dissecting viruses into immunogenic subunits which lack any infectious viral activity. The immunogenicity of the isolated polypeptides may be much lower than that of the intact virus particle; the way in which the subunits are presented to the host greatly influences the response. Further enhancement is possible by aggregating the polypeptides into water-soluble protein micelles.

When the DNA (or RNA in the case of RNA viruses) coding for the immunogenic viral polypeptide has been identified, the gene can be isolated and propagated by inserting natural or synthetic DNA molecules into a suitable vector, using restriction endonucleases (see Chapter 19). The best example of a **recombinant vaccine** is that developed for hepatitis B: the hepatitis B surface antigen gene is transfected into a plasmid vector which is expressed in yeast cells. The vaccine is safe, immunogenic and protective. Similar technology has been used to generate a candidate vaccine for HIV by molecular cloning of the envelope proteins gp160 and gp120, but neither antigen is effective at inducing a neutralizing antibody response. Several other HIV vaccines are currently under evaluation (see Box 7.5).

Recombinant infectious vector vaccines (or hybrid virus vaccines) can be made by inserting viral DNA into an attenuated virus, such as vaccinia, which then replicates in the immunized host. High levels of antibody are obtained to the inserted gene product as well as that of the parent virus. The potential advantages of vaccinia as a vector include low cost, ease of administration by scratching, vaccine stability and a long shelf-life. Against these must be weighed the known risks of adverse reactions with attenuated virus vaccines (see Table 7.10).

The safest form of vaccine is potentially the chemically **synthesized peptide**. When the nucleic acid sequence of the gene coding for an immunogenic protein is known, the amino acid sequence of the peptide can be deduced. However, very few immunogenic epitopes are composed of linear amino acid sequences; they depend on the tertiary or quaternary conformation of the epitope. Consequently, identification of the immunogenic epitopes is a major problem, and attempts to find them have relied largely on predictions, such as computer-based analysis — a hit-or-miss approach.

Genetic immunization using naked DNA (DNA vaccines) incorporated into plasmids shows considerable promise as a simple, novel form of immunization. **DNA vaccines** (also called nucleotide vaccines) are composed of a gene encoding for the relevant antigen incorporated into plasmid DNA which, when injected intramuscularly, induces a strong, sustained humoral and cellular immune response. DNA vaccines are effective in protecting mice against tuberculosis, chimpanzees against hepatitis B and rats against house dust mite allergy.

Immunization with DNA does not carry the risks associated with the use of live vaccines, but there is concern at the possibility of injected DNA causing oncogenic mutations in the recipient's genome or inducing lupus by triggering production of anti-DNA antibodies.

7.8 Cancer immunotherapy

Cancer immunotherapy offers a potentially exciting method of generating an effective anti-tumour immune response. It builds upon the widely recognized concept of immunosurveillance against cancer (Boxes 7.6 and 7.7), which has provided the impetus for immunotherapy.

Most cancers express tumour-associated antigens that are presented by antigen-presenting cells to T cells through either the MHC class I or II pathways. The principles of immunotherapy in cancer are summarized in Box 7.8. Since malig-

---

BOX 7.5 HIV VACCINES: POSSIBILITIES AND PROBLEMS

HIV vaccines under evaluation

- Live attenuated HIV with deleted/mutated nef gene or multiple deletions in several regulatory genes (gp160, gp120)
- HIV envelope proteins (gp160, gp120) in live vectors
- Whole killed HIV
- Gene for envelope proteins inserted into plasmid DNA (see DNA vaccines, section 7.7.6)

Obstacles to the development of an effective HIV vaccine

- Marked variability of HIV and the rapidity with which it mutates
- Inability of most anti-HIV antibodies to neutralize human HIV
- Lack of understanding of the correlates of protective immunity to the vaccine

---

BOX 7.6 CRITERIA FOR THERAPEUTIC TARGETING OF TUMOUR ANTIGENS BY MONOCLONAL ANTIBODIES

(Modified from Harris M. Monoclonal antibodies as therapeutic agents for cancer. *Lancet Oncology* 2004; 5:292–302)

- Antigenic target is stably and homogeneously expressed by tumour cells
- Is expressed negligibly in healthy tissues
- Has little or no soluble form of antigen (to avoid rapid antibody clearance)
- Is easily accessible to the monoclonal antibody

nant melanoma fulfils the criteria for immunotherapy, there has been much interest in developing vaccines containing peptides derived from melanoma-specific antigens such as MAGE or melanocyte differentiation antigens. While tumour regression has been observed in a small number of patients, the overall efficacy of cancer vaccines has, to date, been very limited.

7.9 Novel approaches to autoimmune disease

7.9.1 T-cell vaccines

Traditional methods of immunization concentrate on generating protective levels of antibody. However, some autoimmune diseases are caused by clones of T cells reactive against self-antigens. In rats, experimental autoimmune encephalitis (EAE) can be induced by immunizing them with myelin basic protein (MBP) extracted from the central nerv-

ous system. Virtually all of these rats develop an acute, often fatal, paralytic syndrome mediated by a highly restricted group of T cells, linked by their specificity for a single dominant epitope of MBP. Transfer of these pathogenic T-cell clones into healthy rats induces a florid EAE without the need for immunization with MBP. The different clones of encephalitogenic T cells have structurally similar T-cell receptors (TCRs). These autoreactive T cells can be regarded as pathogens which, when attenuated, can be used as vaccines against autoimmune disease. Rats can be protected against EAE by vaccinating potential recipients with the TCR of the pathogenic T-cell clones. Pretreatment of the autoreactive T cells by chemical or physical methods makes the TCR sufficiently immunogenic to trigger strong, clone-specific, cytotoxic CD8[+] T-cell responses in immunized rats, capable of destroying subsequently infused pathogenic T cells from that clone. Immunization with peptides derived from TCRs of encephalitogenic T cells also induces resistance to EAE. In some animals, however, immunization with TCR peptides has unexpectedly led to enhanced disease activity.

There are additional *problems in extrapolating from these animal experiments to human autoimmune diseases*. First, a prerequisite for the application of TCR peptide immunization is the existence of restricted TCR gene usage by autoimmune human T cells. Second, patients present with disease, not prior to it; and third, it is very difficult to identify and isolate the pathogenic T cell clone. Nevertheless, in the long term, immunization with TCR peptides may prove to be a viable treatment for autoimmune diseases in humans.

7.9.2 Oral tolerance

The concept of using **orally administered antigens** to induce immunological unresponsivenes (oral tolerance) has been known since 1911, when guinea pigs fed with hen egg protein were shown to be resistant to anaphylaxis when challenged later. The mechanisms underlying oral tolerance include clonal deletion or anergy (at high doses) and active suppression mediated by immunosuppressive cytokines such as IL-10 and transforming growth factor-β. Studies in animal models of autoimmune disease were sufficiently encouraging to warrant clinical trials in humans, but the results to date in MS, RA and uveitis have been disappointing.

FURTHER READING

See website: www.immunologyclinic.com

CHAPTER 8

8 Transplantation

8.1 Introduction

Transplantation of living cells, tissues or organs is well established as a routine practice. Cells (e.g. red blood cells, stem cells), tissues (e.g. skin grafting in extensively burned patients), or whole organs (such as kidney, heart, pancreas or liver) may be successfully transferred between genetically dissimilar individuals (**allogeneic grafting**). The outcome depends on the degree of 'matching' of the relevant transplantation antigens of the two individuals and successful therapeutic immunosuppressive measures to prevent rejection. In contrast, grafting of an individual's tissue from one part of the body to another (**autologous grafting**) is always successful, provided there are no surgical setbacks.

Transplantation across a species barrier, i.e. from one animal species to another (**xenogeneic grafting**), has been a focus of renewed interest, in view of the shortage of human organs (see section 8.6).

8.2 Histocompatibility genetics in humans

The surfaces of all human cells express a series of molecules that are recognized by other individuals as foreign antigens. Some antigens, such as those of the rhesus blood group, are irrelevant to the successful transplantation of human organs. In contrast, the **ABO blood group** system on red blood cells and the **human leucocyte antigens** (HLAs) on lymphocytes and other tissues are extremely important in blood transfusion and organ transplantation. HLA antigens are also called 'histocompatibility antigens' since they play a crucial role in determining survival of transplanted organs. They are encoded in humans by a segment of chromosome 6 known as the **major histocompatibility complex (MHC)** (see Chapter 1). Additional antigenic systems (minor histocompatibility systems) play only a minor role in transplantation and are largely ignored.

At least six HLA loci are recognized (Fig. 8.1). The HLA-A and HLA-B loci were the first to be defined and these code for a large number of antigens (see Chapter 1). Together with the HLA-C locus, these MHC class I genes code for products of similar biochemical structure which serve similar functions (see Chapter 1). They are detectable on all nucleated cells in the body. The methods of **tissue typing**, i.e. the detection of HLA antigens, is described in Chapter 19.

In contrast to antigens of the HLA-ABC loci, HLA-D loci antigens are restricted to B lymphocytes, macrophages, epidermal cells and sperm. The antigens of the D loci differ from MHC class I antigens in their chemical structure and

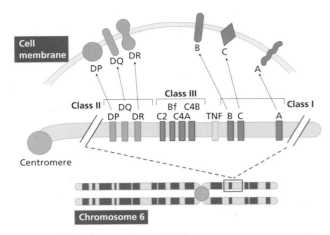

Fig. 8.1 Major histocompatibility complex on chromosome 6; class III antigens are complement components.

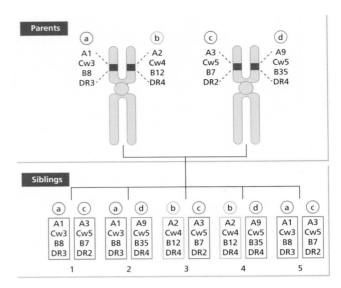

Fig. 8.2 Inheritance of HLA haplotypes in a family. Siblings 1 and 5 are HLA identical. Haplotypes are denoted as a, b, c, d.

interactions with immune cell populations; they are called **MHC class II antigens** (see Chapter 1).

In renal transplantation, **matching** for the *MHC class II antigens is more important than MHC class I antigen compatibility* in determining graft survival. Matching for the ABO blood group system is also important; naturally occurring anti-A and anti-B antibodies can lead to hyperacute rejection of ABO-incompatible kidneys, since A and B antigens are expressed on endothelium.

In bone marrow transplantation, a complete match of chromosome 6 gives the best survival; this is provided by an identical twin or HLA-identical sibling. Mismatched bone marrow invariably induces graft-versus-host disease (GVHD) with reduced survival of the graft (see section 8.5.3). The proximity of the HLA loci means that their antigenic products tend to be inherited together as an 'HLA-haplotype'. Because one haplotype is inherited from each parent, there is a one-in-four chance that two siblings will possess identical pairs of haplotypes (Fig. 8.2).

8.3 Renal transplantation

Kidney transplantation is now widely available for the treatment of end-stage chronic renal failure. Haemodialysis and chronic ambulatory peritoneal dialysis have enabled patients to come to transplantation in a state fit to withstand major surgery. The survival figures for transplanted kidneys have shown progressive improvement due to better immunosuppression with consequent reduction in mortality of patients. A kidney transplant is the treatment of choice for most patients in end-stage renal failure.

8.3.1 Selection of recipient and donor

Criteria for **selection of patients** for renal transplantation

vary between centres. Old age, severe sepsis, osteoporosis, a bleeding tendency or any other contraindication to high-dose steroids make a patient unacceptable as a potential recipient. Once selected, the patient has to wait for a suitable kidney to become available. Two types of donor kidneys are used: those from cadavers and those from living related donors.

The **selection of cadaveric kidneys** is rigorous (Fig. 8.3). In addition to the kidney, the spleen is also removed and

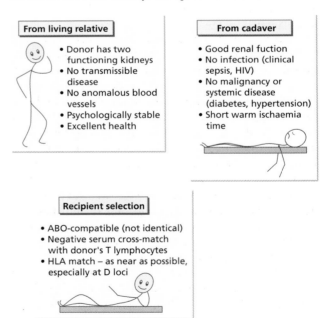

Fig. 8.3 Requirements for successful renal transplantation: selection of donor/recipient.

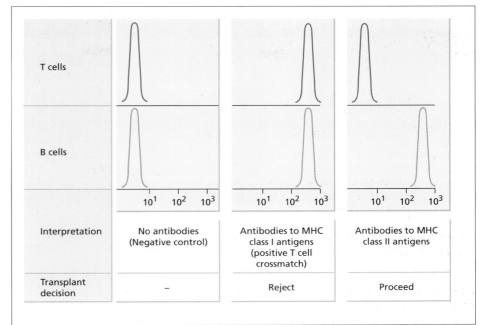

Fig. 8.4 Schematic representation of detection of cytotoxic antibodies in renal transplant recipients by flow cytometric cross-matching. Fluorescence intensity is depicted on the horizontal axis and the number of donor cells on the vertical axis (see Chapter 19 for discussion of flow cytometry). MHC class II antigens are expressed on B cells but not on T cells; MHC class I antigens are expressed on both.

disrupted, and the resulting lymphocyte suspension used to detect MHC class I and class II antigens. *Only patients with an ABO blood group compatible* with the kidney donor are considered suitable recipients; as in blood transfusion, a group O kidney can be transplanted to any recipient. Knowing the ABO blood group and HLA type of a cadaver kidney, the national register of potential recipients is searched by computer to find an ABO-compatible patient who matches the donor at as many loci as possible. Having selected the recipient, the **recipient's serum is then cross-matched against the donor's lymphocytes (Fig. 8.4)**. If the patient has cytotoxic antibodies to donor class I antigens (positive T-cell cross-match), then the kidney is unsuitable for that recipient. Paradoxically, the presence of circulating antibodies to donor class II antigens only may actually be advantageous.

Relatives who are anxious to donate a **live donor kidney** must be screened clinically and psychologically (see Fig. 8.3), and ABO and HLA typed so that the most suitable donor can be chosen. As discussed above, there is a one-in-four chance that a sibling will have the identical HLA haplotype (see Fig. 8.2). Where a compatible donor cannot be found, an attempt is made to choose someone with the least disparity at the HLA-DR locus, as this is the most important locus governing rejection of the graft.

Once the kidneys have been removed from either donor type, they are perfused mechanically with cold physiological fluids. Provided that cooling is begun within 30 min of cessation of the renal blood supply (**warm ischaemia time**), these kidneys have an excellent chance of functioning in the selected recipient. The duration of the perfusion (**cold**

ischaemia time) should be less than 48 h. The transplanted kidney is usually sited in the iliac fossa. Great care is taken with the vascular anastomoses and ureteric implantation. Once the vascular anastomoses are complete, the graft often starts to function immediately.

8.3.2 Post-transplantation period

In the post-transplantation period, the graft and the patient must both be monitored. Renal function may deteriorate immediately after surgery for several reasons (Fig. 8.5). **Acute tubular necrosis** can occur due to low blood pressure in ei-

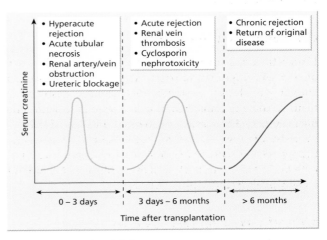

Fig. 8.5 Causes of graft failure.

CASE 8.1 ACUTE REJECTION

An 18-year-old student with end-stage renal failure due to chronic glomerulonephritis was given a cadaveric kidney transplant. He had been on maintenance haemodialysis for 2 months, and on anti-hypertensive therapy for several years. His major blood group was A and his tissue type was HLA-A1, -A9, -B8, -B40, -Cw1, -Cw3, -DR3, -DR7. The donor kidney was also blood group A and was matched for one DR antigen and four of six ABC antigens. He was given triple immunosuppressive therapy with cyclosporin A, azathioprine and prednisolone.

He passed 5 l of urine on the second post-operative day and his urea and creatinine fell appreciably. However, on the seventh post-operative day, his graft became slightly tender, his serum creatinine increased and he had a mild pyrexia (37.8 °C). A clinical diagnosis of acute rejection was confirmed by a finding of lymphocytic infiltration of the renal cortex on fine-needle aspiration. A 3-day course of intravenous methylprednisolone was started. Twenty-four hours later his creatinine had fallen and urine volume increased.

Subsequently, the patient had similar rejection episodes 5 and 7 weeks post-operatively. Both were treated with intravenous corticosteroids, and he has since remained well for over 3 years. Cyclosporin A was discontinued after 9 months but he still takes a daily maintenance dose of immunosuppressive drugs, namely 5 mg prednisolone and 50 mg azathioprine.

ther the recipient or the donor. If this happens, the recipient can be dialysed until renal function recovers; this rarely takes longer than 3–4 weeks. Alternatively, poor renal function may indicate **hyperacute rejection** (see below) or **urinary obstruction**, which must be relieved surgically.

It is crucial to *distinguish rejection from infection*, since the treatment for a bacterial infection is an antibiotic, not an increase in immunosuppressive therapy! Regular core renal biopsies are performed, but the procedure can damage the kidney and should not be done more than once every few weeks. Detection of rejection by **frequent percutaneous fine-needle aspiration** is much less traumatic, gives quick results and allows identification of infiltrating monocytes and increased expression of MHC class II molecules on renal tubular cells in the cortex — features of rejection (Case 8.1).

Immunosuppressive therapy (Table 8.1) is intended to prevent graft rejection and remains an essential component of management. Immunosuppressive drugs are fully discussed in Chapter 7.

Cyclosporin A is a powerful immunosuppressive drug, whose routine use has significantly reduced the number of rejection episodes and consequently the need for high-dose corticosteroids. It has also enabled many patients to be weaned off steroids in the long term. Maintenance immunosuppression varies from centre to centre; low-dose cyclosporin, azathioprine and prednisolone or a combination (triple therapy) may be used to minimize each drug's side-effects. The most frequent side-effects of **cyclosporin A** are nephrotoxicity, hirsutism, gingival hypertrophy and transient hepatotoxicity. *Nephrotoxicity is a major problem* and in vivo levels must be monitored; cyclosporin is stopped after 9–12 months to prevent long-term nephrotoxicity. Furthermore, there is a small but real increase in the risk of developing a lymphoma, especially if antilymphocyte globulin is used as well.

Until recently, azathioprine and corticosteroids were the mainstays of immunosuppressive therapy. Two new drugs have recently been added to the therapeutic armamentarium of the transplant physician. **FK506 or tacrolimus** (see Chapter 7) has been shown to be equally efficacious as cyclosporin. In practice, tacrolimus is used either in preference to cyclosporin in maintenance immunosuppressive regimens or in patients who experience rejection whilst on cyclosporin. **Mycophenolate mofetil (MMF)** (see Chapter 7), a purine-synthesis inhibitor, has replaced azathioprine in most post-renal transplant regimens following its use in three large randomized trials. In the MMF-treated arm, the absence of opportunistic Pneumocystis carinii infection was of scientific and clinical interest since the in vitro growth of Pneumocystis is dependent on inosine monophosphate dehydrogenase, an enzyme inhibited by MMF.

8.3.3 Clinical rejection

Rejection may occur at any time following transplantation. The classification of rejection into early, short term and long term reflects the differing underlying mechanisms (Fig. 8.5).

Hyperacute rejection may occur a few minutes to hours following revascularization of the graft. It is due to pre-

Table 8.1 Drugs used as antirejection therapy in renal transplantation

Prevention of graft rejection	Treatment of acute rejection
Prednisolone	Methylprednisolone
Cyclosporin A	OKT3 or antithymocyte globulin
Azathioprine	
Tacrolimus (FK506)	
Mycophenolate mofetil	

OKT3, Anti-CD3 monoclonal antibody.

formed circulating cytotoxic antibody which reacts with MHC class I antigens in the donor kidney. A similar picture is seen if an ABO-incompatible kidney is inadvertently used. Activation of complement results in an influx of polymorphonuclear leucocytes, platelet aggregation, obstruction of the blood vessels, and ischaemia. The patient may be pyrexial with a blood leucocytosis. Histologically, the microvasculature becomes plugged with leucocytes and platelets, resulting in infarction. The kidney swells dramatically and is tender. Red cells and desquamated tubular cells are often found in the urine. Renal function declines; oliguria or anuria follows. There is no successful therapy and the kidney must be removed. With improved cross-match techniques (see Fig. 8.4), hyperacute rejection has become very uncommon.

Acute rejection occurs within a few weeks or months following transplantation. Early diagnosis is important because prompt treatment with intravenous methyl prednisolone and/or anti-CD3 reverses renal damage. Clinical features may be masked by cyclosporin; a rising serum creatinine and a mild fever may be the only signs. It is important to exclude urinary obstruction or perirenal collections of urine, blood or pus. Histologically, there is a mononuclear infiltrate in the renal cortex, and necrosis of arterial walls; after successful treatment, the inflammatory infiltrate clears (Fig. 8.6). Acute rejection is associated with increased expression of MHC class I and class II antigens in inflamed grafts, and with early infiltration of CD8+ T lymphocytes. Fine-needle aspiration helps to distinguish rejection from cyclosporin toxicity. In a minority of cases, acute rejection may be refractory to treatment, particularly if it involves fibrinoid necrosis of the vessel walls.

Chronic allograft nephropathy results from a number of causes, including rejection and is seen after months or years

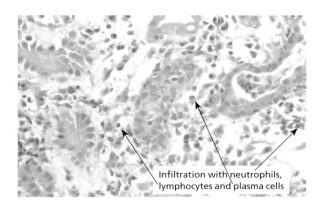

Infiltration with neutrophils, lymphocytes and plasma cells

Fig. 8.6 Acute renal transplant rejection (tubulo-interstitial pattern) showing interstitial oedema and a lymphoid infiltrate with tubulitis, typical of steroid-responsive acute rejection (courtesy of Dr D. Davies, Oxford Radcliffe Hospitals).

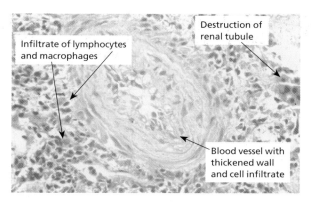

Infiltrate of lymphocytes and macrophages

Destruction of renal tubule

Blood vessel with thickened wall and cell infiltrate

Fig. 8.7 Chronic renal transplant rejection showing intimal proliferation with narrowing of arteriolar lumen (courtesy of Dr D. Davies, Oxford Radcliffe Hospitals).

of good renal function. There is slowly progressive renal failure and hypertension. Dominant histological findings are double contouring of the glomerular basement membrane, hyalinization of the glomeruli, interstitial fibrosis, and proliferation of endothelial cells. Many of these findings are non-specific except for concentric endothelial proliferation in arteries which is characteristically associated with chronic rejection (Fig. 8.7). Occasionally, a short course of steroids may be effective if a renal biopsy shows a predominantly cellular infiltrate, but fibrosis is not reversible. Chronic rejection must be distinguished from recurrence of the original glomerular disease (see section 8.3.6).

8.3.4 Immunopathology of rejection (the allograft response) (Fig. 8.8)

CD4+ T cells play a central role in rejection of allogeneic grafts; such grafts persist without requiring immunosuppression in 'nude' mice and rats, which congenitally lack CD4+ T cells. Furthermore, cyclosporin A, which blocks interleukin (IL)-2 production by CD4+ T cells, prevents rejection.

The rejection process has two parts: an **afferent** (initiation or sensitizing component) and an **efferent** phase (effector component). In the afferent phase, donor MHC molecules found on 'passenger leucocytes' (dendritic cells) are recognized by the recipient's CD4+ T cells, a process called allorecognition. CD4+ T cells are responsible for orchestrating rejection by recruiting a range of effector cells responsible for the damage of rejection — macrophages, CD8+ T cells, natural killer cells and B cells.

Recognition of foreign antigens (allorecognition) can occur in either the graft itself or in the lymphoid tissue of the recipient. **Allorecognition** occurs in one of two ways (Fig. 8.8): either donor MHC may be recognized as an intact molecule on the surface of donor antigen-presenting cells

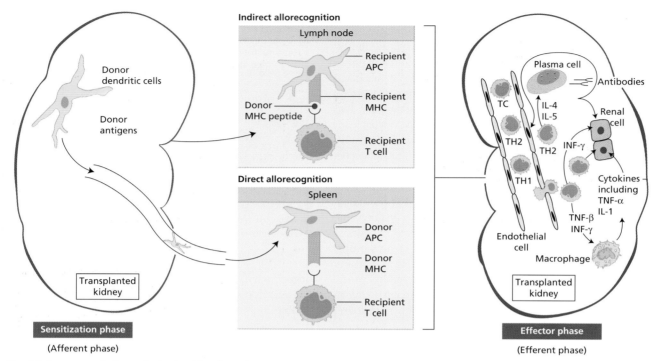

Fig. 8.8 Immunopathology of rejection (the allograft response).

(APC) by the recipient's T cells (direct allorecognition) or a peptide fragment derived from donor MHC may be presented by the recipient's APC (indirect allorecognition).

The direct alloresponse is important for initiating acute rejection, with approximately 2% of recipient peripheral blood lymphocytes responding to a particular alloantigen. The strength of the indirect alloresponse is much weaker, with only about 0.2% of lymphocytes being capable of responding to a particular alloantigen.

8.3.5 Graft survival

Long-term graft survival is closely correlated with the **degree of HLA matching** (Fig. 8.9), particularly at the class II locus. Extrapolation from the graph shows that 50% of fully matched cadaveric grafts will survive approximately 17 years, in contrast to mismatched grafts which survive for only 8 years. While the advent of cyclosporin has minimized the need for a close match at the entire class II locus, it is still important to obtain a good match at the DR locus (but less important at DP and DQ).

Patients who have previously rejected one graft may have **cytotoxic antibodies** which are associated with hyperacute rejection. Efforts to remove or neutralize cytotoxic antibodies with the use of immediate pre-operative immunoadsorption or intravenous immunoglobulin have met with only limited success. Retransplantation is only pos-

sible provided there is a completely negative MHC class I antigen cross-match (see Fig. 8.4), i.e. no relevant cytotoxic antibodies; they may have to wait a considerable time before a second suitable donor kidney is found.

Immunosuppressive therapy leads to generalized suppression; even this frequently fails to maintain the graft. The goal in human transplantation is therefore to induce a state of unresponsiveness (tolerance) to the specific donor antigens, but this has been largely unsuccessful.

8.3.6 Complications (see also Case 7.2)

An important aspect of the management of post-transplant patients is an awareness of their **increased susceptibility to infection** (see Chapter 3). *Death of the patient following transplantation is usually due to infection*, and rarely to graft failure, since, if the kidney fails, the patient can be maintained on haemodialysis (as in Case 8.2). Mortality due to infection has fallen dramatically in the past 15 years. Infections may be bacterial, fungal, viral, protozoal, or mixed and tend to occur at predictable time intervals following transplantation (Fig. 8.10). Infection with CMV is often associated with rejection of the graft. In an attempt to prevent CMV infection, CMV-negative recipients should receive CMV-negative blood products. Excessive immunosuppression has recently led to the emergence of BK polyoma virus in nephropathy; this may account for 1–10% of allograft

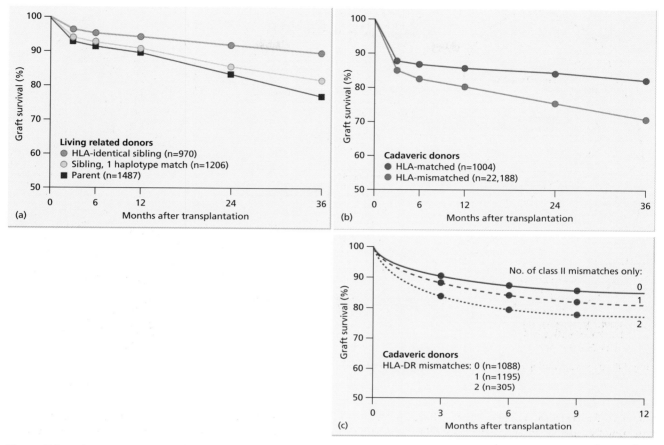

Fig. 8.9 Effect of HLA matching on renal allograft survival rates. (a) Effect of matching on grafts obtained from living related donors. (b) Effect of matching on grafts obtained from cadaveric donors. (c) Effect of different degrees of HLA-DR mismatches on survival of cadaveric grafts. (Data extracted from Suthanthiran M, Strom TB. Medical progress: renal transplantation. N Engl J Med 1994; 331:370.)

failures. Infections in immunosuppressed patients are fully discussed in Chapter 3.

A late complication of renal transplantation is **recurrence of the original disease** (see Chapter 9). This should always be considered in patients in whom there is functional deterioration following long periods of stable graft function. Although glomerulonephritis recurs histologically in about one in four transplants, the *clinical recurrence rate is much less*.

CASE 8.2 PRIMARY CYTOMEGALOVIRUS INFECTION IN A RENAL TRANSPLANT RECIPIENT

A 22-year-old welder was given a cadaveric renal graft after a month of haemodialysis for end-stage renal failure. His immediate post-operative course was uneventful and he was discharged home on maintenance immunosuppressive therapy (cyclosporin A 5 mg/kg, prednisolone 30 mg and azathioprine 75 mg daily).

He was readmitted on the 37th day with general malaise, muscle aches and fever but able to maintain a reasonable urine output (1700 ml/24 h). On examination, he had tender muscles and hepatomegaly; the transplanted kidney was not tender. Investigation showed a leucopenia but a normal serum creatinine.

In view of the leucopenia, azathioprine was withheld for 8 days, and intravenous corticosteroids were substituted. However, his

serum creatinine began to rise and urine output fell, necessitating haemodialysis. Stored pretransplant serum samples showed no evidence of anti-cytomegalovirus (CMV) antibodies or CMV antigen by polymerase chain reaction (PCR) analysis. IgM anti-CMV antibodies were detected in a current serum sample accompanied by a positive PCR signal for CMV antigen. These findings indicated primary CMV infection in the recipient due to transplantation of a CMV-positive kidney into a CMV-negative recipient. He made a complete recovery following prompt treatment with a combination of ganciclovir (a CMV-specific drug) and CMV-specific immune globulin.

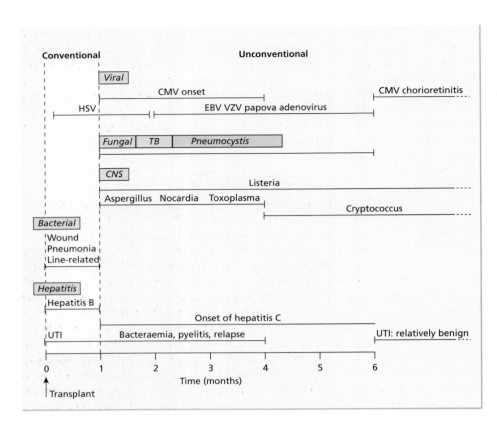

Fig. 8.10 Timetable for the occurrence of infection in renal transplant recipients. (Reproduced with permission Rubin RH. Kidney Int 1993; 44:221–36.) UTI, Urinary tract infection; CMV, cytomegalovirus; HSV, herpes simplex virus; EBV, Epstein–Barr virus; VZV, varicella zoster virus; CNS, central nervous system.

For example, in type II membranoproliferative glomerulonephritis (dense deposit disease), recurrent disease is histologically demonstrable in three-quarters of renal grafts, but less than 10% of graft failure in this group of patients is due to recurrence.

Another late complication is the development of some types of **malignancy** in the recipient (see section 6.5.1). The incidence of lymphoma in transplant recipients is 40 times greater than in the general population, and Kaposi's sarcoma, a major feature of the acquired immune deficiency syndrome (AIDS) (see Case 3.7), also occurs after transplantation. Both are not only more common when severe forms of immune suppression (anti-human thymocyte globulin or monoclonal antibodies) are used but are driven by viral infection — lymphoma due to Epstein–Barr virus (EBV) activation (see Case 7.1) and Kaposi's sarcoma due to the human herpes virus 8. Skin cancers also appear much more frequently in transplanted patients exposed to sunlight.

Transplanted patients also have an increased risk of **acute myocardial infarction**. This may be linked to hypertension, hypertriglyceridaemia or insulin-resistant diabetes, since these conditions are often present before transplantation, and are aggravated by steroids.

8.4 Other types of transplantation

8.4.1 Liver transplantation

The results of human liver transplantation have improved dramatically in the last 10 years (Table 8.2). The liver surgeon faces unique problems; these include the bleeding tendency of a recipient with liver failure and the technically

Table 8.2 Patient survival in various forms of transplantation

Organ	Actuarial survival at				
	1 year	2 years	3 years	4 years	5 years
Liver*	70%	—	—	—	60%
Single lung†	75%	—	> 50%	—	—
Heart and lungs‡	65%	—	55%	—	—
Pancreas‡	90–95%	—	68%	—	—

*Figures from Pittsburgh, USA.
†Harefield Hospital, UK.
‡Worldwide figures.

difficult surgery required to revascularize a grafted liver. However, compared with transplants of other organs, rejection episodes may be milder and require **less immunosuppression**. With the exception of an MHC class I cross-match, HLA matching is not routinely performed, although retrospective studies show a correlation between patient survival and DR compatibility. ABO compatibility is important but livers have been successfully transplanted across the ABO barrier in emergency situations. Recipients with life-threatening disease but some residual liver function are selected since they are best able to withstand major surgery. **Indications** for liver transplantation now include biliary atresia, hepatocellular carcinoma, primary biliary cirrhosis, end-stage hepatitis B and C and alcoholic cirrhosis.

8.4.2 Heart transplantation

Increased experience and the use of cyclosporin have resulted in rapid improvement in survival of heart grafts (Fig. 8.11). Hearts are allocated according to ABO compatibility. HLA matching is not required, although retrospective studies have shown a correlation between graft survival and MHC class II compatibility. The immunosuppressive regimens are the same as those used for kidney transplantation, with some centres opting to use additional induction immunotherapy with monoclonal antibodies such as daclizumab (anti-IL2 receptor). However, unlike renal patients, there is no satisfactory life-support facility (comparable to dialysis) if the donated heart is rejected, so **early diagnosis of rejection** is crucial. To this end, changes in the electrocardiograph are closely monitored; serial endomyocardial biopsies (with increasing use of fine-needle aspirates) show grossly increased MHC class I expression by myocardial cells in early rejection.

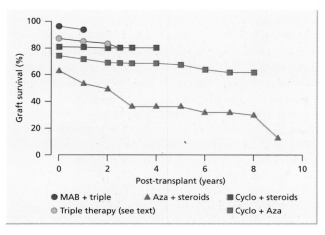

Fig. 8.11 Heart graft survival. Cyclo, Cyclophosphamide; Aza, azathioprine; MAB, monoclonal antibodies. (Data from Sir Terence English, with permission.)

A major post-operative problem is accelerated atherosclerosis in the graft coronary arteries. This is the major **cause of death** in patients who survive more than 1 year; it is estimated that 50% of patients have angiographic evidence of coronary artery disease in the graft after 5 years. Recipients are therefore treated with antithrombotic and anticoagulant agents. CMV infection of the donor heart is another major cause of morbidity and mortality in the first year.

8.4.3 Lung transplantation

Lung transplantation is now a well-established treatment for irreversible and potentially fatal lung disease. The most common **indications** are severe chronic airways disease, cryptogenic fibrosing alveolitis, cystic fibrosis, primary pulmonary hypertension and Eisenmenger's syndrome. Single, bilateral and heart–lung transplantation may be performed, with the last being particularly used when there is severe right-sided heart disease. Current immunosuppressive regimens and refinement of surgical technique gives a 3-year survival of more than 50% in many centres. After the immediate post-operative period, the major causes of death are infection, acute rejection and obliterative bronchiolitis, a process which may have a similar pathogenesis to chronic rejection of the kidney and heart and chronic GVHD.

8.4.4 Pancreatic transplantation

Improvements in surgical technique and better immunosuppression have resulted in 90–95% survival at 1 year of transplanted vascularized pancreatic grafts. In **diabetics** with labile glycaemic control, pancreatic transplantation results in excellent glycaemic control and improved quality of life. Most pancreatic transplants (90%) have been combined with kidney transplants in diabetics with poor renal function. Graft survival correlates with HLA compatibility. In stable non-uraemic diabetics, medical management is preferred to pancreatic transplantation.

Transplantation of isolated pancreatic islets is more hopeful, especially if attempts to reduce their immunogenicity are successful. However, human pancreatic islets are more difficult to prepare than rodent or murine islets and clinical trials have been disappointing so far. Recurrent autoimmunity leading to a recurrence of insulin-dependent diabetes occurs with both pancreatic and isolated islet cell transplants in humans.

8.4.5 Skin grafting

Allogeneic skin grafting in humans is useful in providing skin cover in **severely burned patients**. Although HLA-matched skin survives longer than mismatched skin, HLA typing is not done in practice because the endogenous immunosuppressive effect of severe burns allows prolonged survival of unmatched skin. Although the graft is finally rejected, the short-term protective barrier afforded by covering burns during this time is of enormous benefit to the patient in resisting infection. Skin can be taken from cadavers soon after death and stored in liquid nitrogen until required. Development of skin substitutes and the availability of cultured skin are promising.

8.4.6 Corneal grafting

Corneal transplantation has been routine for over 40 years. Corneas are obtained from cadaveric donors. There is no need to HLA type or systemically immunosuppress the recipient because corneal rejection does not occur unless the graft becomes vascularized. In grafts which do become vascularized, particularly those which follow chemical burns or chronic viral infections, HLA matching significantly improves survival (Chapter 12).

8.5 Haematopoietic stem cell transplantation

The transplantation of haematopoietic stem cells (HSCT) from bone marrow, peripheral blood or cord blood offers the only chance of cure for many patients with a wide range of disorders (Table 8.3). As in other transplant systems, graft rejection is common, but HSCT also has the *unique, and often fatal, complication of GVHD*, in which the grafted immunocompetent cells recognize the host as foreign and mount an immunological attack.

8.5.1 Indications and selection of patients

Theoretically, any abnormality of bone marrow stem cells is correctable by the transplantation of healthy stem cells; such abnormalities include absence of cells (aplastic anaemia), malignancy or functional defects (Table 8.3). **The risks of transplantation** are high and success depends on balanc-

---

Table 8.3 Indications for bone marrow transplantation

1 Severe aplastic anaemia
  Idiopathic
  Iatrogenic
2 Acute/chronic myeloid leukaemia — in first remission
3 Acute lymphoblastic leukaemia
4 Immunodeficiency
  Severe combined immunodeficiency (SCID)
  Chronic granulomatous disease, severe cases only
  Wiskott–Aldrich syndrome
  CD40 ligand deficiency
5 Inborn errors of metabolism

---

ing the severity of the disease against the risks of the procedure.

Ideally, the donor and recipient should be ABO compatible and MHC identical, but there is only a one-in-four chance that two siblings will have identical pairs of haplotypes (see Fig. 8.2). The use of cyclosporin A has enabled bone marrow to be used from HLA-matched but unrelated donors, as well as donors with one haplotype mismatch, such as parents.

8.5.2 Management of the patient

Preparation for transplantation usually begins 10 days before grafting. Measures to **reduce infection risk** include reverse-barrier nursing, decontamination of the skin and gut, the use of appropriate antibiotics and antimycotics. Intravenous feeding and immunoglobulin replacement may be required for those with failure to thrive associated with immune deficiencies.

The **grafting procedure** is straightforward; small amounts of marrow are taken from multiple sites under general anaesthetic. Bone spicules are removed by filtration through graded sieves. Cells can then be given either without fractionation (only in leukaemia—Case 8.3) or after removal of immunocompetent T lymphocytes responsible for GVHD (see Case 8.4). Cells are then transplanted by intravenous infusion. The optimal size of the graft is probably between 10^8 and 10^9 nucleated cells per kg body weight, although fewer cells are needed in immune-deficient infants.

Three major problems dominate the post-transplant period: failure of the graft to 'take', infection and GVHD. **Failure of engraftment** can be due to using insufficient bone marrow cells or rejection of the grafted cells by the host. Patients with some functional immunity (e.g. as in leukaemia in remission or partial immune deficiencies) require immune suppression prior to grafting ('conditioning') to ensure that rejection does not occur. Such patients are pretreated with cyclophosphamide and total body irradiation immediately prior to transplantation. Those patients with no immune function [e.g. severe combined immune deficiency (SCID), see Case 8.4] do not, in theory, require conditioning since they are unable to reject the graft, but some pretreatment is beneficial.

Recombinant growth factors, granulocyte colony-stimulating factor (G-CSF) or granulocyte/macrophage colony-stimulating factor (GM-CSF), are used to shorten the duration of neutropenia post-transplantation and so reduce **infection risk**.

A successful graft is indicated by a rise in the peripheral white cell count and the appearance of haematopoietic precursors in the marrow 10–20 days post-transplantation. The **rate of recovery** is influenced by many factors including prior chemotherapy, conditioning regimen, presence of GVHD and infection. Post-transplant immune reconstitu-

CASE 8.3 BONE MARROW TRANSPLANTATION FOR ACUTE MYELOID LEUKAEMIA

A 22-year-old man was treated for acute myeloid leukaemia (AML) with cyclical combination chemotherapy, and complete clinical remission was obtained after three courses. However, remission in AML is generally short; half the patients relapse within a year and second remissions are difficult to achieve. Bone marrow transplantation after high-dose chemoradiotherapy is therefore considered in young patients with suitable family members. The brother of this patient was HLA identical and willing to act as a marrow donor. The patient was given cyclophosphamide (120 mg/kg) followed by a dose of total body irradiation that is ordinarily lethal. Immediately after irradiation he was given an intravenous transfusion of 10^9 unfractionated bone marrow cells per kg obtained from his brother. He was supported with granulocyte colony-stimulating factor and platelet transfusions during the days of aplasia before engraftment occurred. Methotrexate was administered intermittently to try to prevent GVHD. He was discharged home, well, 7 weeks after transplantation, and remains free of leukaemia 7 years later.

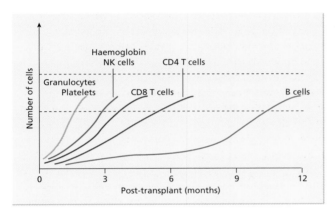

Fig. 8.12 Haematological and immune reconstitution following bone marrow transplantation. Dotted lines represent upper and lower reference ranges.

BOX 8.1 IMMUNOLOGICAL FACTORS UNDERLYING THE DEVELOPMENT OF GRAFT-VERSUS-HOST DISEASE

- Presence of immunocompetent T cells in the graft
- HLA incompatibility between donor and recipient
- Cellular immune deficiency in the host

tion is a lengthy process (Fig. 8.12). Significant impairment of T- and B-cell function is common during the first few months and underlies the increase in susceptibility to infection during this period.

The pace of immunological recovery is slower in recipients of T-cell depleted, HLA-incompatible marrow than in recipients of HLA-identical marrow. While T-cell function usually returns to normal within 6–12 months, B-cell function may take longer. In such cases, replacement immunoglobulin therapy is needed, possibly for life.

8.5.3 Complications and their prevention: graft-versus-host disease and infection

GVHD occurs in most patients who receive allogeneic transplants. The immunological prerequisites for the development of GVHD were stated by Billingham in the 1960s (see Box 8.1). Even in transplants between HLA-identical siblings, differences in minor histocompatibility antigens (small peptides derived from cytoplasmic proteins and presented by the MHC) provoke mild GVHD in 20–50% of cases. As in Case 8.4, the graft can take the form of blood products containing viable T cells. Consequently, the *use of unirradiated blood products in immunosuppressed hosts* (whether due to SCID or drugs) is *fraught with danger* and should be avoided. If blood cells are required, it is essential to ensure that they are irradiated to inactivate all immunocompetent T cells.

GVHD manifests **clinically** as a rash, fever, hepatosplenomegaly, bloody diarrhoea and breathlessness 7–14 days after transplantation. In severe cases, the rash may progress from a maculopapular eruption to generalized erythroderma and exfoliative dermatitis. A skin biopsy (as in Case 8.4) shows lymphocytic infiltration with vascular cuffing and basal cell degeneration. The **mortality** of GVHD is considerable; over 70% of those with severe GVHD and about one-third with mild GVHD will die. Treatment requires an increase in immunosuppression but, once established, GVHD is very difficult to eradicate. Since not all patients have suitable HLA-matched siblings (especially children with congenital immune deficiencies), ways have been sought to prevent GVHD.

Elimination or reduction of the numbers of immunocompetent T cells involves the use of T-cell-specific monoclonal antibodies and complement to lyse mature T cells. **T-cell depletion** of bone marrow can prevent GVHD and so abrogate the need for continuing immune suppression (Table 8.4). However, it is associated with an increased incidence of engraftment failure and/or relapse of leukaemia. This suggests that donor T cells have a role in eliminating leukaemic cells (**graft-versus-leukaemia**). New protocols,

CASE 8.4 GRAFT-VERSUS-HOST DISEASE IN AN INFANT WITH SEVERE COMBINED IMMUNE DEFICIENCY

A 3-month-old boy was admitted to hospital with failure to thrive and a persistent cough. On examination his height and weight were below the third centile. Initial investigations revealed marked anaemia: Hb 50 g/l, white cell count 8.9×10^9/l, platelet count 260×10^9/l. A chest X-ray was reported to be compatible with right lower lobe pneumonia but no organism was identified on blood culture. He was treated empirically with broad-spectrum antibiotics but failed to improve.

In view of his anaemia he was transfused with two units of packed red cells. Six days following transfusion he developed a widespread erythematous maculopapular rash and abnormal liver function tests. A skin biopsy showed diffuse vacuolar degeneration of basal epidermal cells with a mononuclear inflammatory cell infiltrate and aberrant expression of HLA-DR on epidermal keratinocytes. These findings were indicative of GVHD and raised the possibility of underlying immunodeficiency in the baby. Subsequent immunological investigations were diagnostic of SCID: i.e. marked T- and B-cell lymphopenia and hypogammaglobulinaemia.

In the light of this diagnosis, the baby was bronchoscoped and analysis of bronchial secretions revealed Pneumocystis carinii, a common pathogen in babies with defective cellular immunity. The baby was treated aggressively with co-trimoxazole, intravenous immunoglobulin and prophylactic antifungal therapy. Despite his poor outlook, it was decided to perform a single haplotype matched bone marrow transplant from his father. Sadly, this was unsuccessful and the baby died 3 days later from overwhelming sepsis. This was not unexpected, since transplantation in the face of established GVHD and sepsis often proves difficult. GVHD as a result of the use of non-irradiated blood should not occur now that there is greater awareness of SCID, but is included here to demonstrate the obvious similarity of findings between GVHD due to blood T lymphocytes and bone marrow cells.

While the general principles of bone marrow transplantation for leukaemia and SCID are similar, comparison of this case with Case 8.3 highlights some important differences (Table 8.4).

Table 8.4 Comparison of bone marrow transplantation (BMT) for primary immune deficiency with BMT for leukaemia

	Primary immune deficiency	Leukaemia
Age	Infants and young children	Adults
Need for pretransplant conditioning	On theoretical grounds, not required but in practice some conditioning is beneficial	Yes
T-cell depletion of graft	Yes	Yes (but certain degree of GVHD is beneficial in view of its antileukaemia effect)
Complications (infections, GVHD)	Similar	Similar
Pace of immunological and haematological reconstitution	Similar	Similar

GVHD, Graft-versus-host disease.

using incomplete depletion and mild immunosuppression, are currently under investigation to find a balance between GVHD, rejection of the graft and leukaemia relapse. Attempts to separate beneficial effects of graft-versus-leukaemia from GVHD remain experimental, but results are encouraging.

Serious bacterial, fungal and viral **infections** occur despite the elaborate measures aimed at reducing their incidence and severity. Infection with CMV is a common cause of death; evidence of CMV reactivation is seen in 75% of patients who are CMV-positive pretransplant. Patients are divided into two groups in terms of risk of CMV infection (Fig. 8.13).

Recombinant growth factors (G-CSF/GM-CSF) are used to shorten the post-transplant risk period by stimulating rapid maturation of neutrophils. Interestingly, they may also reduce the incidence of non-infective complications, such as GVHD.

8.5.4 Results

The results of HSCT vary according to the **indications** for performing the procedure.

Infants with **SCID** die before they are 2 years old unless marrow can be grafted. As the siblings of infants with SCID

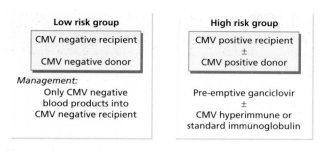

Fig. 8.13 Strategies for cytomegalovirus (CMV) prophylaxis.

are often too young to be bone marrow donors, grafting with incompatible tissue was originally attempted, but nearly always failed due to GVHD. The best results are still obtained when completely matched marrow is used, but T-cell depletion has dramatically improved the outcome if partially matched marrow is used. A **good prognosis** is associated with transplantation within the first 6 months of life and ablative therapy to the recipient's marrow before transplantation to ensure engraftment.

In **aplastic anaemia**, long-term survival following transplantation of selected cases is about 50% compared with only 5% without transplantation. Survival is better in younger patients who are relatively fit at the time of transplantation.

The results of chemotherapy for **acute lymphoblastic leukaemia** are now good, with most patients achieving remission, although only 60% or so are permanently cured (see Chapter 6). Patients (see Chapter 6) now undergo ablative therapy followed by bone marrow transplantation. Survival for this group of patients, who otherwise have a poor prognosis, is now 70% at 10 years, with most patients disease-free. The timing of the transplant in relation to remission remains important.

The technique of **autologous bone marrow transplantation** in leukaemia is established in many centres, although leukaemia relapse remains a problem. This involves cryopreservation of bone marrow taken from the patient during remission. The marrow is then 'transplanted' after total body irradiation has eradicated residual leukaemic cells. The technique has the advantage of eliminating the problem of GVHD but depends on removal of leukaemic cells from the preserved marrow; it is hoped that blast cell-specific monoclonal antibodies can be used selectively to purge the marrow of malignant cells (but not normal stem cells) (see Chapter 7).

8.5.5 Peripheral blood stem cell transplantation

The recognition that pluripotent stem cells can be mobilized from peripheral blood using recombinant G-CSF has led to blood stem cells being increasingly used as an alternative to bone marrow. Recently, there has been much interest in using umbilical cord blood as a source of stem cells in view of its easy availability and the possibility that cord blood-derived stem cells are easier to engraft. Claims that the risk of GVHD is also reduced await confirmation.

8.5.6 Stem cell transplantation for autoimmune disease

Following reports of long-lasting remission of severe rheumatoid arthritis in patients receiving allogeneic bone marrow transplants for drug-induced aplastic anaemia, autologous stem cell transplantation is currently being studied as a possible treatment for severe autoimmune disease, e.g. rheumatoid arthritis, systemic lupus erythematosus. The procedure involves ablating the patient's immune system with the aim of wiping out the cells responsible for autoimmunity. This is followed by infusion of autologous stem cells to repopulate the immune system. Theoretical concerns regarding the reinfusion of autoreactive T cells remain, since T cells are not routinely purged from autologous stem cells.

8.6 Xenotransplantation

Until recently, hyperacute rejection appeared to be an insurmountable barrier to transplantation between species. In the case of pig to primate transplants, this is caused by the presence of preformed IgM antibodies to pig carbohydrate molecules. This problem is now potentially soluble by several novel therapeutic strategies, but there are major problems regarding the ethical and infective issues (risk of transmissible porcine viruses) surrounding xenografts. Long-term immunosuppressive treatment of the recipient will still be required since porcine grafts evoke vigorous T-cell responses in primates.

FURTHER READING

See website: www.immunologyclinic.com

CHAPTER 9

9 Kidney Diseases

9.1 Introduction

Renal disease includes damage to the glomeruli, the tubules or the interstitial tissue. Immunological components are involved in most cases of glomerular damage (glomerulonephritis) and for some forms of injury to the renal tubules and interstitium (tubulointerstitial nephritis), although the precise mechanisms are not always clear. Humoral and cell-mediated immune mechanisms (Box 9.1A,B) play a part in the pathogenesis of nephritis but some common types of glomerulonephritis (e.g. minimal-change disease) and tubulointerstitial disease do not have a clear-cut immune basis.

The terminology of glomerulonephritis is confusing because three descriptive classifications have been in simultaneous use for many years, but none is entirely satisfactory in isolation. There is a clinical classification, describing the commoner modes of presentation; a morphological classification, based on light and electron microscope findings; and an immunological classification, based on the proposed immune mechanism of renal damage.

9.2 Clinical syndromes

Several clinical syndromes are recognized, but with considerable overlap.

Recurrent haematuria may be the first manifestation of renal or extrarenal disease. It can be macroscopic or microscopic. Haematuria of unknown origin requires urological

---

BOX 9.1A WAYS IN WHICH ANTIBODIES CAN INDUCE DAMAGE

- Antibody may react directly with the glomerular or tubular basement membrane

- Antibody may form immune complexes with antigens which subsequently lodge in the kidney

- Antigen may bind with, or be trapped in, the glomerular basement membrane and react with antibody subsequently

- Antibody may induce a vasculitic process that damages the capillary plexus of the glomerulus

BOX 9.1B EVIDENCE THAT T-CELL-MEDIATED MECHANISMS ARE INVOLVED IN PATHOGENESIS OF GLOMERULONEPHRITIS

- Adoptive transfer of sensitized T cells to rats treated with sub-nephritogenic doses of antibody causes glomerular hypercellularity due to proliferation of resident glomerular cells and an influx of mononuclear leucocytes.

- Severe proliferative nephritis can develop after immunization with glomerular basement membrane in bursectomized chickens unable to mount antibody responses

- In humans, T lymphocytes have been found in proliferative and non-proliferative glomerulopathies

- Treatment with cyclosporin is effective in some glomerular disorders

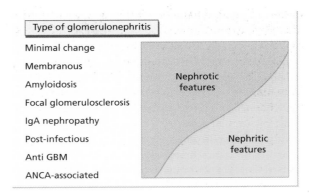

Fig. 9.1 Overlap of nephritic and nephrotic features of various forms of glomerular disease.

(Fig. 9.1). A definite diagnosis leading to a prognosis can be made only by renal biopsy.

9.3 Classifications of glomerulonephritis

An understanding of glomerulonephritis requires a grasp of normal **glomerular structure** (Fig. 9.2a,b). The glomerulus is a unique capillary plexus, fed by an afferent arteriole and drained by an efferent arteriole, supported by a stalk called

investigation to exclude a site of bleeding in the upper and lower urinary tracts.

Persistent proteinuria: a small amount of albumin (up to 30 mg/day) is normally present in urine of healthy adults. Amounts in excess of this are pathological. Excretion of > 300 mg albumin per 24 h is termed 'overt albuminuria', while excretion of amounts between 30 and 300 mg/day is called 'microalbuminuria'. Overt proteinuria is a cardinal sign of established glomerular damage and a risk factor for declining renal function. The higher the level of proteinuria, the faster the development of tubulointerstitial lesions and renal fibrosis and the progression to chronic renal failure. Proteinuria is often discovered by chance when urine is tested for some other reason. Microalbuminuria is used as a marker of early diabetic nephropathy and therapeutic interventions are increasingly targeted at the early microalbuminuric stage in the belief that pathological damage may be modifiable or even reversible at this point.

Nephrotic syndrome is defined as hypoalbuminaemia and oedema resulting from severe proteinuria, usually in excess of 3.5 g/day. In children, this is a common presentation of glomerulonephritis.

Acute nephritis is characterized by sudden onset of haematuria, proteinuria, hypertension and oliguria.

Renal failure may be acute or chronic. Acute renal failure is a period of sudden, severe impairment of renal function, usually triggered by some vascular or inflammatory insult. Chronic renal failure may be the end result of any disorder which destroys normal renal architecture; although there are many causes, about half of cases are caused by some type of glomerulonephritis.

There is a poor correlation between the clinical picture and the underlying morphology. A specific form of glomerulonephritis can show different clinical features in different patients or even in the same patient at different times

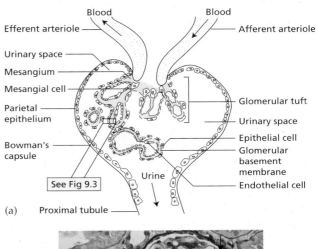

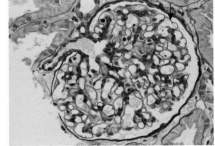

Fig. 9.2 (a) Normal glomerular structure. (b) Normal glomerular histology (PAS stain). The basement membrane is arrowed.

the mesangium. As the afferent arteriole enters the glomerulus, it divides into numerous capillary loops. The wall of the capillary loop (Fig. 9.3) acts as the glomerular filter and is composed of three layers: an inner layer of glomerular endothelial cells, an outer (i.e. urinary side) layer of glomerular epithelial cells, and the glomerular basement membrane between them. Each layer has specialized features distinguishing it from capillary walls elsewhere in the body.

Endothelial cells offer no anatomical barrier to the passage of molecules. The cytoplasm of the endothelial cells forms a thin layer perforated by fenestrations much larger in diameter than macromolecules in the plasma. These openings allow capillary blood to come into direct contact with the glomerular basement membrane.

Glomerular basement membrane (GBM) has unique constituents with restricted isoforms of laminin, type IV collagen and proteoglycans, highly negatively charged molecules which account for the charge-dependent filtration that normally conserves plasma proteins.

Epithelial cells or podocytes are arranged around the capillaries (Fig. 9.3). Epithelial cells are phagocytic. Each cell has multiple foot processes which interdigitate and are partly embedded in the outer layer of the GBM. A thin membrane—called the slit diaphragm—bridges the spaces between the foot processes of the podocytes and is vital for maintaining the barrier to plasma proteins. Several interacting slit diaphragm proteins have been identified and mutations in the genes coding for some of them are associated with inherited forms of nephrotic syndrome, strongly implying that podocytes are vital in preventing proteinuria in healthy people. Disruption of structural slit diaphragm proteins by proteinuria may predispose to apoptosis of podocytes.

The **mesangium**, the central core of tissue in the glomerulus, is made up of mesangial cells separated by an extensive matrix. The mesangial region can take up and dispose of large molecules, particularly immune complexes. The mesangial matrix ultimately drains into renal lymphatics.

9.3.1 Histological classification

Glomeruli are composed of three main cell types—mesangial, endothelial and epithelial—and any or all of these cells may increase in number in response to injury. The term glomerulonephritis must therefore be qualified (Table 9.1) by defining the types of cells affected and whether part or all of the glomerulus is damaged. Classification is based on light microscopy, electron microscopy and immunohistochemistry.

9.3.2 Immune mechanisms of glomerulonephritis

The evidence that human glomerulonephritides are immunological disorders relies heavily on animal experiments. At

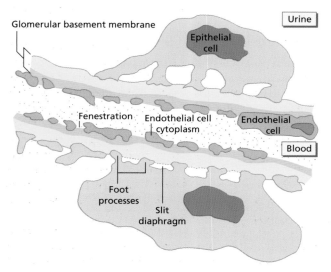

Fig. 9.3 A section across a normal capillary loop (see text for explanation).

Table 9.1 Some descriptive terms used in the morphological classification of nephritis

Extent of damage	
• Diffuse	Involving all glomeruli
• Focal	Involving some glomeruli only
• Segmental	Involving part of a glomerulus while the rest of that glomerulus appears normal
Cellular changes	
• Proliferative	An increase in the numbers of cells within the glomerular tuft. Subgroups exist in which proliferation is predominantly confined to a particular cell type
• Membranous	Thickening of the glomerular capillary wall by abnormal deposits on the epithelial aspect of the basement membrane
• Membranoproliferative	Proliferation of cells **plus** thickening of the glomerular capillary wall
• Crescents	Proliferation of parietal epithelial cells (extracapillary proliferation)

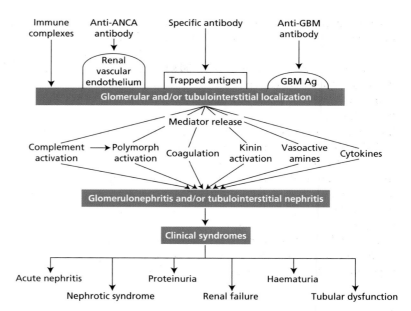

Fig. 9.4 Immunopathological mechanisms involved in clinical syndromes of nephritis.

least two mechanisms are known to induce glomerulonephritis in animals:
• deposition of circulating antigen–antibody complexes within glomeruli — 'immune-complex nephritis'; and
• reaction of circulating antibodies with antigens which are part of the GBM (for instance, 'anti-GBM' nephritis), antigens that have been trapped there or antigenic components of renal vascular endothelium (Fig. 9.4).

After the initiation of glomerular injury, a number of proinflammatory mediator pathways (Fig. 9.4) are activated both in infiltrating cells and in resident glomerular cells and participate in the destructive and restorative processes. Remodelling of extracellular matrix after injury generates signals that differ from those transmitted by normal glomerular matrix and induces activation and proliferation of resident and infiltrating cells in the glomerulus. Haemodynamic changes in remaining functional glomeruli cause hyperfiltration, intraglomerular hypertension and abnormal intravascular shear forces which can worsen glomerular injury. Depending on the cells affected, apoptosis may have a crucial role either in resolution of damage or in causing glomerular scarring.

9.4 Asymptomatic haematuria

Some forms of glomerulonephritis often follow infections of the respiratory tract and usually involve mesangial deposits of IgA.

9.4.1 IgA nephropathy

IgA nephropathy ('mesangial IgA deposition' or 'Berger's disease') is the most common form of primary glomerulone-

phritis in the world. It accounts for about 10% of all cases of primary glomerular disease in the USA, 20% of cases in Europe and 30–40% in Asia. It affects mainly older children or young adults, and **presents typically** as recurrent episodes of macroscopic haematuria occurring after an upper respiratory tract infection or, less frequently, a gastrointestinal or urinary tract infection, or strenuous exercise. Presentation with acute nephritis, hypertension, the nephrotic syndrome or as a chance finding of microscopic haematuria is less frequent. In contrast to poststreptococcal glomerulonephritis (see Case 9.3), the period between infection and haematuria is short, ranging from hours to a few days.

The clinical features are variable and yet the **biopsy findings** are constant and probably persist indefinitely. On light microscopy, the glomeruli show focal and segmental mesangial proliferation and, as the name of the condition implies, prominent deposits of IgA are found in the mesangium of every glomerulus (Fig. 9.5a,b), together with complement components of the alternate pathway. IgA nephropathy can be considered a type of renal limited vasculitis caused by an innate defect in IgA mucosal immunity: repeated exposure to a variety of environmental antigens results in a heightened systemic IgA response, mainly of the IgA$_1$ subclass. Glomerular damage may result from self-aggregation of abnormally glycosylated IgA$_1$ which interacts with mesangial cells. An association is recognized between IgA nephropathy and chronic liver disease, coeliac disease and dermatitis herpetiformis, other disorders linked with immune complexes containing IgA.

Patients presenting with nephrotic-range proteinuria, hypertension or crescents on biopsy are more likely to progress to renal failure. Spontaneous clinical remission occurs in about 10% of patients. Of the remainder, renal survival of

CASE 9.1 IgA NEPHROPATHY

A 14-year-old boy presented with an 18-month history of inter-mittent, painless haematuria, usually occurring after strenuous exercise, but without dysuria or increased frequency of micturition. He also had frequent colds and sore throats and believed that the haematuria also happened at these times. On examination, he appeared fit and healthy; his blood pressure was 120/75. Urine analysis showed microscopic haematuria (3+) and a trace of protein. Intravenous urography, a micturating cystogram and cystoscopy were normal. His haemoglobin, white cell count, blood urea and

creatinine clearance were normal; the urinary protein excretion was 0.95 g/day. Immunoglobulin, CH_{50}, C4 and C3 levels were within normal limits. In view of the duration of haematuria, a renal biopsy was performed. Twelve glomeruli were present: all showed a diffuse increase in mesangial cells with thickening of the matrix. Immunofluorescent examination of the biopsy showed mesangial deposits of IgA and C3 (Fig. 9.5a). The appearances were characteristic of IgA nephropathy.

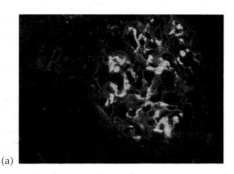

(a)

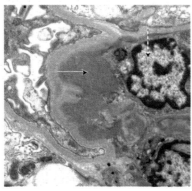

(b)

Fig. 9.5 (a) IgA nephropathy showing IgA deposits in the mesangium on immunofluorescence. (b) Electron micrograph of IgA nephropathy showing an IgA deposit (arrowed) and an adjacent mesangial cell (interrupted arrow).

80–90% at 10 years and 50–80% at 20 years implies that IgA nephropathy is a relatively benign disease with a good **prognosis** but, because IgA nephropathy is so common, it contributes significantly to the population with end-stage renal failure (ESRF) (10–20% of cases). The risk of developing renal failure increases by about 1% per year.

There is no specific **treatment** and trials of immunosuppression and plasma exchange have been controversial. Treatment is limited to those with a poor long-term prognosis. Angiotensin II receptor blockers, angiotensin-converting enzyme (ACE) inhibitors and fish oil supplements

have been used for their renoprotective and antiproteinuria effects, with some benefit.

Mesangial IgA deposition recurs in about 50% of **transplanted kidneys** (see Table 9.8). In contrast, when donor kidneys with occult mesangial IgA deposits are transplanted into patients without previous IgA-related disease, the deposits disappear progressively over a period of 6 months. Spontaneous clearance by the recipient again implies that an abnormal host response is involved in the pathogenesis of IgA nephropathy.

9.4.2 Henoch–Schönlein nephritis

Henoch–Schönlein nephritis (Henoch–Schönlein purpura or anaphylactoid purpura) is a common form of systemic vasculitis in which small blood vessels in a number of organs are involved. It is usually a disease of children, with a peak age of onset between 4 and 10 years. The syndrome is characterized by non-thrombocytopenic purpura of the skin (particularly around joints) (Fig. 9.6), arthralgia, gastrointestinal pain and glomerulonephritis. *Kidney disease is the most important manifestation of HSN and renal failure is the main cause of death.* The overall prevalence of renal disease varies from 40 to 100% but in most patients this is mild; progression to renal failure occurs in fewer than 10%. Those with the most severe clinical presentation have the worst outcome: about 40% of those with nephritic or nephrotic syndromes at onset show long-term impairment of renal function. **Treatment** is largely empirical, controversial and, at best, only partially effective. Steroids seem to control the joint and abdominal pain but have no effect on the skin or renal involvement.

Immunohistology of the **renal biopsy** shows irregular, granular deposits of IgA, C3 and fibrin in the glomeruli. Deposits of IgA and C3 are also found in the skin, even in non-affected areas, and are diagnostic of the condition. As in IgA nephropathy, the available evidence suggests an IgA-dominant immune-complex pathogenesis with complement activation occurring via the alternate pathway. A variety of

CASE 9.2 HENOCH–SCHÖNLEIN NEPHRITIS

A 12-year-old boy presented with a 1-week history of pain in the left loin. This was diagnosed as a urinary tract infection and treated with amoxicillin. One week later, he developed a purpuric rash around the ankles, accompanied by some blistering and superficial necrosis. Shortly afterwards, he developed pain in the left elbow joint. On admission to hospital, he was noted to have haematuria and proteinuria and a blood pressure of 130/90. Over the next month, he suffered further episodes of abdominal colic and purpura. His haemoglobin was 95 g/l with a normal white cell count. Antinuclear antibodies were negative and total haemolytic complement, C4 and C3 levels were normal. Although his blood urea was normal, his creatinine clearance was low at 31 ml/min per m² with proteinuria of 4.5 g/day.

A skin biopsy of a purpuric lesion showed vasculitic changes in the dermis, with IgA and C3 deposition in the blood-vessel walls. A renal biopsy, containing 21 glomeruli per section, showed epithelial crescents and diffuse mesangial hypercellularity in seven glomeruli. On immunofluorescence, granular deposits of IgA and C3 and, to a lesser extent, IgG and properdin were present in the mesangium. The clinical and histological features were those of Henoch–Schön-lein nephritis (HSN). Because of the heavy proteinuria and diminished creatinine clearance, he was treated with cyclophosphamide (as part of an international study of treatment in this condition). Over a 9-month follow-up period, the purpura and episodes of abdominal colic subsided, his creatinine clearance increased to 47 ml/min, but he continued to have moderately heavy proteinuria (3.2 g/day). The prognosis is uncertain.

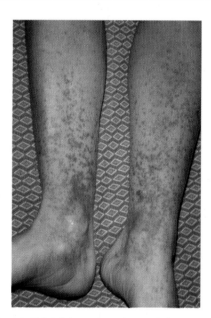

Fig. 9.6 Henoch–Schönlein purpura in an adult.

bacterial or viral antigens could be involved, as there is an association with preceding upper respiratory tract infection. In addition, HSN is a seasonal disease: most patients present during the winter. The clinical and immunological similarity between HSN and IgA nephropathy suggests that IgA nephropathy is a renal limited form of HSN.

9.5 Acute glomerulonephritis

9.5.1 Acute immune-complex nephritis

A single intravenous injection of a foreign protein into a rabbit causes vasculitis, arthritis and glomerulonephritis about 10 days later (**'one-shot' serum sickness**) (Fig. 9.7). This occurs when the amount of circulating antigen is still in excess of specific IgG antibody produced in response to the stimulus (see Chapter 1); the small immune complexes so formed are soluble but become trapped in capillary membranes, particularly in the kidney. Immunofluorescent examination of the kidney shows deposition of the injected antigen, specific antibodies and complement components in an irregular, granular ('lumpy-bumpy') distribution along the GBM. Renal injury is due to the resultant attraction and accumulation of polymorphs in the glomeruli and release of inflammatory mediators.

The symptomatic phase is usually transient and subsides, with complete healing, as the complexes, both soluble and fixed, are cleared in around 2–4 weeks.

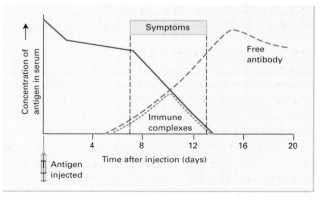

Fig. 9.7 Immune-complex formation in acute serum sickness.

9.5.2 Acute postinfectious glomerulonephritis

Acute poststreptococcal glomerulonephritis is now seldom seen in developed countries. Usually, it is a disease of children aged 2–10 years, but adolescents and adults may be affected. Over 90% of cases are preceded by streptococcal infection of the throat or skin. Patients **typically present** with acute nephritis 7–12 days after a throat infection or about 3 weeks after a skin infection. The diagnosis rests on prior microbiological culture, increasing titres of streptococcal antibodies and a low serum C3 level. Although the ASO titre is high in most cases which follow a throat infection, it is a less consistent finding following skin infection. Firm evidence of streptococcal infection is found in only one-third of patients with acute glomerulonephritis. Postinfectious glomerulonephritis is about 10 times more common in developing countries, with parasitic (malaria, filariasis) and viral (hepatitis B or C) organisms being important aetiological agents.

In adults, postinfectious glomerulonephritis is seen increasingly in immunocompromised adults and in the elderly. It is frequently linked to staphylococcal and Gram-negative bacterial infections, often at multiple sites. The clinical presentation can be insidious and the diagnosis made only after renal biopsy suggests an infectious cause. In contrast to poststreptococcal disease, the destructive glomerular proliferation often persists and the prognosis is poor.

The **histological features** depend on the timing of biopsy. Acute poststreptococcal glomerulonephritis is characterized by the presence of electron-dense deposits ('humps') on the epithelial side of the GBM (Fig. 9.8a,b): these represent the discrete 'lumpy-bumpy' deposits of IgG and C3 found by immunofluorescence along the capillary loop in sites corresponding to the 'humps' (Fig. 9.9). There is also diffuse proliferation of endothelial and mesangial cells and polymorph infiltration of the glomerulus.

Antigenic fragments from nephritogenic strains of streptococci bind to the GBM, so localizing specific antibody to

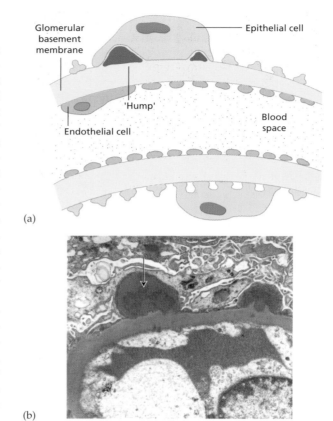

(a)

(b)

Fig. 9.8 (a) Characteristic 'humps' seen in poststreptococcal glomerulonephritis. These are localized, epimembranous, electron-dense deposits found in several forms of acute postinfectious glomerulonephritis. (b) Electron micrograph of acute proliferative poststreptococcal glomerulonephritis showing subepithelial 'humps' (arrow) (see also Fig, 9.13).

this site. After 4–8 weeks, the histological lesions become modified.

The clinical and immunological features of this condition are similar to acute ('one-shot') immune-complex nephritis

---

CASE 9.3 POSTSTREPTOCOCCAL GLOMERULONEPHRITIS

A 9-year-old boy was admitted as an emergency with puffiness of the face, eyes and trunk. A week previously he had complained of a sore throat. On examination, he was mildly pyrexial (temperature 37.5 °C) and hypertensive (BP 170/110). There was periorbital and scrotal oedema. His urine showed proteinuria, haematuria and red cell casts. He was anaemic (Hb 107 g/l) with a normal white cell count and differential. A throat swab grew normal flora but antibodies to streptococcal antigens were present in high titre: antistreptolysin O titre 1600 IU/ml (normal < 300 IU/ml). Serum complement studies done 3 days after admission showed a very

low C3 (0.10 g/l; NR 0.8–1.40) and a normal C4 (0.23 g/l; NR 0.2–0.4). His creatinine clearance was 46 ml/min, serum albumin 29 g/l and urinary protein excretion 1.5 g/day.

These findings were typical of poststreptococcal glomerulonephritis and so renal biopsy was not performed. As anticipated, the serum complement returned to normal in 4 weeks, accompanied by disappearance of the proteinuria and hypertension, although a small amount of microscopic haematuria persisted. The prognosis is good. An unusual feature of this case was the degree of hypertension.

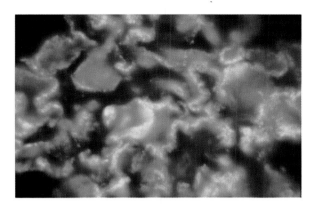

Fig. 9.9 Poststreptococcal glomerulonephritis showing 'lumpy-bumpy' deposits on immunofluorescence. Compare this with anti-glomerular basement membrane nephritis (Fig. 9.15b).

in rabbits. Serum complement C3 is markedly reduced during the early phase, with a gradual return to normal over 6–10 weeks in uncomplicated cases. *A low C3 persisting beyond 12 weeks suggests an different diagnosis* (see section 9.6.2 and Case 9.4).

The **prognosis** of acute poststreptococcal glomerulonephritis is good in children, worse in adults. Almost all preschool children will recover, with less than 1% developing crescentic glomerulonephritis.

9.6 Chronic glomerulonephritis

9.6.1 Chronic immune-complex glomerulonephritis

Immune-complex nephritis is believed to account for the majority of cases of human glomerulonephritis, but certain criteria should be fulfilled for complexes to be considered relevant to the pathogenesis of renal disease (Box 9.2). In practice, however, the diagnosis of immune-complex nephritis usually rests solely on immunofluorescent findings similar to those of experimental models of immune-complex disease.

The **pathogenesis** of experimental immune-complex nephritis is well defined. When rabbits are given repeated intravenous injections of a foreign protein, some develop a

---

BOX 9.2 CRITERIA IN SUPPORT OF AN IMMUNE-COMPLEX-MEDIATED AETIOLOGY OF GLOMERULONEPHRITIS

- Immune complexes are present at the site of tissue damage
- The antigen component of the immune complex is identifiable
- Removal of immune complexes produces clinical improvement

BOX 9.3 EXPERIMENTAL SITUATIONS WHICH TEND TO IMMUNE-COMPLEX DISEASE

- Antigen exposure persists (Table 9.2)
- The host makes an abnormal response
- Local factors, such as C3 receptors or changes in permeability, which promote deposition of circulating complexes
- Complexes are made less soluble

---

chronic progressive glomerulonephritis. Damage depends on producing a state of antigen excess after every injection, which saturates free antibody and generates loads of immune complexes. If animals fail to produce any antibody or, instead, mount a strong humoral response which rapidly eliminates the antigen, they do not develop glomerulonephritis. Affected animals produce non-precipitating, low-affinity antibody which is poor at antigen elimination. Even good antibody producers develop nephritis if the repeated antigen dose is increased to maintain antigen excess.

Reasons for chronic immune-complex disease in humans are not fully understood, but comparisons with this experimental model suggest some specific situations in which this is likely to occur (Box 9.3 and Fig. 9.10). Examples of **persistent antigen exposure** which give rise to immune-complex nephritis are shown in Table 9.2. Chronic infection is the best-recognized source of prolonged antigen exposure.

Variations in host responses are often,due to genetic differences. Associations exist between various forms of glomerulonephritis and certain HLA types which probably reflect linked, partial deficiencies of complement components C4 and C2. Patients with inherited complement defects (see Chapter 3) are unduly prone to immune-complex disease (including nephritis). Classical complement pathway activity is important in preventing the formation of large insoluble immune complexes, whilst the alternate pathway is concerned with disruption of large insoluble complexes. Failure of any of these functions can result in deposition of immune complexes (see Fig. 10.10). Paradoxically, complement both protects against immune-complex disease and yet is a mediator of immune-complex-mediated tissue damage.

The reticuloendothelial system (mononuclear-phagocyte system) is a major mechanism for clearance of complexes (Fig. 9.10, see also Fig. 1.21) and this also applies to the mesangium of the kidney. Clinically troublesome complexes seem to be of intermediate size (Fig. 9.11). Larger complexes, formed in excess of either antibody or antigen, are deposited mainly in the mesangium or, to a lesser extent, between the endothelium and the basement membrane.

Local factors may also be involved in renal damage. Whilst some glomerular damage is due to deposition of circulating complexes, other forms of glomerulonephritis are

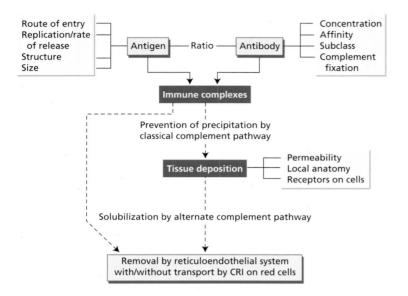

Fig. 9.10 Factors influencing the development of immune-complex disease. CR1, complement receptor 1.

Table 9.2 Examples of immune-complex nephritis in humans

	Antigen*	Associated disease†
Exogenous antigens		
Virus	Hepatitis B virus	Hepatitis B
		Polyarteritis nodosa
	Hepatitis C virus	Mixed essential cryoglobulinaemia
	Cytomegalovirus	Glomerulonephritis
Bacteria	Streptococcus	Poststreptococcal glomerulonephritis
	Streptococcus viridans	Bacterial endocarditis
	Staphylococcus	Shunt nephritis
	Mycobacterium leprae	Lepromatous leprosy
Parasites	Plasmodium malariae	Quartan malarial nephropathy
	Schistosoma mansoni	Schistosoma nephritis
	Toxoplasma gondii	Toxoplasma nephritis
Drugs	Penicillamine	Drug-induced nephropathy
	Gold	
	Foreign serum	Serum sickness
Endogenous antigens		
Autoantigens	Nuclear antigens	Systemic lupus erythematosus
	Renal tubular antigen	Membranous nephropathy
	IgG	Cryoglobulinaemia
	Tumour antigens	Neoplasia

*In many disorders with features suggestive of immune-complex deposition, no specific antigen has been incriminated.
†While immune complexes have been detected in these conditions, other mechanisms may also contribute to tissue damage.

due to formation of complexes in situ. Charged antigens, such as lectins or certain bacterial products, can be trapped electrostatically in the GBM or mesangium and then attract antibody and immune reactants. For instance, DNA binds to the capillary wall and may localize anti-DNA antibodies to this site.

The **diagnosis** of immune-complex nephritis is nearly always made by direct immunofluorescence or immunoper-

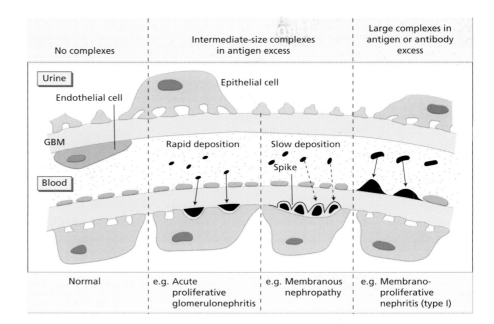

Fig. 9.11 Sites of immune-complex deposition in humans. The size of the complexes and their rates of deposition influence the clinical presentation and eventual renal morphology.

oxidase staining of kidney biopsies. Immunoglobulins and complement may be deposited in tubular basement membrane, interstitial tissue and blood vessels, as well as in the glomeruli. An irregular, interrupted granular or 'lumpy-bumpy' pattern of deposition is characteristic of immune complexes (Fig. 9.9). Deposition may be mainly in the GBM or confined to the mesangium (Fig. 9.12).

9.6.2 Membranoproliferative glomerulonephritis (mesangiocapillary glomerulonephritis)

MPGN is one of the most severe glomerular diseases of late childhood and adolescence. At least two distinct types of MPGN exist (Fig. 9.13; Table 9.3), although the differences are only detectable by electron or immunofluorescent microscopy.

Two-thirds of patients have electron-dense deposits in the mesangium and in the subendothelial space—**type I MPGN**. Immunohistology shows that these contain IgG, IgM, C4, C3 and C1q. Serum C3 levels do not show a consistent pattern and, when complement activation is demonstrated, the classical or alternate pathways or both may be involved. These immune deposits are not specific and can occur in any of the chronic immune complex disorders shown in Table 9.3, but particularly hepatitis B or C, or systemic lupus erythematosus (SLE).

In the remaining one-third, deposits are present within the GBM, as in Case 9.3, giving a 'ribbon-like' appearance—**type II MPGN** ('dense-deposit disease') (Fig. 9.13). In this disease (type II MPGN), there is almost exclusive fixation of C3 along the margin of the dense-deposit material in the me-

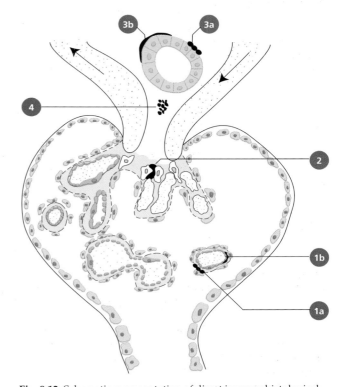

Fig. 9.12 Schematic representation of direct immunohistological staining of renal biopsies. Immune complexes may be present as granular deposits or aggregates in the glomerular capillary loops (1a), mesangium (2), tubular basement membrane (3a) or the interstitium (4). Linear staining is typical of antibodies reacting with antigens present in the glomerular (1b) or tubular (3b) basement membranes.

CASE 9.4 MEMBRANOPROLIFERATIVE GLOMERULONEPHRITIS —TYPE II

A 13-year-old boy had been well until 4 weeks before admission, when he developed a cough, periorbital oedema, ankle swelling, headaches and upper abdominal discomfort. On admission, he was febrile with facial and ankle oedema; there was generalized, super-ficial lymphadenopathy, numerous adventitial sounds in the lungs and hypertension (BP 140/110). His haemoglobin was 72 g/l with a normal white cell count and an erythrocyte sedimentation rate (ESR) of 137 mm/h. His blood urea was high (27.5 mmol/l) with a low serum bicarbonate (13.6 mmol/l) and serum albumin (19 g/l). His creatinine clearance was 45 ml/min per m² with urinary protein loss of 6.7 g/day. His serum CH_{50} was low (14 U/ml; NR 25–45), as was his C3 level (0.20 g/l; NR 0.8–1.4); his C4 level was normal (0.30 g/l; NR 0.2–0.4). A chest X-ray showed several rounded opacities in both lungs. These were presumed to be infective and treated with amoxicillin and flucloxacillin with resolution of the radiological findings.

The association of a low C3 with acute glomerulonephritis sug-gested acute poststreptococcal disease as the most likely diagnosis (see Case 9.1), although no streptococci were isolated and strepto-coccal antibodies were not raised. Over the following 3 weeks, his blood urea fell but the proteinuria and hypertension persisted.

Three months later, he felt better but still had heavy proteinuria with a low serum albumin (22 g/l; NR 35–50). Surprisingly, the serum CH_{50} and C3 levels were still low at 18 U/ml and 0.4 g/l, respectively. This pattern was not consistent with the working diagnosis. It suggested continued complement activation via the alternate pathway, due either to some circulating activating factor or a regulatory defect caused by absence of the inhibitors I or H (see Chapter 1). However, serum levels of I and H were normal. Electrophoresis of fresh serum and plasma showed the presence of C3 breakdown products and his serum was able to break down C3 in normal serum due to the presence of C3 nephritic factor.

C3 nephritic factor shows a strong association with mem-branoproliferative glomerulonephritis (MPGN), but not with acute poststreptococcal glomerulonephritis. Since these conditions have different prognoses, a renal biopsy was performed. This showed 11 glomeruli, all of which were swollen with proliferation of mesangial, endothelial and epithelial cells. On electron microscopy, the capillary loops showed basement membrane thickening with electron-dense deposits within the GBM (Fig. 9.13). On immunoflu-orescence, intense C3 deposition was present in the GBM without immunoglobulin staining. These appearances, together with the finding of circulating C3 nephritic factor, are characteristic of MPGN with dense intramembranous deposits (type II MPGN). Alternate-day prednisolone therapy was started, although this disease nearly always shows a slow progression to chronic renal failure.

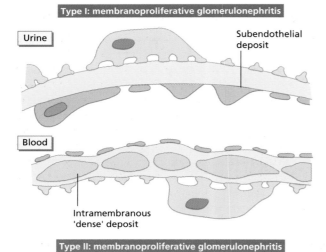

Type I: membranoproliferative glomerulonephritis

Urine

Subendothelial deposit

Blood

Intramembranous 'dense' deposit

Type II: membranoproliferative glomerulonephritis

Fig. 9.13 Membranoproliferative glomerulonephritis. Two major types can be recognized, depending on whether the deposits are subendothelial (type I) or intramembranous (type II).

Table 9.3 A comparison of type I and type II membranoproliferative glomerulonephritis

Feature	Type I	Type II
Acute nephritic episode	Uncommon	Common
Nephrotic syndrome	Common	Common
Serum C3 level	Normal or low	Very low
Genetic association	Not with HLA	HLA-B7
Clinical associations	Hepatitis C Malignancy	Partial lipodystrophy
Recurrence following renal transplantation	Frequent	Invariable

sangium and in the GBM. Serum levels of C3 are low, with normal levels of C1q and C4, implying that complement ac-tivation is occurring via the alternate pathway. Nearly all patients with type II MPGN have circulating C3 nephritic factor (C3 NeF). This is an autoantibody of IgG class which binds to the alternate pathway C3 convertase to create a sta-ble enzyme complex which is resistant to breakdown. As a result, more C3 is cleaved to C3b and this positive-feedback loop continues until most of the serum C3 is consumed.

The role of C3 NeF in MPGN is not clear: its presence is not related to the clinical state of the patient or to the prog-nosis, as some patients with C3 NeF do not develop MPGN. As an IgG antibody, C3 NeF may be transported across the placenta and cause transient hypocomplementaemia in the newborn. However, renal disease does not develop in these children, suggesting that C3 NeF is a marker of MPGN rather than the cause of the renal damage. There is a strong association between type II MPGN and partial lipodystrophy, a condition characterized by loss of subcutaneous fat from the upper half of the body.

These two types of glomerulonephritis show significant clinical differences (Table 9.3). Various types of **treatment** have been tried in both forms of MPGN, with little evidence of any benefit. The overall 10-year survival rate for MPGN, without distinction into subtypes, is about 50%. Prognosis is worse in patients who have a persisting nephrotic syndrome or hypertension or an initial decrease in the glomerular filtration rate. Transplantation is usually successful, although type II MPGN recurs histologically in almost all grafts (see Table 9.8).

9.6.3 Lupus nephritis

Although only 25% of patients with SLE present with renal disease as the first manifestation of lupus, clinical glomerulonephritis occurs in about 50% of cases of SLE at some time, and histological evidence of renal involvement is detectable in nearly all patients, even in the absence of proteinuria. The development of nephritis is closely linked to morbidity and survival in lupus. The **histological appearances** have been classified by the World Health Organization (WHO) according to the pattern and extent of immune deposition and inflammation (Table 9.4). The clinical features of lupus nephritis do not predict the severity of the glomerular lesion on biopsy.

Table 9.4 Modified WHO classification of lupus nephritis

Class 0	Normal
Class I	Light microscopy normal, immune deposits on immunofluorescence involving part of a glomerulus while the rest of that glomerulus appears normal
Class II	A. Mesangial deposits
	B. Mesangial hypercellularity
Class III	Focal segmental proliferative glomerulonephritis (< 50% glomeruli)
	Immune deposits in mesangium
Class IV	As class III but 'diffuse' (> 50% glomeruli)
	Includes membranoproliferative type
Class V	Membranous nephropathy with subepithelial immune complex deposition
	A. Membranous nephropathy (MN) alone
	B. MN plus class II
	C. MN plus class III
	D. MN plus class IV
Class VI	Glomerulosclerosis

The **prognosis** in SLE is not as dismal as was once believed, but the development of renal disease is the strongest predictor of ESRF and early mortality. The 10-year survival in patients with all forms of the disease is over 80%. Patients with ESRF are excellent candidates for renal transplantation. Disease activity post-transplantation is sporadic and infrequent; recurrence of lupus nephritis is rare.

The major causes of death are severe vascular disease and sepsis. Overwhelming infection occurs typically in patients treated with high-dose steroids and other immunosuppressive drugs. While aggressive induction **treatment** reduces renal disease, it increases susceptibility to infection (Chapter 3). No large, prospective randomized trials have been performed in lupus nephritis: most data come from retrospective studies and small trials with an average of 20 patients per treatment arm. Most data suggest that WHO class II nephritis has a benign course, and treatment in the absence of other indications is not usually needed. The outcome and treatment of class V nephritis is hotly debated. The decision to treat active WHO class III and IV lupus nephritis is less controversial. Systematic review of available trials supports treatment with corticosteroids and an immunosuppressive agent, usually cyclophosphamide or azathioprine. The optimum duration of treatment is debated, but continuing treatment for a significant disease-free period of about 2 years is recommended. Cyclosporin is an alternative agent, particularly used in children.

9.7 Rapidly progressive glomerulonephritis

Rapidly progressive glomerulonephritis (RPGN) describes a group of diseases with aggressive glomerular injury which can lead to ESRF within days or weeks if not diagnosed and treated early. The usual pathological lesion is crescentic glomerulonephritis. RPGN constitutes 3–5% of all cases of glomerulonephritis. It is not a single entity but has multiple aetiologies involving several pathogenic mechanisms. Based on the immunological findings, patients fall into three broad groups, as shown in Fig. 9.14. The prognosis is especially grave when over 70% of glomeruli are involved, there are diffuse circumferential crescents, and there is prolonged oliguria.

9.7.1 Anti-glomerular basement membrane disease

Acute glomerulonephritis mediated by anti-GBM antibody accounts for about 1–2% of all cases of glomerulonephritis, but about 20% of cases presenting as acute renal failure due to RPGN. Anti-GBM nephritis is more common in those who possess HLA-DR15 or -DR4. Patients present with nephritis alone or, more commonly, with glomerulonephritis and lung haemorrhage, a combination termed **Goodpasture's syndrome**. However, rapidly progressive nephritis and

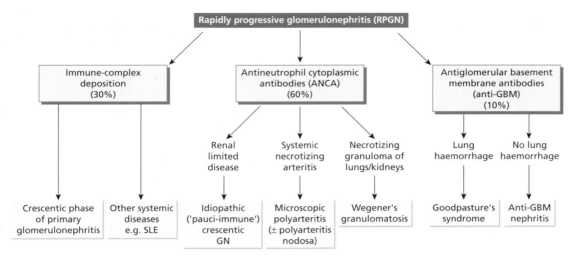

Fig. 9.14 Clinical and immunological classification of rapidly progressive glomerulonephritis.

CASE 9.5 ANTI-GLOMERULAR BASEMENT MEMBRANE GLOMERULONEPHRITIS

A 55-year-old man presented with a 3-week history of malaise, nausea, fever and shivering. Although there were no urinary symptoms, analysis of a mid-stream urine specimen showed microscopic haematuria and proteinuria (2+). There was no cough or haemoptysis and no family history of renal disease or hypertension. On examination, he was mildly pyrexial but there were no vasculitic lesions, oedema or hypertension. Cystoscopy and renal ultrasound showed no cause for his haematuria. Over the next week, his blood urea rose steadily from 10 to 23 mmol/l (NR 2.5–7.5) and the serum creatinine from 164 to 515 μmol/l (NR 60–120). His haemoglobin was 89 g/l with a white cell count of 10.4×10^9/l and a normal differential. His urine contained red cell casts and he rapidly became oliguric. Antinuclear antibodies, including anti-DNA

antibodies, were not detected and serum C3 and C4 levels were normal.

A renal biopsy specimen contained seven glomeruli: four showed focal necrotizing glomerulonephritis with epithelial crescents but the remaining three were normal. On immunofluorescence, linear staining with IgG was present along the glomerular capillary basement membrane (Fig. 9.15b). The patient's serum contained antibodies to GBM (see Chapter 19). The diagnosis was therefore rapidly progressive glomerulonephritis due to antibodies to GBM. Although oliguric, he was treated with high doses of prednisolone and cyclophosphamide, and underwent daily plasma exchanges for 2 weeks, until anti-GBM antibodies were no longer detectable. However, renal function failed to recover: cytotoxic therapy was stopped and regular haemodialysis started.

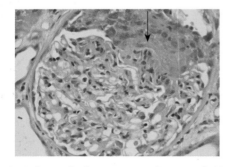

(a)

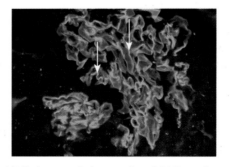

(b)

Fig. 9.15 Anti-glomerular basement membrane nephritis showing (a) a crescent with fibrin necrosis (arrowed) and (b) linear fluorescent staining along the basement membrane (arrowed).

pulmonary haemorrhage can occur in other multisystem disorders such as SLE or Wegener's granulomatosis, so *the combination of renal and lung involvement is not synonymous with anti-GBM disease.*

The target antigen is the α3 chain of type IV collagen, a major constituent of the GBM. **Lung damage** results from antibodies to antigens common to both alveolar and glomerular basement membranes. In Goodpasture's syndrome, res-

BOX 9.4 EVIDENCE THAT ANTI-GBM ANTIBODIES ARE PATHOGENIC

- Linear deposition of IgG reflects binding to regularly spaced antigenic determinants and not deposition as immune complexes
- IgG eluted from the kidneys of patients with anti-GBM nephritis causes identical glomerular damage when injected into monkeys
- Removal of anti-GBM antibodies from the circulation can prevent irreversible organ damage
- Anti-GBM nephritis can recur rapidly in a renal allograft if transplantation is performed while circulating anti-GBM antibodies are still present

BOX 9.5 EVIDENCE THAT ANTI-NEUTROPHIL CYTOPLASMIC ANTIBODIES MAY BE PATHOGENIC

- In vitro, ANCA activate primed neutrophils and react with endothelial cells expressing PR3
- In vitro, ANCA promote recruitment and adhesion between neutrophils and endothelial cells
- ANCA accelerate apoptosis of TNF-primed neutrophils
- Spleen cells from MPO-knockout mice immunized with MPO cause necrotizing, crescentic glomerulonephritis and systemic vasculitis when injected into the immunodeficient Rag 2–/– mouse. Anti-MPO IgG was also able to induce crescentic nephritis

piratory symptoms often precede renal disease by 1 year or longer. Haemoptysis, usually leading to anaemia, is a prominent feature and the sputum typically contains haemosiderin-laden macrophages. Lung biopsies show intra-alveolar haemorrhage and necrotizing alveolitis. There is convincing evidence that anti-GBM antibodies are responsible for the nephritis (Box 9.4).

Although the **cause** is unknown, anti-GBM disease follows upper respiratory tract infections in 20–60% of patients, or exposure to certain hydrocarbons. These agents may damage alveolar basement membrane, generating new and potent antigens able to stimulate autoantibody production. Alternatively, the agent responsible (e.g. a virus) may cross-react with basement membrane antigens. Pulmonary haemorrhage in anti-GBM disease is strongly associated with cigarette smoking.

Aggressive immunosuppressive **therapy**, usually high-dose steroids combined with cyclophosphamide, coupled with intensive plasmapheresis, is the treatment of choice (see Box 9.6). Prompt treatment can lead to long-term recovery, but no improvement in renal function can be expected in patients with established anuria or where crescents involve over 85% of glomeruli. The main risk to life in these circumstances is massive lung haemorrhage. While renal transplantation is successful, nephritis can recur if antibody is still present, so transplantation should be deferred until anti-GBM antibodies are no longer detectable.

9.7.2 Antineutrophil cytoplasmic antibody-associated glomerulonephritis

Serum IgG antibodies reacting with cytoplasmic components of neutrophils and monocytes are a diagnostic marker for active Wegener's granulomatosis (Chapter 11) and reflect disease activity. *Two patterns of antineutrophil cytoplasmic antibody (ANCA) reactivity are important clinically*: generalized cytoplasmic staining (cANCA) and a perinuclear pattern

(pANCA). Most cANCA sera react with a serine proteinase called proteinase 3 (PR3), while most pANCA sera react with myeloperoxidase (MPO). A further pattern is associated with inflammatory bowel disease, particularly ulcerative colitis. Some cANCA/pANCA-positive sera react with neutrophil antigens other than PR3/MPO.

Raised ANCA titres are generally detectable during active disease and rising titres may herald a relapse. There has been debate whether ANCA are pathogenic in vasculitis or simply a marker, but there is mounting evidence that they are pathogenic (Box 9.5).

Patients with ANCA-associated glomerulonephritis are usually aged from 40 to 70 years and most have had a flu-like illness with arthralgia and myalgia a few days or weeks prior to the onset of renal disease or vasculitis. A **spectrum of vasculitis** is seen, ranging from disease limited to the kidneys in about a quarter of cases to a systemic vasculitic process with pulmonary involvement in about half the patients. ANCA-associated glomerulonephritis is now the commonest form of crescentic or rapidly progressive glomerulonephritis. As in Case 9.6, the renal lesion in characterized by few or no deposits of immunoglobulin or complement in the kidney (so-called pauci-immune glomerulonephritis) and by necrosis and crescent formation (Fig. 9.16a).

Over 75% of patients with ANCA-associated glomerulonephritis go into remission following aggressive immunosuppression, although 30–50% relapse within 2 years and require further therapy. Plasma exchange is superior to methylprednisolone in the acute treatment phase. Traditional maintenance **treatment** is with cyclophosphamide for at least 1 year. Overall patient survival is 75% at 1 year and 60% at 5 years. Early deaths are usually due to lung haemorrhage or opportunistic infection.

9.8 Nephrotic syndrome

The three essential features of the nephrotic syndrome are:

CASE 9.6 ANTINEUTROPHIL CYTOPLASMIC ANTIBODY-ASSOCIATED NECROTIZING CRESCENTIC GLOMERULONEPHRITIS

A 64-year-old man presented with a 1-month history of nausea and malaise and a 1-week history of flu-like symptoms, rigors and vomiting. Eight weeks earlier, while on holiday, he developed infected insect bites around his left ankle and was treated with erythromycin. He had no urinary or joint symptoms and no family history of renal disease. On examination, he was pale with mild pitting oedema of both ankles and a blood pressure of 170/90. Analysis of a mid-stream urine specimen showed proteinuria (3+) with microscopic haematuria and granular casts. His haemoglobin was 92 g/l with a white cell count of 17.7×10^9/l and an ESR of 122 mm/h. His blood urea was 42.6 mmol/l (NR 2.5–7.5) and serum creatinine 1094 μmol/l (NR 60–120). Malarial parasites and hepatitis B surface antigen were not detected in his blood. Over the next 72 h, his urine output fell to 30 ml/day with further increases in his blood urea and serum creatinine.

Ultrasound examination showed bilaterally enlarged kidneys but no evidence of obstruction. Serum immunoglobulin levels were normal but C3 (1.56 g/l; NR 0.8–1.40) and C4 (0.46 g/l; NR 0.2–0.4) were raised. There was no paraproteinaemia and no free monoclonal light chains in his urine. Antinuclear, anti-dsDNA, and anti-GBM antibodies were negative. However, the patient's serum contained IgG antibodies which reacted strongly with cytoplasmic antigens of alcohol-fixed neutrophils, producing a granular pattern characteristic of classical antineutrophil cytoplasmic antibodies (cANCA). Further analysis showed antibodies to a neutrophil enzyme called serine proteinase 3 (PR3) by enzyme-linked immunosorbent assay (ELISA) (see Chapter 19).

A renal biopsy was performed to confirm the cause of his rapidly progressive glomerulonephritis. The biopsy specimen contained 30 glomeruli: one-third of these were totally sclerosed and all but one of the remainder showed necrotizing, crescentic glomerulonephritis. Cellular crescents, with extensive tuft necrosis (Fig. 9.16b), were seen in most glomeruli. Immunofluorescence showed no immune deposits in the glomeruli, so-called 'pauci-immune' disease. The diagnosis was that of ANCA-associated, necrotizing crescentic glomerulonephritis.

He was treated with pulse cyclophosphamide (500 mg/m²) and pulse methylprednisolone (1 g daily for 3 days), followed by 60 mg of prednisolone daily. For the next 12 days he required peritoneal dialysis until his renal function improved. He was discharged on maintenance therapy of prednisolone 40 mg/day with pulse intravenous cyclophosphamide at monthly intervals. He continued on this regimen until his cANCA became negative; his treatment was then changed to oral prednisolone and azathioprine.

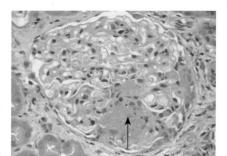

(a)

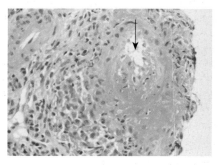

(b)

Fig. 9.16 ANCA-associated glomerulonephritis showing (a) a segmental area of tuft necrosis (arrowed) and (b) vasculitis of a renal arteriole (arrowed).

- marked proteinuria
- hypoalbuminaemia; and
- oedema.

In adults, the proteinuria generally exceeds 3.5 g/day with a serum albumin concentration below 25 g/l. In children, the proteinuria is usually more than 50 mg/kg per day. Although hypercholesterolaemia and hypertriglyceridaemia often accompany the nephrotic syndrome, they are not essential for diagnosis.

Diagnosis of the nephrotic syndrome does not imply any particular renal histology or any specific disease: it reflects an underlying glomerular disease which increases the permeability of the glomerular basement membrane to protein; there are many causes (Fig. 9.17). There are three distinct histological variants of primary nephrotic syndrome: minimal change nephropathy, focal glomerulosclerosis, and membranous nephropathy.

9.8.1 Minimal-change nephropathy

The major features of minimal-change nephropathy (MCN) are exemplified by Case 9.7. It accounts for over 90% of cases of nephrotic syndrome in children and 20% of adult cases (Fig. 9.17). No age is exempt.

CASE 9.7 MINIMAL-CHANGE NEPHROPATHY

An 8-year-old girl presented with a 3-day history of swelling of the legs and puffiness around the eyes following a cold 1 week earlier. She had some mild abdominal discomfort and a headache for 2 days. Examination revealed a generally oedematous girl with ascites and a blood pressure of 120/70. Her height was on the 50th centile but her weight was above the 90th centile. Urinalysis showed marked proteinuria without haematuria. Her haemoglobin, white cell count and urea and electrolytes were normal but there was marked hypoalbuminaemia (11 g/l) and proteinuria (26 g/day). The urinary clearance of IgG relative to that of transferrin was less than 0.1, indicating highly selective proteinuria. Creatinine clearance, CH_{50}, C4 and C3 levels were all normal. A throat swab

grew commensal flora only and the antibody titre to streptococcal antigens was normal.

Highly selective proteinuria in a child with nephrotic syndrome is virtually diagnostic of minimal-change nephropathy. For this reason, renal biopsy was not performed but a trial of steroid therapy (prednisolone 60 mg/day) was started with dramatic effect. Over the next week, her serum albumin rose to 26 g/l and the proteinuria subsided. At discharge, only a trace of proteinuria was detectable but she continued to take 40 mg prednisolone on alternate days for a further 3 months. The nephrotic syndrome did not relapse when steroids were withdrawn.

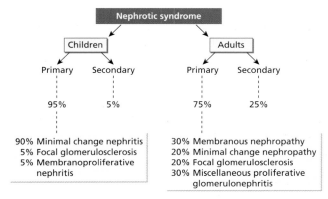

Fig. 9.17 Renal morphology in patients with the nephrotic syndrome. Primary glomerulonephritis is more common than secondary renal disease.

BOX 9.6 EVIDENCE THAT T-CELL-MEDIATED REACTIONS ARE INVOLVED IN MCN

- The condition responds dramatically to corticosteroid therapy
- Hodgkin's disease, lymphoma, leukaemia, thymoma are associated with minimal-change nephropathy
- Spontaneous clinical improvement has been seen following infections that depress cellular immunity, such as measles
- The demonstration of changes in lymphocyte cytotoxicity to human kidney tissue in some patients with MCN
- Cultured T cells from MCN patients synthesize a factor causing transient proteinuria when injected into rats

The **cause and pathogenesis** of MCN are unknown. There is no corresponding animal model. Cell-mediated immune reactions leading to podocyte dysfunction may play an important role (Box 9.6). Mutations in several genes coding for split diaphragm proteins—nephrin and podocin—are known to cause minimal-change nephropathy, severe congenital forms of nephrotic syndrome and some cases of steroid-resistant nephrotic syndrome. Disruption of slit diaphragm proteins is thought to lead to podocyte apoptosis.

The renal **pathology** of MCN shows normal glomeruli on light microscopy and immunohistology but fusion of podocytes on electron microscopy.

MCN responds predictably and consistently to steroids; 95% of patients have a complete remission within 8 weeks. Failure to respond to steroids or the presence of unselective proteinuria challenges the diagnosis of minimal-change disease (see Case 9.4); a renal biopsy is then necessary. Alternate-day steroid **therapy** is less likely to produce a Cushingoid state than daily steroids. The aim is to keep patients

on steroids for 3–4 months: this is associated with a lower relapse rate at 2 years than if steroids are given for a shorter period. About 25% of children have one attack only: the remainder relapse, 50% on more than four occasions, usually as steroids are stopped or the dose reduced. Relapses usually respond to further steroid therapy, but in some frequent relapsers treatment with cyclosporin, cyclophosphamide or levamisole may permit prolonged remission.

MCN has a very good **prognosis**, even when therapy is required for years. The earlier the age at onset of symptoms, the longer the illness persists but death occurs in about 3% of cases only, usually from avoidable complications such as septicaemia, hypovolaemia, thromboembolism or acute renal failure.

9.8.2 Focal glomerulosclerosis

In some cases of the nephrotic syndrome, the picture resembles MCN except that proteinuria is only moderately or poorly selective, hypertension is relatively common and the patient responds poorly to steroids. Subsequent renal biopsies may show focal segmental glomerulosclerosis. Because this disorder involves juxtamedullary glomeruli initially, superficial biopsies of the cortex can be normal. As the disease progresses, more and more glomeruli become sclerosed until the outer cortex is also involved.

The **pathogenesis** of focal glomerulosclerosis, like that of minimal-change disease, is unknown, but mutations in split diaphragm proteins can give rise to an autosomal dominant form of the condition. The incidence of focal glomerulosclerosis seems to be increasing in adults and children and the *prognosis is quite different from minimal change disease*. Progressive renal impairment occurs in 50% of patients. A small number of patients follow a rapidly downhill course and the lesion may recur after renal transplantation. An especially malignant variant of focal glomerulosclerosis occurs in patients with HIV infection. This HIV-associated nephropathy has a strong predilection for African-Americans and runs a fulminant downhill course.

Treatment remains controversial, although up to 20% of patients respond to steroids with complete remission and long-term renal survival. Unfortunately, there is no way of identifying those who will respond.

9.8.3 Membranous glomerulonephritis

About 80% of patients with membranous glomerulonephritis present with a florid nephrotic syndrome; the remainder present with hypertension, poorly selective proteinuria or microscopic haematuria discovered on routine examination of the urine. Membranous glomerulonephritis can occur at any age, with the peak incidence in adults aged between 40 and 70 years. The **characteristic lesion** is uniform thickening of the GBM without proliferation of cells. The lesions uniformly affect every glomerulus, but the degree of membranous thickening is not related to the severity of proteinuria.

The membranous thickening is produced mainly by subepithelial deposits of immune complexes, followed by secondary formation of projections ('spikes') of basement membrane material between the deposits (see Fig. 9.11). The deposits are characteristically granular and may contain C3, IgA and IgM as well as IgG.

About 80% of cases of membranous glomerulonephritis are 'idiopathic' or primary: the causal antigen is never found. The remaining 20%, however, are secondary to another disease or to drugs. The most important causes are drugs (gold, penicillamine, non-steroidal anti-inflammatory drugs, captopril, heroin), infections (hepatitis B or C, malaria, syphilis), SLE, or tumours (carcinoma of the bronchus, breast or colon). Some 10% of patients with membranous nephropathy have an underlying malignancy. It is presumed that nephropathy is the result of either antigenic cross-reactivity between the tumour and an unknown renal antigen or the deposition of tumour antigens in the glomerulus followed by immune-complex formation.

There is considerable evidence that the **pathogenesis** of membranous nephropathy is immunologically mediated (Box 9.7). There is increasing evidence that complexes are formed in situ in the subepithelial space following antigen

---

BOX 9.7 EVIDENCE THAT MEMBRANOUS NEPHROPATHY IS AN IMMUNE-MEDIATED DISEASE

- Immunohistological picture resembles Heymann nephritis, an experimental model induced in rats by immunization with renal tubular autoantigens

- Strong immunogenic associations with HLA-DR3 (Caucasians) or -DR2 (Japanese)

- Presence of IgG, C3 and C4 in the diseased kidney

- Responds to anti-inflammatory/immunosuppressive drugs such as corticosteroids/azathioprine

---

CASE 9.8 MEMBRANOUS GLOMERULONEPHRITIS

A 48-year-old man presented with a 3-month history of intermittent swelling of his ankles and puffiness of his face. There were no urinary symptoms and no family history of renal disease. He was taking no medication. On examination, he was pale and thin with ankle oedema and a blood pressure of 130/80. Investigations showed a normal haemoglobin and white cell count and an ESR of 32 mm/h. His blood urea was 9.1 mmol/l (NR 2.5–7.5), serum albumin 26 g/l with a urinary protein loss of 7.8 g/day and a creatinine clearance of 106 ml/min. His serum immunoglobulin IgM and IgA, C3 and C4 levels were normal, but his IgG was low at 5.1 g/l (NR 7.2–19.0). Antinuclear antibodies, hepatitis B surface antigen

and antibody, and hepatitis C antibody were not detected. There were no free light chains in his urine.

A renal biopsy was done to find the cause of his nephrotic syndrome; this showed no obvious increase in cellularity. However, the basement membrane of all glomeruli showed marked but uniform thickening with numerous subepithelial 'spikes'. Immunofluorescent examination showed granular deposits of IgG and C3 along all the glomerular capillary walls. The biopsy appearances were typical of membranous glomerulonephritis (Fig. 9.9). No specific treatment was given. One year later, he is asymptomatic but still has severe, non-selective proteinuria of 14 g/day.

trapping there. This may explain why serum complement levels are always normal and why circulating immune complexes are not found.

Membranous glomerulonephritis accounts for 30% of nephrotic syndrome in adults. The prognosis of idiopathic disease is variable: one-third of patients undergo spontaneous remission of proteinuria with excellent long-term survival; another third have persistent proteinuria; and the final third progress to renal failure, usually within 10 years of diagnosis.

Treatment of idiopathic membranous nephropathy is controversial and usually reserved for those patients show-

ing definite evidence of renal deterioration. Urinary excretion of β_2-microglobulin is a marker of disease activity and may identify those patients likely to deteriorate relentlessly. In these patients, controlled trials have shown that prednisolone alone is of no benefit but steroids plus chlorambucil may be protective. Cyclosporin has also shown promising results.

9.8.4 Amyloid disease

Amyloidosis is a disorder of protein folding that results in autoaggregation into fibrils. There have been many attempts

---

CASE 9.9 IDIOPATHIC AL AMYLOID

A 52-year-old woman presented with increasing swelling of both legs over a period of 3 months. Fourteen years earlier she had been treated for tuberculosis. On examination, she was pale, with gross bilateral leg oedema extending to the umbilicus and a large infected ulcer on the medial aspect of the right leg. Chest X-ray and electrocardiogram were normal but she had a microcytic anaemia (Hb 75 g/l) with an ESR of 140 mm/h. Her initial biochemical results showed a low serum albumin (14 g/l) and marked proteinuria (12 g/day) but a normal blood urea, serum creatinine and creatinine clearance. Serum electrophoresis showed no monoclonal band. Serum immunoglobulin levels were: IgG 2.2 g/l (NR 7.2–19.0); IgA 1.2 g/l (NR 0.8–5.0); and IgM 1.2 g/l (NR 0.5–2.0). Electrophoresis of a concentrated (× 20) urine sample showed considerable amounts of albumin and gammaglobulin and an M band in the β region. Immunofixation of the serum and urine showed the presence of monoclonal free λ light chains in the urine only.

The presence of urinary monoclonal light chains suggested a possible diagnosis of light-chain myeloma or renal amyloid. A rectal biopsy was performed to look for amyloid deposits: this showed

deposition of small amounts of amorphous material around blood vessels. This material stained strongly with Congo red and showed green birefringence when viewed under polarized light, an appearance which is characteristic of amyloid. A renal biopsy was also performed: striking deposits of amyloid were found in the GBM, in the tubular basement membrane and in the walls of several arterioles.

In view of her past medical history, the amyloid could have been associated with the previous tuberculosis or with the chronic infection of her leg ulcer; this is acute-phase-associated AA amyloid (see Table 9.5). However, antisera to λ light chains stained the material in both biopsies, showing that the amyloid was light-chain-associated (Table 9.5) and thus idiopathic or due to multiple myeloma. The absence of suppression of IgA and IgM levels, the lack of infiltration of the bone marrow and the absence of osteolytic lesions on X-ray excluded the diagnosis of multiple myeloma. Therefore, this was idiopathic AL amyloid. In view of her reasonable renal function, only supportive treatment was given; this consisted of a low-salt, high-protein diet and diuretics. To date, her proteinuria has persisted but has not worsened.

Table 9.5 Protein component of amyloid fibrils

Type of amyloid	Major protein of fibril	Chemically related protein (? precursor) in serum
Light-chain-associated amyloidosis		
Idiopathic	AL	Light chain
Myeloma	AL	Light chain
Other monoclonal gammopathies	AL	Light chain
Acute-phase-associated amyloidosis		
Chronic inflammation/suppuration	AA	SAA
Senile systemic amyloid	ATTR (senile) amyloid	Transthyretin
Haemodialysis-associated amyloidosis	β_2M	β_2M
Transmissible spongiform encephalopathies	Prion protein	?

AA, amyloid A protein; AL, light-chain amyloid protein; β_2M, β_2-microglobulin; SAA, serum amyloid A protein.

to classify amyloidosis. Amyloidosis can be hereditary or acquired and the deposits can be focal, localized or systemic. Hereditary types are very rare though important models for studying pathogenesis. The main clinical problems are the systemic, acquired types. Classifications of these into 'primary' or 'secondary' types and those based on histological grounds or on the pattern of organ involvement have proved unreliable. *The best classification is one based on the nature of the amyloid protein found on biopsy.*

The fibrillary structure confers on amyloid the characteristic staining appearance with dyes such as Congo red or Sirius red or thioflavine T, and its birefringence under polarized light. Many different proteins make up these amyloid fibrils (Table 9.5). **Light-chain-associated amyloidosis (or AL amyloidosis)** is almost always associated with an abnormality of lymphoid cells and excessive production of monoclonal free light chains. About 20% of patients have frank multiple myeloma, but in 70% the immunocyte dyscrasia is more subtle and clonal disease is undetectable in the remaining 10%. Most patients are over 50 years and almost any organ, except the brain, can be involved.

The amyloid protein found in **acute phase-associated amyloidosis (or AA amyloidosis)** is not derived from light chains. This protein is called amyloid A protein (AA). Its circulating serum precursor, serum amyloid A protein (SAA), is an acute-phase reactant with similarities to C-reactive protein. AA amyloidosis occurs in three main types of chronic disease: inflammatory disorders and periodic fever syndromes, local or systemic bacterial infections, and malignant disease. In the UK, rheumatic diseases are the commonest underlying disorders, with about 1% of patients with rheumatoid arthritis or juvenile chronic arthritis developing amyloidosis.

All forms of amyloid also contain **P-component**, which is identical to a plasma glycoprotein called serum amyloid P-component (SAP). SAP does not behave as an acute-phase reactant in humans, although SAP and C-reactive protein belong to the same protein 'superfamily' called pentaxins. SAP binds specifically to all amyloid fibrils as well as to DNA and chromatin, and protects fibrils from proteolysis and digestion by macrophages. Amyloid deposits mostly exert their pathological effects through physical disruption

of normal tissue structure and function, although they may also have a cytotoxic effect by inducing apoptosis.

Case 9.9 shows that the clinical and biochemical picture produced by amyloid deposition in the kidneys has no unique features. Where the **diagnosis** is considered, it is essential that the pathologist is made aware of this possibility so that the appropriate stains are used. However, biopsies do not provide information on the extent of amyloid deposition. This can be achieved by scintigraphy using radiolabelled SAP. The tracer does not accumulate in normal subjects but binds rapidly and specifically to all amyloid fibrils, allowing measurement of the whole-body amyloid load and the tissue distribution of the deposits. Repeat scans are used to monitor the progression of amyloid.

Renal failure is the major cause of death in systemic amyloidosis and this poor prognosis has led to many trials. No **treatment** specifically disrupts amyloid fibrils, although many have been tried. Measures that reduce the supply of the respective amyloid fibril precursor proteins (Table 9.6) can preserve organ function and improve survival. Many patients with underlying B-cell dyscrasias die from amyloidosis of the kidneys or heart before traditional low-dose cytotoxic drugs can produce benefit. More aggressive high-dose chemotherapy, coupled with autologous peripheral blood stem cell transplantation, may prove more beneficial. In such cases, supportive therapy, including dialysis or organ transplantation (heart, kidney or liver), can provide an opportunity for chemotherapy to exert its desired effect on fibril supply.

9.8.5 Other causes of nephrotic syndrome

In adults, the nephrotic syndrome may be secondary to a number of conditions (see Fig. 9.17 and Table 9.2). In the UK, the commonest causes are amyloid disease, SLE and diabetes mellitus, but, elsewhere in the world, chronic parasitic infestation dominates the list of causes. Worldwide, the commonest cause is malaria. In many countries, where 10–30% of the population are carriers of hepatitis B virus, this agent can also cause immune-complex glomerulonephritis and hence the nephrotic syndrome. The nephrotic syndrome may also develop in patients with carcinoma or lymphoproliferative

Table 9.6 Principles of treatment of amyloidosis

Fibril type	Aim of treatment	Example
AL amyloidosis	Suppress monoclonal light-chain production	Chemotherapy for myeloma or immunocyte dyscrasia
AA amyloidosis	Suppress acute-phase response	Immunosuppression, e.g. RA
		Surgery, e.g. osteomyelitis

AA, Amyloid A protein; AL, light-chain amyloid protein; RA, rheumatoid arthritis.

disease and many months may elapse before the underlying malignancy is detected.

9.9 Tubulointerstitial nephropathy

Tubulointerstitial nephropathy (TIN) or 'interstitial nephritis' describes a group of diverse renal disorders with predominant involvement of the renal tubules and interstitial tissue. Immunological mechanisms similar to those causing glomerulonephritis can also cause tubulointerstitial injury. Thus, antibodies to tubular basement membrane, immune complexes and cell-mediated reactions can produce TIN in experimental animals and in man.

In general, there are three types of **functional defect** caused by TIN (Box 9.8).

Clinically, TIN can be divided into acute and chronic forms. Acute TIN is most commonly due to acute bacterial pyelonephritis or to drugs, although Epstein–Barr virus infection has been implicated in some cases. Chronic TIN may be idiopathic or secondary to a wide range of infective, toxic, neoplastic, hereditary or immunological conditions as well as eating disorders. Those conditions in which immunological mechanisms are thought to be involved are discussed in the cases.

9.9.1 Acute drug-induced tubulointerstitial nephritis

Acute TIN is a rare but well-recognized complication of an

increasing list of drugs; these include the β-lactam antibiotics (methicillin, penicillin, ampicillin), sulphonamides, rifampicin, anticonvulsants, cimetidine, diuretics, allopurinol and various non-steroidal inflammatory drugs. Antibiotics and NSAIDs are the most important triggers. Whatever the drug, TIN occurs about 10–15 days after the start of treatment and is not dose dependent. It is characterized by fever, haematuria, proteinuria, arthralgia and a maculopapular skin rash. The majority of patients recover completely, usually within a few days of stopping the drug.

The **mechanism of damage** is unclear but blood and tissue eosinophilia, a rash, lack of correlation with the dose of the drug and the latent period between treatment and symptoms suggest an idiosyncratic or hypersensitivity reaction, possibly mediated by TH2 cells. The interstitial infiltrate consists predominantly of CD4+ T cells, and in vitro lymphocyte transformation responses to the drug have been demonstrated in some patients, supporting this hypothesis. However, circulating antibodies to tubular basement membrane, with characteristic linear IgG staining on immunofluorescent examination of the biopsy, have also been found in some patients. This suggests that the drug, or its hapten, may also bind to components of the tubular basement membrane, forming new antigens.

9.9.2 Multiple myeloma and myeloma kidney

Multiple myeloma (see Chapter 6) is associated with many renal problems (Box 9.9). The most characteristic renal lesion is irreversible chronic renal failure due to **tubular atrophy (myeloma kidney)** with associated acidification and concentration defects. Poor renal function correlates with the presence of light-chain proteinuria. Because of their size, light chains are readily filtered at the glomerulus and catabolized in the proximal tubular cells. When the amount of filtered free light chains exceeds the metabolic capacity of the tubules, two kinds of toxicity occur: first, tubular cells are damaged by intracellular deposits of crystals; and, second, protein precipitates out in the distal tubules and col-

---

BOX 9.8 FUNCTIONAL DEFECTS IN TIN

- Proximal tubular lesion, causing proximal renal tubular acidosis with or without the Fanconi syndrome (phosphaturia, glycosuria and aminoaciduria)

- Distal tubular dysfunction, resulting in distal renal tubular acidosis, hyperkalaemia and salt-wasting

- Medullary dysfunction, causing impaired urine concentrating ability

---

CASE 9.10 ACUTE TUBULOINTERSTITIAL NEPHRITIS

A 37-year-old woman was admitted to hospital with a diagnosis of bacterial endocarditis. Blood cultures grew Streptococcus faecalis. She was treated with intravenous gentamicin and ampicillin with considerable improvement. However, on the 12th day of treatment, she developed a further fever and a macular rash on her trunk and limbs. Her white cell count was normal with an absolute eosinophil count of 0.32×10^9/l. Further blood cultures were negative but her serum creatinine rose from 140 μmol/l (NR 60–120) to 475 μmol/l over the next 3 days, with a rise in the eosinophil count to

0.92×10^9/l. Serum complement levels were normal. A renal biopsy showed marked interstitial oedema and infiltration of tubules by mononuclear cells, neutrophils and eosinophils. A diagnosis of acute TIN, probably drug induced, was made; antibiotics were discontinued and prednisolone started instead. Her serum creatinine rose to a peak of 640 μmol/l but she never became oliguric and did not require dialysis. After 3 days of steroids, her renal function began to improve and the eosinophil count fell.

CASE 9.11 MYELOMA KIDNEY

A 76-year-old man was admitted with a history of progressive weakness over a period of several months. On examination, he was unkempt, thin, pale and acidotic. His blood pressure was 110/60. He was markedly anaemic (Hb 64 g/l) with an ESR of 116 mm/h. His initial biochemical results showed a raised blood urea of 48 mmol/l (NR 2.5–7.5) and a grossly raised serum creatinine of 1910 µmol/l (NR 60–120) but a normal serum calcium. Urinary protein excretion was 2.8 g/day. A diagnosis of chronic renal failure of unknown cause was made. Peritoneal dialysis was started while other investigations were performed; intravenous urography (IVU) was delayed until after urinalysis (see below).

Serum electrophoresis showed a decreased γ fraction with a monoclonal band in the β region. Serum immunoglobulin levels were: IgG 1.4 g/l (NR 7.2–19.0); IgA 24.5 g/l (NR 0.8–5.0); and IgM 0.3 g/l (NR 0.5–2.0). Immunofixation of the serum and urine showed an IgA (λ type) paraprotein in the serum, with monoclonal free λ light chains in the urine. A bone marrow aspirate showed marked infiltration of atypical plasma cells. Radiology of the skeleton revealed osteolytic lesions in the pelvis and skull. A diagnosis of myeloma kidney was therefore made. Despite symptomatic treatment of his renal failure and cytotoxic therapy for myelomatosis, he died from renal failure 5 weeks after admission.

BOX 9.9 RENAL COMPLICATIONS OF MULTIPLE MYELOMA

These include:

- Manifestations of the paraprotein itself, such as proteinuria, myeloma kidney or renal amyloidosis

- Secondary metabolic disturbances, including hypercalcaemia, hyperuricaemia and proximal renal tubular defects

- Adverse effects resulting from investigations (renal failure after intravenous urography) or treatment (drug nephrotoxicity or pyelonephritis)

lects in ducts, forming casts. This is accelerated by dehydration. Other patients with excessive monoclonal light-chain excretion develop renal tubular acidosis and the Fanconi syndrome (phosphaturia, glycosuria and aminoaciduria) or amyloidosis.

The key principles in the prevention and **management** of the renal complications of myeloma are:

- maintenance of adequate hydration and institution of a diuresis if urinary casts are seen
- avoidance of dehydration before diagnostic procedures
- vigorous treatment of any hypercalcaemia or hyperuricaemia; and
- careful monitoring of all potentially nephrotoxic drugs.

Patients whose myeloma responds to chemotherapy are considered for places on maintenance dialysis programmes.

9.9.3 Other immunologically mediated tubulointerstitial nephritides

Immune complexes formed in the circulation may be deposited in the tubulointerstitial tissue of the kidney. In humans, the best example is SLE. Over 50% of renal biopsies from pa-

tients with SLE show evidence of tubulointerstitial immune complexes; these are seen as granular deposits of immunoglobulins and complement along the tubular basement membrane (TBM) or in the interstitium The deposits contain nuclear antigens analogous to those seen in glomerular deposits. The TIN may sometimes be severe enough to cause acute renal failure with minimal glomerular involvement.

Evidence that TIN is also induced by anti-TBM antibodies includes linear deposits of immunoglobulin and complement along the TBM (see Fig. 9.12). In humans, anti-TBM antibodies have been detected in over 70% of patients with anti-GBM nephritis (see section 9.7.1) and in about 20% of patients after renal transplantation, although the importance of anti-TBM antibodies in graft rejection is unknown.

Renal tubular acidosis is often found in association with hypergammaglobulinaemic conditions such as SLE, Sjögren's syndrome, chronic active hepatitis, primary biliary cirrhosis and fibrosing alveolitis. The most common functional defect is an inability to concentrate and acidify the urine. The immunological mechanism responsible for renal tubular acidosis in hypergammaglobulinaemia is not known, but an excess of polyclonal free light chains, normally metabolized in the tubules, may be the cause.

9.10 Chronic renal failure

Glomerulonephritis is a common cause of chronic renal failure (Table 9.7), although there are major differences in causation in different ethnic groups. Because renal biopsies are not always performed in patients with end-stage renal failure, it is difficult to reconstruct a complete picture of the evolution of these disorders. Treatment to halt or reverse the progress of the renal damage remains empirical; management consists mainly of the preservation of surviving nephrons by conservative measures.

Table 9.7 Causes of end-stage renal failure

Cause	Proportion (%)
Chronic glomerulonephritis	20
Diabetes mellitus	30
Hypertension	20
Pyelonephritis/reflux nephropathy	5
Polycystic kidneys	10
Interstitial nephritis	5
Other	15

9.11 Recurrent glomerulonephritis in transplanted kidneys

Glomerulonephritis can recur in the allografted kidney. On average, this happens in about one in four transplants, although the prevalence and severity depend on the original disease (Table 9.8). The graft shows the same lesions that existed in the patient's own kidneys. However, the presence of a form of glomerulonephritis that may recur is not a contraindica-tion to transplantation, since symptomatic recurrence is less frequent.

Table 9.8 Recurrence of original disease in kidney grafts

Original renal disease	Proportion showing histological recurrence (%)*
Focal glomerulosclerosis	30
Henoch–Schönlein nephritis	35
IgA nephropathy	50
Membranoproliferative glomerulonephritis	
Type I	20–30
Type II	50–100
Anti-GBM disease	~1

*Not necessarily associated with clinical disease.

FURTHER READING

See website: www.immunologyclinic.com

CHAPTER 10

10 Joints and Muscles

10.1 Introduction

Immunological mechanisms are responsible for many rheumatological diseases. Although these disorders often present with joint or muscle inflammation, many have multisystem involvement with a particular tendency to involve skin, lungs and kidney. These disorders, which include rheumatoid arthritis (RA), systemic lupus erythematosus (SLE), dermatomyositis, scleroderma and some forms of vasculitis, are often referred to as the 'connective tissue diseases'; this woolly phrase is rather meaningless in pathophysiological terms, but remains in widespread use. Because of the multisystem involvement, discussion of these disorders can also be found in other organ-based chapters. The connective tissue diseases are characteristically associated with non-organ-specific autoantibody production, particularly against components of cell nuclei. These autoantibodies are not necessarily responsible for joint or tissue damage, but are often helpful in diagnosis or prognosis (see Chapter 19).

10.2 Patterns of joint disease

Joint diseases fall into two broad categories: degenerative conditions of cartilage (osteoarthritis) or disorders characterized by inflammation of the joint lining or synovium (**inflammatory arthritis or synovitis**). The diagnosis of a particular form of inflammatory arthritis is only rarely made using a single diagnostic test; notable exceptions being the presence in synovial fluid of uric acid crystals in gout or of bacteria in septic arthritis. Instead, the diagnostic process usually relies heavily upon clinical assessment, with a smaller role being played by various immunological tests (Table 10.1). Most forms of chronic inflammatory joint diseases can be defined using clinical criteria alone, and this, in part, reflects our ignorance of the underlying aetiopathogenesis. The major common patterns of joint inflammation and the common underlying causes are summarized in Table 10.2.

The healthy synovial lining (Fig. 10.1) consists of a single layer of cells overlying loose, well-vascularized stromal tissue. The lining cells are of two kinds: one fibroblastic, which

Table 10.1 Major factors in the assessment of the patient with joint disease

Age/sex
Acute or chronic?
Pattern of joint disease?
  Monoarticular
  Oligoarticular
  Polyarticular
Extra-articular disease?
Rheumatoid factor positive?
Antinuclear antibody positive?

Table 10.2 Common patterns of inflammatory joint disease

Pattern of joint inflammation	Common causes
Monoarthritis	Bacterial infection
	Gout/pseudogout
	Spondyloarthropathy (especially reactive arthritis)
Oligoarthritis	Spondyloarthritis (especially reactive and psoriatic)
	Gout/pseudogout
Polyarthritis	
Symmetrical	Rheumatoid arthritis
	Systemic lupus erythematosus
	Viral arthritis
Asymmetrical	Psoriatic arthritis

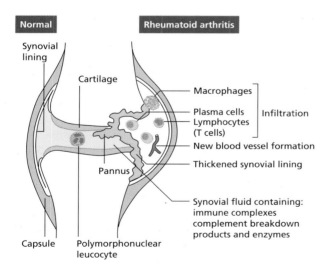

Fig. 10.1 Diagrammatic representation of a joint. One side is normal, the other shows characteristic pathological features of rheumatoid arthritis.

synthesizes the proteoglycans, which act as a lubricant within the joint, and one derived from macrophages, which probably have a scavenging function. Unlike most body surfaces, free passage of intercellular fluid can occur across the synovial membrane, a factor which may explain why antigens tend to be deposited within the joint. The synovial response to injury is relatively limited, and the pathology of most forms of inflammatory arthritis consists of hyperplasia of the lining layer and cellular infiltration of the vascular tissues beneath the lining. Cytokine production in chronic synovial inflammation may also be limited in its variety: most synovial diseases show some response to treatments which block the action of tumour necrosis factor (TNF)-α.

10.3 Arthritis and infection

There are two principal mechanisms whereby microorganisms can cause inflammatory arthritis: direct invasion of the synovium (infective or septic arthritis) or a hypersensitivity response (mediated by T-cell or immune complexes) against microbial antigen deposited within the joint.

10.3.1 Septic arthritis

Pyogenic arthritis can occur in previously healthy joints in immunocompetent subjects, but the risk is greatly increased by previous joint damage or defective immunity, particularly abnormalities of antibody production or neutrophils (the latter being most often a consequence of therapy). Joint damage probably increases the risk of sepsis by allowing increased entry of organisms into the joint. Patients with RA have a particular propensity to joint sepsis, this being partly due to corticosteroid therapy and joint damage, but also related to subtle defects in immunity associated with the disease itself (Case 10.1). The organisms most frequently associated with septic arthritis are summarized in Table 10.3.

Septic arthritis is a medical emergency. Delay in treatment is associated with an increasing risk of severe joint damage and with high mortality in immunocompromised subjects.

Table 10.3 Relative frequency of bacterial causes of septic arthritis in the UK

Staphylococcus aureus	40%
Pneumococcus	10%
Other streptococci	18%
Haemophilus influenzae	7%
Gram-negative bacilli	12%
Gonococcus*	< 1%

*Gonococcal joint infection is much more common in North America and Australia.

CASE 10.1 SEPTIC ARTHRITIS

A 37-year-old woman developed a symmetrical polyarthritis. A test for rheumatoid factor was positive and erosive changes were seen on X-ray, confirming a clinical diagnosis of RA. The arthritis followed an aggressive course with poor response to a variety of disease-modifying antirheumatic drugs and she became increasingly disabled due to severe destructive changes in the knees, wrists and shoulders. A moderate dose of prednisolone was introduced at the age of 42, with some symptomatic improvement in her joints and she was referred to an orthopaedic surgeon with a view to knee replacements. However, 1 month before her orthopaedic appointment she presented to the emergency department with a painful swollen right knee. On examination she was unwell, febrile

(38 °C) and had a hot, red right knee with a sizable effusion. Eighty millilitres of purulent synovial fluid was aspirated from the joint and microscopy of the fluid revealed numerous Gram-positive cocci. A diagnosis of septic arthritis was made on a background of severe RA and steroid therapy. She was treated with high-dose antibiotics and the joint was washed out via an arthroscope. Culture of blood and synovial fluid grew Staphylococcus aureus. She received 6 weeks' antibiotic treatment in total together with vigorous physiotherapy. Her knee, however, was significantly worsened by the infection and she could no longer straighten the leg or walk more than a few yards. Joint replacement was deferred for 6 months to reduce the risk of infection in the prosthesis.

Gonococcal and meningococcal infection can be associated with arthritis. This is most often associated with a subacute septicaemic illness, and organisms can be isolated from the blood and synovial fluid. However, in meningococcal infection, an immune complex-mediated arthropathy can also occur, which usually presents 7–10 days after the onset of infection and is associated with falling levels of meningococcal antigen in serum, rising levels of antibody and evidence of complement consumption, all features suggesting an immune complex-mediated disease.

Lyme disease, which is caused by the tick-borne spirochaete Borrelia burgdorferi, is associated with a chronic large-joint arthritis. This first appears some months after the initial tick bite, and usually has a relapsing and remitting course, but can be persistent and associated with joint destruction. Organisms are difficult to isolate from the joint, but an antibody response can be detected. The arthritis may be partly mediated by hypersensitivity mechanisms but improves after antibiotic treatment, suggesting that live organisms play a role in pathogenesis.

Viral arthritis

Joint and muscle pain is very common in acute viral infections, but inflammatory arthritis is much less common. Infections such as rubella, mumps and hepatitis B can cause a transient arthritis which is probably due to a combination of direct infection and hypersensitivity. This can also occur after immunization with attenuated but live rubella virus. The most common viral cause of arthritis in adults is parvovirus B19 (which in children usually only produces a mild febrile illness with a characteristic 'slapped cheek' rash). This produces a symmetrical, peripheral polyarthritis (clinically similar to early RA), which usually remits within 2 weeks but which can occasionally persist for several months.

Immune-mediated arthritis

The distinction between active infection and immune-mediated arthritis is not always clear-cut, as the above account makes clear. There are other forms of arthritis which appear to be triggered by infection and which follow a subacute, relapsing or chronic course. The most common of these, reactive arthritis, is discussed further in section 10.5. It will also be apparent from the sections on RA, other spondyloarthritides and juvenile chronic arthritis, that attempts have been made to explain most forms of chronic inflammatory joint disease in terms of inappropriate response to an unidentified organism. This model has perhaps been most successfully applied to the spondyloarthritides (see section 10.5). Other disorders in which arthritis is immune mediated include rheumatic fever, which is discussed in Chapter 2, and Henoch–Schönlein purpura, discussed in Chapter 9.

10.4 Rheumatoid arthritis

10.4.1 Diagnosis

RA is a common disease affecting 1–2% of the adult population and is twice as common in women as men. It is most common between the ages of 25 and 55 years, and the most frequent presentation is an insidious, symmetrical polyarthritis, although the disease can begin abruptly. Although systemic manifestations may be present at the outset, they develop more usually as the disease progresses (Table 10.4 and Case 10.3) *The diagnosis of RA is made on clinical grounds*, as illustrated in Case 10.2.

10.4.2 Serology

There is no diagnostic test for RA. Patients with RA fall into two groups: those with usually less severe disease who

CASE 10.2 RHEUMATOID ARTHRITIS

A 37-year-old woman gradually developed painful wrists over 3 months; she consulted her doctor only when the pain and early morning stiffness stopped her from gardening. On examination, both wrists and the metacarpophalangeal joints of both hands were swollen and tender but not deformed (see Fig. 10.2). There were no nodules or vasculitic lesions. On investigation, she was found to have a raised C-reactive protein (CRP) level (27 mg/l) (NR < 10) but a normal haemoglobin and white cell count. A latex test for rheumatoid factor was negative and antinuclear antibodies were not detected.

The clinical diagnosis was early RA and she was treated with ibuprofen. Despite some initial symptomatic improvement, the pain, stiffness and swelling of the hands persisted and 1 month later both knees became similarly affected. She was referred to a rheumatologist.

She was seen 6 months after the initial presentation. By this time she was struggling to work, drive and carry heavy objects. A test for rheumatoid factor was now positive (titre 1/256). X-rays of the feet showed small but definite erosions in two metatarsal heads. She still had a raised CRP (43 mg/l) but normal serum complement (C3 and C4) levels.

This woman had rheumatoid arthritis with some features suggesting a poor prognosis. Her treatment was changed to weekly low-dose methotrexate. This has controlled the arthritis for several years and no further erosions have developed.

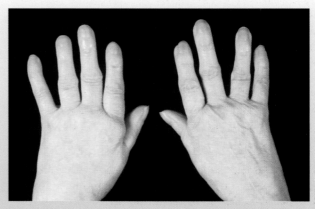

Fig. 10.2 Symmetrical synovitis in early rheumatoid arthritis. With permission from Medical Masterclass: Rheumatology and Clinical Immunology, London: Royal College of Physicians, 2001.

Table 10.4 Extra-articular features of rheumatoid arthritis: the commonest features are marked in bold (adapted from Bacon)

Intrinsic or essential systemic features of rheumatoid disease
   Rheumatoid nodules
   Serositis (pleurisy, pericarditis)
   Vasculitis
   Neuropathy (often caused by vasculitic damage to nerves)
   Felty's syndrome (neutropenia and splenomegaly)
Consequences of chronic inflammation and immune stimulation
   Anaemia
   Weight loss and fever
   Lymphadenopathy
Complications of rheumatoid disease
   Entrapment neuropathy, e.g. carpal tunnel syndrome
   Accelerated atherosclerosis
   Infection
   Amyloidosis
   Cervical myelopathy
Complications of treatment
   Osteoporosis (corticosteroids)
   Accelerated atherosclerosis
   Infection
   Drug-specific side-effects
Associated syndromes (also occur without RA)
   Keratoconjunctivitis sicca
   Interstitial lung diseases
   Episcleritis and scleritis

lack circulating rheumatoid factor (seronegative RA); and a larger group (70%) with more aggressive disease who have, or develop, a rheumatoid factor in the serum (seropositive RA). Extra-articular disease occurs predominantly in this seropositive group. **Rheumatoid factor** is of more value in prognosis than in diagnosis. Rheumatoid factor, in this context, refers only to the IgM antibody which binds aggregated IgG as its antigen (see Chapter 19). Rheumatoid factors of the IgG or IgA class are not clinically helpful, although may play a role in joint inflammation. Antibodies to citrullinated peptides (anti-CCP antibodies—see section 10.4.4) seem to have high specificity for the diagnosis of RA, and their presence predicts a poorer prognosis. However, anti-CCP antibody testing is not yet in widespread clinical use.

Other serological tests are of little value in RA. Antinuclear antibody (ANA) is present in 40%, but is usually of low titre and often of IgM class; such ANAs are found in many other conditions. Serum complement C3 and C4 levels may be normal or raised due to an 'acute-phase' reaction (see Chapter 1). **CRP** (another 'acute-phase' reactant) is also raised, particularly in active RA; this helps to distinguish active RA from active SLE (see Fig. 10.8).

10.4.3 Pathology

The earliest pathological change in RA appears to be an infiltrate of neutrophils and mononuclear cells around small blood vessels in the loose connective tissue beneath the synovium. As the disease progresses, large numbers of T cells, macrophages, B cells and plasma cells accumulate in this tissue and the synovium becomes markedly thickened due to fibroblast proliferation and macrophage migration. The surface area increases and becomes folded into villi. New vessel formation occurs and some blood vessels develop into structures specialized for lymphocyte migration: so-called high endothelial venules (see section 1.7). Secondary lymphoid follicles also develop. In consequence, the histological structure comes to resemble that of an activated lymph node, emphasizing the high degree of immunological activity in RA. Large amounts of synovial fluid can form (especially in large joints), and this contains large numbers of neutrophil polymorphs, which have migrated from the blood.

This chronic inflammatory tissue has several destructive effects upon the joint. First, the hypertrophied lining layer at the margins of the joint (known as **pannus**) erodes cartilage and underlying bone. Second, cytokines induce chondrocytes and fibroblasts to produce enzymes which break down the extracellular matrix. Third, degranulation of neutrophils in the synovial fluid can directly damage the surface of cartilage (Fig. 10.1).

10.4.4 Immunopathogenesis

The immunohistology of rheumatoid synovium suggests that the disease results from an immunological response to an antigen within the joint. The nature of this immunological response and the target antigen remain uncertain. It is, however, clear that joint destruction in RA is driven by activated macrophages (Fig. 10.3), which mediate tissue breakdown directly and also activate other cells in the joint. A large number of inflammatory mediators are produced in RA synovium (Fig. 10.3), and early descriptions of cytokine production in RA talked of a 'cytokine soup', with many different pathways leading to joint damage (and by implication no simple way of inhibiting this process). Some pattern has emerged from this apparent inflammatory chaos with the demonstration that TNF-α, largely derived from macrophages, plays a central role in this inflammatory process (Fig. 10.4): inhibition of this cytokine with neutralizing antibodies reduces the production of most other inflammatory mediators in cell culture. When these antibodies are administered to patients, a dramatic improvement in joint inflammation occurs. The members of the interleukin (IL)-1 family, IL-1α and IL-1β, also play an important role, although less crucial than TNF.

There is probably more than one immunological mechanism leading to macrophage activation in rheumatoid synovium. *The most widely accepted model is a process driven by CD4+ T cells.* The evidence for T-cell involvement in RA is summarized in Table 10.5. However, the model of RA as a

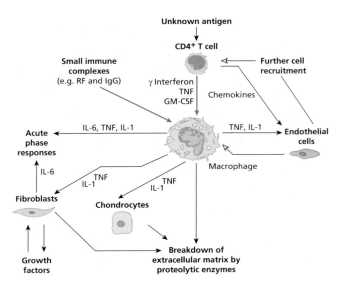

Fig. 10.3 How CD4+ T cells and immune complexes may control the events leading to joint damage in rheumatoid arthritis.

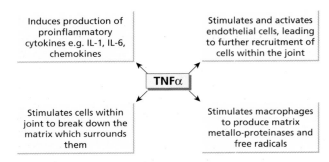

Fig. 10.4 The central role of tumour necrosis factor (TNF)-α in controlling rheumatoid synovial inflammation.

T-cell-driven disease has been criticized, as T-cell cytokines such as IL-2 and interferon (IFN)-γ are hard to detect in RA synovium, in contrast to macrophage-derived cytokines such as TNF-α, IL-1 and IL-6, which are present in abundance. Therapies specifically directed at T cells have also been only partially successful in controlling the disease.

Inflammation driven by antibodies may also be important. Models of RA pathogenesis from the 1960s and 1970s focused on inflammation driven by complement activation induced by immune complexes containing rheumatoid factors and IgG. Rheumatoid factor and other autoantibodies were relegated to a minor subsidiary role with the rise of T-cell models of RA synovitis in the 1980s and 1990s. However, the recent clinical demonstration that depletion of B cells (with an anti-CD20 monoclonal antibody, rituximab—see Chapter 7) dramatically improves the clinical features of RA, suggests that antibody-mediated inflammation may after all play a crucial role in the disease (Table 10.5). There is some evidence that

Table 10.5 Evidence that T and B cells play a central role in the pathogenesis of rheumatoid arthritis (RA)

T cells
- Rheumatoid synovium densely infiltrated with mature T cells (mainly CD4⁺) bearing activation markers
- Disease closely associated with particular MHC class II polymorphism, i.e. DR4
- Therapy directed against T cells (e.g. cyclosporin) modestly effective in treatment
- RA improves with progression of HIV infection
- Most animal models critically dependent upon T cells

B cells
- Rheumatoid synovium contains large numbers of plasma cells
- Disease closely associated with autoantibodies: rheumatoid factor and anti-citrullinated peptide antibodies
- Efficacy of therapy specifically directed against B cells (rituximab)
- B cells also important in animal models

small immune complexes can directly activate macrophages via Fc receptors.

If RA is an immunologically mediated disease, then it should be possible to define the main antigens driving the T- and B-cell responses in the joint. These antigens could be self-molecules expressed in the joint or could be foreign (e.g. bacterial or viral) antigens sequestered in joint tissue. T- and B-cell responses to a number of autoantigens have been described in RA (Table 10.6), but most are not specific for RA and the role of responses against these antigens in the disease is unclear. One of the most plausible autoimmune models of RA would be for the disease to be driven by an immune response against an antigen whose expression is confined to joints, such as type II collagen, the main protein of articular cartilage. However, although immune responses against cartilage and synovial proteins can be found in some patients with RA, these are not found in all and are also found in other diseases. Antibodies against a number of peptides containing the unusual amino acid, citrulline (anti-CCP antibodies)

have recently been found to be highly specific to RA and to predict aggressive and persistent disease. The antigen-driving production of these antibodies, and their role in disease, awaits clarification. Plausible but unproven models of synovial inflammation driven by self-perpetuating rheumatoid factor production have also been proposed.

There is also evidence that macrophage-induced inflammation can become self-sustaining and independent of any triggering immune response: cytokines such as TNF-α produced by macrophages induce further macrophage activation. It is plausible that different mechanisms may predominate at different stages of this chronic disease, with immune mechanisms being key in earlier disease.

10.4.5 Aetiology

In Europeans there is an association between possession of HLA-DR4 and -DR1 and rheumatoid factor-positive RA. This association becomes stronger with increasing severity of disease, and the presence of extra-articular manifestations. Different associations were described in other ethnic groups and a common link to the DR4/DR1 association was not apparent until the detailed structure of DR molecules became known at the amino acid level. This allowed comparison of different DR alleles associated with RA. Almost all alleles associated with RA (HLA-DRB1*0101, 0401 and 0404) have a distinctive five amino acid sequence near the peptide-binding region of the DRβ chain; this sequence is known as the 'shared epitope'. Possession of two copies of the 'shared epitope' (one inherited from each parent) is associated with a high risk of severe disease (Table 10.7). Other genes also appear to be important in determining susceptibility to RA, but the shared epitope association seems to be the strongest. Female sex is an important genetic risk factor, and it seems plausible that this risk is mediated hormonally.

Environmental factors predisposing to RA remain poorly understood. Smoking is a weak risk factor, and use of the oral contraceptive may protect against RA. There is an increased risk of onset of RA in the post-partum period. Many attempts have been made to link RA to infectious agents such as parvovirus, Epstein–Barr virus, mycoplasma and myco-

Table 10.6 Autoimmune responses identified in patients with rheumatoid arthritis (RA)

Autoantigen	Antibodies in RA	T cell response in RA	Specificity for RA
IgG	Yes: rheumatoid factor		No
Type II collagen and other cartilage antigens	Yes: in 10–20%	Yes: in 10–20%	No
Citrullinated proteins (CCP)	Yes	Probably	Yes

Table 10.7 How possession of an HLA-DRB1 allele containing the 'shared epitope' influences absolute risk of developing rheumatoid arthritis (RA) in a Caucasian population. The risk is highest in those who inherit a copy of a different DRB1 gene from each of their parents. Data from Nepom G. Rheum Dis Clin N Am 1992; 18:785

	Approximate risk of developing RA
Total population	1 in 100
Subjects with no copies of shared epitope	1 in 580
DRB1*0401	1 in 35
DRB1*0404	1 in 20
DRB1*0101	1 in 80
DRB1*0401 *and* 0404	1 in 7

bacteria. However, while the idea of RA as a disease either initiated or perpetuated by an immune response against an infection has many attractions, no convincing evidence exists to implicate any known agent (see Chapter 5 for discussion of how infections may trigger autoimmunity).

Many animal models of RA have been developed, centred on both infection and autoimmunity, all with some similarity to the human disease. If nothing else, these models emphasize that the synovial response to injury is limited in scope and most of the above aetiological factors are plausible.

10.4.6 Outcome

Although the outcome of RA is variable and some patients have mild or remitting disease, *it is for most a severe and disabling illness*. Most (70%) of RA patients have many periods of remission and relapse over decades (polycyclic disease). A small proportion (15%) are fortunate to have monocyclic disease and recover over a few years without relapse. Progressive RA, with relentless increase in disability with few partial remissions, occurs in another 15%.

Joint damage begins in the early stages of the disease and once established is effectively irreversible. Five years after diagnosis, one-third of patients are unable to work at all and only one-third are still in full-time work. At 10 years, 10–20% of those affected are highly dependent upon others for self-care. Factors predicting a poor prognosis are detailed in Table 10.8.

It is now also apparent that RA is associated with increased mortality as well as disability. *Life expectancy in RA is reduced by approximately 7 years compared with age- and sex-matched controls*. In severe, disabling RA, the 5-year mortality is around 50%. The causes of these premature deaths are multiple and often not directly attributable to the arthritis, although some patients die of extra-articular disease (Case 10.3) such as vasculitis, amyloid (see Chapter 9) or the side-effects of drug treatment. Patients with RA also show an increased susceptibility to severe or recurrent infection, in both those treated with steroids and those who have not received steroids. The largest single contributor to increased mortality in RA is, however, an increased risk of **ischaemic**

CASE 10.3 PULMONARY FIBROSIS IN RHEUMATOID ARTHRITIS

A 61-year-old man, with a 15-year history of seropositive RA, was admitted with increasing shortness of breath, myalgia and weight loss. He had previously smoked 40 cigarettes a day but had never been exposed to coal or silica dust. On examination, he was pale and thin, with generalized muscle tenderness. Widespread crepitations were heard over both lung fields. His joints were tender and he had subluxation of the metacarpophalangeal joints of both hands. There was bilateral cervical and axillary lymph node enlargement but no splenomegaly. Neurological and cardiac examinations were normal.

Investigations showed a raised CRP (81 mg/l) and a normochromic anaemia (Hb 95 g/l) but a normal white cell count. His serum IgG was raised at 44 g/l (NR 7.2–19.0), although IgA and IgM levels were normal. He had a strongly positive rheumatoid factor titre of 1/1280 (NR < 1/32). There were no detectable antibodies to DNA or to extractable nuclear antigens (ENA) (see Chapter

19) and the serum levels of muscle enzymes were normal. A chest X-ray suggested pulmonary fibrosis. High-resolution computed tomographic scanning of the chest confirmed severe pulmonary fibrosis, with no evidence of any ground glass shadowing (a feature suggesting response to immunosuppression). Pulmonary function tests showed a severe restrictive defect, with an forced expiratory volume in 1 sec/forced expiratory vital capacity of 1.1/1.3. He was too unwell to undergo a lung biopsy.

This man's dyspnoea was rapidly progressive and he continued to deteriorate despite intravenous corticosteroids and cyclophosphamide. At autopsy, both lungs showed severe fibrosis, with the pattern of usual interstitial pneumonia (see section 13.4.3), which is a rare complication of RA with a poor prognosis. The onset of serious complications of RA so long after the initial diagnosis is not unusual.

Table 10.8 Predictors of a poor prognosis in early rheumatoid arthritis

High titre serum rheumatoid factor
Female sex
High levels of acute phase proteins (ESR, CRP)
High levels of disability
Extra-articular disease
Radiological evidence of joint damage
Serum anti-citrullated peptide (anti-CCP) antibodies
Possession of the shared epitope: two copies are worse than one

ESR, Erythrocyte sedimentation rate; CRP, C-reactive protein.

heart disease (IHD). Mortality from IHD in RA is increased by approximately two- to three-fold, a comparable increase in risk to that seen in diabetes mellitus. Similar increased mortality from IHD has also been described in other chronic inflammatory diseases, particularly SLE. The mechanisms underlying this increased risk are unclear, but conventional risk factors alone (such as smoking, hyperlipidaemia and hypertension) cannot explain the increased risk, and corticosteroid treatment and disease-specific factors make substantial contributions.

10.4.7 Management

Although management of RA is a multidisciplinary process, aiming to control the disease and minimize pain and disability, the paramount aim of treatment is the pharmacological limitation of joint inflammation and damage. Joint damage in RA begins early, is effectively irreversible and has a poor outcome: *these are compelling reasons to introduce effective, aggressive treatment early in the disease.*

Recognition of these factors has led to an increasing tendency for early use of disease-modifying drugs, particularly in subjects felt to have a poor prognosis. Methotrexate, leflunomide and sulphasalazine (Chapter 7) are the most commonly used drugs. There is an increasing tendency to use drugs in combination in severe or aggressive disease; these combinations are more effective and no more toxic than single drug regimes. Corticosteroids are widely used, usually being administered directly into inflamed joints, since systemic use can be associated with severe side-effects on long-term use. Patients who fail treatment with methotrexate and similar drugs are now usually treated with anti-TNF agents, such as etanercept and infliximab, which can control RA in 60–70% of patients refractory to other treatments. Anti-TNF agents may have advantages over conventional drugs in early disease, but their use is currently limited by their high cost. It is notable that 30–40% of patients show little or no response to anti-TNF agents, suggesting that inflammatory

mechanisms that are not critically dependent on TNF-α are operating in these patients. Small numbers of patients have been treated with highly aggressive chemotherapy and autologous stem cell transplantation with some success (see section 8.5.6), but the long-term utility of this approach is not yet clear. Dramatic responses in patients with refractory disease have been reported following treatment with the anti-B-cell monoclonal antibody, rituximab. Recombinant IL-1 receptor antagonist (Chapter 1) has also been used to block the action of IL-1α and IL-1β, but the response is not as striking as that seen with anti-TNF agents.

A difficulty with selecting patients for treatment with earlier and more aggressive therapy is identification of patients with a poor prognosis. In order to prevent disability and restore normal life expectancy, treatment needs to be instituted before major joint damage has occurred. However, RA is a very variable disease and even with a combination of genetic, serological and clinical markers (Table 10.8), selection of patients with a poor prognosis is currently imperfect.

10.5 Seronegative spondyloarthritis

This group of disorders includes ankylosing spondylitis, Reiter's syndrome and reactive arthritis, psoriatic arthropathy and enteropathic arthritis.

These syndromes are characterized by absence of rheumatoid factor (seronegative), spinal (spondylo-) involvement and often asymmetrical peripheral arthritis, tending to involve large joints. Inflammation at the insertion of muscles, ligaments or tendons into bone, or enthesitis, is a core feature in these disorders. It has been recognized for many years that enthesitis underlies the spinal involvement. Recent studies of early joint inflammation in spondyloarthropathies using magnetic resonance imaging (MRI) or ultrasound imaging have demonstrated that synovial inflammation also begins with enthesitis at the joint margins. Ossification can occur at the site of enthesitis, and in the spine this can lead to fusion (ankylosis) of adjacent vertebrae. All of these disorders are strongly associated with **HLA-B27**, the association being strongest in subjects with predominantly spinal disease. Most of these disorders show a therapeutic response to anti-TNF agents.

The use of the label 'reactive arthritis' requires comment: while any arthritic process triggered by infection could be reasonably called reactive, the diagnostic label is usually reserved for a form of spondyloarthritis described in more detail below.

10.5.1 Ankylosing spondylitis

Ankylosing spondylitis (AS) is a chronic inflammatory condition of the spine and sacroiliac joints. It is a progressive disease in which restriction of movement is associated

CASE 10.4 ANKYLOSING SPONDYLITIS

A 21-year-old man presented to his local emergency department with acute pain and swelling of one knee. On examination, the joint was tender and restricted in movement. X-ray of the knee showed periarticular osteoporosis. On investigation, he had a raised erythrocyte sedimentation rate (ESR) of 102 mm/h, a mild anaemia (Hb 106 g/l) but no detectable serum rheumatoid factor. The knee effusion was aspirated; the fluid contained a polymorphonuclear leucocytosis but no organisms or rheumatoid factor. No diagnosis was made at this stage but he was treated empirically with diclofenac; his arthritis improved.

Fifteen months later he developed an iritis in his left eye. At this point, a history was also elicited of low back pain and prolonged early morning stiffness dating back to his late teenage years. His peripheral joints were normal but his lumbar spine was rigid and he had some pain and restriction of the neck. X-rays of his lumbar spine and pelvis showed the classic changes of ankylosing spondylitis and tissue typing revealed that he was HLA-B27-positive (see Fig. 10.5). He continues to have widespread spinal discomfort, although daily exercises have reduced the stiffness in his neck. At his last clinic visit he asked whether he should receive an anti-TNF drug.

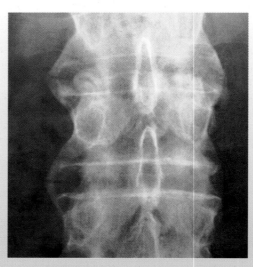

Fig. 10.5 Bamboo lumbar spine in ankylosing spondylitis. With permission from Medical Masterclass: Rheumatology and Clinical Immunology, London: Royal College of Physicians, 2001.

with ossification of the intervertebral ligaments. As in Case 10.4, this disease mainly affects men aged between 15 and 30 years. Four men in 1000 are affected and 5% have a positive family history. Complications are common: 25% develop iritis and 20% have a peripheral arthritis, although either condition may be the sole presenting symptom. Rarer complications include pulmonary fibrosis, aortic incompetence, cardiac conduction defects and amyloidosis.

The association between HLA-B27 and AS is very strong; over 95% of affected individuals are positive for this antigen. The frequency (3–10%) of HLA-B27 in a normal, white population makes a positive test less useful in patients in whom this disease is suspected; the absence of HLA-B27 in a patient makes AS very unlikely, although it does not exclude it.

The precise aetiology is unknown. The association of AS with HLA-B27 is shared with other arthritides which follow infection, such as Reiter's disease (see below). Persistence of specific antigens of the infecting organisms has been demonstrated in joint tissues in these patients. This suggests that AS may also be triggered by infection [possibly in the gastrointestinal (GI) tract] in susceptible HLA-B27-positive individuals. The finding that two-thirds of patients with AS have asymptomatic inflammatory gut lesions supports this, although these may be caused by anti-inflammatory drugs used for therapy.

The relationship of arthritides and HLA-B27 remains uncertain but has been clarified by studies using transgenic

rats. The introduction of the gene for human HLA-B27 into otherwise normal rats results in a multisystem disease resembling AS. The development of this disease is dependent upon exposure to gut commensal organisms, particularly Bacteroides. This model confirmed that the gene is an important predisposing factor.

The most important aspect of treatment is exercise to maintain full mobility, with anti-inflammatory drugs to reduce the pain. Joint replacement and occasionally spinal surgery may be required. *Anti-TNF agents are the only therapies which have been shown to have a significant effect on the spinal inflammation.*

10.5.2 Other seronegative spondyloarthritides

Reiter's syndrome and reactive arthritis (Case 10.5)
Reiter's syndrome and reactive arthritis can be regarded as a spectrum of disease ranging from a multisystem disorder characterized by an inflammatory arthritis, urethritis, conjunctivitis and uveitis and skin changes (Reiter's syndrome) to disease which is confined to the joints (reactive arthritis). Of all the spondyloarthritides, the link to infection is clearest in Reiter's/reactive arthritis: the majority of cases appear to be triggered by either sexually acquired Chlamydia trachomatis infection or by certain bacterial infections of the gut (in particular, Shigella, Salmonella, Campylobacter or Yersinia infection). The overall risk of this syndrome after a trigger-

CASE 10.5 REITER'S DISEASE

A 19-year-old man presented with acute swelling of his right knee and left ankle and extremely painful heels. On questioning, he admitted to a penile discharge and dysuria for 4 days. On examination, he had bilateral Achilles tendonitis and his right knee and left ankle were red, hot and tender. He had aphthous-like mouth ulcers and ulcers around the glans penis. There were no skin lesions and, in particular, no evidence of keratoderma blenorrhagica or subungual pustules.

On investigation, he was found to have a raised ESR (60 mm/h) but a normal haemoglobin and white cell count. A latex test for rheumatoid factor was negative. X-rays of the joints were normal.

Joint fluid aspirated from the right knee showed a polymorphonuclear leucocytosis but no organisms. Gonococci were not cultured from the urethral pus or from the joint fluid but chlamydial DNA was detected by the polymerase chain reaction. Tissue typing showed him to be HLA-B27 positive. A diagnosis of Reiter's disease was made. He was given diclofenac for symptomatic relief of the arthritis and tendonitis. Four days later, he developed bilateral conjunctivitis and some photophobia. However, 6 weeks later he had fully recovered and did not relapse. His chlamydial urethritis was treated with doxycycline and his partner was screened for sexually transmitted infection.

ing infection is around 1%, and HLA-B27 is an important risk factor (80% of patients are B27 positive). The syndrome is commoner in men than women (by about 3 to 1), and tends to affect those under 40 years old.

Bacterial/chlamydial proteins and DNA can be detected in affected joints, but viable organisms have not been found. The arthropathy results mainly from a T-cell response to the sequestered bacterial antigens. Treatment is with intra-articular corticosteroid injections, anti-inflammatory drugs and physiotherapy; antibiotic treatment of the triggering infection has no effect on the arthritis. Most cases remit within a few months, but around 20% (largely B27-positive patients) develop chronic peripheral joint and spinal disease. Severe Reiter's syndrome can occur in human immunodeficiency virus (HIV) infection.

Enteropathic arthritis

Twenty percent of patients with ulcerative colitis develop a mild seronegative inflammatory arthritis, enteropathic arthritis, which affects peripheral joints. Conversely, 5% of patients with ankylosing spondylitis have either clinical ulcerative colitis or Crohn's disease. Inflammatory bowel disease should be considered as an underlying cause in patients with features of a seronegative spondyloarthropathy.

The overlapping clinical features of HLA-B27-related arthropathies suggest that similar immunopathogenic mechanisms are involved.

Psoriatic arthritis

Psoriasis is a common skin disease (see Chapter 11). Two percent of patients with psoriasis develop psoriatic arthropathy; this may affect the peripheral joints or the spine. The psoriasis generally precedes the arthritis by many years; in rare cases where the arthritis comes first, diagnosis may be difficult. A family history of psoriasis is a helpful diagnostic clue and the characteristic nail changes of psoriasis are present in 80% of patients with psoriatic arthritis. Dactylitis is a distinctive feature. Treatment is similar to that for RA, including the use of anti-TNF drugs. The prognosis is usually good, although severe joint destruction can occur.

10.5.3 Other seronegative arthritides

The disorders discussed below do not share clinical and aetiological features with the spondyloarthritides but are sometimes classified with them under the loose (and largely meaningless) banner of seronegative arthritis.

Relapsing polychondritis is a rare, non-hereditary condition characterized by inflammation of cartilage and is often associated with arthritis. Most patients have an episodic, migratory, asymmetrical polyarthritis. A provisional diagnosis of seronegative RA is often made until the characteristic attacks of cartilage inflammation occur, usually in the ears, nose and trachea. The aetiology of this condition is unknown. Cartilage antibodies are found in some patients, and T lymphocytes sensitized to cartilage antigen have been reported in others; however, these changes may be secondary to cartilage damage rather than its cause.

Behçet's disease (Case 10.6) is a chronic, multisystem disorder affecting slightly more men than women. Recurrent, potentially blinding, uveitis with oral and genital ulceration is the commonest clinical feature, but arthritis develops in 45% of patients and is the presenting symptom in 15%. Vasculitis with thrombophlebitis and neurological involvement occurs in 25–30% of cases. There is no diagnostic test and the diagnosis is entirely clinical. No specific treatment is available, although corticosteroids may control symptoms and azathioprine has been shown to reduce progression of visual loss. In severe cases, cyclosporin, tacrolimus and infliximab may be effective. Thalidomide may be useful in refractory orogenital ulceration. There is an association between Behçet's disease and HLA-B51.

CASE 10.6 BEHÇET'S SYNDROME

A 32-year-old man from a Turkish family presented with deteriorating vision and painful swollen knees. Further questioning revealed a 10-year history of relapsing and remitting mouth ulcers and a less severe history of genital ulceration. On examination he had reduced visual acuity associated with a florid retinal vasculitis. Two 1-cm mouth ulcers were found but no active genital ulceration. He had synovitis in both knees. Investigation revealed a raised ESR at 94 mm/h but a normal blood count and negative tests for rheumatoid factor, antinuclear antibodies, cytomegalovirus and HIV infection. A clinical diagnosis of Behcet's syndrome was made. He was treated with high-dose corticosteroids and azathioprine with good response, although his visual acuity remains permanently impaired.

10.6 Chronic arthritis in children (Case 10.7)

Juvenile idiopathic arthritis (JIA) is the generic term for a group of diseases in which an inflammatory arthritis begins before the age of 16 years; there are several distinct syndromes. It is important first to exclude diseases which do not form part of the spectrum of JIA; these include juvenile dermatomyositis, acute rheumatic fever, SLE, post-infective arthropathies and joint disease associated with antibody deficiency or haemophilia.

Chronic arthritis in childhood is divided into six subgroups (Fig. 10.6). Ten percent have a juvenile version of seropositive rheumatoid arthritis. This behaves like the adult disease, and the presence of rheumatoid factor confirms the diagnosis. The condition tends to progress to severe joint destruction with extra-articular complications of RA, such as nodules and vasculitis. A further 15% have enthesitis-related arthritis (ERA), which is closely related to ankylosing spondylitis and the spondyloarthropathies (Fig. 10.5).

The majority (75%) of children with a chronic inflammatory arthritis have seronegative diseases which have no obvious counterpart in adult arthritic disorders, although rarely adults can develop a disorder which is very similar to systemic JIA: this is adult-onset Still's disease.

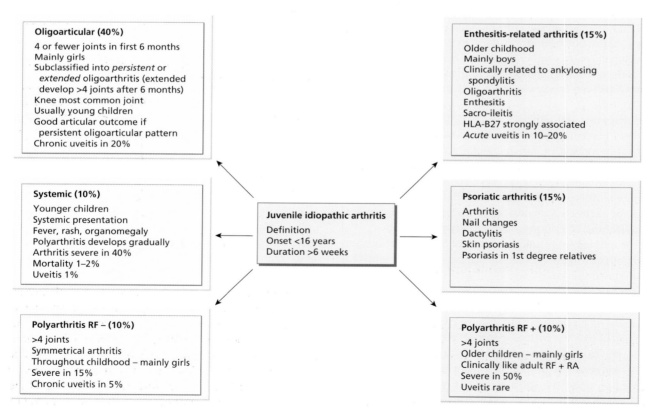

Fig. 10.6 Classification of juvenile idiopathic arthritis. Disorders on the left only occur in childhood, whereas those on the right are childhood equivalents of adult diseases.

CASE 10.7 JUVENILE IDIOPATHIC ARTHRITIS

A 2-year-old girl was taken to her GP because she was unwilling to walk. Her GP found her right knee to be swollen and tender and referred her to an orthopaedic surgeon who was concerned that she may have septic arthritis, although she was systemically well. An X-ray was normal. Synovial fluid was aspirated under general anaesthetic, but was sterile on culture. The pain settled somewhat, although the knee was still swollen on examination. Two months later her left ankle also became swollen and painful. Blood tests showed a raised ESR at 40 mm/h, a negative test for rheumatoid factor and a low-titre (1/40) homogeneous ANA. DNA antibodies were not detected. Serum immunoglobulins were normal. A diagnosis of early-onset pauciarticular JIA was made and she was treated with ibuprofen with a good response. However, 3 months later the knee was still swollen and she was given an intra-articular steroid injection with complete resolution of the synovitis. Her vision seemed normal but ophthalmological screening revealed a severe chronic uveitis which was treated with topical steroids. At the age of 4 her joint disease was in complete remission, but her uveitis remained intermittently active, and she has developed a cataract in the right eye. She remains under long-term ophthalmological follow-up.

The aetiologies of the childhood-specific forms of JIA are poorly understood; no environmental triggers have been identified but a number of genetic associations have been delineated, mainly within the HLA region. These genetic associations further differentiate these disorders from adult forms of arthritis.

Potentially blinding chronic uveitis is a major complication of JIA. This type of uveitis is usually clinically silent until vision is impaired (in contrast to acute uveitis), a common feature of spondyloarthropathies, which is painful. Chronic uveitis occurs predominantly, but not exclusively, in children with oligoarticular JIA. Therefore all children with JIA require screening for this silently progressive condition.

Useful investigations in children with chronic arthritis include the ESR, and acute-phase reactants such as CRP; both increase with disease activity. There is no diagnostic test, although the presence of rheumatoid factor or antinuclear antibodies is helpful in classification. Antinuclear antibodies, directed against histones and other nuclear antigens, but not DNA, are found in a high proportion of cases (Fig. 10.5).

The mechanisms of joint inflammation in the various forms of JIA seem to be similar to those in RA, with similar immunohistology. Treatment is also similar; most cases respond to methotrexate, with a good response to anti-TNF agents in refractory cases.

10.7 Systemic lupus erythematosus

10.7.1 Clinical features (Case 10.8)

SLE is a multisystem disorder which typically affects young women, with a prevalence of around 1 in 2000. It is characterized by the presence of **autoantibodies to nuclear antigens**. The most common presenting feature is arthritis or arthralgia (Table 10.9). Nearly all patients eventually experience joint problems and skin lesions, while about one-half to two-thirds also have pulmonary, renal, neurological or haematological involvement at some time (Table 10.10).

Table 10.9 Presenting features of systemic lupus erythematosus

Features	%
Constitutional symptoms	50
Joints/muscles	62
Skin	50
Blood	8
Brain	15
Kidney	25

Table 10.10 Cumulative organ involvement in patients with systemic lupus erythematosus

Organ/tissue	Patients (%) who eventually develop organ involvement
Skin	80
Joints/muscles	80
Lung/pleura	30
Blood	60
Brain	30
Kidney	40
Heart	15

Atypical and non-specific presentations of SLE often cause difficulty in diagnosis. Pleuropericardial inflammation is common but usually mild and transient; a few patients (10%) have clinical and radiological evidence of diffuse, progressive interstitial lung disease. The renal complications of SLE are described in Chapter 9. Neurological features of SLE (see section 17.6) span the spectrum of neurological and psychiatric disease from headaches to psychosis. Common manifestations include dementia, depression, convulsions, chorea and migraine (see Chapter 17).

Recurrent venous or cerebral arterial thrombosis, thrombocytopenia and recurrent abortions are associated with the presence of the 'lupus anticoagulant' and/or antiphospholipid antibodies. The lupus anticoagulant causes a prolonged clotting time in vitro but thrombosis in vivo. It is often found in association with other autoantibodies to phospholipids, such as anticardiolipin antibodies and false-positive tests for syphilis. The distinction between SLE with antiphospholipid antibodies and the primary antiphospholipid antibody syndrome is discussed in Chapter 16.

In such a varied disease as SLE, it is important to have agreed criteria if comparisons are to be made. The American College of Rheumatology criteria are internationally accepted and were revised in 1982 and slightly modified in 1997 (Table 10.11). *These criteria are designed primarily for use in research rather than everyday clinical work.*

10.7.2 Laboratory findings

Almost all patients with SLE have ANAs, including antibodies to dsDNA. A negative ANA does not completely exclude a suspected diagnosis of SLE, while positive dsDNA antibodies strongly support it. Antibodies to other, extractable nuclear antigens (ENAs) detected by non-fluorescent methods (see Chapter 19) are often present also (Table 10.13;

Table 10.11 American College of Rheumatology criteria for diagnosis of systemic lupus erythematosus (SLE)*

Malar rash
Discoid rash
Photosensitivity
Oral ulcers
Non-erosive arthritis
Serositis (pleuritis/pericarditis)
Renal disease (persistent proteinuria/urinary casts)
Neurological disorder (seizures/psychosis)
Haemolytic anaemia/leucopenia/lymphopenia/
thrombocytopenia
Antinuclear antibody
Antibodies to dsDNA/antibodies to extractable nuclear
antigens/antiphospholipid antibodies

*To establish a diagnosis of SLE, a patient must have four or more of these criteria.

Fig. 10.7). Other laboratory findings are positive in a varying proportion of patients (Table 10.13). In view of the wide range of presenting symptoms and the difficulties of making a definite diagnosis, all patients in whom SLE is suspected should be tested for antinuclear antibodies, including those

CASE 10.8 SYSTEMIC LUPUS ERYTHEMATOSUS

A 26-year-old woman presented with fatigue and painful, stiff knees of 4 weeks' duration. She had a 6-year history of Raynaud's phenomenon, frequent mouth ulcers and had had a blotchy rash and ill-health after a recent holiday in Spain. On examination, she had bilateral effusions in both knee joints, but all other joints were normal. She had no skin lesions, muscle tenderness, proteinuria or fever. A full blood count showed mild thrombocytopenia with a platelet count of 95 (normal $150–400 \times 10^{12}$/l) and lymphopenia (0.7×10^9/l, normal 1.5–4.0). The results of relevant immunological investigations are shown in Table 10.12. On the basis of these findings, a diagnosis of SLE was made and the patient treated with aspirin for her painful knees. She improved over 4 weeks and then remained symptom-free for 5 years. During this time, her antinuclear antibody remained positive at 1/1000, her anti-double-stranded (ds) DNA antibody level varied from 40 to 100 (normal < 25) and her C3 and C4 levels were occasionally low. Later, she developed a bilateral, blotchy rash on her hands and thighs, consistent with active vasculitis. Her Raynaud's phenomenon concurrently became much worse. Following treatment with hydroxychloroquine, the skin manifestations gradually disappeared and the steroids were tailed off.

This patient presented with arthritis and Raynaud's phenomenon. She is unusual in that the arthritis of SLE usually involves

small joints. It is important to note that she remained perfectly well without treatment for 5 years, despite persistently abnormal serology.

Table 10.12 Investigations in Case 10.8 (also see Table 19.6)

C-reactive protein	8 mg/l (normal)
Rheumatoid factor	Negative
Antinuclear antibody	Positive (titre 1/1000; IgG class, homogeneous pattern)
Anti dsDNA-antibodies	80 (< 25)
Antibodies to extractable nuclear antigens	Negative
Serum complement levels	
C3	0.35 g/l (NR 0.65–1.30)
C4	0.05 g/l (NR 0.20–0.50)
Serum immunoglobulins	
IgG	22.0 g/l (NR 7.2–19.0)
IgA	3.8 g/l (NR 2.0–5.0)
IgM	1.2 g/l (NR 0.5–2.0)
Biopsy of normal, sun-exposed skin (lupus band test)	Granular deposits of IgG and complement at dermo–epidermal junction

Table 10.13 Laboratory findings in untreated systemic lupus erythematosus (SLE)*

Immunological test	%	Haematological	%	Others	%
Anti-dsDNA	70–85	Raised ESR	60	C-reactive protein–often normal unless infection	
Antinuclear bodies (high titre; IgG class)	99	Leucopenia	45	Proteinuria	30
Raised serum IgG level	65	Direct Coombs' test positive	40		
Low serum complement C3/C4 levels	60	Lupus anticoagulant	10–20		
		Thrombocytopenia	8		
Antibodies to ENA:					
Sm	30				
RNP	35				
Ro	30				
La	15				
Antibodies to phospholipids	30–40				
Skin biopsy IgG, C3 and C4 deposits in normal skin	75				

*Figures show percentage of patients with positive tests.
ESR, Erythrocyte sedimentation rate; ENA, extractable nuclear antigens; RNP, ribonucleoprotein.

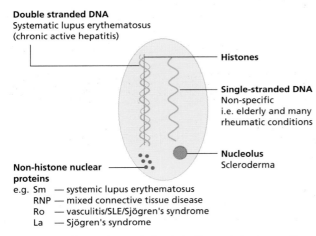

Double stranded DNA
Systematic lupus erythematosus
(chronic active hepatitis)

Histones

Single-stranded DNA
Non-specific
i.e. elderly and many
rheumatic conditions

Nucleolus
Scleroderma

Non-histone nuclear proteins
e.g. Sm — systemic lupus erythematosus
RNP — mixed connective tissue disease
Ro — vasculitis/SLE/Sjögren's syndrome
La — Sjögren's syndrome

Fig. 10.7 Nuclear antigens: their role in diagnosis in rheumatic conditions. DNA + histones = nucleosome.

to dsDNA and ENA, and for antiphospholipid antibodies, as well as having their serum levels of IgG and complement components, C3 and C4, measured.

10.7.3 Differential diagnosis

It is obviously important to distinguish between SLE and RA, since their management differs. The main differentiating features are shown in Fig. 10.8.

10.7.4 Drug-induced systemic lupus erythematosus

Some drug reactions can induce a lupus-like disease. Any of the clinical features of SLE may be found in drug-induced lupus, although renal and central nervous system involvement is rare. The most important diagnostic feature is resolution of the syndrome on withdrawal of the suspected offending drug, even though this may take several months. Most patients with drug-induced lupus have positive ANAs but negative dsDNA binding, negative lupus band tests and normal serum complement levels. The drugs most likely to induce lupus are hydralazine, procainamide, certain anticonvulsants (phenytoin, hydantoins), isoniazid, chlorpromazine, penicillamine and minocycline. Many of these drugs are now little used; **minocycline**, which is very widely used for the long-term treatment of acne, has become the commonest drug to induce this syndrome (Case 5.6).

10.7.5 Management

SLE can be a mild disease, although even when mild, quality of life is often reduced. Patients may require no treatment or only small doses of non-steroidal anti-inflammatory drugs (NSAIDs). The major aims in management are:
• to avoid stimuli which may trigger an exacerbation; and
• to control autoantibody production by immunosuppression.
• to limit damage caused by inflammation.

Flare-up of activity often follows exposure to sunlight or infection; CRP is helpful to detect underlying infection, since disease activity alone rarely stimulates significant CRP synthesis.

SLE is a relapsing and remitting disease, and any immunosuppression required is therefore variable. Corticoster-

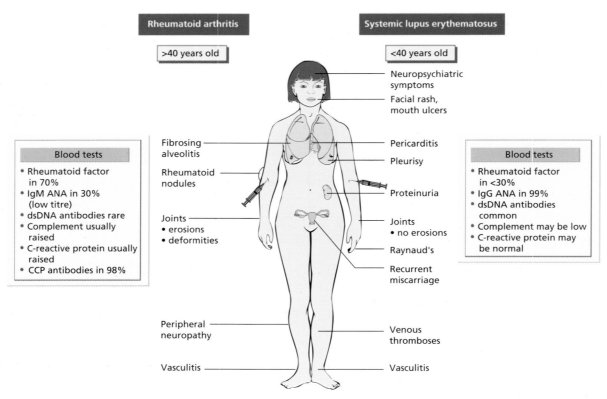

Fig. 10.8 Distinguishing clinical features of rheumatoid arthritis and systemic lupus erythematosus.

oids in moderate doses form the basis of immunosuppression. Skin and joint symptoms respond well to antimalarials such as hydroxychloroquine, which also help prevent relapse. In persistent disease, azathioprine is usually added as a steroid-sparing agent. Most patients can be controlled on a combination of azathioprine, steroids and antimalarials. **Cyclophosphamide**, usually given as intravenous pulses, is widely used in vasculitis, severe cerebral SLE and severe lupus nephritis. Severe, refractory cases may respond to the anti-B cell monoclonal antibody, **rituximab**.

It is important to monitor the activity of SLE by measuring serially the ANA titre, the DNA antibody level and serum C3, C4 and CRP levels (Table 10.14). Anti-DNA antibody levels rise before a major exacerbation of disease and decrease after it. In patients with renal damage, a fall in C4, followed by C3, may be the first indicator of renal damage and may occur 6 months before other features of renal involvement. Routine checks must also be made for proteinuria and renal dysfunction.

10.7.6 Prognosis

The prognosis in SLE has improved considerably over the last 30 years. For all forms of SLE, the 5-year survival figure exceeds 90%, compared with 70–80% in the 1970s. Even in

Table 10.14 Interpretation of serial serological changes in systemic lupus erythematosus

dsDNA antibodies	C3	C4	Interpretation
↑	Stable	Stable	↑Activity — watch for change in clinical state
Stable	↓	↓	Renal involvement should be suspected
↓	↓	↓	
↑/stable	↑	↑	Look for infection — measure C-reactive protein

patients with proven nephritis, the 5-year survival is now over 80%. This reflects improvements in treatment of severe disease such as nephritis. *There is still, however, a considerable late mortality*: survival falls to 80% at 10 years and less than 70% at 20 years. The causes of death differ in early and late disease; in the first 5 years after diagnosis **active SLE** accounts for about one-third of deaths and **infection** for most of the remainder. In later disease, infection is still a significant cause of death but deaths from active lupus are much less common. An increased prevalence of **atherosclerosis**, particularly IHD, accounts for much of the increased mortality in late disease. As in RA, some of this increased risk can be attributed to conventional risk factors and corticosteroid treatment, but there also appears to be a disease-specific risk which is greater in patients with severe or poorly controlled SLE. The risk of atherosclerosis seems much higher in SLE than in RA: the risk of myocardial infarction in women with SLE is around 50 times higher than that in age- and sex-matched controls.

The increased risk of death from infection in SLE is due partly to immunosuppressive treatment, but partly to the disease itself. Secondary complement deficiency (due to consumption of complement in active disease) and functional hyposplenism (due to overload of splenic mechanisms to clear immune complexes) both increase the risk of bacterial infection.

In addition to the continuing late mortality in SLE, there is also a considerable **late morbidity**, due to organ damage, vascular disease and other factors, such as osteoporosis (caused by corticosteroids). This challenge from late mortality and morbidity is also being faced in other severe, life-threatening diseases such as HIV infections and haematological cancers which have seen major improvements in treatment of the underlying disease.

10.7.7 Aetiology and pathogenesis

SLE is largely an antibody-mediated disease with both type II and type III hypersensitivity (see section 1.8 and Chapter 5) *playing major roles in pathogenesis.* There is evidence that tissue damage in many patients is due to deposition of complexes of dsDNA with anti-DNA antibody, although complexes composed of other nuclear and cytoplasmic antigens are also thought to be important. Immunohistological studies of affected tissues show deposition of immunoglobulins and complement and, as noted earlier, there is usually serological evidence for complement turnover and consumption. Antibodies have been eluted from affected tissues (particularly kidney) and are enriched for antinuclear antibodies compared with serum. As might be expected, the inflammatory process is centred around blood vessels, with overt vasculitis (i.e. damage to the vessel wall) in some cases, but also a tendency to cause ischaemic damage by plugging of small blood vessels with large numbers of inflammatory cells. In addition to immune-complex-mediated inflammation, antibodies to red blood cells, platelets and clotting factors can play a direct pathogenic role.

The aetiology of SLE is only partially understood. However, a number of factors contribute (Fig. 10.9). It seems likely that SLE reflects the coincidence of a number of genetic and

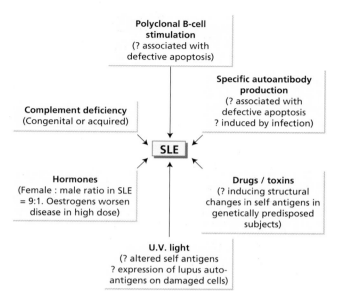

Fig. 10.9 Multiple factors combine in the aetiology of systemic lupus erythematosus.

environmental causes rather than any single aetiological factor.

Complement deficiency

Inherited deficiency of components of the classical pathway of complement (C1, C4 or C2) is associated with a greatly increased risk of developing SLE. This is seen most strikingly in C1q deficiency, in which the risk of severe anti-dsDNA-positive SLE is almost 100%. A similar syndrome is also seen in C1q knockout mice. Metabolism of immune complexes is grossly abnormal in subjects with complement deficiency, with a tendency for deposition in the tissues (Fig. 10.10). These inherited severe complement deficiencies are very rare, and cannot account for more than a handful of cases with SLE. However, partial complement defects are common in SLE: the possession of non-coding or null alleles for C4 is an important genetic risk factor for SLE, and the disease process itself tends to produce a secondary complement deficiency by consumption, and this may in turn perpetuate the disease process. Autoantibodies directed against complement components, especially C1q, have also been described, which may cause further complement deficiency.

Autoantibody production

At one time, it was believed that the plethora of autoantibodies detected in patients with SLE and other connective tissue disease reflected a non-specific polyclonal activation of B cells. However, while a wide variety of autoantibodies are produced, the targets include only a fraction of intracellular molecules and tend to be directed against molecules

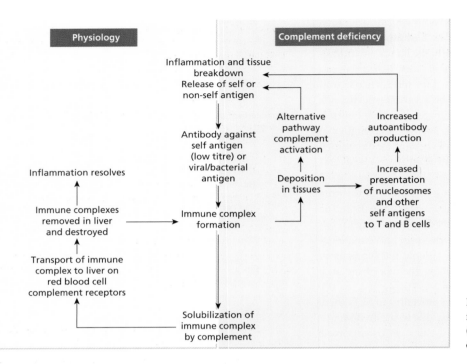

Fig. 10.10 Immune complex metabolism in normal subjects (left) and those with complement deficiency (right).

with a role in transcription and translation of the genetic code. These antibodies increase in affinity for the antigen as the disease progresses, suggesting that their production is driven by that specific antigen. There is some evidence that the primary target of autoantibody production in many patients with SLE is the nucleosome, a subcellular particle formed during cell breakdown by apoptosis and which contains DNA and histones (see Fig. 10.7). Population studies show that antinuclear antibodies usually develop many years before manifestations of disease.

Apoptosis and clearance of damaged cells

Defective apoptosis was implicated in SLE with the recognition that two animal models of spontaneous SLE are due to deficiency of two cell-surface counter-receptors with a key role in triggering apoptosis: Fas and Fas ligand, respectively (see Chapters 1 and 5). Apoptosis triggered through Fas appears to have an important role in deleting autoreactive lymphocytes. Human SLE is not associated with Fas deficiency. Fas deficiency in humans does not cause classical SLE, but does cause a characteristic syndrome comprising red cell and platelet autoimmunity, lymphadenopathy and polyclonal increases in serum immunoglobulins: the autoimmune lymphoproliferative syndrome. Nevertheless, it is plausible that minor defects in apoptosis may contribute to human SLE.

Antinuclear and anti-DNA antibodies are relatively easy to induce in animals by immunization with nucleosomes (see above). This suggests that physiological mechanisms should exist for keeping the nuclear components of dead cells away from the immune system, and that failure of

these mechanisms might lead to the development of SLE. This seems to be another function of apoptosis. C1q binds to apoptotic cells and plays a key role in clearance of these cells. C1q deficiency (whether genetic or acquired) may therefore predispose to lupus by both allowing access of nuclear material to the immune system, and allowing tissue deposition of immune complexes (Fig. 10.10). Acute-phase proteins called pentraxins, which include CRP and serum amyloid P (SAP), can bind to DNA and other nucleosomal particles, which are then cleared by the complement system. SAP gene knockout mice develop a lupus-like illness, and there is some evidence that CRP and SAP production are reduced in some humans with SLE. This suggests a further link between cell death, complement and lupus.

Drugs

A number of drugs can trigger a syndrome resembling SLE (see Chapter 5). Many of these drugs can form conjugates with self-molecules, thus altering their structure and initiating autoreactivity (Chapter 5). Subjects with genetic defects in metabolism of these drugs (particularly those with reduced ability to acetylate these drugs: so-called slow acetylators) are at greatly increased risk of drug-induced SLE.

Ultraviolet light

Sunlight is a well-recognized trigger for both skin and systemic manifestations of SLE. Ultraviolet (UV) light has a number of immunological actions on the skin, but perhaps most significant is induction of apoptosis of keratinocytes. This causes expression of lupus autoantigens (such as Ro and

La) upon the cell surface, where they can gain access to the immune system. Subjects with common genetic polymorphisms reducing their ability to handle UV-induced damage may be particularly liable to develop photosensitivity.

Hormones

SLE is around *10 times more common in women* than in men, and tends to present between the menarche and the menopause. This is due, in part, to the influence of sex steroid hormones: oestrogens can accelerate the disease in animal models of SLE, and reduction in oestrogen levels improves the disease. Similar observations have been made in humans, although sex-specific factors other than oestrogens may also play a role. Surprisingly little is known of the mechanisms underlying these hormonal influences upon immune function.

10.8 Other connective tissue diseases

10.8.1 Mixed connective tissue disease (Case 10.9)

This syndrome was first described in 1972 as an apparently distinct rheumatic disease with a specific diagnostic antibody. The clinical features in the original description included arthritis, polymyositis, pulmonary fibrosis and scleroderma-like changes in the skin. It is now apparent that patients with MCTD also develop some features more commonly associated with SLE (Table 10.15). The length of this list makes some clinicians believe that it is not a separate disease; nevertheless, most patients with MCTD-like symptoms can usefully be grouped together for prognostic and therapeutic purposes. The most important distinguishing feature between MCTD and classic SLE is the relative scarcity of renal and cerebral involvement in MCTD.

Table 10.15 Features of mixed connective tissue diseases

1 **SLE or RA-like features**
   Arthritis (usually mild but can be erosive)
   Constitutional symptoms: fever, malaise
   Lymphadenopathy
   Peripheral neuropathy (particularly trigeminal)
   Erythematous rashes
   Serositis
2 **Polymyositis**
3 **Scleroderma-like features**
   Raynaud's phenomenon — may be severe
   Puffy hands: fingers often sausage-like at presentation
   Abnormal oesophageal motility
   Interstitial lung disease
4 **Antibodies to RNP at high titre**

RNP, Ribonucleoprotein; SLE, systemic lupus erythematosus; RA, rheumatoid arthritis.

The major serological finding is a high titre of antibody against the extractable nuclear antigen, **RNP** (see Chapter 19). The presence of this antibody without other 'lupus' autoantibodies (such as anti-Sm) correlates with the clinical outcome. There is usually a positive ANA, which typically shows a speckled pattern, but antibodies to dsDNA are absent and C3 and C4 levels are normal.

MCTD was once thought to have a better prognosis than SLE because of the relative lack of renal and cerebral involvement. However, longitudinal studies have shown that some patients do develop severe disease with attendant mortality. Pregnancy is uneventful. The response to treatment with corticosteroids is usually reasonable, although steroid-sparing drugs such as azathioprine are often required.

CASE 10.9 MIXED CONNECTIVE TISSUE DISEASE

A 19-year-old typist presented with acute, bilateral arthralgia of her wrists and knees. The pain prevented her from sleeping or typing. On examination, there were no effusions or tenderness of any joints. No diagnosis was made but she was treated symptomatically. Two months later, she developed severe Raynaud's phenomenon, with arthralgia and pronounced sausage-like swelling of her fingers and some proximal muscle weakness. On investigation, she had a low haemoglobin (108 g/l) but a normal white cell count and differential. Her ESR was raised (63 mm/h), and her serum contained ANA (titre 1/160; speckled pattern) (see Chapter 19). dsDNA binding was normal but antibodies to ENA were detected and found to be largely directed against nuclear ribonucleoprotein (RNP); there were no antibodies to the Sm antigen (see Chapter 19). A latex test for rheumatoid factor was negative. Complement levels (C3 and C4) were normal but she had a raised serum IgG of 21.8 g/l (NR 7.2–19.0). X-rays of the hands and knees were normal. There was no proteinuria and her serum creatinine and blood urea were normal. Her creatine kinase was elevated at 2100 IU/ml (normal < 100) and a muscle biopsy showed features of a low-grade myositis.

A diagnosis of mixed connective tissue disease (MCTD) was made and the patient started on prednisolone 40 mg daily. The muscle weakness and joint pain improved dramatically, but attempts to reduce and discontinue the steroids were unsuccessful; muscle weakness returned each time the drug was discontinued. Azathiprine was introduced as a steroid-sparing immunosuppressive. Her Raynaud's phenomenon has slowly worsened and is now associated with progressive sclerodactyly.

10.8.2 Sjögren's syndrome (Case 10.10)

Dry eyes and a dry mouth can occur in otherwise healthy elderly people (around 1–2% of those over 70) and do not appear to be associated with any autoimmune process. However, these features should always raise a suspicion of **Sjögren's syndrome**, particularly in the younger patient. The principal feature of Sjögren's syndrome is autoimmune destruction of exocrine glands, most prominently the lacrimal and salivary glands, but also glands at other sites including the respiratory mucosa and vagina. Sjögren's syndrome can occur as a syndrome in itself, associated with distinctive non-exocrine clinical features and antibodies against Ro and La (primary Sjögren's syndrome: Fig. 10.11) or can occur in association with another connective tissue disease such as RA, SLE or scleroderma (secondary Sjögren's syndrome). Like other connective tissue diseases, Sjögren's has a strong female predominance. The prevalence of Sjögren's is unclear as the symptoms are often mild and hence unrecognized, but the syndrome appears to be at least as common as SLE. It is not clear whether the high prevalence of sicca features in the elderly reflects mild Sjögren's or some other pathology.

The simplest diagnostic test for suspected Sjögren's is the Schirmer test; a slip of sterile filter paper is placed over the lower eyelid. Failure to produce sufficient tears in 5 min to wet 10 mm of the paper suggests defective tear production and in the context of other features of connective tissue dis-

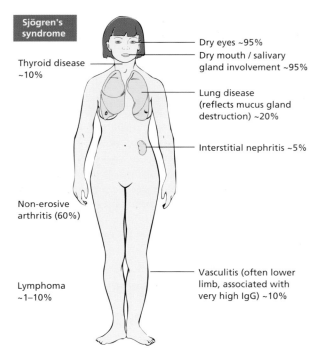

Fig. 10.11 Clinical features of primary Sjögren's syndrome.

ease strongly suggests Sjögren's. Biopsy of glandular tissue involved by Sjögren's (minor salivary glands in the lip being the most accessible) shows a dense lymphocytic infiltrate of

CASE 10.10 SJÖGREN'S SYNDROME

A 38-year-old woman was referred to an oral surgeon for investigation of a dry mouth. She had a sister with arthritis. Examination and investigations were unremarkable except for a raised ESR (42 mm/h). Six months later, she developed a mild conjunctivitis and complained of sore eyes. On testing, rheumatoid factor was now positive (Rose–Waaler titre 1/64); total serum proteins were raised (98 g/l); and immunoglobulin levels showed a raised IgG of 28 g/l (NR 7.2–19.0), with a slightly raised IgM of 2.8 g/l (NR 0.5–2.0) and a normal IgA. Schirmer's test was performed (see section 10.8.2). The test was markedly abnormal as only 3.5 mm of the filter strip in the right eye and 1.5 mm of that in the left eye became wet (see Fig. 10.12).

She was treated with methylcellulose eye drops to prevent corneal ulceration. Over a period of many years, her rheumatoid factor titre steadily increased and ANA and antibodies to the extractable nuclear antigens Ro and La became detectable. Seven years after the development of the dry mouth and dry eyes (together known as the sicca complex), she developed a mild, bilateral non-erosive polyarthritis of her hands, wrists and knees. A diagnosis of Sjögren's syndrome was made. The disease has remained mild. NSAIDs have

been given for the arthritis but have had no effect on the sicca complex.

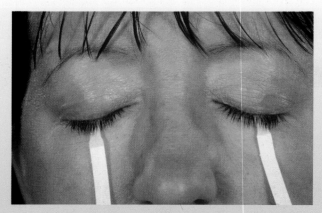

Fig. 10.12 Dry eyes in Sjögren's syndrome demonstrated by Schirmer's test. With permission from Medical Masterclass: Rheumatology and Clinical Immunology, London: Royal College of Physicians, 2001.

largely activated, cytokine-producing CD4⁺ T cells, with marked class II MHC expression on the remaining glandular structures.

Primary Sjögren's is strongly associated with the HLA A1 B8 DR3 haplotype. Environmental causes are unclear, but some evidence exists for infection with an unknown retrovirus.

Therapy of Sjögren's is usually supportive with artificial tears and attention to oral hygiene, since the affected glands are usually irreversibly destroyed at presentation. The prognosis of primary Sjögren's is usually good, but some patients may have problems with extraglandular features (Fig. 10.11) and there is also an increased risk of B-cell lymphoma.

10.8.3 Scleroderma

Scleroderma (progressive systemic sclerosis) is characterized by diffuse fibrosis affecting skin, GI tract, heart and muscle. It is described in detail in Chapter 11; a seronegative polyarthritis develops in 25% of patients, often early in the disease.

10.9 Systemic vasculitis

10.9.1 Polyarteritis nodosa (Case 10.11)

Polyarteritis nodosa (PAN) is characterized by swelling of muscle fibres within the media of medium-sized arteries. This is followed by fibrinoid change and intense infiltration of polymorphonuclear leucocytes. The process results in multiple aneurysm formation (which gives rise to the name 'nodosa'), often with total occlusion of the vessel (Fig. 10.13). The extent of involvement of a particular artery is variable and 'skip' lesions are often present.

The aetiology of the vasculitis is unknown. A small proportion of patients are positive for hepatitis B antigen, regardless of overt clinical hepatitis in the past, whilst a drug reaction or

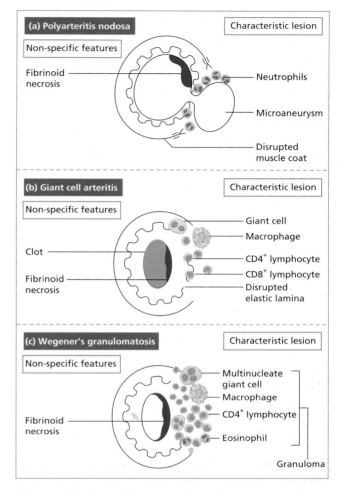

Fig. 10.13 Histology of three types of vasculitis in patients who may present with arthritides/arthralgia or myalgia.

infection may precede PAN. These observations support the view that PAN is triggered by a foreign agent(s), with deposition of the circulating immune complexes in the vessel wall.

CASE 10.11 POLYARTERITIS NODOSA

A 64-year-old man developed diplopia due to a right sixth nerve palsy, lethargy, weight loss and skin lesions on the right leg which were thought to be erythema nodosum. Six weeks later, he presented with aches and pains in his shoulders, which his doctor thought were due to polymyalgia rheumatica. He improved dramatically on steroids, but unfortunately they had to be withdrawn because of hypertension. On investigation, he had an ESR of 104 mm/h, a polymorphonuclear leucocytosis and some proteinuria (1.5 g/24 h) with occasional granular casts. Biopsy of a skin lesion showed non-specific changes. A renal biopsy was normal. No diagnosis was possible.

Four weeks later, he developed profound malaise with fever, marked muscle weakness and anaemia. His haemoglobin was

77 g/l with a CRP of 70 mg/l, a negative direct Coombs' test and a reticulocyte count of 5.4%. His blood urea, serum creatinine and creatinine clearance were normal, as was his serum creatine kinase level. His ANA, dsDNA binding and antineutrophil cytoplasmic antibodies (ANCA) were negative, with normal C3 and C4 complement levels. Biopsy of an affected calf muscle showed a florid arteritis. All the medium-sized arteries showed reduction of their lumens or complete occlusion. On the basis of this muscle biopsy, a firm diagnosis of polyarteritis nodosa was made. The patient was started on 60 mg of prednisolone per day. Over the next few days his temperature fell and his symptoms improved.

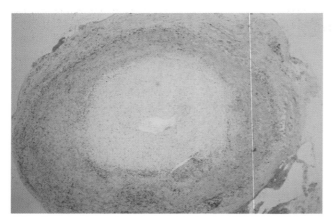

Fig. 10.14 Occluded, temporal artery in giant cell arteritis. The vessel wall is thickened and infiltrated with lymphocytes and macrophages. With permission from Medical Masterclass: Rheumatology and Clinical Immunology, London: Royal College of Physicians, 2001.

The clinical features of PAN are extremely varied (Fig. 10.15) and investigations often unrewarding. Selective renal angiography may show arterial aneurysms but in only 50% of cases. Muscle biopsy is positive in 40% of cases, provided that an affected, tender area of muscle is chosen. It is mandatory to test for circulating hepatitis B surface antigen. Non-specific findings include a raised ESR and CRP, low haemoglobin and a leucocytosis with an occasional eosinophilia. Renal function may be compromised

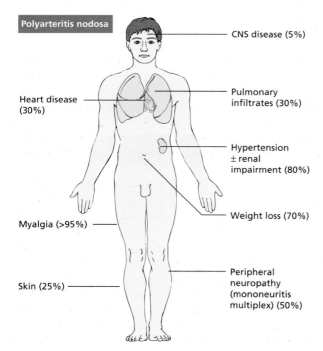

Fig. 10.15 Clinical features of polyarteritis nodosa.

with hypertension, but glomerulonephritis is not a feature. Immunological investigations are unhelpful.

It is important to distinguish PAN from microscopic polyarteritis (MPA) (see Chapters 9 and 11), in which lung involvement may lead to fatal pulmonary haemorrhage. The development of rapidly progressive crescentic glomerulonephritis (typical of Wegener's granulomatosis) and positive ANCA (see Chapters 9 and 19) has led to the view that MPA is related to Wegener's granulomatosis rather than PAN. This is important, not only for treatment (cyclophosphamide as well as steroids) but also for prognosis.

The overall prognosis of PAN depends on the organs involved. Although approximately 60% of patients are alive 5 years after diagnosis, 30% of all patients eventually die of renal failure. Other severe complications include cerebrovascular accidents and malignant hypertension. Treatment with high-dose corticosteroids in the acute stage has improved the prognosis. Cyclophosphamide may be required in severe disease.

10.9.2 Polymyalgia rheumatica and giant cell (temporal) arteritis (Case 10.12)

Polymyalgia rheumatica (PMR) and giant cell arteritis (GCA) are closely related conditions, best considered as part of a spectrum of disease, which are relatively common in the elderly, particularly women. About 1% of over-70-year-olds are affected. PMR alone is the most common, but 20% of patients with PMR also have features of GCA. GCA may also occur without PMR. The disease is rare before the age of 55. The major presenting symptoms of PMR are acute onset of pain and morning stiffness in the muscles of the shoulders and pelvic girdle. Systemic symptoms include malaise, weight loss, depression and anorexia. Severe headaches, pain in the scalp, jaw and tongue and visual loss suggest a diagnosis of GCA (sometimes know as temporal or cranial arteritis). Vascular inflammation in GCA is usually confined to the branches of the external carotid artery. Sudden **blindness** can occur due to occlusion of the posterior ciliary artery, which supplies the optic disc.

Laboratory investigations in this disease are usually nonspecific. The ESR is considerably raised in 95% of patients and the CRP in 90%; temporal artery biopsy is abnormal in only 25–40% of cases, but may be helpful when there is diagnostic uncertainty. The response of polymyalgia rheumatica and temporal arteritis to corticosteroids is dramatic. Because of the risk of blindness, suspected GCA requires immediate treatment with **high-dose prednisolone** 40–60 mg daily, but pure polymyalgia responds to lower doses, often as little as 10–15 mg prednisolone daily. Treatment can usually be reduced and gradually withdrawn over 1–2 years.

The pathological changes in GCA are distinctive: there is an arteritis of large and medium-sized arteries with large

CASE 10.12 POLYMYALGIA RHEUMATICA

A 73-year-old woman presented with sudden pain and stiffness of her shoulder muscles. She had become increasingly depressed over the preceding 3 months, with anorexia and loss of weight. On examination, there was limitation of movement of both shoulders with muscle tenderness; neurological examination was normal. The temporal arteries were extremely tender on palpation. On investigation, her haemoglobin was 101 g/l with a raised CRP of 68 mg/l. A diagnosis of polymyalgia rheumatica and temporal arteritis was made and a temporal artery biopsy taken. Treatment was started immediately with 60 mg of prednisolone daily and within 24 h the patient was markedly improved; she became more alert and her muscle stiffness lessened. The temporal artery biopsy showed a vasculitis with infiltration by lymphocytes, macrophages and giant cells (Fig. 10.9b). Improvement continued over the next few days. Steroids were gradually withdrawn over 2 months but her polymyalgia relapsed a year later and she again improved on steroids.

multinucleate giant cells in the media and around a swollen and fragmented internal elastic lamina (Figs 10.13 and 10.14). The distribution of the arteritis corresponds to the amount of elastic tissue within the vessel; thus, arteries of the head and neck are especially affected, whereas pulmonary and renal vessels are usually spared.

The pathogenesis of temporal arteritis involves infiltration of the vessel wall by CD8$^+$, and to a lesser extent CD4$^+$, T cells and macrophages. There is evidence of both T-cell and macrophage cytokine production and of a cytotoxic T-cell response against cells within the vessel wall. The pathology of polymyalgia rheumatica remains obscure.

There are no real clues as to environmental triggers to temporal arteritis, although some have speculated that UV light may alter the antigenic structure of elastin and other components of the vessel wall. The genetics are better understood: there is a strong association with HLA-DRB1*04, the association being stronger for GCA than PMR alone.

10.9.3 Other vasculitides

Other vasculitides may involve the joints, resulting in arthralgia or arthropathy. In particular, patients with Wegener's granulomatosis commonly present with vague joint pains before developing the more specific clinical features in the respiratory tract, nose or kidneys. The histological features of Wegener's vasculitis are different from those of giant cell arteritis and polyarteritis nodosa (Fig. 10.13). Vasculitis is fully discussed in Chapter 11 (see Table 11.3) and Wegener's granulomatosis is also included in Chapters 9 and 13.

10.10 Inflammatory muscle disease or myositis
(Case 10.13)

The spectrum of autoimmune myositis (Table 10.16) includes muscle inflammation in isolation (primary polymyositis), in association with skin changes and vasculitis (dermatomyositis) or in association with other clinical features of connective tissue disease. Childhood dermatomyositis appears to be a different disease from the adult form with a greater tendency to vasculitis and soft tissue calcification.

Table 10.16 Classification of autoimmune myositis

1 Primary idiopathic polymyositis
2 Primary idiopathic dermatomyositis
3 Myositis with malignancy
4 Juvenile dermatomyositis
5 Myositis as a feature of other autoimmune disease includes myositis occurring in association with systemic lupus erythematosus, scleroderma, etc. and newly defined multisystem disorders such as that associated with Jo 1 antibodies

Myositis usually presents with muscle weakness, principally involving the proximal muscles. Some pain and tenderness may be present, but this is usually mild. Respiratory muscle weakness and swallowing difficulty suggest a poor prognosis. Investigations usually show a raised level of skeletal muscle enzymes (such as creatine kinase), a non-specific finding in many kinds of muscle damage, and electromyography and magnetic resonance scanning provide supportive evidence. A definitive diagnosis is usually made by muscle biopsy which shows damaged fibres and infiltration by lymphocytes. Antinuclear antibodies are present in over 50% of patients with myositis, and specific autoantigens have been linked with patterns of disease, particularly Jo 1, which is associated with myositis, pulmonary fibrosis and sclerodermatous changes.

The pathogenesis of polymyositis and dermatomyositis seems to be different: polymyositis is associated with muscle damage caused by T cells, whereas antibody and complement appear to be more important in dermatomyositis.

The aetiology of myositis is unknown in most cases. There has been much interest in a viral cause, but no convincing evidence has been produced to support this, although transient myositis is well documented after certain viral infections, especially Coxsackie virus. Drugs, particularly statins, may trigger a syndrome resembling myositis, although it is hard to distinguish toxic myopathies from immunologically mediated disease. *Around 10% of cases of adult dermatomyositis are associated with underlying carcinomas*, suggesting that

CASE 10.13 POLYMYOSITIS

A 32-year-old woman with a past history of ulcerative colitis (quiescent for the last 7 years) presented with a dry cough. The cough became productive of clear sputum and she was admitted 2 months later with increasing dyspnoea, myalgia and arthralgia. A clinical diagnosis of fibrosing alveolitis was made and confirmed by transbronchial biopsy. She was treated with prednisolone, which improved her arthralgia, and it became clear that she had a severe proximal myopathy. Serum creatine kinase was found to be very high and a muscle biopsy showed necrosis and a cellular infiltrate compatible with polymyositis. She had a circulating autoantibody to Jo 1 antigen (see Chapter 19).

She recovered eventually, after a stormy course which included treatment with pulsed methylprednisolone, oral azathioprine and three plasma exchanges of 2.5 l. She has persistent myalgia and some arthralgia and remains on 20 mg prednisolone daily.

the tumour is inducing the autoimmune muscle disease. Cancers of the ovary, lung, GI tract and lymphoma are most common in this context.

Treatment is with high-dose corticosteroids, often combined with azathioprine or another immunosuppressive drug. High-dose intravenous immunoglobulin is effective in adult dermatomyositis, but this relapses if treatment is withdrawn. The 5-year mortality from myositis is 10–15%, but long-term morbidity from muscle weakness is much more common and is often severe.

10.11 Hereditary periodic fevers

The hereditary periodic fevers (also know as the **autoinflammatory syndromes**) are a group of genetic disorders of inflammation. All are characterized by episodic fever, often with inflammation involving joints, skin and serosal surfaces. The clinical phenotype and the pattern of inheritance of these disorders have been described for many years, but in the last few years, the genetic basis of all these disorders has been unravelled. The proteins encoded by the affected genes have mainly been found to play a regulatory role in inflammation: pyrin and cryopyrin are intracellular regulators of cytokine production and apoptosis and the 55-kDa TNF receptor modulates the action of TNF. Globally, the most common and serious of these disorders is familial Mediterranean fever (FMF), which has a prevalence of one to five per 1000 among Sephardic Jews, Armenians and some Arabs. If untreated, patients with FMF have a high risk of developing systemic AA amyloidosis. Renal failure due to amyloidosis was a common cause of death in these patients. Treatment with low-dose colchicine decreases the frequency of acute attacks of fever and pain and greatly reduces the risk of amyloid deposition.

The genetics, clinical features and treatment of the five hereditary periodic fevers are summarized in Table 10.17.

FURTHER READING

See website: www.immunologyclinic.com

Table 10.17 Epidemiological, genetic and clinical features of the hereditary periodic fevers

	Familial Mediterranean fever	TNF receptor-associated periodic syndrome (TRAPS)	Hyper IgD syndrome	Muckle Wells syndrome	Familial cold autoinflammatory syndrome
Inheritance	Autosomal recessive	Autosomal dominant	Autosomal recessive	Autosomal dominant	Autosomal dominant
Ethnic distribution	Jewish, Arab, Turkish, Armenian	Irish, Scots plus sporadic families elsewhere	North European	North European	North European
Gene affected	MEFV	TNFRSF1A	MVK	CIAS1	CIAS1
Protein encoded by affected gene	Pyrin	55-kDa TNF-α receptor	Mevalonate kinase (involved in cholesterol synthesis—link with inflammation unclear)	Cryopyrin	Cryopyrin
Duration of febrile episode	1–3 days	> 7 days	3–7 days	1–2 days	

CHAPTER 11

11 Skin Diseases

11.1 Introduction

The skin consists of an impervious horny layer of stratified squamous epithelial cells called keratinocytes (**epidermis**) overlying vascular connective tissue (**dermis**). The epidermis has an important mechanical function as a barrier from the outside world, but also plays a more active role in the skin's response to injury. The **keratinocyte** can synthesize a large number of cytokines and other inflammatory mediators in response to injury or ultraviolet radiation (Fig. 11.1).

These mediators will increase vascular permeability, attract and activate cells of the immune system and induce the expression of adhesion molecules on nearby endothelial cells to allow these cells access to the damaged tissue.

Intertwined with this non-adaptive response to injury is a system for the generation of an adaptive immune response against antigens gaining access via the skin. Around 10% of the cells in the epidermis are a specialized antigen-presenting population known as **Langerhans cells**. These cells have a high capacity for the uptake and processing of anti-

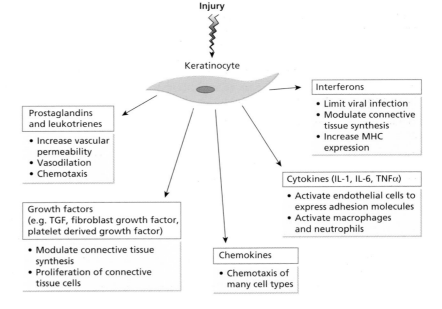

Fig. 11.1 Multiple proinflammatory factors produced by keratinocytes in response to injury. IL, Interleukin; MHC, major histocompatibility complex; TNF, tumour necrosis factor; TGF, transforming growth factor.

gen. Following any insult to the epidermis (such as invasion by microorganisms), they migrate along afferent lymphatics to the paracortex of lymph nodes and during migration they differentiate into dendritic cells with high expression of major histocompatibility complex (MHC) class II and co-stimulatory molecules. They can then activate naive T cells, specific for peptides derived from antigens taken up in the skin, inducing proliferation and differentiation of T cells into effector cells. Most of these then leave the lymph node, enter the blood and then migrate into inflamed skin where they can play a role in eliminating any invading pathogen. This homing of T cells to the skin occurs because they express adhesion molecules specific for receptors found on endothelial cells in inflamed skin (the expression of which is induced by cytokine signals from keratinocytes). This skin-specificity of the T cells is induced by signals from the Langerhans cell-derived dendritic cells. The best characterized T-cell adhesion molecule for homing to skin is known as cutaneous lymphocyte-associated antigen (CLA), which binds to E-selectin on endothelial cells. Skin-homing T cells also express the chemokine receptors CCR4 and CCR10, which selectively bind a distinctive chemokine produced by cutaneous endothelial cells and keratinocytes. This leads to migration and retention of these T cells in the skin. Langerhans cells, keratinocytes, CLA-positive T lymphocytes and local lymph nodes have been regarded collectively as skin-associated lymphoid tissue (SALT). Although this tissue limits infection, it is also responsible for some types of skin disease (see section 11.3).

Unlike the rest of the body, the skin is exposed to ultraviolet radiation (UVR), which has important local and systemic immunological effects (Table 11.1). Chronic UVR exposure leads to skin cancer. The risk of skin malignancy is increased in immunosuppressed patients, especially in skin exposed to high levels of UVR. This suggests that immune mechanisms regulate skin tumour development. UVR exposure depresses Langerhans cell function, reduces in vitro lymphocyte responses and impairs cell-mediated immunity (Table 11.1). These effects of UVR are largely mediated by keratinocyte production of tumour necrosis factor (TNF)-α and other cytokines (Fig. 11.1). Prolonged sun exposure is damaging to the skin immune system.

Autoimmunity and hypersensitivity can cause skin diseases. Skin damage may be triggered by autoantibodies to skin antigens (in the bullous diseases) or by deposition of immune complexes [in systemic lupus erythematosus (SLE)]. T cells are involved in some forms of dermatitis.

11.2 Infections and the skin (Case 11.1)

Bacterial, viral and fungal infections can occur when the physical barrier of the skin is breached, for instance following trauma (especially burns) or widespread eczema, or

Table 11.1 Effects of ultraviolet radiation on the skin

Induces skin cancer formation
Effect on Langerhans cells
- Alters morphology
- Reduces expression of cell-surface receptors
- Reduces ability to present antigen

Effect on lymphocytes
- Alters cell trafficking
- Changes cell populations in peripheral blood (CD4$^+$ lymphocytes ↓; CD8$^+$ lymphocytes ↑)
- Suppresses contact hypersensitivity responses
- Impairs lymphocyte transformation responses to mitogens and antigens
- Alters cytokine production

when immune defences are impaired by systemic or topical immunosuppressive treatment (e.g. corticosteroids and cytotoxic drugs) or by primary immunodeficiency (see Chapter 3). Septicaemic infections, e.g. gonococcal or meningococcal septicaemia, may seed foci of infection into the skin. Certain viruses invade the skin to produce infected lesions (chickenpox or warts), although a reactive, non-infective rash is a more common response to systemic viral infections (e.g. exanthemata of rubella or measles). Recurrent herpes labialis is caused by reactivation of persistent herpes simplex infection and attacks are often provoked by exposure to UV light, probably due to suppression of the skin immune system. Atopics have an increased tendency to herpes labialis, perhaps related to a less effective T-cell response against this virus. Skin granulomas, although rare in developed countries, are most commonly caused worldwide by invading microorganisms such as Mycobacterium tuberculosis, M. leprae or Treponema pallidum.

One of the best examples of the multiple skin manifestations of an underlying infection is human immunodeficiency virus (HIV) (see Chapters 2 and 3). A spectrum of skin problems occurs in HIV-infected individuals (Fig. 11.2). Sometimes these are exacerbations of pre-existing skin disease, such as psoriasis, but more often they are new.

11.3 T-cell-mediated skin disease

T cells play a central role in some of the most common skin diseases: the best understood are contact dermatitis, mediated by TH1 cells, and atopic eczema, mediated largely by TH2 cells. The chronic skin disease psoriasis also appears to be mediated largely by T cells, although the triggering antigen and the mechanism by which T cells induce the characteristic epidermal changes of psoriasis are not fully understood.

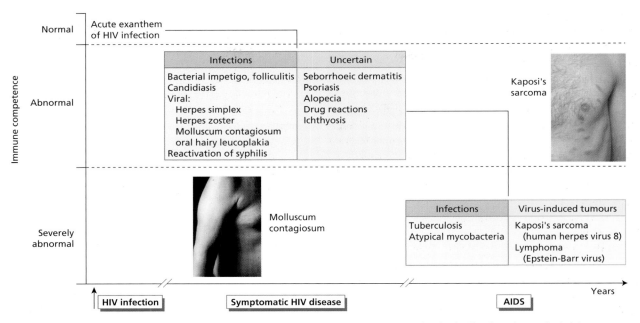

Fig. 11.2 The spectrum of skin disease in human immunodeficiency virus (HIV)-positive individuals. The disorder on the left is molluscum contagiosum and that on the right is early Kaposi's sarcoma.

CASE 11.1 RECURRENT COLD SORES

A 38-year-old woman had been troubled since the age of 8 by recurrent cold sores. Several times each year she would develop a distinctive tingling sensation around her nose or lips, followed several hours later by localized formation of small blisters which crusted, became more painful and gradually cleared over several days. The attacks were often provoked by exposure to strong sunlight. She had a history of troublesome hay fever but was otherwise well. She was able to limit the number of attacks by use of a high-factor sun-block and reduce the severity of each attack by prompt use of aciclovir cream at the onset of symptoms.

11.3.1 Contact dermatitis (Case 11.2)

Contact dermatitis is an inflammatory skin disease caused by TH1-cell-mediated (type IV) hypersensitivity to external agents which come into contact with the skin. It is an important cause of occupational skin disease. The range of potential sensitizing antigens is enormous but, fortunately, a relatively small number of substances accounts for most cases (see Table 11.2). These agents are usually of relatively low molecular weight (< 1 kDa) and are not immunogenic in their own right: instead, they are highly reactive molecules that easily penetrate the epidermis and bind covalently to skin or tissue proteins. The sensitizing chemical is known as a hapten and the protein it combines with as the carrier (see Chapter 1).

The **diagnosis** of contact dermatitis depends on a careful medical history, the distribution of the lesions, and patch testing. In the patch test, a suspected contact sensitizer is applied to normal skin (usually on the upper back) and covered for 48 h. The reaction is read after 2 and 4 days. In a positive response, there is inflammation and induration at the test site. Although there are pitfalls in interpretation, patch-testing is indispensable in the investigation of allergic contact dermatitis.

Contact dermatitis is a prototype of T-cell-mediated hypersensitivity (see Box 11.1). Two phases of pathogenesis are recognized: an induction phase, from the time of initial

---

BOX 11.1 EVIDENCE FOR THE ROLE OF TH1 CELLS (CELL-MEDIATED HYPERSENSITIVITY) IN CONTACT DERMATITIS

- The inflammatory cells found in positive patch tests are CD4+ T lymphocytes which synthesize interleukin (IL)-2 and interferon (IFN)-γ
- Contact sensitivity can be passively transferred to non-sensitized animals by the injection of T lymphocytes from sensitized animals but not by antisera
- In sensitized individuals, contact skin reactions require 48 h to develop, a characteristic of cell-mediated but not antibody-mediated hypersensitivity reactions (see Chapter 1)

CASE 11.2 NICKEL DERMATITIS

A 47-year-old woman presented with a 3-week history of an acute rash which started beneath her watch. Two weeks later, a further patch appeared at the umbilicus. She had previously noted that she could not wear cheap earrings without triggering a rash on her ear lobes. There was no past medical history of note and no personal or family history of atopy. On examination, two patches of dermatitis were seen over the presenting areas. The appearances were sug- gestive of nickel-induced contact dermatitis corresponding to nickel in the watch and on a jeans stud. She was patch-tested to a battery of commonly implicated agents (Table 11.2): strongly positive results were induced by nickel sulphate and cobalt chloride only. The final diagnosis was nickel dermatitis, which cleared spontaneously following avoidance of nickel-containing articles.

Table 11.2 Some agents responsible for allergic contact dermatitis

	Agent	Examples of exposure
Metals	Nickel	Clasps, necklaces, watch-straps
	Chromate	Cement (building site workers)
	Cobalt*	
Medications	'Para'-group chemicals	Benzocaine-type anaesthetics, sulphonamide antibiotics, PABA-containing substances (e.g. sunscreens) and oral hypoglycaemic agents (sulphonylureas)
	Phenothiazines	Phenothiazine-based antihistamines
	Neomycin	Topical antibiotics
Plastics	Epoxyresins, acrylates	Construction industry, glues
Rubber	Accelerators	Tyre industry, rubber gloves, shoes, clothing, household 'grips', etc.
Plants	Poison ivy (USA only)	
	Primula	
	Chrysanthemum	
	Geranium	
Cosmetics	Perfumes	
	Preservatives	
	Lanolin	

*Source of cobalt sensitivity is usually obscure but it may exist as a co-sensitivity with nickel (metal) or chromate (cement).
PABA, Para-amino benzoic acid.

antigen contact to sensitization of T lymphocytes, and an elicitation phase, from antigen re-exposure to the appearance of dermatitis. In the induction phase, Langerhans cells bind the hapten–carrier protein complex and present it, in association with major histocompatibility complex (MHC) class II antigens, to T lymphocytes (Fig. 11.3). Induction of cellular immunity to a contact skin sensitizer can occur within 7–10 days of first contact, but it usually happens after many months or years of exposure to small amounts of antigen. Individual sensitivity varies according to the nature of the chemical, its concentration and the genetic susceptibility of the person exposed. Re-exposure to the relevant antigen triggers the elicitation phase which produces dermatitis. In this phase, effector T lymphocytes carried via the circulation to the skin meet the antigen (composed of hapten complexed to carrier protein) presented by Langerhans cells and other antigen-presenting cells in the epidermis. Activation of T lymphocytes releases cytokines and chemokines, which induce skin inflammation (Fig. 11.3), with recruitment of more T cells and monocytes, keratinocyte proliferation, hyperplasia of the epidermis and consequent protective thickening.

The **management** of contact dermatitis involves two approaches: prevention and treatment. Identification and elimination of the responsible antigen is the most important goal. Unfortunately, many common antigens are ubiquitous and antigen avoidance may be difficult to achieve. Preventative measures in industrial dermatitis depend on the use of protective gloves and clothing, improved ventilation or the substitution of non-antigenic chemicals. Some medicines used to treat skin disease are among the commonest culprits of contact dermatitis (see Table 11.2); they include topical antibiotics and antihistamines. As in atopic eczema, topical corticosteroids are useful therapeutic agents, together with antibacterial measures where indicated.

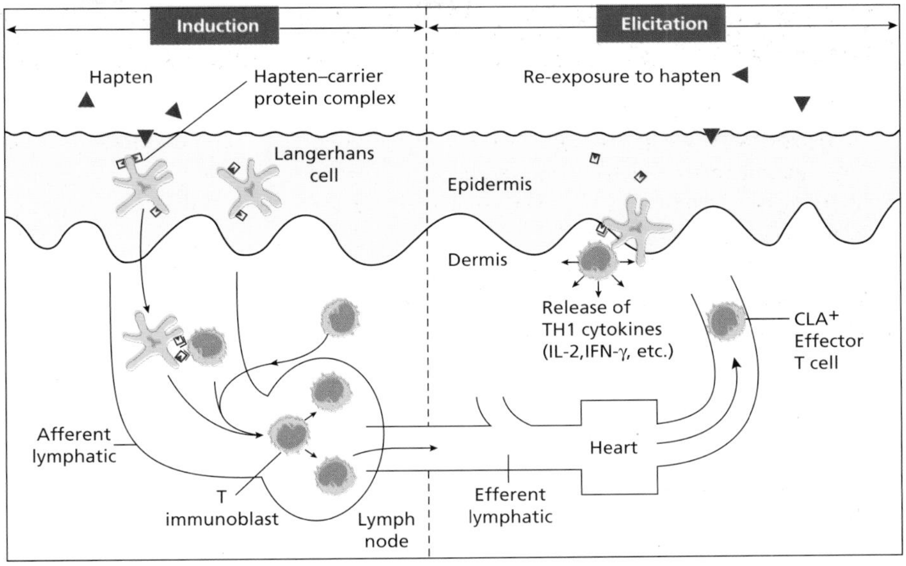

Fig. 11.3 The pathogenesis of allergic contact dermatitis. Langerhans cells bind and present the hapten–carrier protein complex to T lymphocytes (T). Subsequent re-exposure to the hapten triggers a T-cell-mediated (type IV) hypersensitivity reaction in the skin. CLA, Cutaneous lymphocyte-associated antigen.

CASE 11.3 ATOPIC ECZEMA

A 5-year-old boy had developed an itchy rash on his trunk and feet at the age of 18 months. This waxed and waned over the next 3 years and gradually came to involve predominantly his flanks, popliteal and antecubital fossae. He had mild asthma requiring occasional bronchodilators only. His mild atopic eczema was treated with bland emollient creams and occasionally 1% hydrocortisone. His prognosis is good and his skin problems are likely to resolve over the next few years.

11.3.2 Atopic eczema (Case 11.3)

Atopic eczema is a common disorder, occurring predominantly in childhood, which appears to be caused by a TH2 hypersensitivity reaction in the skin. It is usually a mild disorder (as in the case described here) but can sometimes be much more troublesome and on occasions associated with life-threatening complications. The disorder and its pathogenesis are discussed in more detail in Chapter 4.

11.3.3 Psoriasis

Psoriasis is a common skin disease, affecting about 2% of Caucasians. It is less common in sunny climates and in those with pigmented skins. It can present at any age but most commonly appears first at the age of 15–30 years.

The usual clinical form of the condition consists of chronic, raised, red, scaly, round or oval plaques, with sharply marginated edges, mainly occurring on the knees, elbows and scalp. Chronic plaques may remain static for years, resolve spontaneously or progress to involve all the skin, so-called erythrodermic psoriasis. Guttate (drop-shaped) psoriasis may begin with several small lesions 1–2 weeks after a Group A streptococcal throat infection, but these usually resolve spontaneously after a few months. As well as the skin involvement, about 5% of patients develop a seronegative arthropathy (see Chapter 8).

The skin changes in all forms of psoriasis arise because the rate of proliferation and shedding of keratinocytes is both markedly increased and disordered. Normal skin turns over every 4–6 weeks, but this is reduced to less than 1 week in an active psoriatic plaque. These changes in the epidermis are associated with a marked inflammatory infiltrate in the dermis consisting of neutrophils, macrophages and activated T cells (predominantly CD4[+]). Two principal models for the pathogenesis of psoriasis have been proposed. The first suggests that the primary abnormality lies in the keratinocyte, and that the inflammatory infiltrate arises because of mediators produced by the keratinocyte. The second model argues that the keratinocyte proliferation is driven by the cellular infiltrate in the dermis, and in particular by a T-cell-dependent immune response against an unknown antigen (perhaps streptococcal in the case of guttate psoriasis). Evidence is currently strongly in favour of the second model (Box 11.2).

Therapy of psoriasis is usually topical but systemic treatments are used for severe disease. Many older treatments for psoriasis aim to limit keratinocyte proliferation, often using coal-tar-based drugs. More modern treatments involve the

BOX 11.2 EVIDENCE SUPPORTING THE HYPOTHESIS THAT PSORIASIS IS A T-CELL-MEDIATED DISEASE

- Association between psoriasis and HLA-C6 and -DR7
- Relationship with streptococcal infection, which is known to cause other immunologically mediated hypersensitivity disorders
- Worsening of psoriasis in human immunodeficiency virus infection
- Response of psoriasis to therapeutic interventions directed against T cells (such as UV radiation, monoclonal antibodies and ciclosporin/tacrolimus, although the latter drugs also have direct effects on keratinocytes)

follicles. The disease phenotype varies accordingly, from life-threatening disruption of the integrity of the skin to patchy loss of pigmentation. In contrast to the T-cell-mediated diseases described in section 11.3, autoantibodies can be detected in many of these disorders. However, tissue damage in these disorders is probably mediated by both B and T cells.

11.4.1 Bullous skin disease

The bullous skin diseases (which include pemphigus vulgaris, bullous pemphigoid, pemphigoid gestationis and dermatitis herpetiformis) are not common, but they are serious and, so far as pemphigus vulgaris is concerned, may occasionally prove fatal. Immunology has made important contributions to the understanding of these conditions

use of immunosuppressant and anti-inflammatory agents, reflecting the shift towards considering psoriasis as a T-cell-mediated disease. Immunosuppressant therapy can be delivered topically, for example corticosteroids and T-cell-suppressant drugs such as tacrolimus, or physically in the form of UVR. Severe disease often requires the use of systemic immunosuppression, most often with methotrexate or ciclosporin. *Targeted biological therapy is now increasingly used in severe disease (Fig. 11.4), providing confirmation of the role of both T cells and TNF-α in psoriasis.*

11.4 Autoimmune skin disease

The autoimmune skin diseases offer a striking demonstration of the remarkable specificity of autoimmune responses. Many different antigens within the skin can be targeted, including several adhesion molecules, melanocytes and hair

BOX 11.3 EVIDENCE THAT PEMPHIGUS IS AN AUTOIMMUNE DISEASE

- Over 90% of patients have circulating antibodies to desmosomal adhesion molecules, particularly desmoglein 3
- The titre of antibody sometimes correlates with disease activity
- Plasmapheresis reduces antibody titres and disease activity
- Some women with active disease have given birth to children with lesions typical of pemphigus vulgaris
- Pemphigus-like lesions can be produced in mouse and monkey skin by intradermal injections of sera from patients with pemphigus
- IgG fractions from pemphigus sera induce epithelial cell detachment in human skin cultures

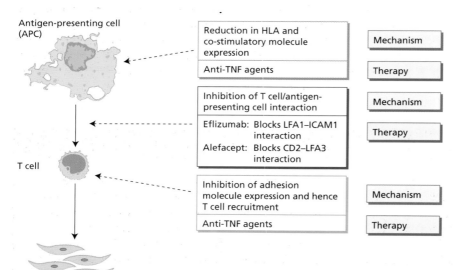

Fig. 11.4 Immunological mechanisms in psoriasis, and how targeted biological therapies may inhibit key steps in pathogenesis.

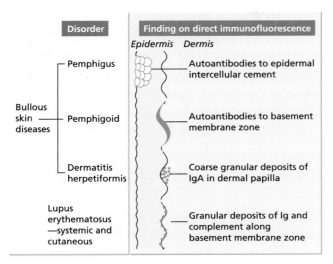

Fig. 11.5 Characteristic findings on direct immunofluorescent examination of skin biopsies.

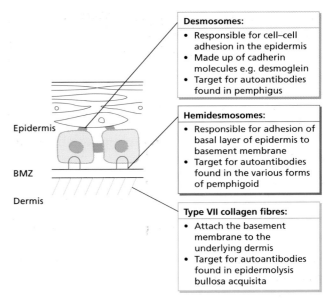

Fig. 11.6 Autoantigens in bullous skin disease. BMZ, basement membrane zone

(Box 11.3), which have characteristic appearances on direct immunohistological examination (Fig. 11.5) and/or serum antibodies detectable by indirect immunofluorescence of human skin. The autoantigens recognized by these antibodies are summarized in Fig. 11.6.

Pemphigus vulgaris (Case 11.4)

This is the most **serious** of the bullous skin disorders and was often fatal before systemic corticosteroids became available. The usual age of onset is between 40 and 60 years, but no age group is exempt. It often begins with ulceration of the oral mucosa, followed by widespread flaccid, weepy bullae. Blisters occur within the epidermis; thus, both the roof and floor of the blister are lined by epidermal cells. The earliest pathological event seems to be dissolution of the intracellular cement substance followed by loss of normal epithelial cell adhesion and detachment of cells (acantholysis). Spontaneous remissions are unusual, although the condition does fluctuate in severity over the years.

In virtually all cases, direct immunofluorescence of perilesional skin is diagnostic (Fig. 11.5): antibodies (IgG class) and complement (C3) react with the cell surfaces of keratinocytes in the epidermis, i.e. at the site of the pathological changes. The main antigenic target is the desmosomal protein, desmoglein 3.

The mainstay of treatment is systemic corticosteroids. The initial dose should be high enough to suppress new blister formation and severe cases may need over 100 mg prednisolone/day. When new blister formation stops, the steroid dose can be quickly reduced to about 40–60 mg/day and more gradually thereafter. Antibody titres may help to gauge the eventual maintenance dose. Azathioprine has a 'steroid-sparing' effect and allows lower maintenance doses of steroids to be used. Plasmapheresis has also proved successful in removing circulating antibodies, especially in steroid-resistant cases.

CASE 11.4 PEMPHIGUS VULGARIS

A 46-year-old woman presented with a generalized, blistering rash of 4 weeks' duration. Her trunk was mainly affected. On examination, there was extensive blistering and large areas of denuded skin. Ulcers were also present in her mouth. The provisional diagnosis was pemphigus vulgaris.

Laboratory investigations showed a normal haemoglobin, full blood count and biochemical profile. Her serum contained antibodies reacting strongly with the cell surfaces of keratinocytes in the epidermis. Direct immunofluorescent examination of a biopsy of normal skin taken from a site adjacent to one bulla showed deposition of IgG around the keratinocytes, giving a 'chicken-wire' appearance (see Fig. 11.5). These findings were characteristic of pemphigus vulgaris. She was treated with 120 mg/day prednisolone initially, reducing to 60 mg/day when new blister formation ceased. She has been regularly followed for 2 years, during which therapy has been gradually reduced to maintenance levels and no new bullae have appeared.

A milder and rarer form of pemphigus, known as pemphigus foliaceus, which tends to spare mucous membranes, is associated with autoantibodies to a different desmosomal protein, desmoglein 1.

Bullous pemphigoid

This condition shows close clinical similarity to pemphigus (hence its name) but the blisters are subepidermal, not intraepidermal. It is most common in people over the age of 60 years and is characterized by the presence of large, tense bullae, usually on the thighs, arms and abdomen.

Direct immunofluorescent staining of perilesional skin is diagnostic; it shows deposition of IgG and C3 as a continuous ('linear') band along the basement membrane zone (see Fig. 11.5). Circulating antibodies to basement membrane zone (BMZ) bind to 230-kDa and 180-kDa hemidesmosomal proteins localized in the lamina lucida and are detectable by indirect immunofluorescence in 75–90% of patients with active disease. In contrast to pemphigus, these autoantibodies are not proven conclusively to be directly pathogenic, since:
1 lesions are not consistently produced in monkey skin or human skin explants by passive transfer of sera from affected individuals;
2 antibodies remain detectable during remission; and
3 their titre does not correlate with disease activity.

The **treatment** of bullous pemphigoid is similar to that of pemphigus vulgaris, except that lower doses of prednisolone and azathioprine are usually sufficient to suppress blistering, and spontaneous fluctuations may sometimes occur.

Pemphigoid gestationis

Pemphigoid gestationis (herpes gestationis) is a rare, blistering skin disease of pregnancy. It resembles bullous pemphigoid in its macroscopic appearance, but the most common finding on direct immunofluorescence is a 'linear' band of C3 at the BMZ. Sera from women with herpes gestationis contain antibodies to the same 180-kDa hemidesmosomal protein which acts as one of the autoantigens in bullous pemphigoid. These antibodies are present at low concentrations and are difficult to detect by conventional indirect immunofluorescence. However, nearly every patient can be shown to have IgG antibodies which 'fix' C3 to normal basement membrane.

Epidermolysis bullosa acquisita

Epidermolysis bullosa acquisita (EBA) is a rare autoimmune blistering disorder with some similarities to the group of inherited blistering disorders known generically as dystrophic epidermolysis bullosa. The bullae in EBA tend to occur in the extremities and to be provoked by trauma. Direct immunofluorescence in EBA shows IgG deposited along the BMZ, but the antigenic target is different from that in the various forms of pemphigoid: the autoantigen appears to be type VII collagen, fibres of which anchor the BMZ to the underlying dermis.

Dermatitis herpetiformis

Dermatitis herpetiformis (DH) is characterized by groups of extremely itchy, small vesicles on extensor surfaces such as the elbows, knees, buttocks, neck and shoulders. Although most patients are aged 20–40 years at diagnosis, any age group can be affected. Like pemphigoid, the bullae are subepidermal, but the immunofluorescent findings are quite different.

Direct immunofluorescence of skin in DH shows deposition of IgA in a granular fashion in the tips of dermal papillae (Fig. 11.5). However, indirect immunofluorescence shows no circulating autoantibodies to skin tissues. Some patients, with large bullae, show linear deposition of IgA instead, but this is now considered to be a different entity (linear IgA bullous dermatosis) because the lesion, the course of the disease, the genetic background and the treatment differ.

Most patients with DH also have an enteropathy indistinguishable from coeliac disease (see Chapter 14): this is usually mild, asymptomatic and demonstrable only by jejunal biopsy. About 70% of patients with DH will have antibodies to gliadin and endomysium in their serum. In DH, as in coeliac disease, there is an increased risk of lymphoma and a markedly increased inheritance of the HLA-B8, -DR3, -DQ2 haplotype. Dietary wheat protein (gluten) is the cause of the enteropathy in DH and the intestinal abnormality improves on gluten withdrawal. The skin lesions are not secondary to the enteropathy, since they can occur in its absence. The skin disease responds to a strict and prolonged gluten-free diet, with disappearance of the granular IgA deposits from the skin, although over 2 years is often needed to control the rash. Reintroduction of dietary gluten causes recurrence of the rash within 3 months, proving that DH is gluten dependent. Despite this close association, the pathogenesis of DH, and the mechanisms underlying the association with coeliac disease, remain obscure. Other treatments are available: dapsone produces prompt improvement in the skin but has no effect on the enteropathy. The mechanism of action of dapsone in DH is unknown.

11.4.2 Vitiligo

Vitiligo consists of patches of skin depigmentation anywhere on the body. These changes result from loss of melanocytes from the epidermis via a process which may be autoimmune. IgG antibodies to melanocytes and, in particular, to tyrosinase, a key enzyme in melanin synthesis, have been found in about 80% of patients with vitiligo and there are strong clinical associations with organ-specific autoimmune diseases, such as thyroid disease, diabetes mellitus, pernicious anaemia and idiopathic Addison's disease.

11.4.3 Alopecia areata

Alopecia is characterized by limited patchy loss of hair (alopecia areata) or loss of all scalp hair (alopecia totalis) or all body hair (alopecia universalis). Alopecia affects children and adults of all ages and races.

Although the aetiology of alopecia areata is unknown, there is evidence that an autoimmune process may be responsible (Box 11.4).

11.5 Systemic diseases with skin involvement

11.5.1 C$\overline{1}$ inhibitor deficiency (Case 11.5)

Hereditary angioedema is caused by deficiency of the inhibitor of the first component of complement (C$\overline{1}$ inhibitor) (C$\overline{1}$ INH) (see Chapter 1). It is the commonest known deficiency of a component of the complement system. Patients suffer from recurrent attacks of skin, laryngeal or intestinal oedema. In contrast to urticaria, localized oedema of the face, limbs and trunk is neither painful nor itchy. Sometimes, however, oedema occurs in the intestinal tract, causing severe abdominal pain and vomiting when the jejunum is involved, or watery diarrhoea if the colon is affected. Laryngeal oedema may be fatal because of airways obstruction. The attacks develop over a few hours and subside spontaneously over 1–2 days. Although often unheralded, episodes may occur after trauma, menstruation, stress or intercurrent infection. Attacks of angioedema are infrequent in early childhood, but exacerbations occur during adolescence and continue throughout adult life.

C$\overline{1}$ INH inhibits activated proteins of several systems, including plasmin and kallikrein as well as activated C1 (C$\overline{1}$). A critical plasma level of C$\overline{1}$ INH, about 30% of normal, is needed to maintain normal inhibitor function. Since C$\overline{1}$ INH is consumed by its interactions with these other enzyme systems, the output of one normal gene cannot maintain plasma levels at 50% of normal in the face of normal or increased

CASE 11.5 HEREDITARY ANGIOEDEMA

Daniel, a 14-year-old boy, presented with a 6-month history of recurrent episodes of swelling of his lips, eyes and tongue (Fig. 11.7). The swellings came on suddenly, grew over a period of 15–20 min, and lasted from 12 to 48 h. They were not itchy but tended to give a prickly sensation. There was no obstruction of airways or abdominal pain during the attacks, which were often associated with intercurrent infection. Urticaria was absent. His sister, aged 21 years, had suffered from an identical problem for 4 years. Physical examination was normal.

The clinical story was typical of angioedema and the family history suggested that this might be hereditary angioedema (HAE). Blood samples taken for complement analysis during remission showed a normal C3 (0.85 g/l), but a rather low C4 of 0.12 g/l (NR 0.2–0.4) and a C1 inhibitor (C$\overline{1}$ INH) level of 0.06 g/l (NR 0.18–0.26); these findings were consistent with the diagnosis of HAE. When the tests were repeated during a subsequent attack of angioedema, the C3 concentration was unchanged but the C4 level was extremely low at 0.04 g/l. Daniel was started on treatment with danazol. Although his C$\overline{1}$ INH level only rose to 0.14 g/l, he

had no further attacks of HAE. What is not clear is why neither parent has a history of HAE, since the condition is inherited in an autosomal dominant fashion.

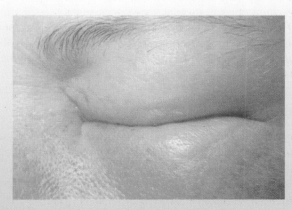

Fig. 11.7 Severe periorbital angioedema.

utilization in the heterozygotes. Plasma C$\overline{1}$ INH levels then fall below the critical threshold, allowing C$\overline{1}$ to act on C4 and C2, generating C2 kinin-like peptides (see Chapter 1), which produce angioedema. The diagnosis rests on finding low levels of C$\overline{1}$ inhibitor functionally or antigenically. In active disease, uninhibited C$\overline{1}$ cleaves C4 and C2, causing increased turnover and low levels of these components. A low serum C4 and normal C3 thus provide a useful screening test for this condition. Two forms of the disease exist: in the commoner form (85%) a low level of C$\overline{1}$ inhibitor is found, but in the rarer type (15%) a functionally defective protein is synthesized with apparently 'normal' serum levels of a non-functioning inhibitor. In the patient with angioedema, a low C4 level with a normal immunochemical C$\overline{1}$ inhibitor concentration indicates the need for a functional assay. A normal C4 level during an attack of angioedema excludes the diagnosis of hereditary angioedema.

All patients should carry a medical card stating the diagnosis and a contact doctor. Symptoms fail to respond to antihistamines or steroids. An acute attack can be treated by infusion of pure C$\overline{1}$ INH or fresh plasma to increase serum levels of the inhibitor (Fig. 11.8). Treatment with a modified androgen, danazol, has been effective in stimulating synthesis of functional C$\overline{1}$ inhibitor. The long-term use of this drug may be limited by troublesome side-effects. These include acne, cholestatic jaundice, virilization of females and suppression of endogenous testosterone production in males. The protease inhibitor, tranexamic acid, is a fairly effective prophylactic agent; it probably functions by restricting activation of the various other enzymes with which C$\overline{1}$ inhibitor reacts, so minimizing its consumption.

Deficiency of C$\overline{1}$ inhibitor can also occur secondary to underlying disorders: the most frequent association is lymphoproliferative disease, although cases have also been described in association with autoimmune haemolytic anaemia and chronic infection. An autoantibody to C$\overline{1}$ inhibitor has been described which blocks its function. In some cases, circulating paraproteins may activate C1, with consumption of the inhibitor, resulting in very low levels of C1, C2 and C4. As in the hereditary form, danazol has proved successful in some cases. Steroids are helpful in those patients with autoantibodies to C$\overline{1}$ inhibitor. Treatment of the underlying disease, where feasible, may also stop the attacks.

11.5.2 Vasculitis

Vasculitis is a diagnosis which rests on histological evidence of **inflammation of blood vessels**. The diversity of clinical lesions seen in vasculitis is extensive (Box 11.5).

Many agents can induce vasculitis (Table 11.3), although the incriminating evidence is often circumstantial. Removal of the drug or treatment of the infection may clear the vasculitis but this is not proof of causation. In most cases, no cause

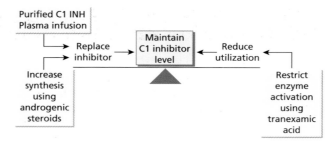

Fig. 11.8 Principles underlying the treatment of C$\overline{1}$ inhibitor deficiency.

is found. A search must be made for systemic involvement in patients who present with cutaneous vasculitis. However, the disorder is confined to the skin in many cases (Case 11.6).

Immunopathogenic mechanisms may be responsible for vasculitis. Some forms of vasculitis are caused by deposition of circulating antigen–antibody complexes in blood vessel walls. A vasculitic skin rash is a common feature of acute ('one-shot') experimental serum sickness. Acute serum sickness is a self-limiting process: resolution occurs spontaneously as the injected antigen is cleared. However, when an endogenous source of antigen (i.e. an autoantigen) is available, or the antigen is replicating (e.g. a microorganism), circulating antigen is produced on an intermittent or

BOX 11.5 FACTORS AFFECTING CLINICAL LESIONS OF VASCULITIS

- The severity and type of vessel wall damage
- The size of the vessels affected
- The organ(s) supplied by these damaged vessels

Table 11.3 Some causes of vasculitis

1	Drugs	
2	Infections	
	• Bacterial	Streptococci
		Mycobacterium tuberculosis
		Gonococci
		Bacterial endocarditis
	• Viral	Hepatitis B
		Infectious mononucleosis
3	Injection of foreign protein	'Serum sickness'
4	Autoimmune diseases	Systemic lupus erythematosus
		Rheumatoid arthritis
		Chronic active hepatitis
		Ulcerative colitis
		Wegener's granulomatosis
		Kawasaki's syndrome
5	Cryoglobulinaemia	Lymphoproliferative disease
		Hepatitis C

CASE 11.6 URTICARIAL VASCULITIS

A 41-year-old woman presented with itchy lumps on her legs of 5 weeks' duration. The lumps lasted 4–5 days. She had a history of asthma from childhood and was being treated with an array of drugs. As far as she knew, she had never 'reacted' to any of these drugs. On examination, her legs showed palpable, purpuric lesions and areas of urticaria. General examination was otherwise normal. The skin lesions were those of urticarial vasculitis.

Investigations showed a low haemoglobin (107 g/l) with a hypochromic blood film. Her white cell count was 12.2 × 10⁹/l, with a raised eosinophil count of 1.56 × 10⁹/l; the erythrocyte sedimen-

tation rate was 45 mm/h. Serum immunoglobulins were normal but her complement levels were low: C3 was 0.55 g/l (NR 0.8–1.4) and C4 was 0.15 g/l (NR 0.2–0.4). Antinuclear and anti-dsDNA antibodies, antineutrophil cytoplasmic antibodies, cryoglobulins and rheumatoid factor were not detected. Biopsy of an acute lesion showed histological features of vasculitis, with deposition of C3 in the deep dermal blood vessels on direct immunofluorescence. She was treated empirically with prednisolone. Her vasculitis improved considerably but no underlying cause was ever found.

---

continuous basis; the result may be chronic immune-complex-induced injury (see Chapter 9). The best examples of this are nuclear antigens in SLE and hepatitis B antigen in some cases of polyarteritis nodosa or hepatitis C antigens in mixed cryoglobulinaemia. In most other cases of vasculitis, positive direct immunofluorescence on fresh lesions is the only evidence of an immune-complex-mediated pathogenesis (Box 11.6).

Some forms of systemic vasculitis are strongly associated with circulating **antineutrophil cytoplasmic antibodies** (ANCA). These disorders show no evidence of immune-complex deposition or complement consumption. The sensitivity of ANCA in the diagnosis of classical Wegener's granulomatosis is high (75–100%), but lower in patients with limited disease (60–70%) and only 35% in patients in remission. The pathogenesis of Wegener's granulomatosis is largely unknown, although the clinical pattern suggests that an inhaled antigen may be responsible. In other conditions, such as erythema nodosum, direct assault by T lymphocytes on vascular antigens may induce vessel damage (type IV hypersensitivity), since activated T lymphocytes and macrophages are the predominant infiltrating perivascular cells.

There is no entirely satisfactory classification of vasculitis. For many years, histopathologists have based their schemes on the **size** and **site** of the vessels involved or the presence or absence of **granulomas** (Table 11.4); on the other hand,

Table 11.4 Classification of vasculitis

	Granuloma	
Vessel size	Present	Absent
Large	Giant cell arteritis Takayasu arteritis	—
Medium	Churg–Strauss syndrome	Polyarteritis nodosa
Small	Wegener's granulomatosis	Micropolyarteritis Henoch–Schönlein syndrome Hypersensitivity (cutaneous) vasculitis

clinicians have recognized clinical syndromes, such as Henoch–Schönlein syndrome or polyarteritis nodosa. The more important conditions are discussed in other chapters according to the site at which they make a major clinical impact, for example Henoch–Schönlein syndrome in renal diseases (see Chapter 9), polyarteritis nodosa and SLE in rheumatic diseases (see Chapter 10) and Wegener's granulomatosis in chest diseases (see Chapter 13).

11.5.3 Cryoglobulinaemia (Case 11.7)

Cryoglobulins are immunoglobulins which form precipitates, gels or even crystals in the cold. Pathological cryoglobulinaemia occurs as a primary disorder or secondary to another disease. The clinical features are caused by the vasculitis following destruction of small blood vessels, but the severity of symptoms depends on the concentrations of the relevant proteins and the temperature at which cryoprecipitation occurs. Since some cryoglobulins can precipitate at temperatures above 22 °C, blood should be collected in prewarmed (37 °C) syringes and taken directly to the labo-

BOX 11.6 PROOF OF INVOLVEMENT OF A SPECIFIC ANTIGEN IN THE PATHOGENESIS OF VASCULITIS

- The causative antigen is part of the circulating immune complex
- Antigen, as well as antibody, is fixed in blood vessels within vasculitic lesions
- Injection of preformed antigen–antibody complexes induces tissue damage

CASE 11.7 MIXED CRYOGLOBULINAEMIA

A 45-year-old woman presented with ankle oedema due to nephrotic syndrome. In the preceding 5 years, she had experienced several episodes of a purpuric, erythematous, papular rash on the legs, accompanied by a bilateral arthropathy of the knees and ankles. A biopsy of the rash had shown features of vasculitis which had responded to systemic steroids. She now had a non-selective proteinuria of 10 g/day and a creatinine clearance of 74 ml/min. Serum alanine aminotransferase (ALT) was increased at 140 U/ml (NR < 50). Rheumatoid factor was detectable to a titre of 1/1280 but antinuclear antibodies were negative. Hepatitis B surface antigen was absent but antibodies to hepatitis C and hepatitis C viral RNA were detected in her serum. The serum immunoglobulins, measured at room temperature, were: IgG 2.10 g/l (NR 7.2–19.0); IgA 0.85 g/l (NR 0.8–5.0); and IgM 2.80 g/l (NR 0.5–2.0). Comple-

ment levels were abnormal, with a C3 of 0.80 g/l (NR 0.8–1.4) and a C4 of 0.02 g/l (NR 0.2–0.4). The very low C4 level raised the suspicion of cryoglobulinaemia. A warm sample of her serum contained a mixed cryoglobulin, composed of a monoclonal IgM and polyclonal IgG. A skin biopsy showed scattered deposits of IgM, IgG and C3 in dermal blood vessels. The histology of a renal biopsy showed membranoproliferative glomerulonephritis: on direct immunofluorescence, granular deposits of IgM and IgG were seen along the epithelial basement membrane. The final diagnosis was mixed cryoglobulinaemia secondary to chronic hepatitis C infection with cutaneous vasculitis, arthropathy and membranoproliferative glomerulonephritis. No risk factors for hepatitis C infection were identified.

ratory. 'Routine' interdepartmental transport arrangements operating in most hospitals are totally unsatisfactory.

Immunochemical analysis of cryoprecipitates allows their classification into three types.

Type I cryoglobulins (25%) are monoclonal proteins, usually IgM, which have no recognizable antibody activity. They have an inherent tendency to cryoprecipitate as the

paraprotein concentration increases. In most cases, there is an underlying malignant disease, usually Waldenström's macroglobulinaemia, lymphoma or myeloma. Symptoms are due to hyperviscosity and sludging of cryoprecipitates in cold extremities.

Type II cryoglobulins (25%) are of a mixed type in which the monoclonal protein (usually IgM) has antibody specifi-

CASE 11.8 SUBACUTE CUTANEOUS LUPUS ERYTHEMATOSUS

A 34-year-old woman presented with a 2-year history of a waxing and waning rash on her neck and arms. She had noticed that the rash was likely to flare following exposure to bright sunlight. Her general health was good, although in the last few months she had developed flitting pain and stiffness in the small joints of her hands. She had no history of Raynaud's phenomenon, mouth ulcers or eye trouble. On examination, there was an extensive skin rash involving the neck and arms and extending onto the face. The rash was red, raised above the surrounding skin and tended to form ring-like patterns with scaly margins (Fig. 11.9). There was no evidence of vasculitis and there were no other abnormal physical signs. The skin appearances were those of subacute cutaneous lupus erythematosus (SCLE); there was no clinical evidence of systemic involvement.

Laboratory investigations showed a normal haemoglobin, white cell count, blood creatinine and urinalysis. Antinuclear antibodies were detected at a titre of 1/100 and antibodies to Ro were detected by precipitation. Serum C3 and C4 levels were normal. A biopsy of affected skin on the neck showed typical changes of SCLE. Direct immunofluorescence demonstrated granular deposits of C3 and IgG along the basement membrane zone in the affected skin. She was treated with sunscreens, topical steroids and hydroxychloroquine. Over a period of several months, the skin lesions became less frequent but still flared after sun exposure.

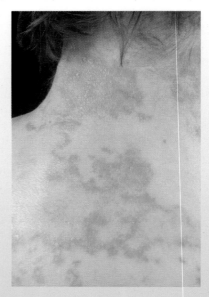

Fig. 11.9 Typical changes of subacute cutaneous lupus erythematosus on the neck.

city directed against the Fc portion of IgG, that is, rheumatoid factor activity. Cryoprecipitation occurs when complexes of IgM–anti-IgG antibody are formed. This type is strongly associated with chronic hepatitis C infection but may occasionally be found in B-cell malignancy or SLE. As in Case 11.7, patients typically present with features of 'immune-complex disease', such as diffuse vasculitis, arthritis and glomerulonephritis.

Type III cryoglobulins (50%) are of mixed polyclonal type in which olyclonal or oligoclonal IgM rheumatoid-like factors react with IgG. About one-third of cases are associated with hepatitis C. The remainder are associated with rheumatoid arthritis, SLE, polyarteritis nodosa or chronic infection (e.g. hepatitis B). Small amounts of type III cryoglobulins are found in many inflammatory conditions and are usually of no particular significance.

The treatment of cryoglobulinaemia is generally directed towards management of any recognized underlying disorder. Common-sense measures such as avoidance of cold environments and wearing warm clothing are helpful, but plasmapheresis and immunosuppression may be required.

11.5.4 Lupus erythematosus (Case 11.8)

The clinical features of lupus erythematosus (LE) range from a severe disease involving many organs, including the kidney, joints, brain and skin (SLE) (see Chapter 10), to a benign, chronic, purely cutaneous form, called discoid lupus erythematosus (DLE). Between these ends of the spectrum, all variations can occur. While it may be artificial to distinguish SLE from DLE, there are important clinical, immunological and prognostic differences between these forms of LE (Table 11.5).

The skin lesions of DLE are usually distinctive but, in cases of difficulty, immunological investigations are often helpful. Direct immunohistological examination of biopsies from areas of sun-exposed, normal skin (the lupus band test) (Fig. 11.5) is usually negative (Table 11.5). The prevalence of transformation from DLE to a systemic disease is around 10% or less.

A third form of clinically distinct cutaneous lupus is subacute cutaneous LE. Although subacute cutaneous LE (SCLE) and DLE have features in common, there are definite differences (Table 11.5). SCLE is non-scarring, less persistent, more widespread and more frequently complicated by alopecia than is DLE. Patients with SCLE often have a mild systemic illness characterized by joint pains and fever, but severe central nervous system and kidney disease are uncommon. Patients with this form of cutaneous LE have antibodies to the cytoplasmic antigen Ro (or SS-A) (see Chapter 19).

11.5.5 Systemic sclerosis (Case 11.9)

Systemic sclerosis is a chronic fibrosing disease of unknown aetiology. It can affect the skin, blood vessels, musculoskeletal system and many internal organs. Since indurated and thickened skin is the most striking feature of the disease, the term scleroderma is often used as a synonym for systemic sclerosis. Sclerodermatous changes may be localized or generalized, and generalized scleroderma can be further classified (Fig. 11.10) into **limited systemic sclerosis**, in which cutaneous and internal involvement is relatively limited (although Raynaud's phenomenon is often severe) and **diffuse systemic sclerosis**, in which skin and visceral involvement is usually extensive and sometimes life-threatening. Limited systemic sclerosis was formerly

Table 11.5 Characteristic features of the different forms of cutaneous lupus erythematosus (LE)

	Discoid LE	Subacute cutaneous LE	Systemic LE
Usual age of onset, years	30–40	< 40	< 40
Skin features	Oedematous plaques with scaling and follicular plugs Scarring Face, ears, scalp	Widespread Symmetrical Non-scarring erythematous plaques Upper chest, back, shoulders	Almost anything
Systemic features	None	Joint pains, fever, malaise	Almost any organ affected
Antinuclear antibodies present in	25%	80%	95%
dsDNA antibodies present in	0%	30%	70–85%
Anti-Ro antibodies present in	< 5%	70%	30%
Predominant HLA type	B7	B8, DR3	B8, DR3
Positive direct immunofluorescence of:			
Lesional skin	90%	40%	90%
Normal, sun-exposed skin	0%	20%	75%

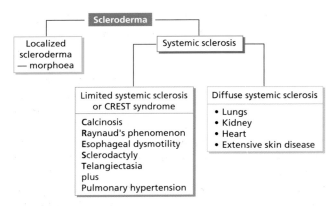

Fig. 11.10 Classification of scleroderma.

known as the CREST syndrome (this acronym is explained in Fig. 11.10).

Systemic sclerosis usually presents between the ages of 45 and 65; women are affected four times more frequently than men. It is a rare disorder with a prevalence of around 1 in 10 000. The prognosis depends upon disease severity, but the overall 10-year survival rate in diffuse disease is about 40%. **Renal failure** and malignant hypertension were his-

torically the major causes of death, but the incidence of this complication has declined with improved treatments for hypertension, particularly angiotensin-converting enzyme (ACE) inhibitors. **Pulmonary fibrosis** has now become the most feared complication in diffuse disease. Limited systemic sclerosis is a more benign disorder with a 10-year survival of 60–70%, although severe Raynaud's phenomenon is a major cause of morbidity in this group. There is also a risk of **pulmonary hypertension** developing many years into the disease, with significant associated mortality.

Diagnosis of systemic sclerosis is largely clinical, supported by biopsy of skin and other organs and assessment of the microcirculation in the hands by nailfold microscopy and thermography. Several patterns of autoantibody production are seen in systemic sclerosis, some of which are useful diagnostic or prognostic markers (Table 11.6). Antibodies to Scl-70 (an enzyme, topoisomerase 1, important in controlling coiling of DNA superhelices) are found almost exclusively in patients with systemic sclerosis, where, particularly in association with HLA-DR52a, they are associated with subsequent development of pulmonary fibrosis. Anticentromere antibodies are strongly associated with limited systemic sclerosis (sometimes also known as the CREST syndrome). Other patterns of autoantibody production are less clearly

CASE 11.9 SYSTEMIC SCLEROSIS

The patient first developed Raynaud's phenomenon in her early 20s. In cold weather, her hands and toes became white and painful and then turned blue; when the circulation returned, it was accompanied by extreme redness and pain (see Fig. 11.11). Several years after developing Raynaud's phenomenon, she noticed some tethering and thickening of her skin, starting in the hands but eventually affecting her face and mouth. On one occasion, an ulcer on her right index finger discharged 'tiny pieces of chalk'. At the age of 54, she developed dysphagia: she could swallow food only if she took fluids with it. At the age of 56, diarrhoea became a problem. Barium studies showed pseudodiverticulae typical of systemic sclerosis, a hiatus hernia, an atonic oesophagus and stomach, and a dilated, distorted proximal jejunum.

When reassessed at the age of 59, her heart, chest and abdomen were normal. She showed marked sclerodactyly and typical skin changes of scleroderma. Soft-tissue, calcified nodules were present on her fingers, forearms and over the patellae. Telangiectasia was evident on the hands, face and lips. Over the following 2 years she became increasingly short of breath, with marked ankle oedema and worsening of the diarrhoea. Lung function tests showed a restrictive defect with a reduction in transfer factor. A computed tomography scan of the thorax showed no evidence of pulmonary fibrosis but an electrocardiogram and echocardiogram

suggested right-ventricular strain secondary to pulmonary hypertension associated with limited systemic sclerosis. There was no biochemical evidence of renal or liver disease.

She has taken part in controlled trials of new treatments for systemic sclerosis: none has worked. She has now been referred to a specialist pulmonary hypertension unit for assessment as to whether she might benefit from treatment with bosentan, an endothelin 1 antagonist.

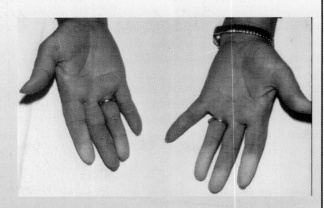

Fig. 11.11 Raynaud's phenomenon in limited systemic sclerosis.

Table 11.6 Autoantibodies in systemic sclerosis

	Frequency (%)
Any antinuclear antibodies	80
• Anticentromere antibody:	
Limited disease	90
Diffuse disease	5
• Antinucleolar antibody	40
• Anti-Scl-70 antibody	25
• Anti-RNP antibody	10
• Anti-Ro antibody	<5
• Anti-dsDNA antibody	0
Rheumatoid factor	25–33

associated with different patterns of disease, although some subtypes of nucleolar autoantibodies, such as those directed against RNA polymerase types I–III, may be associated with severe disease. Conventional immunofluorescence cannot distinguish these subtypes of antinucleolar antibody. The presence of any of these patterns of autoantibody production is predictive of the development of scleroderma in subjects presenting with Raynaud's phenomenon.

The pathology of the skin and affected organs is characterized by marked deposition of extracellular matrix, often centred around blood vessels, together with abnormalities of the vessels themselves: vessels are often obliterated by intimal proliferation. Inflammatory changes are not usually severe and C-reactive protein is not raised.

The pathogenesis of systemic sclerosis is poorly understood, but vascular, immunological and fibrotic abnormalities have been identified (see Fig. 11.12). An assumption is usually made that scleroderma is primarily an immunological disease, but definitive proof of this is lacking. There is certainly no evidence that any of the autoantibodies associated with scleroderma plays any direct role in the pathogenesis of systemic sclerosis. The origin of these antibodies and the reasons for their disease specificity are obscure, although

there is some evidence that free-radical-induced damage (as might occur in the recurrent ischaemia of Raynaud's phenomenon) makes many of these molecules highly immunogenic.

T cells may play an important role in scleroderma. Circumstantial evidence for this comes from the observation that a scleroderma-like disorder may occur in chronic graft-versus-host disease, which is thought to be largely T-cell mediated. In scleroderma itself, activated CD4[+] T cells are found in early lesions and in vitro experiments suggest that these T cells may activate dermal fibroblasts (either directly or indirectly via endothelial cells or macrophages) to increase production of collagen and other matrix proteins. Regardless of the stimulus, scleroderma fibroblasts develop marked abnormalities in function with a sustained increase in production of connective tissue proteins. There is some evidence that **transforming growth factor (TGF)-β** is a key mediator of fibrosis. This potently fibrogenic cytokine is expressed at high levels in tissue from systemic sclerosis and fibroblasts from patients with the disease express abnormally high levels of TGF-β receptors. Signalling through these receptors induces synthesis of collagen and other matrix proteins, but also induces further production of TGF-β. This semi-autonomy of scleroderma fibroblasts may explain two puzzling features of the disease: first, the very poor response to immunosuppression and, second, the minimal evidence of inflammation in many involved tissues.

The aetiology of systemic sclerosis is also poorly understood. Weak genetic associations have been identified with various HLA alleles, the strongest association being between HLA-DR52a and lung fibrosis in scleroderma (the risk of lung disease is 17 times greater in patients with this allele). Scleroderma tends to occur in geographical clusters, suggesting unknown environmental risk factors. A small proportion of cases have been associated with exposure to environmental toxins, particularly vinyl chloride. The similarities between systemic sclerosis and chronic graft-versus-host disease led to the development of the microchimerism hypothesis. Microchimerism develops when small

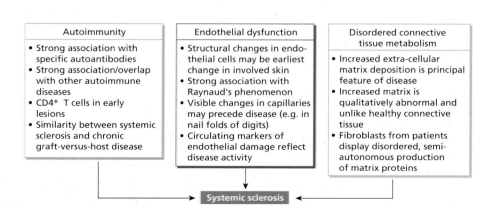

Fig. 11.12 Three major factors in the pathogenesis of systemic sclerosis.

numbers of fetal or maternal cells cross the placenta during pregnancy and then persist in the mother or child, respectively. Fetal cells can be detected in the blood and tissues of some normal healthy women up to decades after the birth of these children. It has been suggested that delayed onset of an immune response against these chronically engrafted cells might lead to systemic sclerosis. Some evidence exists that the burden of microchimeric cells may be higher in systemic sclerosis, but the significance of this elegant hypothesis is as yet unclear.

Treatment is largely limited to management of complications (ACE inhibitors for hypertension, vasodilators for Raynaud's, the endothelin-1 antagonist bosentan for pulmonary hypertension, etc.). Immunosuppression plays no current role in management of the skin changes, although may be of limited use in pulmonary fibrosis. A great variety of antifibrotic drugs and immunomodulatory drugs have been used with almost uniformly negative results. Much current therapeutic research revolves around inhibition of the action of TGF-β and other fibrogenic mediators.

FURTHER READING

See website: www.immunologyclinic.com

12 Eye Diseases

12.1 Introduction

The eye is a fragile and complex organ, whose physiological function is intolerant of any distortion in structure. Immunological defence mechanisms within the eye need to strike a delicate balance between exclusion or rapid elimination of invading pathogens and the need to minimize excessive inflammation within the eye which might disrupt transmission of light or impair retinal processing. For this reason, the eye relies heavily upon mechanical or physical barriers to infection.

Immunologically, the eye can be divided into two major compartments: the conjunctival sac and the globe (Fig. 12.1).

Conjunctival sac

The conjunctival sac has similar defence mechanisms to the skin and upper respiratory tract mucosa and is affected by similar diseases (Table 12.1). The conjunctival sac is the main site for entry of antigen into the eye. The major physical barriers to antigen entry are blinking and the free flow and drainage of tears. These physical factors are supplemented by antimicrobial factors within tears such as IgA and lysozyme. The conjunctiva can respond briskly to local irritation or injury, being highly vascular and containing mast cells. As in other sites, persistence of inflammation within the eye leads to the accumulation of chronic inflammatory cells, i.e. activated T and B cells and macrophages.

The globe

The anatomy of the globe is summarized in Fig. 12.1. Two

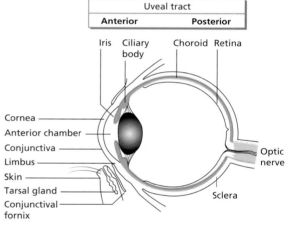

(a)

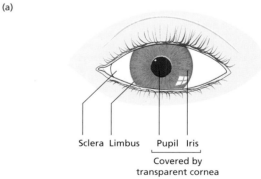

(b)

Fig. 12.1 Anatomy of the eye. (a) In lateral section (only the lower eyelid is shown). (b) Frontal view (left side).

Table 12.1 Conjunctivitis and types of hypersensitivity

Disease	Mechanism of hypersensitivity	Aetiology
Seasonal conjunctivitis	IgE-mediated (type I)*	Grass pollens + other antigens
Vernal conjunctivitis	Above plus TH2 cells	Air-borne allergens
Atopic keratoconjunctivitis	Atopic (probably TH2 cells)	Ocular equivalent of atopic dermatitis
Cicatrizing conjunctivitis (pemphigoid)	Antibody on conjunctival basement membrane (type II)	Autoimmune
Stevens–Johnson syndrome	Immune complex (type III)	Drug-reaction or unknown
Sarcoidosis	Granuloma (type IV)	Unknown
Contact dermatoconjunctivitis	Cellular immune reactions (type IV)	Drugs, cosmetics, contact lens solutions

*Types I–IV refer to the Gell and Coombs' classification; see Chapter 1.

principal types of tissue are present: avascular tissues (cornea, lens, vitreous and sclera) and highly vascular tissues (the uveal tract, the posterior part of which is closely associated with the retina). Historically, the globe was regarded as invisible from the immune system (**immunologically privileged**, Chapter 5) because of a lack of lymphatic drainage, the presence of an **endothelial blood–eye barrier**, and the avascular nature of much of the globe's contents. This physical separation of the eye and the immune system is important in preventing autoimmune disease within the eye, but it is now known that active suppression of immune responses is also of major importance in limiting inflammation within the globe.

Antigens can potentially enter the globe via the sclera, cornea, optic nerve or via the uveal tract. The tough physical barrier of the avascular tissues can exclude most antigens provided conjunctival function is normal. The uveal tract, however, is highly vascular and has the capacity for trapping blood-borne antigens or microorganisms, a property that is shared with other highly vascular structures such as the glomerulus. As in the kidney, this is limited by the presence of tight junctions between uveal endothelial cells, which usually limit extravasation of cells or plasma. This blood–eye barrier may, however, break down in response to injury of many kinds.

If antigen does gain access to the globe, immune responses to that antigen are likely to be reduced or inhibited. Multiple mechanisms underlie this **down-regulation**: immunosuppressive cytokines such as transforming growth factor (TGF)-β are present within the eye, but cells throughout the cornea absorb endothelium and also express high levels of a protein called Fas ligand (FasL), which will bind to any cells expressing its receptor, Fas, and trigger apoptosis in the Fas-bearing cells. Since Fas is richly expressed upon most cells which migrate into sites of inflammation, such as activated T cells, macrophages and neutrophils, this mechanism limits inflammation within the eye. FasL/Fas interactions also

Table 12.2 Systemic immunological diseases and the eye

Conjunctiva	Reiter's syndrome
	Sarcoidosis
	Pemphigus/pemphigoid
	Sjögren's syndrome
Cornea	Sjögren's syndrome
	Systemic vasculitis
Uveal tract and retina	Sarcoidosis
	Spondyloarthropathies
	Ankylosing spondylitis
	Reiter's syndrome
	Psoriatic arthritis
	Enteropathic arthritis
	Systemic lupus
	Juvenile idiopathic arthritis
	Behçet's disease
Sclera	Systemic vasculitis
	Rheumatoid
	Wegener's

help to maintain tolerance within the eye, since autoreactive T cells entering the eye are deleted. Disruption of this process may contribute to autoimmune and hypersensitivity disease within the eye.

Immunological diseases of the eye fall into two groups: the eye may either be the sole target of local immunological mechanisms or it may be one of many tissues involved in a systemic process (Table 12.2). The symptoms and signs of inflammation involving different parts of the eye are summarized in Fig. 12.2 and these diseases are discussed below.

12.2 Conjunctivitis

Conjunctival inflammation is very common. The major causes are infection and hypersensitivity reactions (see Table 12.1).

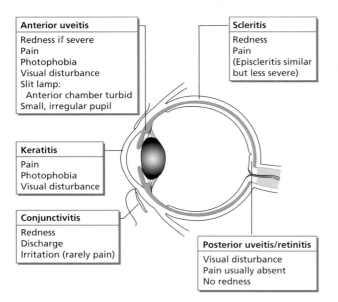

Fig. 12.2 Symptoms and signs of eye disease.

12.2.1 Conjunctival infection (Case 12.1)

The case emphasizes the importance of mechanical barriers in protecting the eye from infection. Failure of blinking and loss of the tear film will inevitably lead to severe infection even in the absence of any immunological defect. **Bacterial infection** can also follow trauma to the eye and can be the sequel to other forms of ocular inflammation, such as viral infection. Local immune responses do have some role to play: patients with antibody deficiency can develop bacterial conjunctivitis, usually caused by Haemophilus influenzae (also commonly responsible for respiratory tract infections in these patients).

Infection is the most important cause of conjunctivitis worldwide. The commonest organism involved is Chlamydia trachomatis, an intracellular bacteria-like agent which causes trachoma; over 400 million people suffer from this condition. They show a profound local immune response to the organism. Specific antichlamydial antibodies are found in tears and serum, but the concentration is not related to the outcome. Treatment requires systemic and topical antibiotics and the prognosis, if treated in the early stages, is excellent. Where treatment is unavailable, trachoma commonly causes blindness, especially if accompanied by superadded bacterial infection.

The commonest viral cause of conjunctivitis is **adenovirus**. Another virus causing conjunctivitis is **herpes simplex**. Primary infection occurs in childhood and is usually asymptomatic; if inflammation does occur, it is usually confined to the skin, conjunctiva and superficial cornea, where the actively replicating virus causes typical herpetic ulcers. Secondary herpes infection results in keratitis (see below).

12.2.2 Allergic conjunctivitis (Case 12.2)

The various forms of allergic conjunctival disease are summarized in Table 12.1. Seasonal and perennial conjunctivitis are extremely common disorders. Allergic conjunctivitis is discussed in more detail in Chapter 4.

12.2.3 Autoimmune conjunctivitis

All types of hypersensitivity may damage the conjunctiva (Table 12.1). Specific autoantibodies directed against conjunctival antigens are involved in the pathogenesis of ocular pemphigoid (cicatrizing conjunctivitis) and pemphigus.

12.2.4 Stevens–Johnson syndrome (Case 12.3)

This is a severe form of erythema multiforme, which produces ocular changes in 50% of patients. *Early diagnosis of*

CASE 12.1 CONJUNCTIVAL INFECTION

A 22-year-old man was involved in a motorcycle accident and suffered a severe closed head injury which produced diffuse cerebral injury and a fracture of the left temporal bone. He was admitted to a neurosurgical intensive care unit and required artificial ventilation for 17 days. A tracheostomy was performed to assist with ventilation. He gradually became independent of the ventilator, and regained consciousness and was eventually transferred to the neurosurgical ward. He was noted to have a left facial nerve palsy (caused by the fracture) and to be restless and confused, but no other focal neurological defect was identified. The facial nerve palsy impaired his ability to blink on the left. While unconscious both his eyes had been taped shut to prevent injury and infection. Attempts were made to tape the left eye shut on the ward, but he persistently removed the dressing. Three days after his transfer to the ward the left eye was noted to be red with crusted swollen lids. The cornea was hazy and he was photophobic. A clinical diagnosis was made of conjunctivitis and keratitis secondary to exposure. Swabs taken from the eye grew Pseudomonas aeruginosa. He was treated vigorously with topical antibiotics and the eyelids were temporarily sutured together. Despite this, he suffered considerable corneal scarring with loss of visual acuity in the left eye.

CASE 12.2 ALLERGIC CONJUNCTIVITIS

A 23-year-old student vet presented with a history of intermittent redness and itching of the eyes, associated with some swelling of the eyelids. These episodes occurred only when he was involved in small-animal work, particularly when handling rabbits. Each episode lasted for several hours and several recent episodes had been associated with sneezing and running of the nose, but no wheeze. He had also noticed that large, itchy weals developed on his skin if he was scratched by a rabbit. He had a history of mild hay fever. Skin-prick testing showed a marked positive response to rabbit proteins and moderate levels of rabbit-specific IgE were found in his blood. A diagnosis of allergic conjunctivitis and rhinitis due to rabbit hypersensitivity was made. He was able to limit the problem by taking a non-sedative antihistamine on the days when he was likely to be exposed to rabbits.

CASE 12.3 STEVENS–JOHNSON SYNDROME

A 17-year-old girl was admitted as an emergency with a 3-day history of severe ulceration of her lips, 'sticky' eyes, sore feet, diffuse itching and an erythematous rash. Following a major epileptic fit 8 days previously, she had been put on carbamazepine. On admission, she was pyrexial with extensive haemorrhagic ulceration of the mouth, which became too sore even to take fluids. A clinical diagnosis of Stevens–Johnson syndrome was made and she was treated immediately with systemic corticosteroids (45 mg daily). She improved symptomatically, but when an ophthalmologist was asked to see her 3 weeks later she was found to have severe conjunctival ulceration and punctate keratitis. The conjunctival ulcerations required 'rodding' to prevent adhesion of the raw surfaces and she was also treated with topical antibiotics to prevent infection. Unfortunately, she then developed cicatricial entropion (inward-turning eyelids), with resulting corneal trauma. The lid deformity was surgically corrected and further corneal ulceration prevented by an extended-wear contact lens. Another late complication of this syndrome is obliteration of the conjunctival sac, leading to 'dry eye', corneal scarring and even blindness.

ocular involvement is imperative. The syndrome is probably caused by immune complexes (type III reaction) involving a drug or microorganism (Table 12.1). The severe conjunctivitis, presumably caused by deposition of immune complexes in conjunctival vessels, leads to ulceration, secondary keratitis and infection. Long-term ocular complications, as in Case 12.3, are common. Treatment of the ocular complications may be disappointing, although intensive, short-term, topical steroids help to reduce inflammation and prevent conjunctival ulceration, and topical antibiotics are used to prevent superinfection.

12.2.5 Other causes of conjunctivitis

T-cell-mediated TH1 immune (type IV) mechanisms are involved in allergic contact dermatitis (see Chapter 11) and **contact dermatoconjunctivitis** (Table 12.1). The condition is characterized by erythematous, indurated lesions on the eyelids. There is less conjunctival injection than in immediate reactions. Ophthalmic contact sensitizers include almost all topical drugs (such as antibiotic drops or atropine-like compounds), cosmetics and even contact lens solutions.

Conjunctivitis may also be a feature of other systemic diseases such as **Reiter's syndrome** and **sarcoidosis**. Seventy-five percent of patients with Reiter's syndrome (see Chapter 10) develop conjunctivitis (see Fig. 4.2), while 15% also have an iridocyclitis. Uveitis (30%) is commoner than conjunctivitis (5%) in patients with sarcoidosis (see Chapter 13).

12.3 Keratitis

Recurrent **herpes simplex stromal keratitis** is probably due to a cell-mediated hypersensitivity reaction rather than to active virus infection. Epithelial cells may be damaged during the primary infection, so that T lymphocytes become sensitized to persistent viral antigens or virally altered corneal antigens. Topical steroids may be required to prevent permanent scarring and blindness.

Marginal ulcers are sometimes seen in response to **staphylococcal infection**, particularly in younger patients, and are thought to be due to deposited antigen–antibody complexes.

Marginal ulcers also occur in vasculitides, particularly rheumatoid vasculitis and Wegener's granulomatosis. An important complication is the **peripheral corneal melting syndrome**, which can lead to corneal perforation with prolapse of the uveal tissue — an ocular emergency. Systemic immunosuppression may be helpful but corneal grafting may be necessary.

Keratoconjunctivitis sicca is inflammation resulting from insufficient lacrimal gland secretions. The patient complains of sore or gritty eyes, and tear secretion is deficient when measured by Schirmer's test (see Chapter 10). Dry eyes are common in the elderly, but in some patients the dry eyes are accompanied by a dry mouth (due to involvement of salivary glands) and by arthritis (Sjögren's syndrome). Treatment of dry eyes is difficult, as dryness is experienced only when the lacrimal glands are severely damaged. Artificial tears are usually the only option.

The damaged cornea can be replaced with a cadaveric graft (see Chapter 8). Although it is antigenic, the cornea is a poor inducer of allogeneic immune responses (see section 12.1). In avascular grafts, major histocompatibility complex (MHC) compatibility is irrelevant, and over 90% of those which remain avascular are successful. However, rejection of a corneal graft is associated with revascularization, and MHC matching may then be important; well-matched grafts can survive despite revascularization.

12.4 Scleritis

The episcleral tissue is that between the fascia of the eyeball and the sclera itself. Inflammation of episcleral tissue, **simple episcleritis**, is common, particularly in young women. It is a benign condition and resolves in 3–4 weeks. The cause is unknown but an autoimmune process has not been excluded. **Nodular episcleritis** is a more protracted disease; about 30% of patients have an associated systemic rheumatic disease (usually rheumatoid arthritis).

Inflammation of the sclera, **scleritis**, is a severe and painful disease which can lead to blindness. It occurs in association with severe systemic vasculitic diseases, such as rheumatoid arthritis, polyarteritis nodosa, Wegener's granulomatosis, relapsing polychondritis or systemic lupus erythematosus.

12.5 Uveitis (Case 12.4)

Uveitis, or inflammation of the uveal tract, describes a common group of conditions which can be classified into **anterior, posterior and pan-uveitis**. Anterior uveitis includes iritis and cyclitis. Posterior uveitis usually refers to choroiditis, but retinitis or retinal vasculitis are often part of the same pathological process and are discussed here together with choroiditis. Since the inflammation in uveitis extends beyond the uveal tract into the lens, vitreous and retina, the more general term **intraocular inflammation** has been proposed, but this is not in widespread use.

All parts of the uveal tract can be affected by either acute or chronic inflammation, and uveitis can occur as a purely ocular process or as a manifestation of systemic disease. As outlined in section 12.1, the highly vascular uveal tract has great potential for trapping blood-borne antigen, immune complexes and microorganisms.

12.5.1 Anterior uveitis

Acute anterior uveitis can occur in association with several systemic diseases, most notably sarcoidosis and the seronegative spondyloarthropathies (see Chapter 10). The latter are strongly associated with the possession of the

CASE 12.4 BEHÇET'S DISEASE

A 21-year-old man from a Turkish family presented with a painful left eye for 2 days associated with blurred vision. He also gave a 3-month history of relapsing and remitting ulceration of his mouth and scrotum. Three days later the right eye also became involved.

Ophthalmological examination showed a florid anterior uveitis of such severity that neutrophils in the anterior chamber settled out to form a fluid level visible to the naked eye: a hypopon (Fig. 12.3). There was no posterior uveitis at this stage. A clinical diagnosis of Behçet's disease was made. He was treated with oral and topical (ocular and mucosal) corticosteroids and a low dose of colchicine. The eye changes and ulceration gradually settled.

However, 3 months later he developed painless deterioration of vision in the left eye and was found to have a severe retinal vasculitis. This was treated aggressively with oral corticosteroids and azathioprine with little response. Despite treatment with ciclosporin, mycophenolate mofetil and infliximab over the following year, he also developed vasculitis in the right retina. He then presented with a left hemiparesis due to cerebral vasculitis. His treatment was switched to pulsed intravenous cyclophosphamide. This gradually controlled the ocular inflammation and he has developed no further neurological symptoms. His vision remains severely impaired.

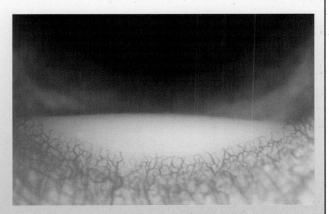

Fig. 12.3 Hypopyon due to severe anterior chamber inflammation in Behçet's disease. Slide courtesy of Mr N. P. Jones.

HLA allele B27. This HLA allele (found in around 5% of the healthy population) is also present in about 50% of patients with recurrent anterior uveitis with no evidence of systemic disease, suggesting that common disease mechanisms may underlie many cases of uveitis, regardless of associated systemic disease (Fig. 12.4). Over half of the UK cases of uveitis have no underlying disease, i.e. **idiopathic uveitis.**

Inflammation of the anterior uvea involves a breakdown of 'the blood–aqueous humour barrier' so that there is outpouring of serum proteins and inflammatory cells into the anterior chamber (see Fig. 12.2). The inflammatory exudate, which can be seen by slit-lamp microscopy, may form small deposits on the back of the cornea (keratic precipitates—Fig. 12.5). The back of the inflamed iris may become stuck to the lens (posterior synechiae), producing an irregularly shaped pupil and increased pressure in the posterior chamber (secondary glaucoma).

An animal model of experimental allergic uveitis (EAU) is provoked by distant immunization with a well-defined retinal autoantigen and is mediated by CD4$^+$ T cells and macrophages. *However, once uveitis has occurred, any inflammatory*

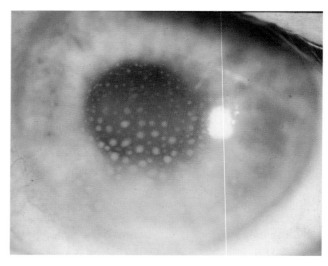

Fig. 12.5 Keratic precipitates cover the posterior surface of the cornea in a patient with granulomatous uveitis (slide courtesy of Mr N. P. Jones).

agent can trigger a recurrence. It is possible that slight changes in vascular permeability in the eye, like those in the kidney, encourage the deposition of immune complexes or antigen.

Mild recurrent anterior uveitis is usually self-limiting and symptomatically treated with local steroids and mydriatic agents under ophthalmic supervision.

In contrast to acute anterior uveitis, chronic anterior uveitis is painless and presents with insidious loss of vision, due to a combination of raised intraocular pressure and cataract formation. This can occur without systemic disease but most notably occurs in children with juvenile idiopathic arthritis, particularly in those with early-onset disease involving a small number of joints and who have antinuclear antibodies (about 50% of children with this pattern of arthritis have uveitis). *Ophthalmological screening of children with juvenile chronic arthritis is essential, as early detection and treatment can prevent blindness in this silent, insidiously progressive disease.*

12.5.2 Posterior uveitis

Posterior uveitis (or choroiditis) (Fig. 12.4) is also painless and presents with visual impairment. This can occur as one of a group of idiopathic disorders confined to the eye, but more often occurs secondary to infection or systemic inflammatory disease. The inflammatory process is often centred on blood vessels, particularly when acute (Fig. 12.6). It is appropriate to consider choroiditis, choroidoretinitis and retinal vasculitis under the same heading.

Acute choroidoretinitis occurs in several connective tissue diseases, most notably Behçet's disease and systemic lupus erythematosus. Vigorous immunosuppression may

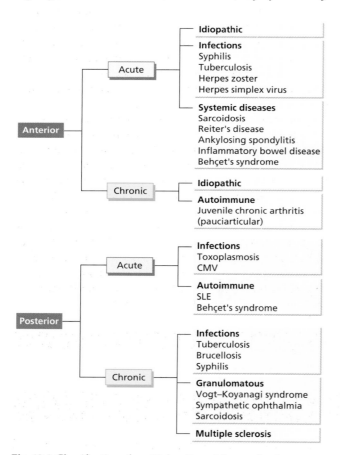

Fig. 12.4 Classification of uveitis by site and time scale of symptoms (post-trauma or surgery cases not included).

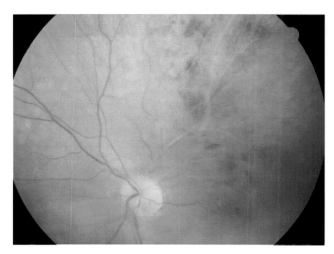

Fig. 12.6 Retinal vasculitis showing vascular occlusion and haemorrhage from damaged vessels (slide courtesy of Mr N. P. Jones).

be sight-saving in these disorders. However, similar ocular changes may be seen in infection, which should be excluded before immunosuppression is used.

A particularly devastating form of acute choroidoretinitis is caused by cytomegalovirus infection in patients with severe defects in cellular immunity, particularly in advanced HIV infection. This is difficult to treat and often blinding.

Chronic posterior uveitis can occur in a number of chronic infections, in sarcoidosis and in Vogt–Koyanagi syndrome (uveitis and vitiligo). Granuloma formation occurs in several of these disorders and it seems likely that TH1-cell-mediated hypersensitivity underlies their pathogenesis. A mild chronic posterior uveitis also occurs in multiple sclerosis. This is not of any clinical consequence but is of interest in showing that the disease process in multiple sclerosis is not confined to the central nervous system.

The suspicion of an associated systemic disorder depends on the pattern of the uveitis (bilateral, granulomatous site) and on a careful clinical history and examination. 'Uveitis investigations' are unrewarding, as there are no specific tests.

12.5.3 Uveitis following trauma (Case 12.5)

Lens-induced uveitis occurs about 2 weeks after surgery to

the lens or may be seen spontaneously in eyes with mature disintegrating lenses. Lens damage may release 'hidden' antigens and the subsequent uveitis is believed to be due to the immune response to those antigens. Although injection of sterile lens antigens into the eye has a minimal effect, any natural adjuvants present (such as bacterial antigens) potentiate the immune reaction. Animal experiments suggest that lens-induced uveitis is caused by local production of specific antibodies to denatured lens antigens, which cross-react with native uveal antigens. Antibodies to lens proteins are also found in the eye and circulation in human disease. The disease is usually confined to the traumatized eye, except in elderly patients, when spontaneous leakage of lens protein may provoke a bilateral reaction.

Sympathetic ophthalmia is a devastating bilateral, progressive granulomatous uveitis following penetration or perforation of one orbit. Uveitis in the non-traumatized eye is thought to be due to an autoimmune response to antigens liberated from the other eye. A severely traumatized 'blind' eye should be removed within 2 weeks of injury to avoid risk of a sympathetic reaction in the intact eye. A choroiditis is the first sign, but granulomatous inflammation eventually involves the whole tract. Animal experiments suggest that a penetrating injury releases minute doses of retinal antigens into the subconjunctival space with drainage to the local lymph node where autosensitization occurs.

Treatment is difficult but ciclosporin A may limit progression.

Sympathetic ophthalmia is often used as a striking example of how self-tolerance can break down when self-antigen from an 'immunologically privileged' site gains access to the immune system. Theoretically sympathetic ophthalmia could complicate any invasive surgical procedure on the eye. However, the extreme rarity of this disorder after both surgery and trauma (fewer than five cases per year in the USA) emphasizes how powerfully the eye suppresses inappropriate immune responses by the mechanisms outlined in section 12.1. Sympathetic ophthalmia has been associated with similar HLA alleles to the Vogt–Koyanagi syndrome, suggesting some similarities in the immunopathogenesis of these two forms of granulomatous uveitis.

FURTHER READING

See website: www.immunologyclinic.com

CASE 12.5 LENS-INDUCED UVEITIS

A 73-year-old woman had a left-sided extracapsular cataract extraction and lens implant, although the cortical lens material was never completely removed. She made an uneventful post-operative recovery but 2 weeks later developed a severe uveitis in the same eye. Two years after the operation, she still has to use topical steroids to suppress the uveitis. The presumed diagnosis is lens-induced uveitis.

CHAPTER 13

13 Chest Diseases

13.1 Introduction

Antigen can enter the respiratory tract either in the inspired air or via the circulation. Organisms that enter through the airways may be killed by local defence mechanisms, persist in the lung with damaging consequences (such as bronchiectasis or fibrosis) or invade the systemic circulation to cause septicaemia. Since all the blood from the right side of the heart passes through the pulmonary bed, the respiratory tract is also exposed to circulating organisms, immune complexes and toxic substances from distant sites.

The respiratory tract can be crudely but usefully divided into **two** anatomical, functional and pathological compartments: the **airways** (from the nose to the terminal bronchiole) and the **air spaces** (or alveoli). The airways are protected from inhaled microorganisms and other potentially injurious particles by multiple mechanical factors, backed up by soluble antimicrobial proteins and rapid recruitment of neutrophils and other inflammatory cells (Fig. 13.1). Access to the alveolar compartment is therefore usually limited to very small inhaled particles (< 5 µm diameter) (see Fig. 4.4) and organisms or antigen carried via the pulmonary circulation. Particles and organisms gaining access to the alveoli encounter further protective mechanisms such as the surfactant proteins (which have a complement-like function) and alveolar macrophages. **Alveolar macrophages** are responsible for ingesting, killing and degrading foreign mate-

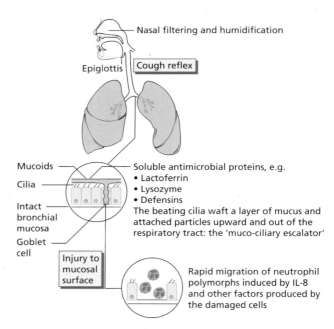

Fig. 13.1 Non-specific protective mechanisms in the airways.

rial, both living and dead. Although their action in removing organisms from the lower respiratory tract is crucial, their reaction to inert materials can sometimes cause pulmonary damage. Viable alveolar cells can be recovered by bronchoalveolar lavage (BAL). Macrophages comprise about 90% of the cells in BAL fluid, while lymphocytes (mostly T cells) constitute about 10%. Cigarette smoking increases the cell yield by four- to five-fold and the macrophages are seen to be filled with tars and silicates. The proportion of neutrophils (10–20%) is increased in smokers compared with non-smokers (2–5%), and a greater number are activated. The supernatant BAL fluid contains a high concentration of neutrophil elastase, which may play a role in the lung destruction seen in chronic bronchitis and emphysema.

Antigen-specific immune components are also found in the respiratory tract. **Bronchial-associated lymphoid tissue (BALT)** forms part of a common mucosal immune system (see Chapter 14). Unlike gut-associated lymphoid tissue, BALT does not form discrete structures in healthy subjects, but develops in response to repeated or persistent infection or other injurious stimuli such as smoking. Under these circumstances, BALT becomes organized in follicles and consists mainly of B cells, but distinct sites of collections of T cells are found on the periphery of these follicles. Epithelium overlying the BALT is devoid generally of cilia and goblet cells but displays membranous projections into the lumen, suited to selective antigen sampling, like its counterpart in the intestine — the M cell (see Chapter 14). Antigens are transported into the follicle where they can stimulate an antigen-specific T- and B-cell response. Subsequently, IgA precursor B cells migrate into lymphatics. Bronchial IgA-bearing cells recirculate through both gut and lungs, so dispersing antigen-sensitive cells.

There are also large numbers of less organized lymphocytes in the lung within the pulmonary vasculature, in the lung interstitium and in the bronchoalveolar space.

Although relatively few lymphocytes are seen on routine sections, when calculated for the whole lung, lymphocyte numbers are comparable to the circulating blood pool, i.e. about 10×10^9 lymphocytes.

Plasma cells producing IgE and IgG are also found in the bronchial tract. The physiological reason for the presence of IgE cells in the lung is unknown; it may even be an evolutionary accident, since the respiratory tract is a foregut derivative and IgE has a role in expulsion of intestinal parasites. While its physiological function is unclear, IgE is implicated in immediate (type I) hypersensitivity mechanisms (see Chapter 4) responsible for allergic asthma and hay fever.

We have considered respiratory diseases under four headings: infection, granulomatous disease, interstitial lung disease and vasculitis. Allergic diseases, which constitute the major immunological airways diseases, are considered in Chapter 4.

13.2 Respiratory infections

Infectious processes within the respiratory tract usually affect either the airways (e.g. rhinitis, sinusitis, laryngitis, bronchitis) or alveoli (pneumonia), although pneumonia can develop as a consequence of airways infection, particularly the small airways (bronchopneumonia).

Most respiratory tract infection reflects an interaction between virulent microorganisms and a relatively normal respiratory tract, whose protective mechanisms have been overcome either by the organism or by other injurious factors such as smoking or malnutrition. The respiratory tract is, however, also the most common site for infection to develop in immunodeficient subjects, and *compromised immunity must be considered in all patients who present with serious, persistent, unusual or recurrent infection.*

13.2.1 Infection in the immunocompetent host

The airways are a major target for **viral infection** (Table 13.1), manifested most typically as the common cold, caused by many different viruses. These viruses usually replicate better in the cooler upper airways than at normal body temperature. Infection is probably cleared largely by virus-specific cytotoxic T cells.

Table 13.1 Respiratory infections classified according to site and pattern of infection.

Site	Organism	Incidence and pattern of infection	Predisposing factors
Upper respiratory tract	Viral	Common — colds	
	Bacterial	Less common — sinusitis	Physical damage Viral infection Immune dysfunction
Lower respiratory tract	Viral	Pneumonia — rare in adults Bronchiolitis due to respiratory syncytial virus common in children	Immune dysfunction
	Bacterial	Common	Age Smoking Immune dysfunction

Bacterial infection of the airways is less common and often occurs as a result of *suppression of defence mechanisms by prior viral infection*. The transient susceptibility of the airways to infection induced by some viral infections is only partially understood but includes physical factors such as inhibition of ciliary function and damage to the airway epithelium (e.g. influenza), and more subtle immunological mechanisms such as reduced expression of MHC molecules (adenoviruses) and inhibition of cytokine production [e.g. measles inhibits interleukin (IL)-12 production]. The most striking example is **influenza A**, which can lead to devastating pneumonia, usually caused by Staphylococcus aureus, in debilitated patients. However, the most important causes of pneumonia in the immunocompetent host are bacterial (Table 13.1).

Bacterial pneumonia is a common problem. It accounts for up to 10% of hospital admissions in developed countries and carries a considerable mortality: in the UK, pneumonia causes 10 times as many deaths as all other infectious diseases together. While most of these deaths occur as a final event in debilitated patients, some previously healthy children and adults also die of pneumonia in spite of seemingly appropriate antibiotic therapy. The most devastating consequences of pneumonia are seen in developing countries. Each year, about 5 million children die of pneumonia before they are 5 years old. In South American countries, for instance, infant mortality from pneumonia and influenza is approximately 30 times greater than in the USA. Pneumococcal infections account for the majority of bacterial pneumonias and carry a mortality rate of 6–30%.

13.2.2 Infection in the immunocompromised host (Case 13.1)

Serious or recurrent infection does not always reflect disordered immunity (Table 13.2). The abnormal mucosal environment in cystic fibrosis is a potent predisposing cause for infection,

Table 13.2 Important non-immunological causes of recurrent or severe infection

Airway obstruction
• Tumour
• Foreign body (e.g. peanuts in children)
• Inflammatory/fibrotic (e.g. in tuberculosis)

Mucociliary dysfunction
• Cystic fibrosis (abnormal mucus)
• Ciliary dyskinesia (genetic defect in ciliary proteins)
• Squamous metaplasia (due to smoking)

as is bronchial obstruction due to factors ranging from tumours to plugging by mucus. Recurrent bronchial inflammation from many causes, particularly when associated with obstruction, leads to the development of bronchiectasis: dilated, damaged bronchi which themselves predispose to further infection, thus amplifying and perpetuating the process. *However, there are certain infections or patterns of infection which should always lead to the consideration of underlying immunodeficiency (Fig. 13.2).* Some of these infections (such as Pneumocystis pneumonia) are virtually always associated with underlying immunodeficiency, whereas chronic sinopulmonary infection is associated with antibody deficiency in only 5% of cases. Nevertheless, the highly treatable nature of many immunodeficiency states (particularly antibody deficiency) makes investigation mandatory (see Chapter 3).

In adults, secondary causes of immunodeficiency are more common than primary ones and should be excluded first (see Chapter 3). An insidious pneumonic illness with dry cough, dyspnoea and fever may be caused by Pneumocystis carinii, cytomegalovirus (CMV) or atypical mycobacterial infection and should raise the possibility of acquired immune defi-

---

CASE 13.1 PNEUMONIA AND CHRONIC LYMPHATIC LEUKAEMIA

A 65-year-old man was admitted with bilateral lower-lobe pneumonia. He had felt exhausted for 6 months and had lost 3 kg in weight. He did not smoke. He was clinically anaemic but had no finger clubbing, lymphadenopathy or splenomegaly. On investigation, he had a low haemoglobin (92 g/l) and a raised erythrocyte sedimentation rate (ESR) (84 mm/h). The white cell count was very high (98×10^9/l) and 95% of these were lymphocytes. The platelet count was normal. Serum immunoglobulins were all low: IgG 3.2 g/l (NR 7.2–18.0), IgA 0.6 g/l (NR 0.8–5.0) and IgM 0.3 g/l (NR 0.5–2.0); no paraprotein bands were seen.

A provisional diagnosis of pneumonia complicating chronic lymphatic leukaemia was made and confirmed by surface marker

studies, which showed that 98% of peripheral lymphocytes were monoclonal B cells (see Chapter 6).

Sputum cultures grew Haemophilus influenzae. Treatment with amoxycillin resulted in rapid clearing of the pneumonia but, in view of his high lymphocyte count and mild anaemia, he was started on chlorambucil to control the lymphoproliferation. He lacked detectable serum antibodies and failed to make IgG antibodies to pneumococci on immunization; furthermore, all three major classes of serum immunoglobulins were low. Prophylactic IgG replacement therapy was started at a dose of 0.4 g/kg body weight per month.

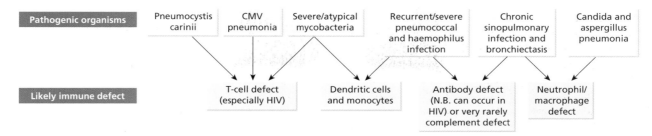

Fig. 13.2 Patterns of respiratory infection associated with specific immunodeficiencies. CMV, Cytomegalovirus; HIV, human immunodeficiency virus.

ciency syndrome (AIDS) (see Chapter 3). Opportunistic viral, fungal and protozoal infections are common in patients with AIDS or iatrogenic defects in cell-mediated immunity, but they also suffer from common bacterial infections. Patients with AIDS frequently have infections with several microorganisms simultaneously.

13.3 Granulomatous diseases

The granulomatous diseases are a heterogeneous group of disorders with differing aetiologies, clinical presentations, histological characteristics and responses to therapy.

13.3.1 Formation of a granuloma

A **granuloma** is a histological structure made up largely of macrophages which have differentiated into epithelioid cells and often also fused to form multinucleate giant cells. Granulomas form in the presence of an antigen or foreign substance which cannot be easily broken down or eliminated and they can be regarded as a mechanism for containing and possibly destroying that antigen or foreign body. Granuloma formation is frequently associated with increased deposition of fibrous tissue. This fibrosis is often the most troublesome

feature of granulomatous diseases. Granulomatous diseases can be both infective and non-infective (Fig. 13.3).

The most important **immunological pathway** leading to granuloma formation involves CD4+ T-cell-dependent activation of macrophages (type IV hypersensitivity). The presence of a suitable intracellular antigen, such as mycobacterial cell wall, induces the production of IL-12. This cytokine then stimulates the development of a TH1 T-cell response, with production of cytokines such as such as interferon (IFN)-γ. The process appears to be sustained and perpetuated by IFN-γ, IL-12 and other cytokines, in particular tumour necrosis factor (TNF)-α, produced by both T cells and macrophages themselves (Fig. 13.4). The key role of TNF-α in sustaining this process is shown by the effects of anti-TNF agents on granuloma formation. This is useful therapeutically in the treatment of Crohn's disease and sarcoidosis, but also contributes to the increased risk of tuberculosis following use of these treatments. Epithelioid cells also produce fibrogenic cytokines such as transforming growth factor (TGF)-β and can synthesize the active form of vitamin D from inactive precursors. Active vitamin D plays an important role in stimulating macrophage differentiation within the granuloma. In some granulomatous disorders, sufficient active vitamin D can be produced to cause hypercalcaemia.

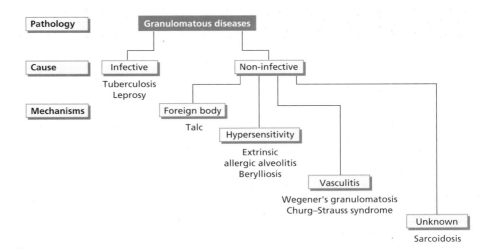

Fig. 13.3 A classification of granulomatous lung diseases.

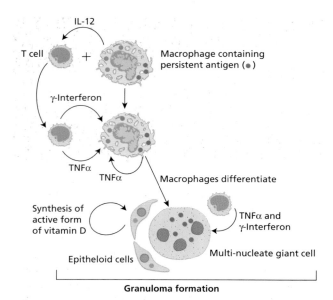

Fig. 13.4 Mechanisms of T-cell-dependent granuloma formation.

Granulomas also form in some diseases dominated by a TH2 pattern of cytokine production such as schistosomiasis and the Churg–Strauss syndrome, though the mechanism in these disorders is less clear.

13.3.2 Tuberculosis (Case 13.2)

The global impact of infection with Mycobacterium tuberculosis is enormous. *Around one-third of the world's population is infected with the tubercle bacillus and about 3 million people die every year from the consequences of this infection.* The greatest part of this burden of disease falls upon the developing world. Tuberculosis is a disease driven by poverty and poor nutrition. Immunosuppression associated with HIV infection has combined with these older risk factors to increase the incidence of tuberculosis across the developing nations (Table 13.3). The impact of tuberculosis in Western Europe and North America is minimal by comparison, and has fallen considerably over the last 50 years. However, even in the

Table 13.3 Risk factors for developing tuberculosis

1 Poverty and malnutrition
2 Close contact with patients with active infection
3 Immunosuppression (especially HIV infection and anti-tumour necrosis factor drugs)
4 Prolonged residence in countries with high prevalence of tuberculosis
5 Genetic predisposition

western world, the downward trend in cases of tuberculosis has stopped and in many places started to increase. This is due to a combination of HIV infection, increased mobility of populations across the world and worsening pockets of poverty even in the richest of nations. Other immunosuppressive factors should not be forgotten, particularly poor nutrition and the immunosuppressive effect of other infections such as measles. Vitamin D deficiency (due to diet or lack of exposure to sunlight) may be an important cofactor, reflecting the regulatory role of this vitamin within granulomas. Genetic factors may also play a significant role in determining the outcome of exposure to M. tuberculosis, and the intensity of exposure to the organism is also important: high levels of exposure may overwhelm even vigorous immune responses.

Mycobacterium tuberculosis is a slow-growing bacterium with an inert, waxy cell wall. It produces no toxins and causes disease only by its stimulation of the body's immune defence mechanisms coupled with an inexorable increase in numbers. The organism is rapidly taken up by macrophages upon entering the body. Most of those infected then develop a brisk TH1-pattern immune response leading to local granuloma formation in an area of lung and the draining lymph node. This contains and effectively eliminates the organism, although the immune system alone may never be able to clear M. tuberculosis completely and, once infection has occurred, the organism remains in a latent form even when disease does not develop. In a smaller proportion, the T-cell

CASE 13.2 PULMONARY TUBERCULOSIS

A 23-year-old man presented with a 4-week history of coughing, breathlessness and malaise. He had lost 4 kg in weight, but had no history of night sweats or haemoptysis. He had returned from holiday in Pakistan 2 months earlier. On examination, he was mildly pyrexial (37.8 °C) but had no evidence of anaemia or clubbing. Crepitations were audible over the lung apices; there were no other physical signs. His haemoglobin and white cell count were normal but the C-reactive protein (CRP) was 231 mg/l. The chest X-ray showed bilateral upper- and middle-lobe shadowing but no hilar enlargement. Sputum was found to contain acid-fast bacilli and Mycobacterium tuberculosis was subsequently cultured. A Mantoux test was strongly positive. A diagnosis of pulmonary tuberculosis was made. The patient was treated with isoniazid and rifampicin for 6 months, together with pyrazinamide for the first 2 months. He was allowed home on chemotherapy when his sputum became negative on direct smear. The chest X-ray is now much improved.

response is still brisk but less effective and the granulomatous response only partially contains the organism. An area of localized but progressive granulomatous inflammation develops which slowly enlarges and often cavitates due to a necrotic process called caseation, which is typical of tuberculous granulomas and which distorts surrounding structures by fibrosis. The immune response to M. tuberculosis may wax and wane over time: latent disease can reactivate and become clinically evident if the TH1 response becomes diminished by factors such as malnutrition, HIV infection or immunosuppressive drug treatment. Treatment with an anti-TNF agent such as infliximab may more specifically reduce resistance to reactivation.

If the T-cell response is defective, or skewed towards a TH2 pattern, then the organism reproduces freely in macrophages, and disseminated disease may develop. This is **miliary tuberculosis** (Fig. 13.5), where many organs are involved by small collections of macrophages packed with mycobacteria with only partial evidence of granuloma formation. This is associated with marked systemic ill-health, due to cytokine release from macrophages. Cytokine release is driven partly by the ineffective T-cell response and partly by the direct effect of the mycobacterial cell wall on macrophages.

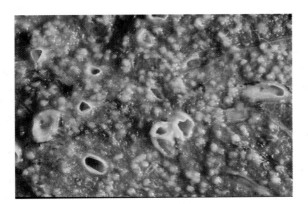

Fig. 13.5 Cut section of lung from a patient who died from miliary tuberculosis. Note the 2–5-mm nodules scattered through the lung tissue. 'Miliary' means 'resembling millet seeds'.

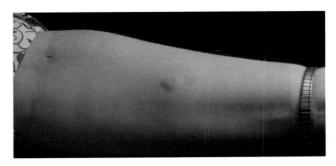

Fig. 13.6 Strongly positive Mantoux reaction 96 h after the intradermal injection of antigen from Mycobacterium tuberculosis.

Improvement in diet and living conditions, and more recently control of HIV infection, are the major public health measures which reduce the impact of tuberculosis. Prophylactic immunization with an attenuated form of mycobacterium, bacillus Calmette–Guérin (BCG), has a significant but less important role in controlling the disease. It is particularly valuable in protecting high-risk groups, such as hospital personnel and tuberculosis contacts. The presence of a T-cell response to M. tuberculosis can be established clinically by injecting mycobacterial antigen intradermally and assessing the delayed skin reaction at 48–72 h (the basis of the **Heaf and Mantoux tests**: Fig. 13.6). This is useful in assessing prior immunity before immunization, and may also be a helpful diagnostic pointer in active disease.

13.3.3 Sarcoidosis (Case 13.3)

Sarcoidosis is a multisystem, granulomatous disorder most commonly affecting young adults of either sex. It is uncommon after the age of 40.

Clinically, there are two types (Table 13.4): **acute** sarcoid and **insidious-onset** sarcoid. Bilateral hilar lymphadenopathy alone is asymptomatic and may be a chance finding on chest X-ray. Acute sarcoid presents as erythema nodosum with or without arthralgia; this form is particularly common in Scandinavia and common in the UK. Most patients, how-

---

CASE 13.3 SARCOIDOSIS

A 36-year-old man complained of breathlessness on exercise for 6 months. He also had mild chest tightness and stiff joints but no skin or eye problems. There was no family history of chest disease and he had never been abroad. He had been immunized with BCG as a schoolboy. On examination, he had no clubbing and no abnormal chest signs. Investigations showed a normal haemoglobin (143 g/l), white cell count (4.4×10^9/l) and differential (27% lymphocytes, 70% neutrophils), a mildly raised CRP (23 mg/l) and increased serum levels of angiotensin-converting enzyme (ACE). A serum biochemical profile, including serum calcium, was otherwise normal. A chest X-ray showed fine, diffuse radiological shadows, predominantly in the mid zones, and bilateral hilar lymphadenopathy. Lung function tests were normal and a Mantoux test was negative. A clinical diagnosis of sarcoidosis was made. Since he had pulmonary infiltration on X-ray, he was treated with corticosteroids to good effect.

Table 13.4 Systemic involvement in sarcoidosis (with incidence in each group of patients)

Acute sarcoidosis
Fever
Malaise
Arthralgia
Iritis
Erythema nodosum
Bilateral hilar nodes on chest X-ray (100%)
Radiological pulmonary infiltrates

Insidious sarcoidosis
Breathlessness due to alveolitis
Lymphadenopathy — common
Hepatic involvement — often subclinical (20–85%)
Hypercalciuria/hypercalcaemia (10–50%)
Anterior uveitis (10–35%)
Skin lesions — plaques/erythema nodosum (10%)
Pulmonary infiltrates on chest X-rays
    Late stages show fibrosis only
    Bilateral hilar nodes (uncommon)
Neurosarcoid

ever, have a more insidious disease; this form is about 10 times more prevalent in Afro-Caribbeans than in most other ethnic groups.

The **diagnosis** of sarcoidosis depends on the clinical and radiological picture and the histology of any lesions which can be biopsied. Historically, the Kveim test was used to establish a diagnosis of sarcoidosis. In this test, a small amount of Kveim antigen (derived from splenic tissue of patients with sarcoidosis) was injected intradermally and the site of injection biopsied 6 weeks later; typical granulomatous changes were found. The test is now seldom performed due to concerns regarding the safety of injecting human tissue into patients.

Tuberculosis is an important differential diagnosis of sarcoidosis. Curiously, the Mantoux or Heaf test is nearly always negative in active sarcoidosis, even in subjects known to have a previously positive test, and then becomes positive again as the sarcoidosis goes into remission or is treated. The immunological basis for this phenomenon is unknown.

Other laboratory tests are of little value in diagnosis or predicting disease evolution, although it is important to exclude hypercalcaemia due to uncontrolled vitamin D synthesis. Histologically, sarcoid granulomas are no different from granulomas in many other diseases. Epithelioid and giant cells are found focally, with little or no evidence of necrosis. Persistent lesions may become fibrotic and irreversible.

The **immunopathology** of sarcoidosis is consistent with a TH1-cell response to an unknown persistent antigen. There is often evidence of B-cell activation, with a polyclonal increase

in immunoglobulin production. Macrophage production of IL-12 and the expression of IL-12 receptors are increased in sarcoidosis, which seems likely to drive granuloma formation. Lung cells from patients with a better prognosis and self-limiting disease seem to produce higher amounts of the immunosuppressive cytokine TGF-β than those who progress. Sarcoidosis seems to occur on a variety of genetic backgrounds, with no clear HLA association yet identified. However, in subjects with sarcoid who possess HLA-DR3, there is evidence of very restricted usage of T-cell antigen receptors, consistent with response to a specific antigen. The nature of this antigen remains obscure. The similarities between sarcoid and tuberculosis have led to speculation that sarcoid is due to some form of mycobacterium, but no consistent evidence has been found to support this.

Inhalation of beryllium dust can produce lung disease (berylliosis), which is histologically identical to sarcoidosis. Berylliosis is strongly associated with the possession of a specific amino acid (glutamate) at position 69 in the β chain of HLA-DP. This amino acid lies within the antigen-binding groove and may affect binding of beryllium ions, possibly complexed with a self-peptide. There is no evidence that sarcoidosis is caused by beryllium exposure, but berylliosis does provide an instructive example of how a granulomatous disease can develop in response to a simple inert antigen, without invoking an infectious process.

The **prognosis** of sarcoidosis depends on whether or not granulomas or fibrosis develop in vital organs. Those who present with acute disease have an excellent prognosis after treatment and 90% recover within 3 months, although the chest X-ray changes may take a further 3 months to resolve. Insidious-onset sarcoid can proceed to generalized sarcoidosis; those who present with exertional dyspnoea or non-productive cough often have a better prognosis than asymptomatic cases, because they receive treatment. About 5% of patients with sarcoidosis die from their disease.

Treatment depends upon the severity of disease. Many patients improve spontaneously, but those with pulmonary infiltrates and evidence of granulomata in vital organs, such as the nervous system or lungs, should receive steroid therapy. Corticosteroids also correct the hypercalcaemia.

13.4 Interstitial lung disease

There are many causes of non-infectious inflammation of the airspaces and connective tissue of the lung, which can be classified under the general banner of interstitial lung disease (or parenchymal lung disease) (Table 13.5). Many of these disorders have a strong immunological contribution to their pathogenesis. Although this classification usually excludes specific infection, *infection can both mimic and complicate interstitial lung disease, and should be considered part of the differential diagnosis.*

Table 13.5 Major causes of interstitial lung disease and pulmonary fibrosis

Connective tissue diseases
Inorganic dusts
- Asbestos
- Silica

Hypersensitivity to known inhaled antigens
- Extrinsic allergic alveolitis
- Berylliosis

Drug hypersensitivity/toxicity
- Cytotoxic drugs (e.g. bleomycin)
- Paraquat poisoning
- Drugs associated with eosinophilic pneumonia (e.g. nitrofurantoin)
- Methotrexate

Pulmonary eosinophilia
Granulomatous diseases
- Sarcoidosis
- Tuberculosis

Idiopathic interstitial pneumonias

Almost all forms of interstitial lung disease can lead to **pulmonary fibrosis** (see Table 13.5), an end-stage of disease which is effectively irreversible and associated with severe disability and significant mortality. *Regardless of the initial cause, the pathogenesis of the fibrotic process may be similar in many disorders characterized by pulmonary fibrosis*: injury and/or stimulation of alveolar macrophages leads to production of cytokines such as TGF-β and chemotactic chemokines. Fibrogenic cytokines such as TGF-β induce fibroblasts both to proliferate and to synthesize large amounts of extracellular matrix proteins (such as collagens). Chemokines recruit bone-marrow-derived fibrocytes from the blood, which then produce large amounts of matrix proteins.

In some interstitial lung diseases, for example sarcoidosis, it is clear that the fibrotic process is driven by immunologically mediated chronic inflammation. Immunosuppressive and anti-inflammatory treatment is therefore effective in limiting progression of lung fibrosis. The assumption that chronic inflammation always precedes fibrosis led to widespread use of immunosuppressive treatment in some forms of pulmonary fibrosis, often with little or no clinical response. However, it is now clear that pulmonary fibrosis can develop and progress without any evidence of preceding chronic inflammation, which challenges current concepts of how immunological processes lead to tissue damage. This pattern of fibrosis may still be driven by immunological processes: similar patterns of fibrosis without inflammation may be seen in other diseases in which there is strong evidence for an autoimmune pathogenesis, especially systemic sclerosis. Potential strategies for therapeutically limiting fibrosis include inhibition of fibrogenic cytokines such as TGF-β or, if recruitment of circulating fibrocytes plays a dominant role in fibrosis, inhibition of chemokine action and cell recruitment. Until such strategies are available, severe established pulmonary fibrosis can be treated only by lung transplantation.

13.4.1 Pulmonary eosinophilia (Case 13.4)

The pulmonary eosinophilias are a group of disorders characterized by lung pathology (manifest as fleeting shadowing on the chest X-ray) and blood eosinophilia ($> 0.4 \times 10^9$/l). These can be further divided into bronchopulmonary and pneumonic types (Fig. 13.7). Bronchopulmonary eosinophilia is usually due to infection with Aspergillus fumigatus in asthmatic patients but the pneumonic type, which consists of pneumonia and a blood eosinophilia, has several causes.

Allergic bronchopulmonary aspergillosis (ABPA) typically occurs in chronic asthmatics, but is also increasingly recognized to complicate cystic fibrosis. Inhaled spores of A. fumigatus germinate and grow in the bronchi, behaving as an insoluble, particulate immunogenic stimulus which

CASE 13.4 ALLERGIC BRONCHOPULMONARY ASPERGILLOSIS

A 54-year-old woman presented with a 5-year history of a cough productive of mucopurulent sputum. On several occasions she had coughed up plugs of mucus. Courses of antibiotics had proved ineffectual. She had suffered from asthma for over 20 years and had a daughter with asthma. On examination, a few crepitations were audible in the left axillary region but the chest X-ray was apparently normal. She had a blood eosinophilia (1.05×10^9/l; normal $< 0.4 \times 10^9$/l). The total serum IgE was 325 IU/ml (normal < 125 IU/ml). Skin tests showed immediate (type I) hypersensitivity to cat fur, grass pollen and Aspergillus fumigatus. Her serum also contained strong precipitating antibodies ('precipitins') to this mould. At bronchoscopy, the left lingular bronchus was plugged with golden, tenacious mucus. This was aspirated and sent for culture; Aspergillus fumigatus was subsequently grown. Her allergic bronchopulmonary aspergillosis was treated with bronchial lavage and a 10-day course of oral corticosteroids. She has subsequently remained symptom-free on a low-dose steroid inhaler and the antifungal agent, Itraconazole, in the spore season (September–December).

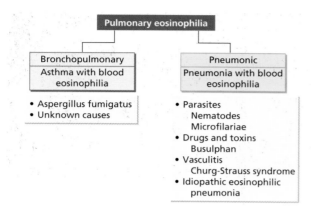

Fig. 13.7 Classification and causes of pulmonary eosinophilia.

triggers specific antibody production and TH2-dependent release of interleukins, especially IL-5: these recruit eosinophils into the airways and adjacent alveoli to cause eosinophilic consolidation. Attacks are characterized by paroxysms of coughing, with the production of large, well-formed casts. There may be areas of lung collapse and bronchiectasis due to plugging of a bronchus by casts. A typical cast contains inspissated mucus, often with fungal hyphae; the production of fungal casts is diagnostic. In their absence, however, skin testing with Aspergillus antigen shows immediate (type I) and late (type III) reactions in 90% of cases and precipitating antibodies to Aspergillus are detectable in the serum, as in Case 13.4.

The aim of **treatment** is to remove these plugs. If the plugs are not expectorated, bronchoscopy is required to remove them because residual casts result in bronchiectasis. Systemic steroids may be needed to suppress the immunopatho-

logical response to A. fumigatus; they cause rapid clearance of shadows and reduce the rate of recurrence. Antifungal therapy may speed recovery and reduce the risk of relapse.

Pneumonic eosinophilias, which are not associated with asthma, are of gradual onset and characterized by lassitude, night cough, shortness of breath and chest X-ray shadowing. With this insidious onset, many cases do not present until irreversible pulmonary fibrosis is established. There are several causes, but globally helminth infection is the most common cause (Fig. 13.7). A TH2 response against the parasitic worm drives the development of eosinophilia, with IL-5 playing a central role in eosinophil production. There are two major patterns of pneumonic eosinophilia associated with parasitic infection: first, an acute form, which occurs soon after infection as helminths migrate through the lung—this is known as **Loefler's syndrome**. Second, a more chronic syndrome known as **tropical pulmonary eosinophilia**. This occurs in filariasis, presents insidiously and may lead to pulmonary fibrosis. The serum IgE level is raised in those with parasitic eosinophilic pneumonia, and specific IgE against the infecting helminth may be present.

Acute and chronic **idiopathic eosinophilic pneumonia** may occur in the absence of any triggering infection or other external trigger. Treatment is with corticosteroids (Fig. 13.8).

In the rare **hyper-eosinophilic syndrome**, eosinophilic infiltration of tissues seems uncontrolled and occurs without evidence of preceding inflammation or allergy. Men aged 20–50 years are affected predominantly, and tissue damage is most obvious in the heart (producing a cardiomyopathy) and in the central nervous system. The eosinophil proliferation is usually polyclonal, although eosinophilic leukaemia can sometimes develop. In some cases, a clonal proliferation of TH2 cells may cause hyper-eosinophilia.

CASE 13.5 EXTRINSIC ALLERGIC ALVEOLITIS: FARMERS' LUNG

A 36-year-old farmer was admitted as an emergency with headache, fever, shortness of breath, a non-productive cough and myalgia. These symptoms came on suddenly. He had no features of upper respiratory tract infection, although he had had similar symptoms 3 weeks previously and had been treated with antibiotics. On examination, he had a tachycardia of 120/min, a temperature of 38 °C and bilateral widespread crepitations. His chest X-ray showed faint mottling in the middle and lower zones of both lung fields, but no hilar enlargement. He had a high white cell count (15 × 10⁹/l). A Mantoux test was negative. Lung function studies showed a restrictive defect.

His serum contained precipitating antibodies (see Chapter 19) to Micropolyspora faeni and Aspergillus fumigatus. The probable diagnosis was farmers' lung, a variety of extrinsic allergic alveolitis

caused by hypersensitivity to antigens found in mouldy hay. In retrospect, his earlier bronchial 'infection' was almost certainly a similar episode. His symptoms and X-ray changes gradually improved, although he continued to have exertional dyspnoea for 3 weeks. This man depended on his farm for his livelihood and was therefore reluctant to consider changing his job. He was strongly advised to dry his hay before storage or to let someone else handle the hay! Six weeks after discharge, he returned with acute symptoms after feeding hay to his cattle. He had had no immediate shortness of breath, but 5 h later had again experienced acute fever, malaise, shortness of breath, a cough and myalgia. This episode convinced him that there was a relationship between hay and his illness; his wife has fed the animals and handled the hay for the last 6 years and the patient (and his wife!) have remained well.

Fig. 13.8 High-resolution computed tomography scans of the lungs of a patient with chronic eosinophilic pneumonia. (a) Scan on the left shows patchy ground-glass shadowing indicating active disease. (b) Scan on the right taken 3 months later after corticosteroid treatment shows resolution of most of the changes.

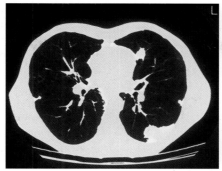

(a)

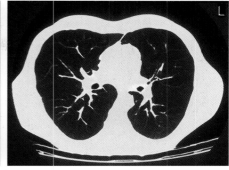

(b)

13.4.2 Extrinsic allergic alveolitis

Extrinsic allergic alveolitis (EAA) results from immune reactions in the alveoli to a variety of **inhaled organic materials** (Table 13.6). In the USA, the condition is known as 'hypersensitivity pneumonitis'. The clinical presentation may be acute, subacute or chronic. Patients exposed to high concentrations of the inhaled antigen usually present with acute disease (as in Case 13.5), whereas those who are chronically exposed to relatively small doses of antigen over a prolonged period are more likely to develop insidious disease (Case 13.6). In the UK, the commonest cause of EAA is budgerigar fanciers' lung; in the USA, humidifier lung.

Early **histological** lesions show a mononuclear cell infiltration in the alveoli. This often proceeds to granuloma formation with surrounding infiltration by macrophages, plasma cells and CD8⁺ T lymphocytes. EAA is therefore a differential diagnosis in any granulomatous or infiltrative condition of the lungs. In the subacute stage, obliterative bronchiolitis may also be present and permanent lung

Table 13.6 Common antigens involved in some varieties of extrinsic allergic alveolitis*

Antigen	Source	Disease
Microorganisms		
Micropolyspora faeni	Mouldy hay	Farmers' lung
Thermactinomyces candidus	Contaminated humidifiers	Humidifier lung
Thermactinomyces sacchari	Mouldy sugar cane	Bagassosis
Aspergillus clavatus	Mouldy barley	Malt workers' lung
Animal proteins		
Pigeon serum proteins	Pigeon droppings	Pigeon-breeders' disease
Budgerigar or parrot serum proteins	Budgerigar or parrot droppings	Bird fanciers' lung
Chicken proteins	Chicken droppings and urine	Feather pluckers' disease
Rat serum proteins	Rat urine	Rodent handlers' lung

*This list is not intended to be exhaustive: there are many other examples.

CASE 13.6 EXTRINSIC ALLERGIC ALVEOLITIS: BIRD FANCIERS' LUNG

A 41-year-old woman presented with gradual weight loss, lethargy and breathlessness on exertion of 4 months' duration, with intermittent mild wheezing and a cough. She was a non-smoker who bred budgerigars as a hobby. On examination, there were scattered crepitations throughout both lung fields but finger clubbing was absent. On investigation, she had a normal haemoglobin, white cell count and CRP. A chest X-ray showed a diffuse, generalized haziness in both lower zones but pulmonary function tests were normal. A Mantoux test was negative. Precipitating antibodies to budgerigar antigens were present in her serum.

A laboratory diagnosis of extrinsic allergic alveolitis due to hypersensitivity to budgerigar serum proteins (bird fanciers' lung) was made. The patient gave away her birds, and her symptoms regressed over a few months. Eight years later, her serum still contains antibodies to budgerigar serum proteins but she is asymptomatic — and birdless.

damage due to interstitial fibrosis may occur after repeated exposure. The precise **pathogenesis** is unclear, but immunofluorescent studies of lung biopsies during the early stages have shown deposits of antigen, IgG, IgM, IgA and C3 in the lesions, consistent with an immune-complex-mediated (type III) mechanism. Activated T cells (both CD4 and CD8) are also present and it seems likely that type IV hypersensitivity is also involved, particularly in cases with granuloma formation and fibrosis.

The clinical features of **acute EAA** often resemble infection and this possibility should be considered in all patients who present with an 'acute atypical pneumonia'. Systemic symptoms are typical and occur about 6 h or more after exposure to the dust. The attacks can subside rapidly but recur on further exposure. In many cases, the causal agent may not be appreciated. It is only by careful charting of the relationship between jobs and symptoms that work-related hypersensitivities are suspected. **Chronic EAA** is more common and often presents with gradual exertional dyspnoea and a dry cough, accompanied by anorexia, weight loss and malaise.

It is seen most commonly with low but near-continuous exposure, for instance where a single caged bird is responsible. Interstitial diffuse pulmonary fibrosis may have already developed in these patients at the time of presentation.

13.4.3 Idiopathic interstitial pneumonias (Case 13.7)

The **idiopathic interstitial pneumonias (IIPs)** are a group of disorders characterized by varying degrees of inflammation and fibrosis of the lung parenchyma. They are diagnoses of exclusion, made only when extrinsic allergic alveolitis and other causes of pulmonary fibrosis (see Table 13.5) have been ruled out. The IIPs are often considered as autoimmune disorders, although the evidence for autoimmunity is largely circumstantial, based upon the occurrence of most patterns of interstitial pneumonia in the connective tissue disorders (Table 13.7). There are several distinct patterns of IIP (Table 13.8). All present with a similar clinical picture of progressive exertional breathlessness and dry cough, with the commonest age of onset being 40–50 years. Examina-

CASE 13.7 IDIOPATHIC PULMONARY FIBROSIS

A 57-year-old man complained of malaise, anorexia and increasing exertional breathlessness for 4 months. When pressed, he admitted that the dyspnoea had been present for 2 years but he had attributed this to smoking 30 cigarettes a day. He had been treated for two episodes of 'bronchitis' in the preceding winter. On examination, he had finger clubbing and widespread crepitations in his chest but no arthropathy, cyanosis or skin lesions. Investigations showed a normal haemoglobin and white cell count but a raised ESR (80 mm/h).

All serum immunoglobulin levels were raised; IgG was 24 g/l (NR 6.8–19.0), IgA 9.7 g/l (NR 0.8–5.0) and IgM 12.0 g/l (NR 0.5–2.0). No paraprotein was detected. His serum contained antinuclear antibodies (titre 1/160) and rheumatoid factor (titre 1/64). A chest X-ray showed diffuse fine shadowing throughout both lung fields, especially in the lower zones, consistent with diffuse pulmonary fibrosis. A high-resolution computed tomography (HRCT) scan showed extensive established fibrosis with no evidence of ground-glass shadowing (see Fig. 13.9). This was supported by results of lung function tests. A video-assisted thorascopic lung biopsy showed extensive non-uniform fibrosis and minimal inflammation: characteristic appearances of usual interstitial pneumonia. Since no other cause was found, a diagnosis of idiopathic pulmonary fibrosis was made. The histology, CT findings and the rapid clinical progression suggested a poor prognosis. A trial of oral corticosteroids, cyclosporin and azathioprine had no beneficial effect. He was referred for lung transplantation but died from respiratory failure before a suitable organ became available.

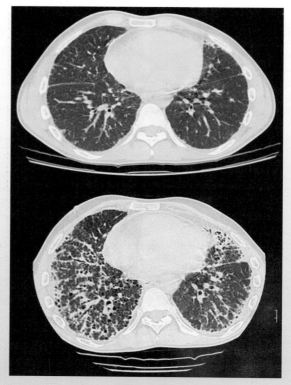

Fig. 13.9 High-resolution computed tomography scan showing (top) established fibrosis at diagnosis with relentless progression over 1 year despite aggressive immunosuppressive therapy (bottom).

Table 13.7 Evidence that the idiopathic interstitial pneumonias (IIPs) may be immunological disorders

Association with autoimmune diseases
All forms of IIP occur in connective tissue diseases, rheumatoid arthritis and systemic sclerosis
Circulating autoantibodies
50% of patients have:
  Antinuclear antibodies (but no significant dsDNA binding)
  Rheumatoid factor (often low titre)
Bronchoalveolar fluid may contain
↑ Lymphocytes (up to 15%)
↑ Macrophages—often 'activated' and containing ingested immune complexes
Histology
Lymphocytic infiltration involving CD4$^+$ > CD8$^+$ T cells
Expression of MHC class II antigens on alveolar epithelial cells
Immunoglobulin and complement deposition in early stages only

tion reveals widespread inspiratory fine crackles, and clubbing is often present. The various forms of IIP are defined histologically, and biopsy (usually thorascopic) is the best way to make a definitive diagnosis. Making a correct diagnosis is critical, since the response to therapy and prognosis varies enormously. The various types of IIP can also be distinguished on HRCT scanning, although this is less reliable than histology. One of the most important prognostic features on HRCT is **'ground glass' shadowing**, the presence of which may predict a response to corticosteroids.

The **aetiology** of the IIPs is unclear. Genetic factors do not appear to make a major contribution. The risk of IIP is increased two- to five-fold by exposure to environmental factors which may injure the lung, such as smoking and occupational exposure to wood, stone and metal dusts, and there is some evidence that infection (for example, Epstein–Barr virus) may act as a trigger. Two rarer forms of IIP, desquamative interstitial pneumonia and respiratory bronchiolitis with interstitial lung disease, occur almost exclusively in smokers, and improve with smoking cessation.

Idiopathic pulmonary fibrosis (IPF), sometimes called cryptogenic fibrosing alveolitis in the UK, is the most common and serious of the IIPs, with a prevalence in the UK of around 1 in 5000 adults. The presentation is usually with insidiously progressive breathlessness. The mean survival following diagnosis is very poor at 3-5 years.

HRCT usually shows patchy, peripheral basal fibrosis with no ground glass shadowing. **Histology** shows damaged alveoli and patchy fibrosis, becoming more extensive and developing a 'honeycomb' appearance as the disease progresses. This appearance is known as Usual Interstitial Pneumonia, which is also sometimes used as a diagnostic label instead of IPF.

There is some evidence that immunological processes underlie the pathogenesis of IPF: activated T cells with a TH2 phenotype can be found in affected tissue and, even in the absence of an associated connective tissue disease, there is an association with autoantibody production. However, IPF exemplifies the pattern of fibrosis outlined above, whereby extracellular matrix is laid down with no evidence of preceding inflammation. It is not clear how an immunological mechanism might drive this process.

Table 13.8 Epidemiology, histology, treatment and outcome in the idiopathic interstitial pneumonias

	Relative frequency, %	Histology	Response to immunosuppression	Outcome
Idiopathic pulmonary fibrosis	55	Fibrosis	Minimal	50–70% mortality at 5 years
Non-specific interstitial pneumonia	25	Cellular infiltrate with some fibrosis	Reasonable (better if less fibrosis on biopsy)	Reasonable. 10% mortality at 5 years
Smoking-associated interstitial pneumonia	15	Mainly cellular infiltrate, little fibrosis	Usually good (key intervention is smoking cessation)	Good with treatment
Cryptogenic organizing pneumonia	3	Mainly cellular infiltrate, little fibrosis	Good	Good with treatment
Lymphocytic organizing pneumonia	< 1	Mainly cellular infiltrate, little fibrosis	Good	Good with treatment
Acute interstitial pneumonia	< 1	Fibrosis	Poor	> 50% mortality. Survivors may recover completely

Given the lack of inflammation, it is perhaps not surprising that IPF should show little or no response to conventional immunosuppression. Nevertheless, given the bleak prognosis, patients with IPF are often subjected to a period of intense immunosuppression with high-dose corticosteroids and a drug such as azathioprine. If a good response occurs, this may indicate that the diagnosis of IPF is wrong and the patient has a more treatable disorder such as non-specific interstitial pneumonia. Some attempts at anti-fibrotic treatment have been made: the cytokine IFN-γ suppresses synthesis of collagen and other matrix proteins, and also inhibits TH2 cytokine production. Early trials of IFN-γ in IPF appeared to show a significant clinical response, but a larger randomized trial showed no convincing evidence of any benefit. Single-lung transplantation is now an effective treatment in selected patients with relentlessly progressive disease. Patients receiving a transplant are 75% less likely to die than equivalent patients on the transplant waiting list. The disease does not recur in the transplanted lung.

Non-specific interstitial pneumonia (NSIP) accounts for around a quarter of patients with IIP and is a more benign, treatment-responsive disorder than IPF (Table 13.8). This responsiveness to immunosuppressive drugs correlates with significant inflammatory changes on biopsy, and the presence of ground glass shadowing on HRCT. Although the overall prognosis of NSIP is much better than that of IPF, there is considerable heterogeneity in outcome: histologically, more fibrosis and less inflammation signifies a poorer prognosis. NSIP is the pattern of IIP most strongly associated with connective tissue disease.

13.5 Pulmonary vasculitis

The lungs are a major site of involvement in systemic vasculitis, reflecting the highly vascular nature of the pulmonary bed. Pulmonary vasculitic syndromes often produce alveolar inflammation (particularly when the vasculitis involves small blood vessels at the alveolar level) and can cause pulmonary fibrosis.

The most devastating form of pulmonary vasculitis involves small vessels at the alveolar level and presents with diffuse and often overwhelming **pulmonary haemorrhage**. This life-threatening emergency occurs particularly in **Goodpasture's syndrome**, **microscopic polyarteritis** and occasionally in **systemic lupus erythematosus (SLE)**. Pulmonary haemorrhage usually occurs in parallel with rapidly progressive glomerulonephritis (reflecting small-vessel involvement in the kidney). These disorders are discussed in more detail in Chapter 9. In the granulomatous vasculitides, Wegener's granulomatosis and the Churg–Strauss syndrome, the respiratory tract is a major target organ; these disorders are discussed below.

13.5.1 Wegener's granulomatosis

The characteristic feature of this condition is a **necrotizing granulomatous vasculitis**. It is one of many forms of vasculitis involving the lung.

Although most patients have pulmonary involvement, this can be asymptomatic; multiple nodules are sometimes seen on a chest X-ray taken for other reasons. The clinical features can be divided into those caused by local granuloma formation (such as the changes in the lungs, the paranasal sinuses and the nasopharynx) and those due to vasculitis in other organs (namely glomerulonephritis, keratoconjunctivitis, polyarthralgia and cutaneous vasculitis) (Fig. 13.10).

The **diagnosis** depends on the clinical features and histopathological identification of the typical necrotizing vasculitis and granuloma. Nasal mucosa is easily biopsied, but occasionally open lung biopsy is required. A renal biopsy should be performed if there is evidence of kidney involvement. Antibodies directed against a neutrophil cytoplasmic antigen (cANCA: see Chapter 19) are found in over 90% of patients with active Wegener's granulomatosis and in about 40% of patients in remission. cANCA in Wegener's usually have specificity for a cytoplasmic enzyme called proteinase 3 (PR3). The finding of ANCA in sputum and BAL fluid suggests that these antibodies are produced in the respiratory

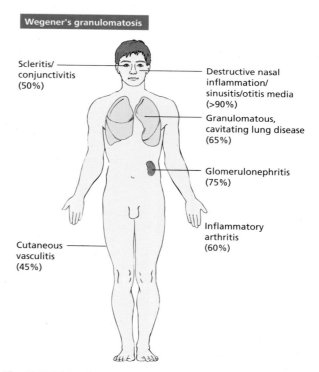

Fig. 13.10 Major clinical features of Wegener's granulomatosis.

tract of such patients. ANCA antibodies and raised CRP levels are helpful in diagnosis and assessment of disease activity.

Untreated Wegener's granulomatosis is rapidly fatal, with a mean survival of 5 months and a 5-year survival of < 10%. *The treatment of choice is prednisolone plus cyclophosphamide.* The remission rate with careful treatment is approximately 90%, and about 50% of patients sustain this remission for over 5 years.

The **Churg–Strauss syndrome (CSS)**, or allergic granulomatosis, refers to a related but rare multisystem disorder in young adults with a diagnostic triad of asthma and systemic vasculitis associated with marked peripheral eosinophilia. ANCA reactivity is found less frequently and is of less diagnostic value. Without treatment, the mortality of CSS may be as high as 50% within 3 months of diagnosis. Fortunately, the condition usually responds well to corticosteroid therapy. Cyclophosphamide may further improve the outcome In severe cases.

13.6 Connective tissue disease and the lung

Connective tissue diseases frequently involve all parts of the respiratory system: pleura, airways, lung parenchyma and pulmonary vessels (Table 13.9). Although lung disease causes symptoms in a significant minority of these patients, subclinical pleural disease and/or mild pulmonary fibrosis are present in more than 50% of patients with rheumatoid arthritis (RA). Although NSIP and IPF are the two most common patterns of interstitial lung disease in connective tissue disorders, all forms of IIP can occur. The response to treatment and prognosis mirrors, in general, that seen in IIP occurring in isolation. 'Isolated' pulmonary hypertension (that is, not secondary to interstitial lung disease or pulmonary thromboembolism) occurs particularly in limited systemic sclerosis (see Chapter 11). Lung disease secondary to treatment of connective tissue disease is also common. Infection may complicate all forms of immunosuppressive treatment, with the pattern of infection reflecting the nature of the immunosuppressive drug: for example, bacterial, viral and Pneumocystis infection with the T- and B-cell-suppressing drug cyclophosphamide, tuberculosis with anti-TNF agents. *Methotrexate, the most commonly used drug for the treatment of RA, can cause interstitial lung disease, usually with a picture resembling NSIP.*

13.7 Cardiac disease

Immunological disease processes involving the heart and great vessels can be classified according to either their cause or the anatomical structures involved (Table 13.10 and Fig. 13.11). Some disorders selectively involve one tissue within the heart, whereas others can involve all structures, i.e. **pancarditis** (e.g. in rheumatic fever or SLE).

13.7.1 Pericarditis

Inflammation of the pericardium presents primarily with pain but sometimes with the haemodynamic consequences of a pericardial effusion or pericardial fibrosis. The pericardium is structurally very similar to the pleura and these two tissues are often involved by the same disease processes (e.g. in RA and SLE). Chronic inflammation of the pericardium can be asymptomatic: over 40% of patients with RA have evidence of pericardial disease at post-mortem, but symptomatic pericarditis occurs in less than 10% during life.

13.7.2 Myocarditis

Myocardial inflammation presents primarily with heart failure or disruption of the cardiac rhythm due to damage to the conducting system. Worldwide, the most important immunological disease process affecting the myocardium is **Chagas' disease**, caused by Trypanosoma cruzi.

Although autoimmune mechanisms lead to myocardial involvement in rheumatic fever, bacterial infection hardly ever causes myocardial disease directly, with the notable exception of the carditis associated with **Lyme disease**, due to

Table 13.9 Patterns of lung disease in the major connective tissue diseases

	Rheumatoid arthritis	SLE	Myositis	Systemic sclerosis
Pleural disease	Common	Common	No	Rare
Interstitial lung disease	Yes—NSIP and IPF pattern	Rare	Yes—NSIP and IPF pattern	Yes—usually IPF pattern
Isolated pulmonary hypertension	No	No	No	Yes
Intrapulmonary nodules	Common	No	No	No
Respiratory muscle weakness	No	Yes—usually diaphragm	Yes	No
Vasculitis/pulmonary haemorrhage	No	Yes but rare	No	No

NSIP, Non-specific interstitial pneumonia; IPF, idiopathic pulmonary fibrosis.

Table 13.10 Classification of immunological cardiac disease according to cause

Infection	Autoimmune	Alloimmune	Infiltrative
Direct result of infection	*Local*	*Acute*	Sarcoidosis
Chagas' disease	Postmyocardial injury	Acute rejection	Amyloid
Lyme disease	?Atherosclerosis		
Viral carditis	?Cardiomyopathies	*Chronic*	
		Chronic vascular rejection	
Hypersensitivity to	*Systemic*		
infectious agent	SLE		
Rheumatic fever	RA		
Chagas' disease	Scleroderma		
Viral carditis			

SLE, Systemic lupus erythematosus; RA, rheumatoid arthritis.

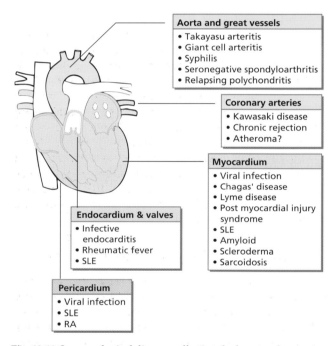

Aorta and great vessels
• Takayasu arteritis
• Giant cell arteritis
• Syphilis
• Seronegative spondyloarthritis
• Relapsing polychondritis

Coronary arteries
• Kawasaki disease
• Chronic rejection
• Atheroma?

Myocardium
• Viral infection
• Chagas' disease
• Lyme disease
• Post myocardial injury
  syndrome
• SLE
• Amyloid
• Scleroderma
• Sarcoidosis

Endocardium & valves
• Infective
  endocarditis
• Rheumatic fever
• SLE

Pericardium
• Viral infection
• SLE
• RA

Fig. 13.11 Immunological diseases affecting the heart and great vessels.

direct invasion of the myocardium by the spirochaete, Borrelia burgdorferi. Recognition of this condition is important, as there is an excellent response to antibiotics.

Viral infection may also cause myocarditis, particularly viruses that have a tropism for muscle such as the Coxsackie family. This is usually transient. The involvement of viruses in the most common form of chronic myocardial disease, dilated cardiomyopathy, is less certain. Plausible hypotheses and animal models have been developed implicating viral infection in triggering a chronic T-cell-mediated autoimmune process directed against myocardial antigens.

However, evidence that this mechanism plays a role in most patients with dilated cardiomyopathy is lacking.

Autoimmune processes have a more clearly defined role in the postmyocardial injury syndromes (e.g. Dressler's syndrome), which occur 1–2 weeks after cardiac surgery or myocardial infarction. An autoimmune response occurs to sequestered cardiac antigens released as a result of cardiac damage (analogous to the development of sympathetic ophthalmia after eye injuries, Chapter 12).

13.7.3 Endocarditis

Endocardial inflammation presents principally with cardiac valve dysfunction: usually valvular incompetence, but sometimes stenosis or embolism from the damaged valve. The most significant long-term consequence of **rheumatic fever** (see Chapter 2) is valve damage due to endocardial involvement. The likelihood of endocardial inflammation is greatly increased by factors that lead to endothelial damage within the heart, in particular turbulent flow around a structurally abnormal heart valve, damaged by previous rheumatic endocarditis. This endothelial damage allows antigen (including bacteria) and antibody to gain access from the circulation.

Colonization of heart valves by bacteria leads to **infective endocarditis**. This can be a devastating acute infection leading to rapid valve destruction (usually associated with infection with Staphylococcus aureus), but more often occurs in a subacute form where an antibody response against organisms of low virulence leads to a multisystem immune complex disease associated with glomerulonephritis, vasculitis and complement consumption.

13.8 Coronary artery disease (Case 13.8)

Vasculitis of the coronary arteries can occur as a rare feature of many forms of systemic vasculitis affecting medi-

CASE 13.8 KAWASAKI'S DISEASE

A 2-year-old girl became unwell and feverish. She was seen by her GP who felt she had a chest infection and prescribed a broad-spectrum antibiotic. She remained persistently unwell over the next 2 days and was admitted to hospital. On admission she was febrile (38.2 °C), looked ill and had enlarged lymph nodes in her neck and a blotchy red rash on her limbs. Her chest was clear and ear drums normal. Systemic infection was suspected. Investigations showed a raised white cell count (24×10^9/l, 90% neutrophils), a platelet count of 600×10^9/l and a CRP of 143 mg/l; however, a chest X-ray was clear, urine and cerebrospinal fluid (CSF) contained no cells on microscopy and subsequent blood, urine and CSF cultures were sterile. She remained unwell over the next 4 days and over this time developed marked swelling and redness of the hands and feet. Kawasaki's disease was suspected and this diagnosis was confirmed by an echocardiogram which demonstrated aneurysms of the right and left anterior descending coronary arteries. She was treated with high-dose (2 g/kg) intravenous immunoglobulin (IVIG) and oral aspirin and her fever subsided over the next 48 h. Over the next 2 weeks she developed striking peeling of the skin over the hands and feet. A repeat echocardiogram showed that the coronary arteries had improved but localized dilation was still apparent. The best results of IVIG treatment are seen when given early in the course of disease, before aneurysms have developed. She remains under long-term cardiological follow-up.

um-sized or large arteries (e.g. polyarteritis nodosa, giant cell arteritis) but occurs most notably as the most serious clinical feature of **Kawasaki's disease**. The cause of Kawasaki's disease is unknown, but there is some evidence that bacterial superantigens play a pathogenic role. Prompt treatment with aspirin and intravenous immunoglobulin abates the systemic symptoms but, more importantly, reduces morbidity and mortality from the coronary artery disease.

A very different pattern of immunologically mediated coronary artery disease occurs in the recipients of heart transplants. Progressive intimal fibrosis occurs which can occlude the coronary arteries. This process of **chronic rejection** is more likely to occur if there is substantial HLA mismatch between donor and recipient and if episodes of acute rejection have occurred. There is some evidence that CMV infection may act as a cofactor in this process. A comparable process occurs in vessels in transplanted kidneys, and there are also similarities with chronic graft-versus-host disease and scleroderma. In all these disorders immunological mechanisms appear to lead to fibrosis without significant evidence of inflammation. The underlying mechanisms are unknown.

The most common cause of coronary artery disease is **atherosclerosis**. The pathogenesis of atherosclerosis involves inflammatory mechanisms as well as lipid accumulation and thrombosis. It has been hypothesized that immunological processes might play a role in progression of the vascular changes, perhaps involving an immune response against sequestered bacterial or viral antigens in the vessel wall or an autoimmune response against lipoproteins damaged by free radicals. No strong evidence exists to support these hypotheses at present.

Although the evidence that atherosclerosis itself is an autoimmune disease is limited, there is clear evidence that *some chronic immunological diseases increase the risk of developing atherosclerosis and its consequences.* In patients with SLE, the risk of myocardial infarction may be increased as much as 50 times above that of age- and sex-matched controls. This increase in risk is not wholly attributable to conventional risk factors such as hypertension and serum cholesterol, or treatments such as corticosteroids. The risk seems to be higher with increased activity and severity of the underlying disease. The mechanisms are unknown, but plausible hypotheses argue that the increased production of cytokines in these disorders up-regulate adhesion molecules and procoagulant factors on endothelial cells, which facilitates the process of atherogenesis.

13.9 Diseases of the great vessels (Case 13.9)

Inflammation of the aortic wall or **aortitis** can occur as a feature of a number of disorders (see Fig. 13.11). Most of these disorders affect principally the proximal aorta with a variable amount of distal disease. The consequences of aortitis are twofold: first, aortic dilation and even aneurysm formation may occur, leading to stretching and incompetence of the aortic valve, and more rarely aortic rupture or dissection. Second, stenotic lesions may develop in the branches of the aorta, either at their junction with the aorta or more diffusely along the length of the branching vessels.

Takayasu's disease is a granulomatous vasculitis of the aorta and its branches, usually occurring under the age of 40 and more commonly in women. It presents with the consequences of occlusion or stenosis of the aortic branches: neurological symptoms, vascular insufficiency in the arms, hypertension due to renal artery stenosis and features of systemic illness including fever, malaise, weight loss, arthralgia and myalgia. Blood tests are of no specific help in making the diagnosis, which is often delayed. Aortography and mag-

CASE 13.9 TAKAYASU'S ARTERITIS

A 23-year-old typist was referred to a rheumatologist with a 3-month history of cramp-like discomfort, which occurred reproducibly with any task involving the left arm. She was otherwise well, smoked five cigarettes per day and her only medication was a combined oral contraceptive. Examination revealed no abnormality in the neck or arm. A provisional diagnosis of tendonitis was made and she was treated with physiotherapy without benefit. Her ESR was found to be mildly elevated at 30 mm/h (normal < 10) but no cause was identified for this.

Two months later she was admitted to hospital following an episode of right-sided weakness associated with speech disturbance. She had a very mild right hemiparesis (which resolved over the next 6 h), a left-sided carotid bruit and a mild fever (37.7 °C). Her blood pressure was 165/90, taken from the right arm. Investigations included a CRP of 31 mg/l, normal creatinine, cholesterol 4.8 mmol/l

(normal < 5.7), negative ANA, ANCA, cardiolipin antibodies, lupus anticoagulant and normal immunoglobulins. An ECG and echocardiogram were also normal. Three days after admission she asked why the nurses had such great difficulty measuring her blood pressure in the left arm, and used the right instead. Further assessment revealed that the radial and brachial pulses were almost impalpable on the left. Doppler ultrasound studies indicated an arterial systolic pressure of 80 mmHg in the left arm. An aortogram showed long, tapering tight stenoses of the left common carotid and subclavian arteries, with less severe lesions in the left renal artery. A diagnosis of Takayasu's arteritis was made and she was treated with high-dose corticosteroids. Her ESR returned to normal and subsequent ultrasound studies showed partial resolution of the carotid and subclavian stenoses.

netic resonance imaging can be used to confirm the diagnosis. The response to steroids is often reasonable, but surgery or angioplasty may be required where structural changes do not respond to immunosuppression.

FURTHER READING

See website: www.immunologyclinic.com

14 Gastrointestinal and Liver Diseases

14.1 Introduction

14.1.1 Normal immune mechanisms

The gastrointestinal tract is the largest immunological organ in the body. Over 90% of the exposure of the human body to microorganisms occurs at the mucosal surface of the gastrointestinal tract and over 400 bacterial species inhabit the average human gut. The gut is protected by several **non-specific mechanisms** (Fig. 14.1). Epithelial cells form an important physical barrier via their intercellular tight junctions and turn over rapidly (every 24–96 h). Any injury to the epithelial barrier results in rapid migration of adjacent viable epithelial cells to cover the denuded area, a process called 'restitution', while lymphocytes and macrophages migrate out through pores in the basement membrane to provide temporary host protection. The acid pH of the stomach is a formidable chemical barrier to many organisms and bacterial overgrowth is a consequent complication in patients with achlorhydria due to atrophic gastritis. Any change in the normal microflora of the intestine also allows pathogenic bacteria to flourish: an example is pseudomembranous colitis caused by the toxin-producing bacterium Clostridium difficile in patients given certain antibiotics.

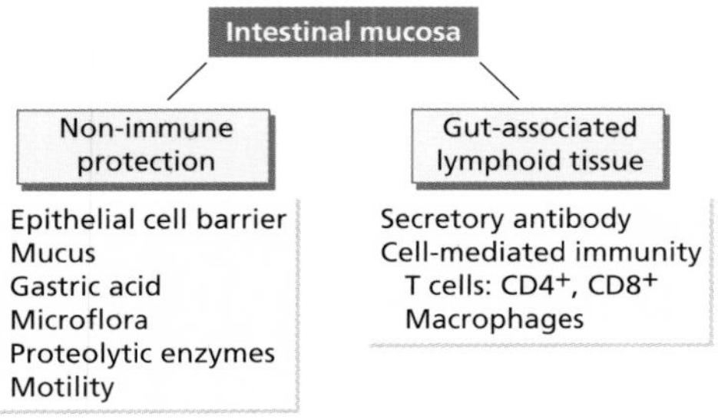

Mucosal immune responses involve the gut-associated lymphoid tissue (GALT). Lymphocytes are found at three sites within the mucosa (Fig. 14.2 and Box 14.1).

GALT is divided into two functional compartments: an afferent arm — Peyer's patches — where interaction occurs between luminal antigen and the immune system; and an effector arm — the diffusely distributed intra-epithelial and lamina propria lymphocytes.

Peyer's patches are covered by specialized epithelium (follicle-associated epithelium). Some of these epithelial cells have surfaces which seem folded under the scanning electron microscope (Fig. 14.3). These microfold, or M, cells sample and actively transport particulate antigens from the lumen into the 'dome' area, where priming of both T and B lymphocytes occurs. Within Peyer's patches are specialized

Fig. 14.1 Protection of the intestinal mucosa.

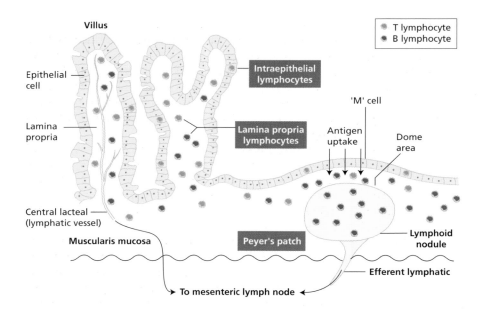

Fig. 14.2 Organization and structure of gut-associated lymphoid tissue (GALT).

BOX 14.1 SITES OF LYMPHOCYTES IN THE GUT

- Organized lymphoid aggregates (Peyer's patches) beneath the epithelium of the terminal small intestine
- Lymphocytes within the epithelial cell layer (intra-epithelial lymphocytes)
- Lymphocytes scattered, with other immunocompetent cells, within the lamina propria

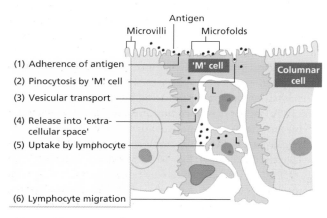

Fig. 14.3 The stages involved in the transport of antigen by the M cell from the intestinal lumen into the extracellular space where it is taken up by dendritic cells and T lymphocytes (L).

T cells that induce immature IgM-bearing B lymphocytes to switch isotype to IgA.

Primed B lymphoblasts, committed mainly to producing IgA class antibody, migrate from Peyer's patches, via the lymphatics and mesenteric lymph nodes, to the thoracic duct and hence into the circulation (Fig. 14.2). These cells return preferentially to the lamina propria, a process called 'homing'. Once back in the gut, they mature into IgA plasma cells and are responsible for local and secretory immune defences. The number of IgA-producing cells in the lamina propria far exceeds the numbers producing IgM, IgG or IgE.

The IgA coating the epithelium is specially adapted for its function. IgA plasma cells produce monomeric IgA, which is converted into a dimer by a smaller 'joining' peptide (J chain), also produced by the plasma cells. The polymeric immunoglobulin receptor is synthesized by epithelial cells and is essential for transport of **secretory IgA** into the lumen of the gut (Fig. 14.4). The receptor binds the dimeric IgA, the complex is endocytosed and transported through the cytoplasm to the luminal surface of the cell where proteolysis of

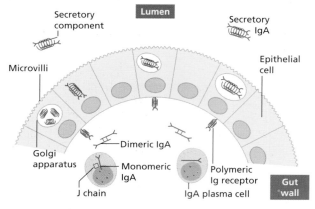

Fig. 14.4 Synthesis and transport of secretory IgA through the gut epithelial cells into the gut lumen.

the polymeric Ig receptor occurs. As a result, the IgA dimer is released into the gut attached to a 70-kDa proteolytic fragment of the receptor, now called secretory component. Secretory component stabilizes the secretory IgA molecule and protects it from proteolytic attack by enzymes in the gut.

Secretory IgA neutralizes viruses, bacteria and toxins, prevents the adherence of pathogenic microorganisms to gut epithelium and so blocks the uptake of antigen into the systemic immune system — a role termed 'immune exclusion'.

There is a similar **migration pathway for T lymphocytes** whereby T blasts from mesenteric nodes 'home' both to the epithelium and to the lamina propria. **Intraepithelial lymphocytes (IEL)** express both non-rearranged innate immune receptors and rearranged adaptive immune receptors and have been conserved throughout vertebrate evolution. Peripheral blood T cells rarely express the human mucosal lymphocyte antigen 1 (HML-1) but nearly all IEL do (Fig. 14.5). HML-1 (CD103) is an adhesion molecule of the β_7-integrin family. It is important in the homing of IEL, allowing IEL to bind via HML-1 to its ligand, E-cadherin, expressed on epithelial cells. IELs are not a homogeneous population: they comprise at least three different T-cell phenotypes. The major population is CD8$^+$ and shows increased expression of the γ/δ form of the T-cell receptor compared with peripheral blood lymphocytes. Another population expresses the α/β form of the T-cell receptor, while the third subset expresses both CD4 and CD8 and is not found elsewhere in lymphoid organs. In experimental models, some IELs are cytotoxic and some have natural killer cell activity, functions important in the control of enterovirus infection. IELs also seem to have a role in controlling epithelial cell barrier function, i.e. 'restitution'. However, the functions of IEL in humans are unknown.

Large numbers of lymphocytes, natural killer cells, mast cells, macrophages and plasma cells are seen in the **lamina propria**. T and B lymphocytes are both found, but T cells predominate in a ratio of about four to one. These T cells do not proliferate well after stimulation of the T-cell receptor, yet

produce large amounts of the cytokines interleukin (IL)-2, IL-4, interferon (IFN)-γ and tumour necrosis factor (TNF)-α. Such lymphocytes express at least two molecules essential for homing to the gut: $\alpha_4\beta_7$ integrin and the chemokine receptor CCR9. MAdCAM-1 (see section 1.2.5), the ligand for $\alpha_4\beta_7$, is expressed widely in gut mucosal vessels and is the predominant adhesion molecule in the intestinal lamina propria.

Many similarities exist between the mucosal lymphoid tissues of the gut and organs such as the bronchus, breasts, salivary glands and uterine cervix. Lymphoblasts from any of these sites will repopulate all mucosa-associated lymphoid tissue in irradiated animals, with a slight selective preference for the organ of origin. If antigen is fed to lactating females, specific IgA antibodies appear in the milk, and gut-derived lymphoblasts home to breast tissue, lungs and parotid glands as well as back to the gut. There is evidence, therefore, of a **common mucosal immune system**. This has at least one important implication: it may eventually prove possible to provide immune protection at one mucosal site by immunization at another.

14.1.2 Spectrum of the intestinal immune response

Ingestion of antigens can lead to a local or systemic immune response, or oral tolerance (specific immune unresponsiveness).

The gut can mount **a local immune response** to an antigen independent of a systemic response. For example, immunization against poliomyelitis with oral attenuated Sabin vaccine typically gives better protection than the injected killed Salk vaccine, even though both induce serum antibodies of IgG and IgA class. Local IgA antibody, produced in response to the oral vaccine, partly blocks uptake of pathogenic virus into the circulation. The disadvantage of the oral vaccine is that the attenuated but still living virus can cause poliomyelitis in immunocompromised recipients.

A range of macromolecules and particles are absorbed by the intestine into the portal or systemic circulations, via either the glandular epithelium covering the villus or the specialized M cells. Up to 2% of a dietary protein load can appear antigenically intact in the circulation. Sinusoidal phagocytes (Kupffer cells) of the liver destroy much of the antigen, but enough passes through the liver to stimulate **systemic antibody production**, particularly in the spleen. Antibody formed in the spleen goes directly into the portal circulation to complex with incoming antigen. Circulating immune complexes of IgA and dietary antigens are regularly found in normal people after meals.

A unique feature of the mucosal immune system is its ability to down-regulate immune responses to dietary antigens — **oral tolerance**. In animal models, oral feeding of an antigen followed by systemic antigenic challenge results in

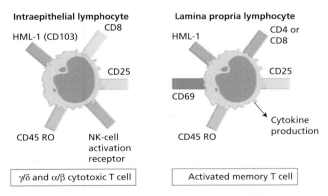

Fig. 14.5 Typical phenotypes of gut lymphocytes. CD69, activation marker; CD25, activation marker; CD45 RO, memory cell marker.

Table 14.1 Some examples of immunological involvement in intestinal disease

1 *Infection* with virulent organism	Gastroenteritis
2 *Immunodeficiency*, e.g. primary or secondary	Chronic infection with enteropathogens
	Intestinal tumours
3 *Autoimmunity*, e.g. gastric atrophy	Pernicious anaemia
4 *Hypersensitivity* to dietary antigen	Coeliac disease
	Food allergy

marked reduction of antibody levels and cell-mediated immunity compared with animals not fed the antigen first. This has led to attempts to treat autoimmune diseases in humans by feeding autoantigens to patients (see Chapters 5 and 7).

Normally the intestinal immune system steers a delicate course between the undesirable extremes (Table 14.1) of immune incompetence, with resulting vulnerability to ingested pathogens [for instance, the gastrointestinal consequences of human immunodeficiency virus (HIV) infection] and hypersensitivity, with damage each time the relevant antigen is eaten (e.g. coeliac disease).

14.2 Infection and the gut

14.2.1 Infection and the gut

Infections of the gastrointestinal tract can be life-threatening. For example, the intestinal tract is a major target of HIV infection. About half of all patients with HIV infection will have gastrointestinal involvement at some time and the pathophysiological consequences are a cause of serious morbidity. Diarrhoea, malabsorption and weight loss are the most common manifestations and, in Africa, this wasting syndrome is frequently called 'slim disease'.

HIV infects lymphocytes and macrophages within the gut. HIV is thought to exert its effect on the gut both directly, through infection of intestinal cells, and indirectly, through impairment of the intestinal immune response, with consequent chronic infection with enteropathogens and the development of intestinal tumours such as lymphoma or Kaposi's sarcoma (Fig. 14.6). The principal change in the small intestine is a partial villous atrophy detectable early in the natural history of HIV infection. Breast-feeding may transmit HIV in humans, suggesting that the intestine is an important portal of entry for HIV.

Enteropathogens causing intestinal infections are of the same types as in immunocompetent subjects (Fig. 14.7), but the clinical symptoms produced by these infections are chronic, lasting for the duration of the patient's life. Treatment of these infections remains a major problem, since some of the organisms cannot be eradicated by available antibiotics.

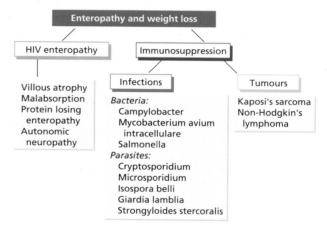

Fig. 14.6 Gastrointestinal manifestations of HIV infection.

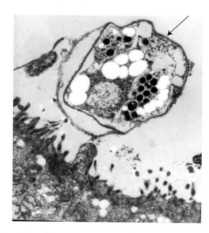

Fig. 14.7 Scanning electron micrograph of Cryptosporidial infestation (arrowed) of the intestine.

14.3 Gastritis

14.3.1 Atrophic gastritis and pernicious anaemia

The gastric mucosa contains several cell types: parietal cells producing acid and intrinsic factor, chief cells producing pepsinogen, epithelial cells, mucus neck cells and endocrine

CASE 14.1 PERNICIOUS ANAEMIA

A 67-year-old widow presented with gradually increasing tiredness, exertional dyspnoea and ankle swelling. Two years earlier she had been found to be anaemic and had been treated with oral iron without symptomatic improvement. She had lost 6 kg in weight, but denied any history of anorexia, dyspepsia or blood loss. On examination, she was very pale and had signs of congestive cardiac failure.

Laboratory investigations showed a very low haemoglobin of 54 g/l with a reduced white cell count of 3.7×10^9/l (and a platelet count of only 31×10^9/l). A blood film showed marked macrocytosis with a mean cell volume of 112 fl. Bone marrow examination revealed marked megaloblastic erythropoiesis with abundant iron stores. Serum vitamin B_{12} was 40 ng/l (NR 170–900) but serum folate, serum iron and total iron-binding capacity were normal. Her serum contained strongly positive gastric parietal cell antibodies of IgG class (Fig. 14.8) and blocking antibodies to intrinsic factor (see below). Antibodies to thyroid microsomal antigen were also found, although the patient was clinically and biochemically euthyroid.

The patient had pernicious anaemia and was therefore started on intramuscular injections of hydroxycobalamin at 3-monthly intervals. Four days after the first injection, her reticulocyte count rose to 16%.

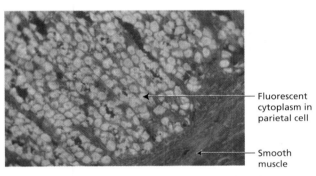

Fluorescent cytoplasm in parietal cell

Smooth muscle

Fig. 14.8 Gastric parietal cell antibodies detected by indirect immunofluorescence (see Chapter 19).

cells. Chronic inflammation of the gastric mucosa (gastritis) is relatively common, and associated with atrophy of gastric glands and loss of specialized secretory cells (Fig. 14.9). Two main types of gastritis are recognized (Table 14.2). Type A is immunologically mediated: type B gastritis is not autoimmune but caused by Helicobacter pylori infection. Autoimmune gastritis is associated with other organ-specific autoimmune disease, both in a given patient and in families (Table 14.3).

Pernicious anaemia (PA) is characterized by megaloblastic anaemia due to malabsorption of vitamin B_{12}, itself secondary to deficiency of intrinsic factor secretion and gastric atrophy. Most patients are over 60 years old and women are affected more often than men (ratio 3 : 2). About 2% of people over 60 years old have undiagnosed PA. There is no specific clinical picture. The most common presenting features are tiredness and weakness (90%), dyspnoea (70%), paraesthesia (30%) and a sore tongue (25%). Although neurological features are relatively rare (about 5%), involvement of the posterior and lateral columns of the spinal cord (subacute combined degeneration) is a serious complication which may not reverse on vitamin B_{12} treatment.

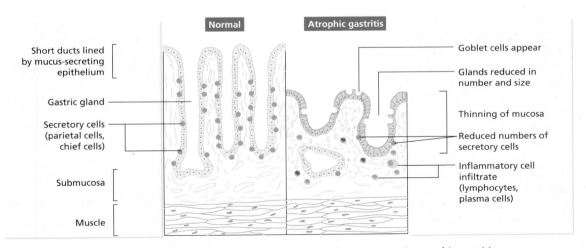

Normal | Atrophic gastritis

Short ducts lined by mucus-secreting epithelium

Gastric gland

Secretory cells (parietal cells, chief cells)

Submucosa

Muscle

Goblet cells appear

Glands reduced in number and size

Thinning of mucosa

Reduced numbers of secretory cells

Inflammatory cell infiltrate (lymphocytes, plasma cells)

Fig. 14.9 Schematic representation of normal gastric mucosa and the histological changes seen in atrophic gastritis.

Table 14.2 Types of gastritis

Feature	Type A	Type B
Association	Pernicious anaemia	Helicobacter pylori infection
Antral inflammation	Antral-sparing (fundus and body affected)	Antritis (fundus and body also affected)
Antral gastrin cell counts	High	Low
Serum gastrin level	High	Low
Intrinsic factor production	Low	Normal
Acid production	Low (achlorhydria)	Normal or low
Gastric autoantibodies:		
Parietal cell	Present	Absent
Intrinsic factor	Present	Absent
Other autoimmune disease	Often present	Absent
Risks of malignant disease	Gastric carcinoma (3 × risk) B-cell gastric lymphoma	Gastric carcinoma (2–6 × risk)

Table 14.3 Features of pernicious anaemia (PA) consistent with an autoimmune aetiology

1 Presence of autoantibodies to:
  • Gastric parietal cell canaliculi (90%)
  • Intrinsic factor (70%)
  • Thyroid antigens (50%)
2 In vitro inhibition of parietal cell function and inhibition of intrinsic factor by autoantibodies
3 Association with other autoimmune disorders:
  • Autoimmune thyroid disease
    Thyrotoxicosis
    Hashimoto's thyroiditis
    Myxoedema
  • Autoimmune adrenalitis (Addison's disease)
  • Insulin-dependent diabetes mellitus
  • Primary ovarian failure
  • Vitiligo
  • Idiopathic hypoparathyroidism
  • Myasthenia gravis
4 Occurrence of PA/other autoimmune conditions in relatives:
  • First-degree relatives, especially females (30% have PA)
  • Concordance in monozygotic twins
5 Good experimental response to immunosuppressive drugs:
  • Increased absorption of vitamin B_{12}
  • Some regeneration in parietal cells

Over 90% of patients with PA produce an antibody to a parietal cell antigen other than intrinsic factor. This antibody, **gastric parietal cell antibody** (GPC Ab), is commonly detected by indirect immunofluorescence (see Chapter 19) and its molecular target is the gastric proton pump (H^+, K^+ ATPase) contained within the membranes of the secretory canaliculi. These antibodies are unlikely to be pathogenic in vivo because gastric H^+ K^+ ATPase is not accessible to circulating autoantibodies. GPC Ab is found in nearly all patients with PA and provides a useful screening test, but because GPC Ab can be present in other diseases, diagnosis depends on the demonstration of intrinsic factor antibodies (Table 14.4).

Evidence from mouse models suggests that TH1-type $CD4^+$ T cells initiate the autoimmune gastritis. Transfer of $CD4^+$ T cell clones that recognize the β subunit of gastric H^+ K^+ ATPase into naive mice results in gastritis and serum antibodies to the target antigen. Transfer of autoantibodies and $CD8^+$ T cells has no such effects. Whether this mechanism is also responsible for gastritis of PA in humans is not known.

Intrinsic factor (IF) is a 60-kDa glycoprotein produced by gastric parietal cells. It binds avidly to dietary vitamin B_{12} and the B_{12}–IF complex is carried to the terminal ileum where it is absorbed after binding to intrinsic factor receptors on ileal cells. *Malabsorption of vitamin B_{12} in patients with PA is due to intrinsic factor deficiency* and two mechanisms are responsible. First, the progressive destruction of parietal cells leads to failure of IF production. The severity of the gastric lesion correlates with the degree of impairment of IF secretion. Second, patients with PA produce autoantibodies which impair absorption of the B_{12}–IF complex in the ileum. Two types of **IF antibody** are recognized (Fig. 14.10). Blocking antibody is directed towards the combining site for vitamin B_{12} on IF. Binding antibody reacts with an antigenic determinant on IF distinct from the B_{12} combining site: this antibody can react either with free intrinsic factor or with the B_{12}–IF complex to inhibit absorption (Fig. 14.10). Binding antibody rarely occurs without blocking antibody. Blocking antibody is readily detected in serum by radioimmunoassay (see Chapter 19), but large amounts of free B_{12} in the circulation (e.g. after a vitamin injection) can produce a false-positive result.

Table 14.4 Occurrence of gastric autoantibodies

Condition	Parietal cell antibody	Intrinsic factor antibody
Pernicious anaemia	*Serum* 90%	
	IgG — 65%	Blocking type 70%, IgG
	IgA — 25%	Binding type 35%
	Gastric juice 70%	
	IgA	Blocking type 85%, IgA
Relatives of patients with PA	30%	< 1%
Other autoimmune disease:		
Thyroid disease		
Diabetes mellitus	20%	5%
Addison's disease		
Iron-deficiency anaemia	25%	< 1%
Healthy adults		
Females > 60 years	10%	< 1%
Females < 20 years	2%	< 1%
Clinical value	*Screening test*	*Diagnostic test*

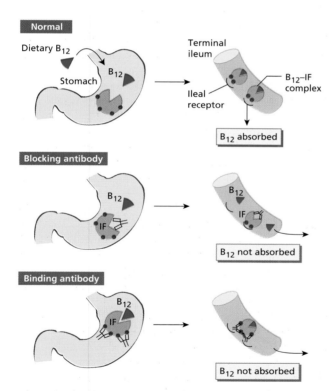

Fig. 14.10 Types of intrinsic factor antibody and their effect on vitamin B_{12} absorption. IF, Intrinsic factor.

Although IF antibodies are found more frequently in the gastric juices than in the sera of patients with PA (Table 14.4), it is more convenient to test sera. Antibodies to IF are specific and rarely occur in the absence of overt or latent PA.

14.4 Food-induced gastrointestinal disease

14.4.1 Food allergy

Doctors and the public have different perceptions of food allergy. Up to 20% of 'food-allergic' adults believe their symptoms to be food dependent, although the objective confirmation of prevalence is nearer 1%. A limited number of foods are responsible for most cases of true food allergy and the case history provides most of the diagnostic clues. Some patients have acute, life-threatening anaphylactic reactions, e.g. peanut allergy, while others have localized gastrointestinal reactions with diarrhoea, bleeding and failure to thrive, e.g. children with 'cow's milk protein intolerance'.

There are circumstances where patients experience distressing food-related symptoms that cannot be confirmed by objective tests or food challenge. Many of these cases have atypical or non-specific symptoms and involve foods rarely implicated in allergic reactions. It is inappropriate to label such patients as having food allergy without evidence of an immunological reaction to a food.

Food allergy and intolerance is discussed more fully in Chapter 4.

14.4.2 Coeliac disease

Coeliac disease, or gluten-sensitive enteropathy, is a relatively common small bowel enteropathy resulting from immunological hypersensitivity to ingested gluten (the storage protein of wheat and related cereals) in genetically susceptible individuals. Coeliac disease is most prevalent in Europeans and rare in Chinese or Afro-Caribbean people.

CASE 14.2 COELIAC DISEASE

A 35-year-old school cook presented to her dentist with a 30-month history of a sore mouth and tongue; she was treated with triamcinolone oral paste without improvement. Three months later she developed loose stools and generalized but vague abdominal pain. On questioning, she had felt tired for 2 years and had lost 8 kg in weight during the preceding 6 months despite a good appetite. During her second and third pregnancies she had developed moderate folic acid-deficiency anaemia. There was no family history of gastrointestinal disease and no abnormalities were found on examination.

Laboratory investigations showed a macrocytic anaemia but normal white cell, platelet and reticulocyte counts. The blood film showed many Howell–Jolly bodies (fragments of nuclear material within red blood cells) (Fig. 14.11), suggestive of hyposplenism. Bone marrow examination revealed active erythropoiesis with early megaloblastic features but no stainable iron. The appearances

were those of a combined deficiency of iron and folate/vitamin B₁₂; laboratory tests confirmed this (Table 14.5). In view of the blood film and the malabsorption of fat, coeliac disease was the most likely diagnosis. Her serum was positive for IgA antibodies to endomysium and to tissue transglutaminase, strongly supporting the clinical diagnosis. A jejunal biopsy was performed: this showed a convoluted pattern of stunted villi under the dissecting microscope, and subtotal villous atrophy with marked increase in intraepithelial lymphocytes and chronic inflammation in the lamina propria (Fig. 14.12).

The patient was started on a strict gluten-free diet with folic acid, iron and calcium supplements. One year later, she had put on 4.8 kg. A repeat jejunal biopsy showed improvement in villous architecture. This improvement following gluten withdrawal confirmed the diagnosis of coeliac disease and the patient will continue her gluten-free diet for life.

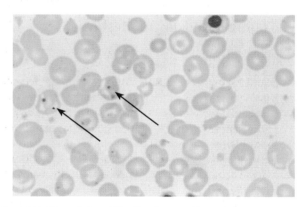

Fig. 14.11 Howell–Jowell bodies (arrowed) in a blood film.

Population screening surveys based on autoantibody testing have suggested a worldwide prevalence rate around 1 in 250 people.

The characteristic **histological lesion** in untreated cases is the loss of normal villi with a marked increase in the numbers of intra-epithelial T lymphocytes, particularly those expressing the γ/δ T-cell receptor (Figs 14.12 and 14.13); the infiltrate resolves following treatment with a gluten-free diet, suggesting that the intestinal damage may be caused by a local cell-mediated reaction to gluten. Within the lamina propria there is a mixed-cell infiltrate of plasma cells, stimulated CD4⁺ lymphocytes, macrophages, mast cells and basophils.

Table 14.5 Laboratory investigation in Case 14.2

Investigations of anaemia			Investigations of malabsorption		
Analyte	Value	NR	Analyte	Value	NR
Hb	107	120–160 g/l	Serum albumin	27	35–50 g/l
Mean cell volume	102	80–90 fl	Serum calcium	2.22	2.33–2.60 mmol/l
Serum iron	5.9	14–29 μmol/l	Serum phosphate	0.74	0.80–1.45 mmol/l
Iron-binding capacity	85	45–72 μmol/l	Serum alk. phosphatase	70	20–85 IU/l
Serum folate	1.0	2–13 μg/l	Serum IgG	8.2	7.2–19.0 g/l
Red cell folate	52	165–600 μg/l	Serum IgA	3.9	0.8–5.0 g/l
Serum vitamin B₁₂	197	160–900 ng/l	Faecal fat excretion	25	<17 mmol/day
			Serum endomysial antibodies (IgA class)	Positive	
			Anti-tissue transglutaminase (IgA class)	Positive	

(a) Low power

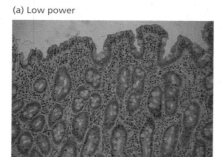

(b) High power

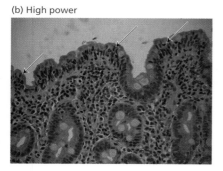

Fig. 14.12 Typical histological features of coeliac disease shown in (a) low and (b) high power. Intraepithelial lymphocytes are arrowed.

Two factors are obviously important in the **pathogenesis** of coeliac disease (Fig. 14.14): exposure to gluten and a genetic predisposition to react to it. A unique 33 amino acid gluten peptide (33mer) is thought to initiate the disease because it encloses several, in part overlapping, HLA-DQ2 binding and T-cell-stimulating epitopes that are resistant to intestinal proteinases. This peptide undergoes deamidation by an enzyme—tissue transglutaminase—in the small intestine and is then endocytosed and processed by antigen-presenting cells to three epitopes that preferentially bind to HLA-DQ2 or -DQ8 and are subsequently recognized by T-cell receptors of CD4[+] T cells. These activated T cells generate IFN-γ and other cytokines and are believed to cause the villous atrophy and crypt hyperplasia characteristic of coeliac disease. There are several strands of supporting evidence: (i) the mucosal damage is similar to that seen in experimental animal models involving T-cell-mediated injury and in the enteropathy of graft-versus-host disease (see Chapter 8); (ii) gluten-specific, HLA-DQ2 and -DQ8-restricted T cells have been isolated from the small intestines of coeliac patients; and (iii) T-lymphocyte infiltration of the small bowel epithelium is seen within hours of gluten exposure.

Coeliac disease runs in families: 10–20% of first-degree relatives, 40% of HLA-identical siblings and around 75% of monozygotic twins have the condition. In Europeans, coeliac disease is strongly associated with inheritance of the histocompatibility antigens HLA-DQ2 and HLA-DQ8: most coeliac patients carry these risk alleles but they are also found in 20% of the general population. Consequently, it is likely that at least one other, non-HLA-linked gene on the long arm of chromosome 5 is involved in determining disease susceptibility. The absence of complete concordance in identical twins implies that other factors are involved, presumably environmental. Whatever these factors are, patients with coeliac disease remain sensitive to gluten for the rest of their lives.

Patients with coeliac disease and gluten sensitivity can **present** in many ways (Fig. 14.15): only a few present with typical intestinal features of diarrhoea or malabsorption, and the diagnosis may be overlooked for months or years, as in Case 14.2. A jejunal biopsy is the only essential diagnos-

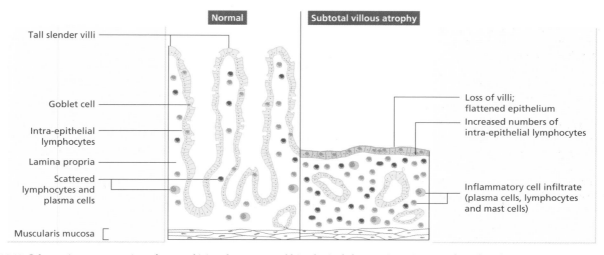

Fig. 14.13 Schematic representation of normal jejunal mucosa and histological changes in patients with coeliac disease.

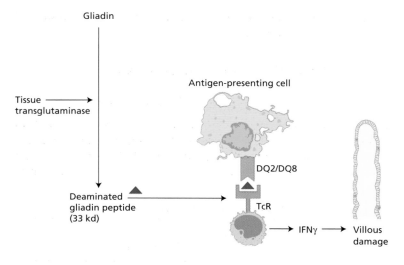

Fig. 14.14 Proposed pathogenesis of coeliac disease. TcR, T-cell receptor.

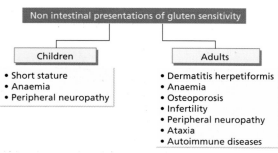

Fig. 14.15 Non-intestinal but increasingly common clinical presentations of coeliac disease.

Table 14.6 Immunological features of coeliac disease

Circulating antibodies
IgA antibodies to tissue transglutaminase and endomysium
IgA/IgG antibodies to gliadin

Mucosal lesion
Infiltration by immunocompetent lymphoid cells

Genetic factors
Familial
Associated with HLA-DQ2 or -DQ8

Associated autoimmune disorders
Dermatitis herpetiformis
Extrinsic allergic alveolitis
Endocrine disorders: thyroid disease, Addison's disease, diabetes mellitus
Rheumatic disorders: systemic lupus erythematosus, rheumatoid arthritis, Sjögren's syndrome

Immunological complications
Hyposplenism
Development of lymphoma

tic test of coeliac disease. However, **immunological tests** are extremely useful and are of two types:
• antibodies against gluten or gliadin extracts; and
• IgA antibodies against 'endomysium' of primate oesophagus or human umbilical cord are in fact detecting tissue transglutaminase, an 85-kDa tissue repair enzyme capable of cross-linking glutamine-rich proteins such as gliadin and believed to be important in the pathogenesis of the disorder (see above).

The diagnostic specificity and sensitivity of IgA antibodies to endomysium or tissue transglutaminase is almost 100%. Consequently, they can be used to screen populations at risk because of heredity, extraintestinal features or associated disorders (Table 14.6). These tests show that coeliac disease is underdiagnosed. While immunological tests cannot substitute for a diagnostic biopsy, they can be used to select those patients in whom a biopsy is needed.

Coeliac disease is **a premalignant condition**: the risk of T-cell lymphoma is 50-fold higher than in the general population. There is also an increased frequency of carcinoma of the jejunum, oesophagus and pharynx. Treatment with a gluten-free diet reduces significantly the likelihood of subsequent small-intestinal malignant disease. It is not known

why malignancy occurs, but the oncogene *c-myc* is found in maturing jejunal enterocytes, particularly in untreated coeliac disease. Persistent stimulation by gluten may therefore lead to malignant proliferation of lymphoid tissue.

Dermatitis herpetiformis (DH) is a bullous skin eruption that is associated with a coeliac-like lesion of the jejunum in almost all patients (see Chapter 11). The intestinal morphology improves on a gluten-free diet and, if the diet is strict enough, the skin lesion may also remit. The genetic background of DH is similar to coeliac disease; there is a high prevalence of HLA-DQ2 or -DQ8. Biopsy of the skin lesions shows deposition of IgA and C3 below the epithelial basement membrane; these lesions probably represent damage by IgA immune complexes originating in the intestinal mucosa following gluten ingestion.

14.5 Autoimmune enteropathy

Rare children have a severe and extensive enteropathy which is not due to coeliac disease, cow's milk protein intolerance, or other recognized forms of food-related intestinal disease. Some of these individuals have an autoimmune enteropathy, characterized by protracted diarrhoea, often associated

with organ-specific autoantibodies and a family history of autoimmune disease.

14.6 Inflammatory bowel disease

14.6.1 Crohn's disease and ulcerative colitis

Ulcerative colitis and Crohn's disease are chronic inflammatory disorders of the gastrointestinal tract, with a tendency to remit and relapse (Table 14.7). Ulcerative colitis affects only the colon, and is confined to the mucosal layer.

Table 14.7 Some differences between ulcerative colitis and Crohn's disease

	Ulcerative colitis	Crohn's disease
Disease site	Colon	Any part of gastrointestinal tract
Inflammation	Mucosal	Transmural, granulomatous
Cytokine profile	TH2	TH1
ANCA positivity	50–80%	5–20%
Genetic factors	HLA-DR2	Chromosome 16: NOD2
		Chromosome 12: IFN-γ
		Other loci on chromosomes 6 and 14
Concordance in monozygotic twins	6–14%	45%
Risk in first-degree relatives	× 10	× 30
Smoking	Protective	Harmful

CASE 14.3 CROHN'S DISEASE

A 30-year-old woman was admitted with a 4-week history of increasing bloody diarrhoea and abdominal pain; she had lost 3 kg in weight. She smoked 25 cigarettes a day. On examination, she was not clinically anaemic but had a temperature of 37.8 °C. She was tender over the right iliac fossa, and had a number of hypertrophic tender anal skin tags which she thought were haemorrhoids. Sigmoidoscopy to 15 cm showed a red, granular mucosa with mucopus and contact bleeding. Laboratory investigations showed a low haemoglobin (108 g/l) with a raised C-reactive protein (CRP) (67 mg/l) but a normal white cell count. Urea and electrolytes, serum vitamin B$_{12}$, folate, iron, ferritin and iron-binding capacity were normal. Her total serum proteins were 54 g/l (NR 62–82) with a serum albumin of 29 g/l (NR 35–50). Antibodies to neutrophil cytoplasmic antigens (ANCA) were not detected. Faecal examination and culture revealed no ova or Campylobacter. Clostridium difficile toxin was absent from the stools.

The rectal biopsy taken at sigmoidoscopy showed a small area of ulceration of the surface epithelium with considerable mucopus. Many crypt abscesses were present. The lamina propria contained a heavy infiltrate of lymphocytes, plasma cells and macrophages. Several non-caseating granulomas (Fig. 14.16) were present in

the muscular layer. The appearances were those of Crohn's disease affecting the colon. A small bowel barium examination showed extensive areas of fissuring ulceration interspersed with areas of apparently normal mucosa—skip lesions. She was treated with corticosteroids and a 3-month course of metronidazole with symptomatic improvement. She was strongly advised to stop smoking but refused to heed this advice.

Over the next 2 years, her symptoms worsened, with an anal fistula, persistent diarrhoea and colicky lower abdominal pain despite prednisolone 15 mg per day. She was weaned off prednisolone and started on budesonide, but then developed spondyloarthropathy of the left hip, both knees and her left wrist. Because of her limited response to steroids, she was given an intravenous infusion of a monoclonal antibody to TNF—infliximab (see Chapter 7). Clinically, she improved and her bowels were open two or three times each day and without nocturnal diarrhoea. This remission lasted nearly 3 months before her profuse diarrhoea and abdominal pain returned. She has now had four infusions of infliximab, each inducing symptomatic improvement of several months' duration. She still smokes.

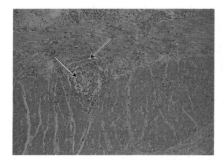

Fig. 14.16 A typical granuloma (arrowed) in the muscular layer of the bowel in Crohn's disease shown in low power.

Crohn's disease, on the other hand, may affect any part of the gastrointestinal tract from mouth to anus, although the ileocaecal region is most frequently involved. It can affect the colon alone and then must be distinguished from ulcerative colitis (UC) and other diseases causing segmental colitis, such as tuberculosis, intestinal lymphoma, lymphocytic or collagenous colitis, the latter being associated with long-term use of non-steroidal anti-inflammatory drugs. The diagnosis of both conditions is made by endoscopy, biopsy and radiology. **Immunological tests** have little part to play in the routine assessment of inflammatory bowel disease (IBD), although acute-phase proteins (such as orosomucoid and CRP) are useful in monitoring disease activity and its response to treatment. Antibodies to ANCA have been demonstrated in the sera of patients with IBD, particularly UC. The staining pattern of these antibodies is distinct from those of cANCA and pANCA (Chapter 19), but the target antigen is unknown. Several clinical features of IBD indirectly suggest an immune-mediated pathogenesis, including the occurrence of aphthous ulceration, iritis, erythema nodosum and arthritis, the association with disorders such as ankylosing spondylitis or primary sclerosing cholangitis, and their response to immunosuppressive drugs.

Histologically these diseases are distinct. Transmural inflammation in Crohn's disease involves lymphocytes, plasma cells and eosinophils, and there is granuloma formation (Fig. 14.16). The mucosa in UC is infiltrated with neutrophils as well as plasma cells and eosinophils. With increasing severity of disease, there is ulceration with loss of goblet cells and formation of crypt abscesses. Compared with normal intestine, diseased bowel shows intense expression of major histocompatibility complex (MHC) class II antigens on epithelial cells, and on lymphatic and vascular endothelium, while T lymphocytes and macrophages infiltrating the diseased lamina propria express activation markers such as CD25 (IL-2 receptor), as in other types of inflammation.

The **pathogenesis of Crohn's disease** is complex but related to three interacting factors: genetic susceptibility, gut microflora and immune-mediated tissue injury (Fig. 14.17).

Intestinal inflammation arises from abnormal immune reactivity to bacterial flora in the intestines of patients who are genetically susceptible. There is considerable evidence that **genetic factors** contribute to the pathogenesis of Crohn's disease but have a more dominant role than in UC (Table 14.7). Siblings of patients have a much higher risk of developing Crohn's disease (× 30) or UC (× 10) than the general population. In Crohn's disease, the concordance in monozygotic twins is 45%, so environmental factors must also operate: most (70%) patients with Crohn's disease are smokers, while those with UC (5%) are not. Crohn's disease is a polygenic disorder. Mutations in the nitric oxide dismutase (NOD)2 gene on chromosome 16 have been conclusively linked to about a fifth of cases of Crohn's disease. NOD2 expression is restricted to monocytes and is believed to act as a cytosolic receptor for pathogenic components of gut bacteria. A defective NOD2 gene makes its bearer susceptible to Crohn's disease, but this is only one of several genes linked to this condition (Fig. 14.17). Genetic manipulation of cadherins in mice disrupts intercellular tight junctions and leads to chronic intestinal inflammation, while deletion of specific cytokine genes (IL-10 'knockout' mice) results in a Crohn's-like disease in the presence of normal luminal flora. Crohn's disease seems to be driven by activated TH1 cells secreting IL-12, TNF-α and IFN-γ in response to bacterial exposure. The main mediators of tissue damage are matrix metalloproteinases generated in response to this cytokine release. T effector cells also show increased resistance to apoptosis, so perpetuating the inflammatory process. There is also much evidence for the role of intestinal microflora in Crohn's disease, but claims that infection by Mycobacterium tuberculosis or measles virus triggers the disease have not been substantiated..

Studies of intestinal inflammation in humans and animals suggest that UC results from environmental factors triggering a loss of tolerance to intestinal flora in genetically susceptible individuals. Several pieces of evidence implicate environmental factors: cigarette smoking or early appendicectomy seem to be protective, while lack of breastfeeding and treatment with NSAIDs increase the risk of developing UC. The retrograde gradient of UC lesions mirrors the bacterial concentration gradient in the colon and inflammation can occur in the ileal pouch after surgical anastomosis, 'pouchitis', which responds to treatment with metronidazole.

Current understanding of the likely pathogenesis of Crohn's disease has led to some newer **approaches to management** (Fig. 14.17). Monoclonal antibody to TNF-α—infliximab—is a safe and effective treatment for resistant or fistulating Crohn's disease (Case 14.3). About 50–65% of patients respond beneficially to infusion of infliximab and 20–30% patients go into remission, allowing infliximab to be used as maintenance therapy in some cases. Antibodies to α_4-integrins can block T-lymphocyte migration from the

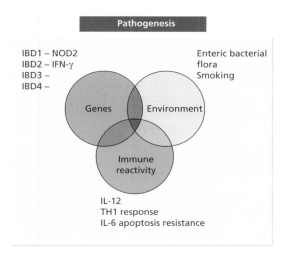

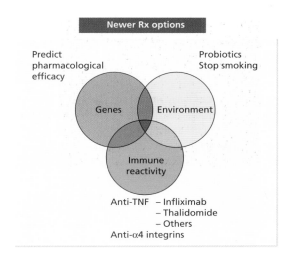

Fig. 14.17 Current understanding of the aetiology and pathogenesis of Crohn's disease and new approaches to treatment.

circulation into inflammatory foci, while cytokine-targeted treatment with anti-IL-12 and anti IL-6 receptor induces apoptosis. Alteration of the gut microbial environment by probiotics and cessation of smoking are also beneficial in some patients. In contrast, no innovative treatments have been developed to treat UC.

14.7 Viral hepatitis

Viral hepatitis is an infection of the liver caused by one of a range of specific hepatitis viruses (Table 14.8). Other viruses, such as Epstein–Barr virus, cytomegalovirus, herpes simplex virus and rubella, also cause hepatitis

14.7.1 Hepatitis A

Hepatitis A (Table 14.8) is caused by a small RNA picornavirus which replicates in the gut and liver. Hepatitis A virus causes a mild or unnoticed illness in children or young adults. The **diagnosis** can be confirmed either by demonstrating virus in the faeces or by detecting a rise in specific antibodies (Fig. 14.18). Antibody tests are usually more reliable because the virus has often been eliminated completely before the patient seeks medical attention. Sera collected within a few weeks of the onset of symptoms contain anti-hepatitis A antibody which is almost exclusively IgM; its presence indicates recent infection.

Table 14.8 Comparison of major features of hepatitis A, B, C and E

	Hepatitis type			
	A	B	C	E
Type of virus	RNA	DNA	RNA	RNA
Incubation period (days)				
Average	30	70	50	40
Range	15–45	50–180	15–150	15–60
Transmission				
Blood inoculation	+	+++	+++	–
Faecal–oral	+++	+	–	+++
Sexual	–	++	+	–
Vertical (transplacental)	–	+++	+	–
Age of patient	Any—usually young	Any	Any	Any—usually young adults
Severity of infection	Mild	Occasionally severe	Mild	Mild but can be fulminant in pregnancy
Chronicity	Very rare	Common	Very common	Rare
Extrahepatic features	Rare	Common	Rare	Rare
Development of hepatoma	Very rare	Common	Common	Rare

CASE 14.4 HEPATITIS A

An 18-year-old man presented with a 10-day history of anorexia, nausea and upper abdominal discomfort. Two weeks earlier, he had experienced some mild arthralgia in his fingers which lasted for 2 days. He normally smoked 20 cigarettes and drank two to three pints of beer each day, but had done neither for several days. He had noticed that his urine was much darker than normal. There was no significant medical history. On examination, he was afebrile but jaundiced. There were no needle tracks on his arms. His liver was just palpable and tender.

Hepatitis was diagnosed and confirmed by routine investigations. His serum bilirubin was 48 μmol/l (NR 1–20) with raised liver enzyme levels [aspartate transaminase 895 IU/l (NR 5–45); alanine transaminase 760 IU/l (NR 5–30)], and an alkaline phosphatase of 128 IU/l (NR 20–85). A monospot test for infectious mononucleosis was negative. Hepatitis B surface antigen (HBsAg) was also negative but he had detectable IgM antibodies to hepatitis A virus. He was managed conservatively at home. There is no active treatment for hepatitis A infection, although rest may be beneficial. The clinical and biochemical evidence of hepatocellular damage subsided over the next 4 weeks but he continued to feel vaguely unwell for several months. A further blood sample after 6 months showed IgG antibody to hepatitis A.

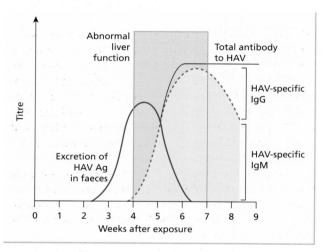

Fig. 14.18 Humoral immune response in acute hepatitis A virus (HAV) infection. Ag, antigen.

The **pathogenesis** of liver cell damage in viral hepatitis is not known. The virus itself may be cytopathic or the immune response to the virus may result in the destruction of infected hepatocytes, as postulated for hepatitis B. The younger the patient, the milder the infection tends to be. Most patients with hepatitis A make a full recovery, and progression to chronic hepatitis or cirrhosis is extremely rare.

Epidemiological control of hepatitis A is largely dependent on high standards of personal hygiene and proper disposal of sewage. Person-to-person spread is common in close communities. In countries where disposal of sewage is primitive, hepatitis A is endemic, as shown by a major outbreak involving 1.2 million people in China in 1988. For travellers or close contacts of affected patients, human normal immunoglobulin provides about 90% protection against hepatitis A for a period of 4–6 months. For long-term protection, hepatitis A vaccine gives over 97% protection against infection and lasts at least 10 years.

14.7.2 Hepatitis B

Hepatitis B is one of the most widespread infections in humans and the commonest cause of worldwide liver disease. In general, the prevalence is low in cold, developed countries and high in hot, developing countries. Hepatitis B virus may be spread by several routes (see Table 14.8), but over half of the patients in Western countries give a history of inoculation. **Transmission** has occurred in minute quantities of infected blood or blood products by the use of shared or unsterile syringes, unsterile needles in tattooing and acupuncture, or by surgical or dental procedures. The rate of transmission by needlestick injury may be as high as 20–30% compared with a transmission rate of 3% for hepatitis C and 0.3% for HIV. Hepatitis B virus is also transmitted sexually, particularly in those with multiple sexual partners. Mothers positive for hepatitis B have a high risk of infecting their infants in pregnancy. The earlier in life a person is infected, the more likely he or she is to become a carrier: virtually all babies infected in the neonatal period become chronic carriers and this is the predominant route of transmission in countries where hepatitis B is endemic. It has been estimated that there are about 300 million carriers in the world. In the UK, about 0.1–0.3% of the general population are believed to be carriers, but in tropical Africa, China and South-East Asia this proportion rises to 8–35%.

Electron microscopy of serum infected with hepatitis B reveals three types of particle: spheres, filaments and virions (Dane particles) (Fig. 14.19). HBsAg is found on the surfaces of all three types of particle. A second antigen is associated with the core (HBcAg), while a third, called hepatitis Be antigen (HBeAg), is located within the core of the virus particle.

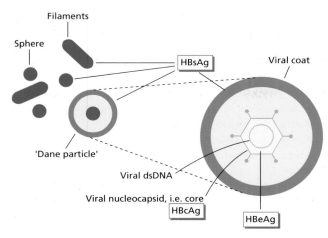

Fig. 14.19 Schematic diagram of the three morphological types of particle found in hepatitis B. Only the Dane particle is infective.

Acute hepatitis B infection may go unnoticed or be associated with vague symptoms only. Typically, however, infection leads to the appearance of HBsAg in the blood two or more weeks before abnormal tests of liver biochemistry or the onset of symptoms (Fig. 14.20). HBsAg remains detectable usually until the convalescent phase. Because it appears soon after HBsAg and is closely associated with the inner core (HBcAg) and viral DNA, HBeAg is a good measure of infectivity. IgM antibody to core antigen (IgM anti-HBcAg) appears early on and is a reliable marker of current acute infection, whereas IgG anti-HBcAg indicates previous infection. Clinical recovery and clearance of the virus is associated with the disappearance of HBeAg and then HBsAg, with subsequent detection of their respective antibodies during convalescence (Fig. 14.20). In practice, the diagnosis of hep-

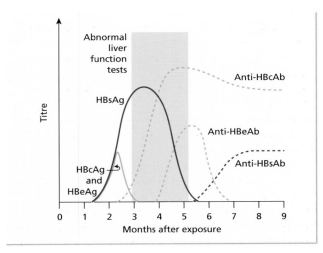

Fig. 14.20 Humoral immune responses in acute hepatitis B infection.

atitis B infection is usually confirmed by detecting HBsAg in sera collected during the acute phase of the illness, or by showing a rising titre of antibody to HBcAg. Patients with acute hepatitis B do not need treatment.

Patients with HBsAg persisting in the serum for over 6 months are defined as carriers. They may be of high or low infection risk to others depending on the presence or absence, respectively, of HBeAg. Overall, the **transmission** rate following inoculation injury with HBsAg-positive material is about 3–5%. If the patient is also HBeAg positive, the transmission rate rises to over 20% but is only 0.1% if the patient is HBe antibody positive. These risks are important to healthcare workers: in the UK, workers who are HBe-antigen positive cannot carry out invasive 'exposure-prone' procedures on patients. Consequently, all healthcare workers in developed countries are immunized with hepatitis B vaccine.

Elimination of infection in acute hepatitis B involves immunological lysis of infected cells and removal of infective virus particles. Cytotoxic CD8+ T cells are responsible for destroying the infected hepatocytes, while antibody-dependent mechanisms neutralize extracellular virus particles and so prevent the spread of infection to other liver cells. Hepatitis B is not directly cytopathic; liver injury is the result of the immune responses of the host to these antigens on the cell surface.

Acute fulminant hepatitis is associated with abnormally rapid clearance of HBsAg and HBeAg, implying an excessive, self-damaging immune response. In contrast, immunocompromised patients usually develop subclinical disease associated with viral persistence.

Three main forms of **chronic carriage of hepatitis B** are recognized: chronic active hepatitis, chronic persistent hepatitis and carriage with relatively normal liver histology. About 10% of previously healthy adults and over 90% of babies born of HBeAg-positive mothers become chronic carriers (Fig. 14.21). Most of these show chronic active hepatitis on liver biopsy. In contrast, HBsAg carriers who give no history of previous symptomatic hepatitis usually have chronic persistent hepatitis or relatively normal liver histology. This group of carriers were probably infected during the neonatal period, when the relative immaturity of the immune system can lead to tolerance of HBsAg (Fig. 14.22). Their response to other organisms, met at a later age, is completely normal.

Extrahepatic complications are probably the result of deposition of circulating immune complexes composed of viral antigens and host antibodies. Some complexes, particularly those formed in antigen excess, can be deposited in the kidney and cause glomerulonephritis. Complexes formed in antibody excess are large and usually present as vasculitic lesions. HBsAg has been found in blood and vascular lesions in some patients with polyarteritis nodosa (see Chapter 10) or mixed essential cryoglobulinaemia (see Chapter 9).

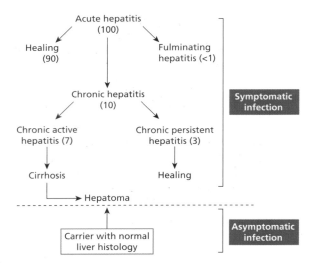

Fig. 14.21 Outcome of hepatitis B infection. Percentages of patients shown in brackets.

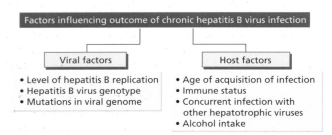

Fig. 14.22 Factors influencing outcome of chronic hepatitis B virus infection.

Primary hepatocellular carcinoma (hepatoma) is a common tumour in countries with a high prevalence of hepatitis B carriers. Carriers are about 100 times more likely to develop hepatoma than non-carriers. A raised level of serum α-fetoprotein (AFP) is found in 30–95% of hepatoma patients (depending on the series) and provides a useful diagnostic marker because of its negative predictive value (see Chapter 19).

The aims of **therapy** are a reduction in the level of viraemia and improvement in hepatic function. Current treatment is based on IFN-α and lamuvidine. IFN-α, given for over 3 months, is an effective treatment for about 30% of patients with chronic hepatitis B infection. Those patients with low concentrations of hepatitis B virus DNA in their sera are six times more likely to respond than those with high concentrations. Remissions are usually of long duration and followed by loss of HBeAg, HBsAg and other evidence of residual virus replication. Lamuvidine, a nucleoside analogue, inhibits the viral enzyme reverse transcriptase and has replaced IFN-α as first-line therapy because of its good safety profile. When given for 12 months, lamuvidine low-

ers concentrations of HBV DNA in most patients and is associated with an improvement in liver histology and a fall in liver enzymes to normal. Viral replication commonly returns when lamuvidine is stopped and drug resistance occurs in two-thirds of patients after 4 years. The combination of lamuvidine with interferon does not increase the response rate. Adefovir, a nucleotide analogue, inhibits viral reverse transcriptase even in mutant hepatitis B virus and is used in patients who have developed resistance to lamuvidine.

Liver transplantation has been performed in patients with cirrhosis due to hepatitis B; long-term survival has been poor, with recurrence of hepatitis B in 80% of the grafts, although post-transplantation prophylaxis with lamuvidine and hepatitis B immunoglobulin cuts the reinfection rate to 10% and extends the 5-year survival rate to about 80%.

Several preventative measures have been taken to reduce the incidence of hepatitis B infection:
• high-risk carriers are prevented from performing 'exposure-prone' procedures;
• the incidence of post-transfusion hepatitis B has been greatly reduced by screening potential blood donors for HBsAg;
• 'hepatitis B immunoglobulin', obtained from convalescent patients, is of prophylactic value for individuals following single acute exposure to blood from HBsAg-positive patients; and
• active immunization is recommended.

Hepatitis B vaccine is available as a genetically engineered surface antigen introduced into a yeast vector (see Chapter 7). The vaccine is safe and effective; the protection rate is over 80% in adults and 90% in neonates, although several factors are associated with a suboptimal response (Box 14.2). The duration of protection is at least 2–5 years in most people but depends on the antibody titre attained. If hepatitis B and its consequences are to be eradicated, worldwide immunization is needed. In some endemic countries, all newborn babies are immunized with hepatitis B vaccine and given hepatitis B immunoglobulin simultaneously — so-called active/passive immunization. The cost of the vac-

BOX 14.2 FACTORS ASSOCIATED WITH A SUBOPTIMAL RESPONSE TO HEPATITIS B VACCINE

• Age
• Genetic predisposition—low response in HLA-B8, -DR3
• Alcoholism
• Obesity—higher protection if vaccine given into deltoid rather than buttock
• Immunosuppression—including HIV infection
• Virus 'escape' mutants—natural virus may differ from vaccine

cine is an impediment to global vaccination schemes, but the World Health Organization recommends routine hepatitis B vaccination for countries that can afford to buy the vaccine and have a carrier rate of over 2.5% of the population.

14.7.3 Hepatitis C

During the 1970s, it was established that many cases of post-transfusion hepatitis were due neither to hepatitis A nor to hepatitis B infection. The viruses responsible were initially called non-A, non-B (NANB) hepatitis viruses but it is now known that nearly all cases of post-transfusion hepatitis are caused by hepatitis C virus (HCV), an RNA virus. HCV is a highly variable agent with six major genotypes and over 100 subtypes, many of which are grouped geographically.

Although hepatitis C was first identified and characterized in association with blood transfusions, this route of **transmission** accounts for only a small proportion of cases of hepatitis C in the UK. A history of parenteral drug abuse is the most common risk factor, with about 70% of drug abusers being positive for hepatitis C antibody, compared with about 0.2% of blood donors. Healthcare workers appear to have a slightly increased risk. Sexual and perinatal transmission have been described but are comparatively inefficient routes with a 5% risk of infection from a partner or mother with hepatitis C.

Hepatitis C infection is **characterized clinically** (see Table 14.8) by an incubation period of around 50 days. Acute infection is usually mild and asymptomatic. Only 10% of patients become jaundiced and it is rarely a cause of fulminant hepatic failure. Hepatitis C infection has a complex natural history, not yet fully defined (Fig. 14.23). About 60–80% of patients will develop chronic hepatitis and 10–20% are at risk of developing cirrhosis, often 20–30 years follow-

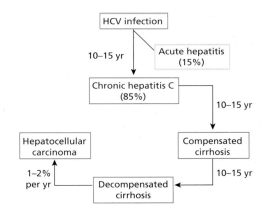

Fig. 14.23 Outcome of hepatitis C infection.

ing infection, and hepatocellular carcinoma after a further 10 years. Chronic hepatitis C is frequently associated with extrahepatic features such as mixed cryoglobulinaemia, glomerulonephritis, seronegative arthritis and cutaneous vasculitis.

Hepatitis C virus uses several strategies to evade the host immune response: (i) the high HCV replication rate can outpace the normal immune response; (ii) studies suggest that CD8+ T cells become 'stunned' and unable to produce IFN during the peak of viraemia; (iii) HCV 'counterattacks' several components of the cellular immune response by promoting CD95 (Fas)-induced apoptosis of virus-specific cytotoxic T cells.

Typical **histological features** of hepatitis C include lymphoid aggregates in portal areas, reactive epithelial changes of bile ducts and moderate lymphocytic infiltration of hepatic parenchyma. Although the cellular immune response of the host is rather weak in the chronic phase of hepatitis

CASE 14.5 HEPATITIS C-INDUCED LIVER DISEASE

A 29-year-old man was noted to have abnormal liver function tests on routine 'well-man' medical screening in the private health sector. Apart from an episode of cellulitis and septic arthritis aged 24 years, he had been fit and well. He had no symptoms of liver disease and his GP notes showed no record of jaundice. Liver function testing, subsequently repeated twice, showed a mild chronic hepatitis with serum alanine transaminase levels of 140–210 IU/l (NR 0–50), and normal serum levels of alkaline phosphatase, bilirubin and albumin. He had no detectable antibodies to smooth muscle or mitochondria. Virus serology showed no evidence of exposure to hepatitis A or B. However, he was positive for hepatitis C antibody but negative for hepatitis C virus RNA by polymerase chain reaction (PCR). He underwent a liver biopsy which showed normal liver

architecture. There was mild non-specific portal tract inflammation but no piecemeal necrosis or fibrosis.

The source of his chronic hepatitis C liver disease was uncertain. He denied any use of intravenous drugs and had received no transfusions of blood or blood products. However, he was adorned with tattoos on his limbs and trunk. Tattooing carries a risk of transmitting hepatitis C of up to 3% in the West. It has been suggested that up to 40% of current carriers were infected by tattooing. The risk is increased by multiple tattooing, work by an amateur tattooist, and if the tattooist is hepatitis C positive.

He was told that his chronic hepatitis was likely to progress only slowly and over decades provided he abstained from alcohol, but that his liver biopsy would need to be repeated every 2 years or so as an indicator of the potential need for antiviral therapy.

C, liver-infiltrating, activated, HCV-specific CD4$^+$ and CD8$^+$ TH1 lymphocytes are the main factor in the development of liver fibrosis and cirrhosis.

The **diagnosis** of hepatitis C infection depends on demonstrating rising antibody titres (anti-HCV) or viral RNA by PCR. Evidence of hepatitis C infection can be found in 60–95% of cases of transfusion-associated NANB hepatitis and in about 50% of cases of NANB hepatitis with no transfusion history. The introduction of screening of blood donors for anti-HCV in the early 1990s reduced the frequency of transfusion-associated hepatitis considerably.

Treatment with IFN-α restores transaminase levels to normal and improves liver histology in 50% of patients treated for 6 months. Unfortunately, half of the initial responders promptly relapse. Overall, only 10–20% of unselected patients have a sustained improvement for 6–12 months after IFN therapy: several factors may contribute to a favourable response (Box 14.3). Ribavirin has a limited effect if used alone, but in combination with IFN it doubles the response rate to about 40%. Pegylated interferon, interferon coupled to polyethylene glycol, has a long half-life and needs to be given only once a week rather than three times weekly for interferon. The combination of pegylated interferon and ribavirin clears hepatitis C infection in up to 55% of cases. Efficacy varies with the HCV genotype: up to 80% of patients infected with genotypes 2 and 3 respond successfully.

Hepatitis C recurs in patients following **liver transplantation**, but appears to progress less rapidly than hepatitis B in this situation. Although hepatitis C has never been cultured, the genome has been cloned and the development of a protective **vaccine** is a realistic goal. The antigenic differences imply that a polyvalent vaccine will be needed.

14.7.4 Other hepatitis viruses

Hepatitis D (delta) virus is an incomplete RNA virus which can only replicate in the presence of hepatitis B virus. Hepatitis D is found wherever hepatitis B is endemic and is spread by the same routes. Simultaneous co-infection with hepatitis B and hepatitis D is usually self-limiting, but can be associated with more severe acute hepatitis and increased morbidity. Superinfection of an HBsAg-positive, chronically infected person with hepatitis D virus leads to an increased prevalence of chronic active hepatitis and cirrhosis compared with hepatitis B infection alone.

Hepatitis E virus is an enterically transmitted RNA virus (see Table 14.8). It is endemic in Asia, Africa, the Middle East and Central America. Outbreaks in China and India have affected many thousands of people, usually young adults. Hepatitis E runs a self-limiting course in most people, but fulminant hepatitis can occur in pregnant women with fatality rates of 25% in women infected in the third trimester. Surviving infants seem to be unaffected and chronic hepatitis does not occur.

Hepatitis G virus — or GB virus (GBV) from the initials of an American surgeon infected with a non-A, non-B, non-C, non-D virus — is a parenterally transmitted agent. Co-infection with hepatitis B and C can occur, but hepatitis G does not cause clinical hepatitis on its own. It is found in about 2% of blood donors and around 20% of patients who receive regular blood products.

Seronegative hepatitis is the term for remaining cases of non-ABCDEG hepatitis and accounts for up to 10% of acute hepatitis. Such cases often have more severe jaundice and higher levels of serum transaminases, but usually recover completely. The route of transmission is unknown.

14.8 Autoimmune liver diseases

14.8.1 Chronic active hepatitis

By definition, chronic hepatitis is a chronic inflammation of the liver which lasts for more than 6 months. On the basis of the liver biopsy appearances, two broad categories are recognized — chronic persistent hepatitis and chronic active hepatitis.

Chronic persistent hepatitis is characterized by non-specific inflammation of the portal zones of the liver only. Some cases follow of complicate viral hepatitis (particularly hepatitis B and hepatitis C), alcohol, drug hypersensitivity or chronic inflammatory bowel disease. In contrast to chronic active hepatitis, immunological investigations are normal, progression to cirrhosis is rare, treatment with corticosteroids is unnecessary and the overall outlook is excellent.

Chronic active hepatitis is also marked by the presence of a mononuclear cell infiltrate in the portal areas, but this also extends into the parenchyma to produce necrosis of individual periportal hepatocytes ('piecemeal necrosis'). As the disease progresses, piecemeal necrosis extends, from the portal tracts to the central veins ('bridging necrosis'), eventually causing cirrhosis.

CASE 14.6 AUTOIMMUNE HEPATITIS

A 43-year-old woman presented with a 5-month history of weight loss (6 kg), anorexia, irritability and generalized pruritus. On examination, she was icteric with numerous spider naevi, scratch marks, palmar erythema and hepatosplenomegaly. Investigations showed a low haemoglobin (95 g/l) with a normal white cell count but an erythrocyte sedimentation rate of 140 mm/h. The prothrombin time was prolonged but urea and electrolytes, calcium and phosphate concentrations were normal. Although the serum albumin was normal (41 g/l), the total serum proteins were raised at 93 g/l (NR 62–82) with a raised serum bilirubin of 34 μmol/l (NR 1–20), alanine transaminase of 152 IU/l (NR 5–30), and aspartate transaminase of 164 IU/l (NR 5–45). The alkaline phosphatase level was normal (83 IU/l). Her serum immunoglobulins showed an increased IgG level of 44 g/l (NR 7.2–19.0) with normal IgA and IgM levels. No paraprotein was present on serum electrophoresis.

Antinuclear antibodies (of IgG class) were strongly positive to a titre of 1/10 000 and antibodies to dsDNA were positive (60% binding; normal < 30%). Her serum was positive for antibodies to smooth muscle (Fig. 14.24) to a titre of over 1/1000 (see Chapter 19). HBsAg and hepatitis C antibody were absent and alphafoetoprotein (AFP) was not detected. The immunological picture strongly favoured a diagnosis of autoimmune hepatitis. She was therefore started on prednisolone (30 mg/day) and vitamin K, with dramatic improvement. Her serum bilirubin, transaminases and prothrombin time returned to normal over the next fortnight. A diagnostic liver biopsy was performed: this showed chronic active hepatitis with cirrhosis (see below). She was continued on prednisolone (15 mg/day) and is fully reassessed every 6 months, including a repeat liver biopsy, as appropriate.

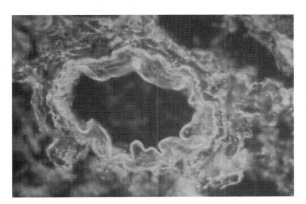

Fig. 14.24 Smooth muscle antibodies staining actin in a blood vessel.

Chronic active hepatitis (CAH) also has several, widely different aetiologies, such as hepatitis B, hepatitis C, alcohol, drugs (minocycline, isoniazid, nitrofurantoin), Wilson's disease and α_1-antitrypsin deficiency. In cases where no aetiological agent is found, an autoimmune basis is suspected. Autoimmune hepatitis and CAH associated with hepatitis C virus infection are the major recognized forms in Western countries

Characteristically, **autoimmune hepatitis** (Table 14.9) affects young to middle-aged women, many of whom (60%) have associated autoimmune disorders such as haemolytic anaemia, diabetes mellitus, thyroiditis, fibrosing alveolitis and glomerulonephritis . Smooth-muscle antibodies (SMA) are not specific for autoimmune hepatitis and are found as a temporary phenomenon in many patients with viral infections, particularly infectious hepatitis. However, high-titre

IgG antibodies to smooth muscle are classically found in autoimmune hepatitis. The target antigen is actin, a cytoskeletal protein. Antibodies to liver and kidney microsomes (LKM) occur in a proportion of patients, mainly children. The antigen recognized by LKM antibodies is a human cytochrome P450, also found in a recombinant antigen—cytochrome mono-oxygenase CYP2D6—which shows molecular mimicry with a component of hepatitis C. Similar antibodies, directed against different isoenzymes of the cytochrome, have been found in cases of drug-induced hepatitis. A distinct form of LKM-positive autoimmune hepatitis has been recognized in association with autoimmune polyendocrinopathy-candidiasis-ectodermal dysplasia (APECED) (Chapter 15).

Liver injury results from T-cell-mediated damage to genetically predisposed hepatocytes. Aberrant expression of MHC class II molecules on the surfaces of hepatocytes facilitates expression of normal liver cell membrane constituents to antigen processing cells which stimulate the clonal expansion of autoantigen-sensitized cytotoxic T cells which infiltrate liver tissue and release tissue destructive cytokines. The reasons for aberrant HLA expression are unclear, but may be triggered by genetic factors, viral infection or drugs.

Treatment of autoimmune hepatitis is currently aimed at suppressing the effector mechanisms of this self-damaging response. Randomized, controlled trials have shown that prednisolone induces clinical remission and prolongs life. Liver histology shows less inflammatory activity but cirrhosis cannot be reversed. The addition of azathioprine enables lower doses of prednisolone to be used or even withdrawn, while maintaining the patient in remission. The 10-year sur-

Table 14.9 Major features of autoimmune chronic active hepatitis

Feature	Autoimmune hepatitis
Proportion of all cases of CAH in the UK*	50–80%
Sex	Female > male (6 : 1)
Age at onset	10–30 years
	40–60 years
Associated autoimmune disease	Common
Smooth-muscle antibodies	Positive 85%
	High titre
Antinuclear antibodies	Positive in 80%
Anti-DNA antibodies	May be positive
Antimitochondrial antibodies	Positive 25%
Antibodies to liver and kidney microsomes	Positive 4% (especially children)
Serum immunoglobulins	IgG ↑↑
HLA type	HLA-B8: aggressive disease in younger patients
	HLA-DR4: extrahepatic features
Response to steroids	Good
Risk of hepatoma	Low

vival rate is 90% for autoimmune hepatitis patients without cirrhosis but only 50% when cirrhosis is present.

For patients with cirrhosis, liver transplantation gives good survival rates (90% at 5 years), although milder disease may recur in the graft despite intensive immunosuppression.

14.8.2 Primary biliary cirrhosis

Primary biliary cirrhosis (PBC) is a chronic progressive disease characterized by progressive destruction of small intrahepatic bile ducts with portal inflammation leading to fibrosis and cirrhosis. About 25–50% of patients are asymp-

CASE 14.7 PRIMARY BILIARY CIRRHOSIS

A 62-year-old woman presented with a 6-week history of generalized itching and progressive shortness of breath. She also had a dragging feeling in the right upper quadrant of her abdomen. There was no history of weight loss, anorexia or jaundice. She smoked 25 cigarettes a day. On examination, she had many scratch marks but no xanthomas, xanthelasmas or jaundice. A large right-sided pleural effusion was present, with smooth, firm moderate enlargement of the liver. She was thought to have a bronchial carcinoma with hepatic secondaries.

Investigations showed a haemoglobin of 131 g/l, a normal white cell count and an erythrocyte sedimentation rate of 93 mm/h. Prothrombin time, urea and electrolytes, calcium, phosphate, total proteins, serum albumin and serum bilirubin were normal. However, the alkaline phosphatase was 1050 IU/l (NR 20–85), aspartate transaminase 166 IU/l (NR 5–45), and alanine transaminase 121 IU/l (NR 5–30). HBsAg and hepatitis C antibody were not detected. A chest X-ray confirmed the right pleural effusion but

showed no evidence of malignancy or tuberculosis. The pleural effusion was aspirated three times; on each occasion, malignant cells were absent, culture was non-contributory, the fluid had the characteristics of a transudate and pleural biopsies were normal.

During her stay in hospital, however, the patient became obviously jaundiced, with a rise in serum bilirubin from 8 to 32 μmol/l. She also developed ascites and a palpable spleen. In view of her progressive obstructive jaundice she underwent a laparotomy; no surgically correctable cause could be found but a liver biopsy was taken. This showed the typical changes of primary biliary cirrhosis. Immunological tests were first performed at this stage—rather late! Antimitochondrial antibodies were present (Fig. 14.25) to a titre of 1/10 000. Serum immunoglobulins showed a polyclonal rise in IgM to 6.20 g/l (NR 0.5–2.0) with normal IgG and IgA levels. She was given cholestyramine to control her itching and ursodeoxycholic acid therapy. In the 4 years since diagnosis she has been reasonably well.

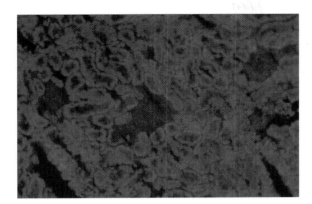

Fig. 14.25 Antimitochondrial antibodies by indirect immunofluorescence.

tomatic at diagnosis, and this phase can last for many years. Symptomatic patients usually present with pruritus (50%), right upper quadrant pain (25%) or symptoms of hepatic decompensation (20%) (Fig. 14.26). Characteristically, the disease affects middle-aged women; 5% have affected relatives. Clustering of cases has also been reported. The reported incidence ranges from 5 to 20 per million people per year and seems to be increasing.

As in Case 14.7, the diagnosis of PBC may be overlooked at first. However, **antimitochondrial antibodies** (AMA) provide a vital diagnostic test. About 95% of patients with PBC have circulating AMA by either immunofluorescence (Fig. 14.25) or ELISA. Several AMA staining patterns are recognized on indirect immunofluorescence: the M2 type is the most important marker of PBC. The target antigen is known to be the E2 component of pyruvate dehydrogenase, a mitochondrial enzyme. There is no evidence that AMA are responsible for the pathogenesis of PBC: in animals at least, experimental induction of antibodies to the pyruvate dehydrogenase complex fails to trigger PBC, while in hu-

mans there is no correlation between serum antibody titre and liver damage. Mitochondrial antibodies are also found in a small proportion of patients with CAH or cirrhosis of unknown aetiology.

The characteristic **histological lesion** in the early stages is the presence of granulomas in the portal tracts with destruction of middle-sized bile ducts (Fig. 14.27). The damaged ducts are surrounded and infiltrated typically by CD4+ T lymphocytes, with a further surrounding infiltrate of CD8+ T cells at the periphery of the portal tract, the site at which cirrhosis develops eventually. Copper is retained in the liver in chronic cholestasis and its demonstration is useful in diagnosing late-stage PBC.

The **pathogenesis** of bile duct damage in PBC is unclear. Bile ducts in PBC patients express increased densities of adhesion molecules, MHC class II antigens, IL-2 receptor and pyruvate dehydrogenase compared with normal ducts, and so represent potential targets for the infiltrating activated T cells (CD4+ and CD8+). There are similarities between PBC and chronic graft-versus-host disease (see Chapter 8), which is known to be mediated by cytotoxic T cells. Unlike CAH, PBC is not definitely associated with inheritance of any particular histocompatibility antigens. 'Clustering' of reported cases implies that an environmental agent is somehow involved. This agent, possibly a microorganism such as Chlamydia or a retrovirus, may damage intrahepatic bile ducts and trigger an autoimmune response in a susceptible individual.

The course of PBC is characterized by insidious progression to an almost invariably fatal hepatic cirrhosis. In asymptomatic patients with positive antimitochondrial antibodies and normal liver enzyme concentrations but his-

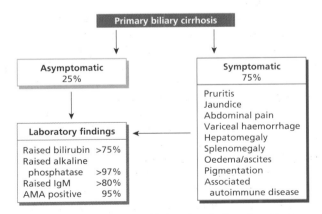

Fig. 14.26 Clinical features and laboratory findings in patients with histologically proven primary biliary cirrhosis. AMA, antimitochondrial antibody.

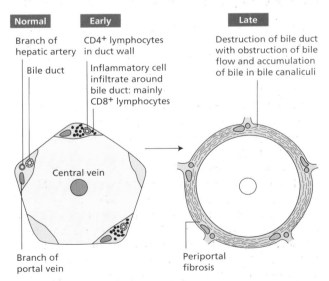

Fig. 14.27 Schematic representation of histological features of early and late stages of primary biliary cirrhosis.

tological features of early PBC, 75% become symptomatic and 40% show histological progression over a 10-year follow-up period. In symptomatic people with abnormal liver function tests, the median survival time from diagnosis to death is about 10–15 years, and less (5–7 years) in those with advanced histological disease. Despite this poor prognosis, the long natural history makes adequate prospective studies of **therapy** difficult to do. Patients are treated symptomatically: for instance, pruritus usually responds to cholestyramine. Several randomized controlled trials have shown that ursodeoxycholic acid (UDCA), an endogenous tertiary bile acid, is effective in improving liver biochemistry and reducing AMA titres. The drug reduces the risk of developing oesophageal varices and cirrhosis, but a meta-analysis of eight placebo-controlled trials reported no difference in overall death rates between UCDA-treated and placebo-treated patients. The mechanism of action of UDCA and its effect on long-term progression seems multifactorial: it appears to reduce aberrant MHC class II expression on hepatocytes, reduce cytokine progression and induce apoptosis. Current studies are evaluating UDCA in combination with newer immunosuppressive agents such as mycophenolate (see Chapter 7). Standard immunosuppressive drugs such as corticosteroids, azathioprine, methotrexate and ciclosporin are ineffective in PBC.

Liver transplantation remains the only effective therapy for patients with end-stage PBC. Indications for transplantation are either symptomatic disease or signs of end-stage liver disease. Results are good, with 5-year survival in excess of 80%. PBC recurs in the allograft with a cumulative risk of 30% at 10 years.

14.8.3 Associated syndromes

About 80% of patients with PBC have associated autoimmune disorders (Box 14.4). Most have **Sjögren's syndrome** (see Chapter 8). This combination of cholestasis, dry eyes, dry mouth and pancreatic hyposecretion classifies PBC as a 'dry gland' or 'sicca' syndrome. Some patients show a mixed picture of PBC with CAH. These hybrids are histologically similar to CAH but are positive for AMA and have raised serum transaminase and alkaline phosphatase levels. About one in three patients with cryptogenic cirrhosis is positive for smooth-muscle, mitochondrial or nuclear antibodies. It has been suggested that these cases represent an end stage of autoimmune liver disease, where the destruction of liver cells or bile duct epithelial cells has 'burnt out', leaving the patient with cirrhosis.

Sclerosing cholangitis is a chronic cholestatic liver disease characterized by an obliterative inflammatory fibrosis of the biliary tract. It can lead to biliary cirrhosis, liver failure and carcinoma of the bile ducts. It may be primary or secondary to bile duct stones or bile duct surgery. Primary sclerosing cholangitis (PSC) usually presents insidiously with jaundice and hepatosplenomegaly in young adults. The cause is unknown but there is a close association with inflammatory bowel disease, especially ulcerative colitis (Box 14.5). About 5% of patients with ulcerative colitis develop PSC, typically those with pancolitis. Conversely, 50–75% of patients with PSC have colitis. There is no specific treatment. Liver transplantation is the only option and PSC is now the second most common indication for liver transplantation in the UK.

14.8.4 Alcohol-induced liver disease

Alcoholic liver disease is common and found in 15–20% of those who abuse alcohol. Several factors contribute to the liver damage. Alcohol and its metabolites are directly hepatotoxic and cause ultrastructural changes within hours of ingestion. Progression to hepatitis and cirrhosis occurs in some subjects even after cessation of intake, implying that host factor(s) influences susceptibility. Many of the immunological features of alcohol-induced disease (Box 14.6) are common to other types of liver injury and probably result from dysfunction of the mononuclear phagocytes of the liver (Kupffer cells).

BOX 14.4 ASSOCIATED SYNDROMES IN PATIENTS WITH PRIMARY BILIARY CIRRHOSIS.

- Sjögren's syndrome
- Sicca syndrome
- Autoimmune thyroid disease
- Systemic lupus erythematosus
- Scleroderma
- CREST syndrome
- Rheumatoid arthritis
- Fibrosing alveolitis
- Renal tubular acidosis

BOX 14.5 IMMUNOLOGICAL FEATURES IN PRIMARY SCLEROSING CHOLANGITIS

- Associated with HLA-B8, -DR3/-DR52
- Hypergammaglobulinaemia
- Positive antineutrophil cytoplasmic antibodies (ANCA) in 70% of patients—associated with a more severe course
- Increased expression of HLA class II antigens on biliary epithelial cells
- Associated with other diseases
  Ulcerative colitis
  Primary antibody deficiency

BOX 14.6 EVIDENCE FOR IMMUNOLOGICAL INVOLVEMENT IN ALCOHOLIC LIVER DISEASE

- The mononuclear cell infiltrate is composed mainly of T lymphocytes
- Reports of an increased prevalence of circulating autoantibodies, including antibodies to dsDNA, in patients with alcoholic hepatitis and/or cirrhosis
- Antibodies reacting with acetaldehyde-altered liver cell membrane antigens are present in some patients
- Lymphocytes from these patients are cytotoxic to hepatocytes in vitro
- Women who are HLA-B8 positive are especially susceptible

Table 14.10 Basic distinctions between directly toxic and hypersensitivity drug reactions

	Directly toxic	Hypersensitivity
Susceptibility	All subjects	Some subjects
Dose related?	Yes	No
Onset following first exposure	Immediate (hours–days)	Delayed (days–weeks)
Onset following second exposure	Immediate	Less delayed (days)

14.8.5 Drug-induced liver disease

A number of drugs can damage the liver; some drugs (or their metabolites) are directly hepatotoxic, while others induce a hypersensitivity reaction (Table 14.10).

Hypersensitivity reactions occur in only a minority of patients exposed to these drugs and the severity of the reaction is not dose related. The drug or a metabolite may combine with a component of the liver cell membrane or denature a 'self' antigen; in either case a 'new' antigen may be formed which is no longer tolerated as 'self'. However, successful attempts to prove immunological hypersensitivity to a drug are rare. The immunological features are usually non-specific, for example α-methyldopa, oxyphenisatin (a constituent of many laxatives) and isoniazid may all induce hepatitis. Although the reaction usually subsides when the drug is stopped, some patients progress insidiously to a form of chronic active hepatitis which is indistinguishable from the 'autoimmune' type and is often accompanied by circulating antibodies to nuclei, smooth muscle or liver and kidney microsomes. Deliberate rechallenge would clearly be unethical. In cases of halothane hepatitis, rechallenge has been inadvertent. The reaction may occur 1 or 2 weeks after the first operation, or earlier after subsequent exposure. Pyrexia and eosinophilia may precede the appearance of jaundice. Some patients, exposed to halothane on a number of occasions, have eventually lost their hypersensitivity; it is not known whether this was due to faster handling of the toxic metabolite (enzyme induction) or to the development of immunological tolerance.

FURTHER READING

See website: www.immunologyclinic.com

15.1 Introduction

Endocrine cells may be localized in a defined glandular structure such as the adrenal gland, or distributed throughout a non-endocrine organ such as the stomach. Functional disorders of endocrine glands result from **overactivity**, with excessive production of the hormone, or from **atrophy**, with failure to produce the relevant hormone. There are many causes of glandular dysfunction but autoimmunity to endocrine tissues is one of the commonest.

Most autoimmune endocrine disorders are clinically silent until they present with features of insufficiency of the affected organ. At this stage the gland is often irreversibly damaged with little prospect of recovery even if the autoimmune process were arrested. Current treatment of many of these diseases therefore centres around replacement of hormones. The long period of silent inflammation and glandular destruction, which can last for many years, offers a window during which progress of these diseases could potentially be reversed. However, detection and treatment of preclinical endocrine autoimmunity is currently confined to experimental studies involving small numbers of first-degree relatives of subjects with polyendocrine syndromes and autoimmune diabetes who are at increased risk of developing the condition.

15.2 Mechanisms of endocrine autoimmunity

Autoimmune reactions may be directed against endocrine cells, their receptors, hormones or receptors on target cells (Fig. 15.1).

Since the first report of autoimmune thyroid disease in 1957, autoimmune diseases of every endocrine organ and virtually all endocrine cells have been described.

Autoantibodies to endocrine cells are organ specific and detected only by tests using antigen from the specific endocrine gland involved (Chapter 19). This contrasts with non-organ-specific diseases (such as systemic lupus erythematosus), where non-organ-specific antigens (such as nuclear antigens) are present in all organs and tissues of the body. A feature of **organ-specific autoimmunity** is that several autoantibodies to endocrine glands may be found in a single patient; this patient may have clinical evidence of one or many endocrine disorders or may be asymptomatic.

There are several mechanisms of autoimmune damage (Fig. 15.1) and more than one mechanism may occur in a given disease. Evidence suggests that both T cells and antibodies often work in parallel to produce autoimmune endocrine disease. As a broad generalization, T cells (both CD4 and CD8) are responsible for glandular destruction and antibodies act via mechanisms discussed below to disturb

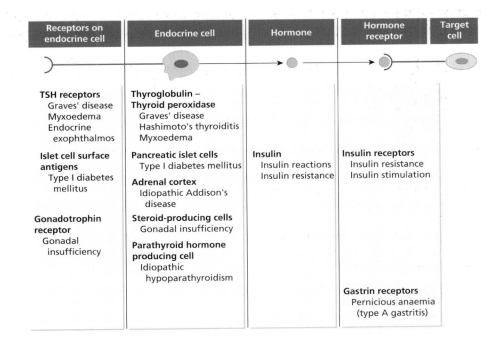

Fig. 15.1 Examples of autoantibodies in endocrine and other organ-specific autoimmune diseases.

the physiological function of the gland. Thus, in the autoimmune syndromes caused in neonates by transplacental transfer of IgG, the disturbance in endocrine physiology is transient and disappears with a time course consistent with the half-life of IgG (around 3 weeks), without any significant residual damage in the target organ.

Antibodies can influence the function or growth of an endocrine gland through its trophic hormone receptors. Stimulating and blocking antibodies are well recognized, as are antibodies that selectively influence cell growth. Patients may have a mixture of receptor antibodies, some of which stimulate and some of which block the receptor. Shifts from one type to the other explain why some patients fluctuate from overactivity to underactivity of the gland.

15.3 Thyroid disease

Several thyroid antigens are recognized, including thyroglobulin, thyroid peroxidase (thyroid microsomal antigen), Na^+ I^- symporter (responsible for iodine uptake by thyroid cells), surface and other cytoplasmic thyroid antigens. The most widely available and clinically useful antibody tests are those for **thyroid peroxidase** (see Chapter 19) (Table 15.1).

15.3.1 Thyrotoxicosis (Case 15.1)

Thyrotoxicosis is a common condition with a prevalence of about 20 per 1000 of the population. It can occur at any age, but the incidence peaks in the third and fourth decades. It is about five to 10 times more common in women than men.

Thyrotoxicosis is most commonly due to **Graves' disease** or to local hyperactive single or multiple nodules in the thyroid gland. The presence of autoantibodies to thyroid microsomal antigens confirms an autoimmune process, i.e. Graves' disease (see Table 15.1). Those patients who have high titres of these autoantibodies are the ones most likely to proceed to myxoedema.

Strong evidence that a circulating factor was responsible for Graves' disease was discovered over 40 years ago. Both thyroid-stimulating hormone (TSH) and sera from patients with Graves' disease stimulated thyroid secretion, but the sera had a more prolonged duration of action. This

Table 15.1 Prevalence and relative strength of antibodies to thyroid peroxidase commonly detected in various thyroid diseases

Clinical presentation	Antibodies to thyroid peroxidase
Thyrotoxicosis	
Graves' disease	Positive (low titre)
Hot nodules	Negative
Goitre	
Hashimoto's thyroiditis	Positive (high titre)
Simple goitre	Negative
De Quervain's thyroiditis	Transient positive
Carcinoma	Negative
Thyroxine deficiency	
Primary myxoedema	Positive
Normal population	Positive (5–10%)

CASE 15.1 GRAVES' DISEASE

A 29-year-old woman presented with a 3-month history of increased sweating and palpitations with weight loss of 7 kg. On examination, she was a nervous, agitated woman with an obvious, diffuse, non-tender, smooth enlargement of her thyroid, over which a bruit could be heard. She had a fine tremor of her fingers and a resting pulse rate of 150/min. She had no evidence of exophthalmos. A maternal aunt had suffered from 'thyroid disease'.

On investigation, she had a raised serum T3 of 4.8 nmol/l (NR 0.8–2.4) and a T4 of 48 nmol/l (NR 9–23). Measurement of her thyroid-stimulating hormone showed that this was low normal, 0.4 mU/l (NR 0.4–5 mU/l). The biochemical findings pointed to primary thyroid disease rather than pituitary overactivity. Circulating antibodies to thyroid peroxidase (titre 1/3000; 200 IU/ml) were detected by agglutination. A diagnosis of autoimmune thyrotoxicosis (Graves' disease) was made. She was treated with an antithyroid drug, carbimazole, to control her thyrotoxicosis, and surgery was not required.

was due to an IgG antibody to the TSH receptor on the surface of human thyroid cells (Fig. 15.2). Almost all patients with Graves' disease have TSH receptor antibodies which stimulate the thyroid cell (**thyroid-stimulating antibodies**) (Figs 15.2 and 15.3).

The autoimmune thyroid is characteristically infiltrated by T lymphocytes: both CD8+ and CD4+ cells are present. These T cells express a more limited number of T-cell receptor genes (see Chapter 1) than do peripheral blood T cells from the same patient; the implication is that intrathyroid T cells are less diverse because they are enriched for T cells specific for thyroid-derived peptides.

Two of every 1000 pregnant women are thyrotoxic; occasionally such pregnancies result in **neonatal Graves' dis-**

ease. This is due to transplacental transfer of thyroid-stimulating IgG from mother to fetus. The neonatal disease can be severe. Affected babies have a goitre, exophthalmos, feeding problems, pyrexia and tachycardia and may develop heart failure unless treated promptly. Spontaneous recovery gradually occurs over 2–3 months, as the maternal IgG is metabolized at a rate consistent with its half-life (i.e. 3 weeks).

The levels of thyroid antibodies in patients with Graves' disease and Hashimoto's thyroiditis (see section 15.3.2) tend to fall during pregnancy and rebound afterwards. Many pregnant women without overt thyroid disease develop fluctuations in thyroid autoantibodies, with transient disturbances of thyroid function—**post-partum thyroiditis**. The prevalence of the disorder is about 5–10% of all preg-

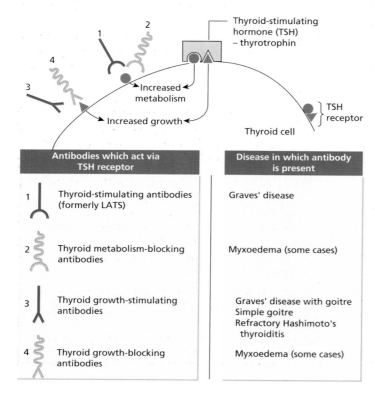

Antibodies which act via TSH receptor	Disease in which antibody is present
1 Thyroid-stimulating antibodies (formerly LATS)	Graves' disease
2 Thyroid metabolism-blocking antibodies	Myxoedema (some cases)
3 Thyroid growth-stimulating antibodies	Graves' disease with goitre Simple goitre Refractory Hashimoto's thyroiditis
4 Thyroid growth-blocking antibodies	Myxoedema (some cases)

Fig. 15.2 Surface of a thyroid cell showing actions of the primary antibodies in autoimmune thyroid diseases. LATS, Long-acting thyroid stimulator.

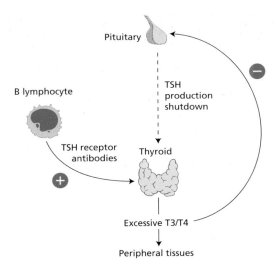

Fig. 15.3 Pituitary–thyroid axis in Graves' disease.

nancies. Thyroid dysfunction in the year following pregnancy should be treated cautiously, although the proportion of women with post-partum thyroiditis who later develop overt autoimmune thyroid disease is unknown.

The degree of thyrotoxicosis in Graves' disease is not related to the size of the goitre; indeed, 10% of patients do not have an enlarged thyroid. Thyroid growth-stimulating immunoglobulin (TGI) has been demonstrated in the sera of patients with Graves' disease with goitre, and in some patients with toxic multinodular goitres and non-toxic goitres. In contrast to the thyroid-stimulating immunoglobulins (TSI) which cause hyperthyroidism, these antibodies correlate with goitre size but not with the overproduction of T3 and T4.

Half of the patients with Graves' disease develop **exophthalmos**; this may precede, coincide with or follow the hyperthyroid phase. It may even occur occasionally in euthyroid patients or in association with Hashimoto's thyroiditis or primary myxoedema. Smoking is a strong risk factor. Exophthalmos is the result of two pathological processes: a myositis affecting the eye muscles and a proliferation of retro-orbital tissue. The myositis is accompanied by infiltration of lymphocytes. The sera from affected patients contain antibodies which bind to eye muscle extract; some of these antibodies cross-react with other orbital antigens as well as thyroid antigens. The TSH receptor seems to be aberrantly expressed in the inflamed orbital tissue, suggesting that an immune response to this antigen may also contribute to the eye disease. In patients with severe exophthalmos and optic nerve compression ('**malignant exophthalmos**'), high-dose steroids are of value, sometimes coupled with other immunosuppressive drugs. If there is deterioration, surgical

decompression is indicated. Irradiation of the orbit is also used, although the benefits are uncertain.

A few (3–5%) patients with Graves' disease develop **pretibial myxoedema**; they tend to have exophthalmos as well. Pretibial myxoedema refers to well-demarcated, subcutaneous thickening of the antero-lateral aspects of the legs; these areas do not pit on pressure, and are shiny and reddish brown in appearance. The development of pretibial myxoedema is not related to the duration or extent of the hyperthyroidism. Its pathogenesis is unknown, although, as in thyroid eye disease, aberrant expression of the TSH receptor has been described in the affected tissue.

Genetic factors are important in the aetiology of Graves' disease. A positive family history of hyperthyroidism is found in around 50% of patients and there is 50% concordance in monozygotic twins but less than 5% in dizygotic twins. HLA-DR3 and polymorphisms of the CTLA-4 gene (see Chapter 1) are both strongly associated with Graves' disease in Caucasians, and together contribute about 50% of the genetic susceptibility in this ethnic group. Genetic associations in other ethnic groups are less well defined. **Environmental** triggers of Graves' disease remain obscure. Some limited evidence exists for infection with a retrovirus in thyroid tissue in patients with the disease. There is also an association between the onset of Graves' disease and psychological stress. Treatment of multiple sclerosis with the lymphocyte-depleting monoclonal antibody Campath-1H can induce Graves' disease in around 10% of those treated, possibly by depleting an inhibitory T-cell population (see Chapter 5).

Graves' disease can be treated successfully by antithyroid drugs, radioactive iodine or surgery. Immunosuppressive therapy to reduce levels of the causative antibodies has not therefore proved necessary (see Box 15.1).

BOX 15.1 INDIRECT EVIDENCE IMPLICATING IMMUNOLOGICAL MECHANISMS IN THE PATHOGENESIS OF GRAVES' DISEASE

- Thyroid infiltration by T lymphocytes (both CD4+ and CD8+ cells) and plasma cells

- The presence of circulating autoantibodies to thyroid antigens, especially the TSH receptor. Antibodies to the TSH receptor cause stimulation of cultured thyroid cells

- An increased risk of thyroid disease in first-degree relatives of patients with Graves' disease

- Associations with other autoimmune diseases, including myasthenia gravis, pernicious anaemia and rheumatoid arthritis

- Transient Graves' disease in the neonates of pregnant women with Graves' disease

CASE 15.2 HASHIMOTO'S THYROIDITIS

A 39-year-old woman presented with a large, painless swelling in her neck. The enlargement had been a gradual process over 2 years. She had no other symptoms and felt generally well. On examination, her thyroid was diffusely enlarged and had a rubbery consistency. There were no signs of thyrotoxicosis or of thyroid failure.

Thyroid function tests showed that she was euthyroid; T3 was 1.2 nmol/l (NR 0.8–2.4), T4 was 12 nmol/l (NR 9–23) and TSH was 6.3 mU/l (NR 0.4–5 mU/l). However, her serum contained high-titre antibodies to thyroid peroxidase (1/64 000; 4000 IU/ml).

This patient had Hashimoto's thyroiditis. The goitre was huge, and she was treated by partial thyroidectomy; the goitre did not recur, and the patient has remained euthyroid for 12 years.

15.3.2 Hashimoto's thyroiditis (Case 15.2)

Hashimoto's disease is much more common in women than in men and is probably the commonest cause of goitre in the UK. At presentation, 75% of patients are euthyroid, 20% are hypothyroid, and the remaining 5% are hyperthyroid and have a disease which closely resembles Graves' disease (known as 'Hashitoxicosis'). *About 50% of patients eventually become hypothyroid due to destruction of the thyroid gland.* Hashimoto's thyroiditis is familial and associated with other organ-specific autoimmune diseases.

The **pathogenesis** (Box 15.2) of Hashimoto's thyroiditis involves T cells specifically sensitized against thyroid antigens, with an uncertain contribution from thyroid growth-stimulating antibodies. The goitre results from a combination of marked lymphocytic infiltration of the gland together with some degree of hypertrophy of thyroid tissue. The cellular infiltrate consists mainly of $CD8^+$ and $CD4^+$ T cells and some B cells which can form lymphoid follicles. These cells display activation markers and a range of cytokines can be detected in the inflamed tissue. Destruction of thyroid cells probably occurs by Fas-mediated apoptosis triggered by cytotoxic T cells (see Chapter 5). T cells responsive to thyroid antigens (particularly thyroid peroxidase and thyroglobulin) can be detected in both blood and thyroid tissue.

The **differential diagnosis** of Hashimoto's thyroiditis includes simple goitre and subacute (de Quervain's) thyroiditis. The latter usually presents with bilateral painful tender enlargement of the thyroid gland, a low-grade fever and general malaise. **De Quervain's thyroiditis** may be of infective origin, since the condition often follows a viral illness. Antibodies to thyroid antigens are usually transient and of low titre; high-titre antibodies to thyroid microsomes suggest considerable thyroid damage, and the patient may ultimately develop myxoedema. About 70% of the patients with this rare subacute thyroiditis have the HLA antigen B35, suggesting that susceptibility to this disease is also partly governed by the major histocompatibility complex but by a different region from other autoimmune endocrine diseases.

15.3.3 Idiopathic thyroid atrophy (myxoedema) (Case 15.3)

The term myxoedema describes the severe form of hypothyroidism in which deposition of mucinous substances leads to thickening of the skin and subcutaneous tissues, but is often used as a label for hypothyroidism in general. There are several causes (Fig. 15.4). **Idiopathic thyroid atrophy**, like Hashimoto's thyroiditis, is more commonly found in women. Thyroid biopsies show a lymphocytic infiltration, fibrosis and atrophy. Conventional antithyroid antibodies are present in roughly the same proportion of patients as in Hashimoto's thyroiditis (see Table 15.1).

The **pathogenesis** of idiopathic thyroid atrophy is interesting. Just as there are antibodies which stimulate thyroid cell metabolism (in Graves' disease) and those which stimulate growth (in simple and Hashimoto's goitre), so there are antibodies in idiopathic thyroid atrophy that block both growth and metabolism (see Fig. 15.2). Growth-blocking antibodies can occur in the absence of function-blocking antibodies. These appear to be primary antibodies which react with TSH receptors or other membrane sites and the reason for their production is unknown. Maternal growth-blocking

BOX 15.2 EVIDENCE FOR AN AUTOIMMUNE PATHOGENESIS IN HASHIMOTO'S THYROIDITIS

- T cells specific for thyroid antigens are present in the circulation. T-cell clones derived from these cells can kill cultured thyroid cells
- Demonstration of serum autoantibodies which stimulate or block the growth and division of thyroid cells
- Thyroid infiltration by T lymphocytes (both $CD4^+$ and $CD8^+$ cells) and plasma cells
- Induction of experimental, cell-mediated autoimmune thyroiditis by injection of thyroid antigens
- Association of other autoimmune diseases in given individuals and in families

CASE 15.3 PRIMARY MYXOEDEMA

A 41-year-old woman complained to her doctor that she 'always felt cold', and that she had become increasingly clumsy. Although she made no other complaint, her husband had noticed increasing physical and mental lethargy in his wife in recent months. One of her sisters had thyroid disease and her mother suffered from pernicious anaemia. On examination, her skin was dry, her voice was hoarse and her hair was coarse and brittle. Her pulse rate was 58/min, with a blood pressure of 140/70. Her tendon reflexes showed a markedly delayed relaxation phase.

Clinically, she had hypothyroidism and this was confirmed by thyroid function tests; her serum T3 was 0.4 nmol/l (NR 0.8–2.4), T4 was 4 nmol/l (NR 9–23), and TSH was 12.1 mU/l (NR 0.4–5 mU/l). High titres of autoantibodies to thyroid peroxidase were found in the patient's serum to a titre of 1/128 000 (6400 IU/ml). This patient therefore had primary myxoedema and she was treated with replacement doses of L-thyroxine.

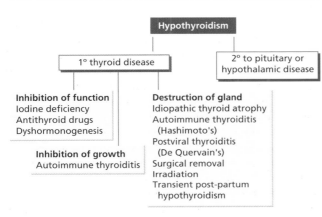

Fig. 15.4 Causes of hypothyroidism.

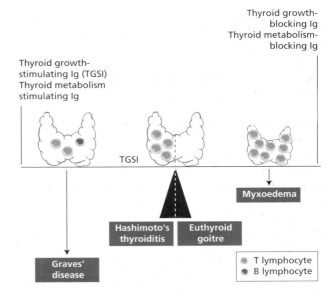

Fig. 15.5 Autoimmune thyroid disease. The clinical state depends on the balance between immunological mechanisms operating at any one time.

antibodies may play a part in the failure of the thyroid to develop in utero, so leading to athyreotic cretinism.

Like Graves' disease, the genetic predisposition to autoimmune hypothyroidism and Hashimoto's thyroiditis is linked to polymorphism within the HLA locus and the CTLA-4 gene. Unlike Graves' disease, there is no strong association with HLA-DR3, but instead a range of relatively weak associations with various HLA polymorphisms, which differ with ethnic group.

Environmental triggers are uncertain. Smoking, infection, and exposure to high and low levels of iodine have all been linked to hypothyroidism. Treatment with certain drugs (for example, lithium and interferon-α) can induce autoimmune hypothyroidism. Exposure to environmental radiation (e.g. following the Chernobyl disaster) has been associated with an increased incidence of thyroid autoimmunity, but the significance of this for sporadic thyroid disease is unclear. The high prevalence of subclinical thyroid autoimmunity in Western populations (see Table 15.1) suggests that environmental triggers must either be very widely distributed among the population or that no specific external trigger exists. This would be consistent with current models of autoimmunity, whereby autoimmune responses could po-

tentially develop after disruption of a target organ by many different inflammatory processes.

Autoimmune thyroid disease shows that the clinical state depends on the balance between the effects of sensitized T cells and autoantibodies against target antigens (Fig. 15.5). In this respect, autoimmune thyroid disease serves as a model for other autoimmune endocrine states.

15.4 Diabetes mellitus

15.4.1 Classification of diabetes mellitus

Diabetes is divided into **insulin-dependent diabetes mellitus (IDDM or type 1)** and **non-insulin-dependent diabetes mellitus (NIDDM or type 2)**. The contrasting features of these types are shown in Table 15.2. Type 1 diabetes can

Table 15.2 Types of diabetes mellitus

Features	Type I	Type II
Prevalence	1 : 3000 population	3 : 100 population
Age at onset	Usually < 30 years	Usually > 40 years
Speed of clinical onset	Acute	Insidious
Associated with autoimmune disorders	Yes	No
Islet cell antibodies	Yes	No
Other autoantibodies	Sometimes	No
Percentage of cases of diabetes mellitus	10–20%	80–90%
HLA association	DR3 and DR4	No

be subdivided further into two main forms: type 1A, usually of childhood onset and characterized by immunologically-mediated destruction of the β-cells of pancreatic islets, and type 1B, where severe β-cell destruction occurs in the absence of any obvious immune response directed against the pancreas. Antibodies against islet cells can be detected in type 1A but not type 1B diabetes. Confusingly, the term type 1b diabetes has also been used in the past, especially in the UK, to describe a subset of autoimmune diabetes of adult onset and often associated with other autoimmune diseases (see section 15.10).

15.4.2 Immunopathogenesis of diabetes mellitus

Like thyroid disease, diabetes mellitus is an organ-specific autoimmune disease and is associated with other organ-specific autoimmune diseases such as thyrotoxicosis. *Insulin production fails in autoimmune diabetes because of a specific immune response directed against the insulin-producing β-cells in the pancreatic islets of Langerhans.* Histological studies show extensive immune infiltration of the islets by activated CD8 and CD4 T cells and macrophages, reduction in the number of β-cells and relative sparing of the glucagon-producing α-cells. β-Cells show expression of both class II MHC and co-stimulatory molecules, indicating that they may present autoantigens to CD4+ T cells. Cellular infiltration of the islets, and consequent β-cell damage, may precede overt diabetes by many years, sometimes decades; the presence of subclinical β-cell destruction is suggested by the presence of circulating ICA, activated T cells and impaired glucose tolerance long before clinical diabetes develops (Fig. 15.6).

Numerous **autoantigens** have been identified in autoimmune diabetes. Antibody responses, and to a lesser extent T-cell responses, against these antigens have been studied in detail. Those most closely linked to the disease include islet cell cytoplasmic enzymes—particularly glutamic acid decarboxylase (**GAD**) and **IA-2** (a tyrosine phosphatase) and **insulin** itself. Islet cell antibodies (**ICA**) detected by immunofluorescence are probably made up of a mixture of

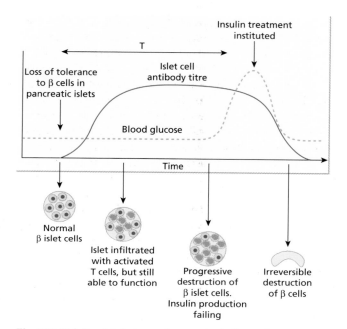

Fig. 15.6 Relationship between immunologically mediated damage to islet cells, islet cell antibodies as a marker of this process and blood glucose. The time interval 't' represents the window of opportunity for immunological intervention to prevent diabetes.

antibodies reacting against GAD and several other cytoplasmic antigens. The relationship between these autoimmune responses and islet cell damage is not well defined, but the recurrence of diabetes following pancreatic transplantation between IDDM-discordant identical twins, histological studies and evidence from animal models suggest that β-cells are probably killed by cytotoxic T cells, with autoantibodies playing a more minor role.

Among the numerous potential autoantigens, GAD has been the subject of particular interest. Antibodies to GAD were first described in the neurological condition called '**stiff man syndrome**', which is often associated with IDDM and ICA. Antibodies to GAD are highly predictive of subsequent development of IDDM, and T- and B-cell responses to GAD have been shown to be of major pathogenic importance in an animal model of diabetes.

Genetic factors make a considerable contribution to the risk of developing type 1A IDDM. An unaffected identical twin of a newly diagnosed diabetic has an approximately 45% chance of subsequently developing the disease, compared with a risk of 0.4% in the general population. A substantial proportion of this genetic predisposition can be accounted for by associations with specific MHC polymorphisms. Around 95% of diabetics from north European ethnic groups possess HLA-DR3 or -DR4 (compared with around 45% of healthy subjects), and around 40% of Caucasian type 1A diabetics are DR3/DR4 heterozygotes (compared with only 2.5% of healthy subjects). Studies of HLA genes at the molecular level showed that this association with HLA-DR is secondary to a stronger link with certain HLA-DQ variants: particularly the DR3, DQ2 or DR4, DQ8 haplotypes. A critical factor seems to be the amino acid at position 57 in the HLA-DQβ chain. Genetic variants of DQB which encode the amino acid aspartate at this position seem to confer protection against IDDM, whereas variants encoding other amino acids increase the risk. The HLA-DR3 and -DR4 association arises because, in north European populations, these DR alleles are linked to DQB alleles which do not encode aspartate. The mechanism behind this very specific molecular association is not known, but amino acid 57 in HLA-DQβ lies in the 'antigen-binding groove' and could potentially influence binding of a critical autoantigenic peptide. No genetic associations have been identified for type 1B diabetes.

Although this is the strongest and most clearly defined association between a gene and risk of diabetes, detailed studies of large numbers of families suggest that interactions between **10–15** genes are important in controlling the onset of IDDM. The locus with the second strongest linkage to IDDM is a non-coding region of the insulin gene; polymorphisms in this region may influence how strongly the insulin gene is expressed in the thymus.

The observation that more than 50% of non-diabetic identical twins of newly diagnosed diabetics do not ultimately develop diabetes shows that **environmental** factors also play a role in triggering this disease. This is further emphasized by a marked global increase in incidence of IDDM over the last decade, and the seasonal variation in diagnosis, with autumn and winter peaks. Models of environmental causation of IDDM have centred around infectious agents, although exposure to cow's milk or other food proteins has also been suggested as risk factors. A small number of cases of diabetes can be temporally linked to specific infections, particularly with viruses which are known to have a tropism for the pancreas such as mumps and coxsackie. Similarities have been noted between the sequence of certain coxsackie virus proteins and ICA such as GAD, suggesting a potential for autoimmunity triggered by molecular mimicry (see Chapter 5). However, the only infection which has been unequivocally linked to type 1 diabetes is congenital rubella, which is now very rare. Most newly diagnosed diabetics, however, show no consistent relationship with any specific infection. It should be noted that current models of autoimmunity (Chapter 5) do not require a specific trigger, and that autoimmune disease could potentially follow a variety of inflammatory insults to the target organ.

Because IDDM is immunologically mediated, attempts have been made to prevent IDDM by immunotherapy. Attempts to stop β-cell destruction have involved intensive immunosuppressive therapy (e.g. ciclosporin or monoclonal antibody) started at diagnosis, when probably less than 10% of functioning β-cell mass remains. Not surprisingly, success in inducing remission of diabetes has been limited. Controlled trials have shown the efficacy of ciclosporin in maintaining remission for at least the first year after the onset of disease in about 25% of newly diagnosed diabetics. Uncertainty about the long-term safety and efficacy of ciclosporin limits its use. An alternative approach would be to induce specific tolerance to major ICA. It is not known whether this could be achieved in human IDDM, but animal experiments suggest that administration of autoantigen by particular routes (especially via mucosal surfaces) can alter the immune response to that antigen, and both prevent and arrest the course of IDDM.

Pancreatic transplantation has been limited by multiple surgical problems, together with the need for immunosuppression to prevent rejection. Strategies are under development which might allow specific transplant of islet cells in a form resistant to immunological attack.

Type II diabetes is not associated with ICA. This type of diabetes shows a strong familial tendency, but no association with autoimmunity or with any particular HLA type. However, over 10% of adult patients initially treated by diet or oral hypoglycaemic drugs do have ICA in their sera at presentation. Often these patients eventually require insulin therapy to achieve satisfactory diabetic control; therefore, they are latent type 1 diabetics.

15.4.3 Complications of diabetes mellitus

Infection is a major complication of diabetes mellitus. The mechanism of increased susceptibility to infection is not fully understood, although poorly controlled diabetics have defects in neutrophil function which reverse following adequate insulin therapy. The pattern of infection seen in poorly controlled diabetes is consistent with a neutrophil defect, with a high incidence of staphylococcal and fungal infection.

CASE 15.4 DIABETES MELLITUS

A 26-year-old pregnant woman attended the antenatal clinic regularly. She had no family history of diabetes. At 24 weeks' gestation she was found to have asymptomatic glycosuria. A glucose tolerance test showed that not only was her fasting blood glucose raised but she had poor glucose tolerance. Gestational diabetes was diagnosed and the patient was admitted for diabetic control. This was achieved on oral hypoglycaemic agents alone and the patient was instructed to check her urine daily. The pregnancy was uneventful and a normal, 3.8 kg baby was born. The patient's glucose tolerance returned to normal in the puerperium; however, her serum, which was found to contain antibodies to pancreatic islet cells at the time of diagnosis, remained positive. Nine years later, after yearly checks, the patient developed overt diabetes mellitus.

The long-term complications of diabetes mellitus involve diseases of major arteries (leading to atheroma) or of capillaries (microangiopathy). Microangiopathy is responsible for the retinal and glomerular lesions of diabetes. In developed countries, diabetic retinopathy accounts for much of the acquired blindness in young and middle-aged adults. Retinopathy is rarely found within 5 years of diagnosis, but more than one-third of patients are affected 15–20 years after diagnosis. Long-term control of blood glucose and other cardiovascular risk factors (such as hypertension and serum cholesterol) reduces the incidence and severity of these complications.

15.4.4 Are immunological tests useful? (Case 15.4)

Immunological tests have no part to play in the clinical diagnosis of diabetes mellitus. The autoantibody response to islet cell antigens does, however, powerfully predict the risk of developing IDDM in first-degree relatives (Fig. 15.7): the risk of diabetes increases dramatically with the number of antigens targeted by the antibody response. If antibodies are detected against three major antigens, development of diabetes is virtually certain to develop over the next few years. The titre of ICAs is also important in determining outcome: among relatives of patients with IDDM, over 50% of those with high-titre ICAs develop IDDM compared with less than 10% of those with low-titre antibodies. In a population sample of school children, those positive for ICA were about 500 times more likely to develop IDDM over a 10-year period than children negative for serum ICA. At present, there are no safe and effective immunological interventions to prevent islet cell destruction in those individuals at high risk of diabetes. However, once such therapies are available, the case for clinical screening programmes will become very strong.

15.5 Adrenal disease

Primary adrenocortical hypofunction, or **Addison's disease**, is an uncommon disease which affects six in every 100 000 of the population. Some cases of Addison's disease are due to destruction of the adrenal cortex by tuberculosis, other granulomatous diseases or carcinoma (primary or secondary); the majority (75–80%) of cases, called idiopathic Addison's disease, are autoimmune in origin, i.e. autoimmune adrenalitis.

15.5.1 Autoimmune adrenal disease (Case 15.5)

Over three-quarters of all cases of Addison's disease are due to an autoimmune adrenalitis which affects the adrenal cortex but spares the medulla. Like other autoimmune endocrinopathies, it is more common in women and reaches a maximum incidence between 40 and 50 years of age. Patients' sera should be tested for all organ-specific autoantibodies, as 40% of patients have at least one other autoimmune endocrinopathy (Table 15.3). The presence of autoantibodies may predict future onset of the disease, so that replacement therapy (or other relevant treatment) can be started promptly.

Evidence for immune involvement in idiopathic Addison's disease is shown in Box 15.3. The presence of antibodies to cytoplasmic adrenal cortex antigens in this disease sug-

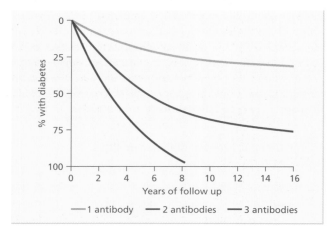

Fig. 15.7 The relationship between the number of autoantibody specificities directed against insulin, IA-2 and/or GAD detected in the serum of first-degree relatives of patients with type 1 diabetes, and subsequent development of diabetes. Those patients with three antibodies develop diabetes fastest.

CASE 15.5 ADDISON'S DISEASE

A 12-year-old girl presented with vague abdominal discomfort for 6 months. She had noticed occasional diarrhoea but had not passed any blood. She admitted to weight loss (6 kg) and anorexia. On examination, she was obviously pigmented, although she thought this was sun induced; however, her buccal mucosa and gums were also brown. There were no other physical signs.

She had a low cortisol level and her response to the adrenocorticotrophic hormone in a Synacthen test was poor. A diagnosis of adrenal cortical failure was made. X-ray of her abdomen showed no calcified areas in either adrenal gland, and her serum contained antibodies to adrenal cortex, consistent with a diagnosis of Addison's disease due to autoimmune adrenalitis. Her serum also contained antibodies to pancreatic islet cells and thyroid microsomes. In view of her young age at presentation and these serum antibodies, she will be followed at yearly intervals to see if she develops other autoimmune endocrinopathies (see below).

Table 15.3 Association of 'idiopathic' Addison's disease with other endocrine diseases

Associated autoimmune disease	Patients (%) with other organ involvement
Thyroid diseases	19
Diabetes mellitus	15
Ovarian failure	8
Hypoparathyroidism	4
Pernicious anaemia	2

BOX 15.3 EVIDENCE FOR IMMUNE INVOLVEMENT IN IDIOPATHIC ADDISON'S DISEASE

- Association with other autoimmune diseases
- Presence of autoantibody to steroid cells of adrenal cortex, especially to 21α-hydroxylase, and high incidence of other organ-specific autoantibodies
- Diffuse lymphocytic infiltration of adrenal cortex
- Evidence of cell-mediated immunity to adrenal cortex antigens
- Adrenal failure produced experimentally in animals by immunization with adrenal tissue, with transfer by lymph node cells

gests immune involvement, since fewer than 5% of patients with adrenal damage due to tuberculosis have this antibody. Cell-mediated immunity to adrenal tissue can be demonstrated in about 60% of patients with 'idiopathic' Addison's disease. Circulating antibodies to corticotrophin receptors have also been detected which block adrenocorticotrophic hormone (ACTH)-induced adrenal cell growth in vitro; such antibodies are probably pathogenic autoantibodies.

One of the key enzymes in steroid biosynthesis, 21α-hydroxylase, seems to be the major target autoantigen in adrenal autoimmunity.

15.6 Parathyroid disease

Some cases of parathyroid failure, usually in childhood, are due to organ-specific autoimmunity. These are often accompanied by Addison's disease, premature ovarian failure or pernicious anaemia. Vitiligo may precede autoimmune hypoparathyroidism. Autoantibodies to cytoplasmic parathyroid tissue are detected in 30–70% of patients with idiopathic hypoparathyroidism.

15.7 Gonadal disease

15.7.1 Oophoritis

Primary amenorrhoea or premature menopause are often described in women with autoimmune disease, particularly 'idiopathic' Addison's disease, myxoedema or hypoparathyroidism. Histologically, the ovaries show lymphocytic infiltration (oophoritis), as do the other target organs in autoimmune endocrinopathies. These women sometimes have **steroidal cell antibodies** which react with Leydig cells, ovarian granulosa and theca interna cells. The presence of such antibodies predicts ovarian failure, especially in patients who have Addison's or other autoimmune disease and yet still have normal menstrual function. Sera from other women with a premature menopause inhibit the binding of follicle-stimulating hormone (FSH) to its receptor. The pathogenic significance of ovarian antibodies in autoimmune oophoritis remains to be determined.

15.8 Infertility

15.8.1 Immunology of infertility

Five to 15% of infertile couples show evidence of sperm antibodies. These antibodies may be produced by the man, the woman or both.

Experimental male animals can be made sterile by active or passive immunization against testicular or seminal antigens. In man, damage to the seminal tract by surgery, accidental trauma, occlusion or infection may trigger autoimmunity to testicular and seminal antigens. For example, antisperm antibodies appear in the serum in 50% of vasectomized men within 6–12 months of surgery. Antisperm antibodies seldom appear in seminal plasma following vasectomy, as local antibody production occurs proximal to the operation site. High titres of antisperm antibodies may appear in the semen after reversal by vasovasostomy and affect the success of the reversal.

15.9 Pituitary disease

Compared with other endocrine organs, autoimmune disease of the pituitary is rare. Patients who have multiple autoimmune endocrine diseases occasionally have antibodies that stain normal human pituitary gland, but the significance of these is unclear.

15.10 Autoimmune polyendocrine disease

The close relationship between different autoimmune endocrine diseases is clear from preceding discussions. They may overlap not only in individual patients but also in other members of a family. The association of at least two autoimmune endocrinopathies in a single patient is known as **autoimmune polyendocrine** disease.

Three principal patterns of autoimmune polyendocrine disease have been identified, although not all cases fit neatly into this pattern. These syndromes show a strong tendency to aggregate within families, although sporadic cases do occur. Families with so-called **type I polyglandular syndromes** have autoimmune failure particularly of the parathyroids, adrenal cortex and gonads together with chronic mucocutaneous candidiasis. This autosomal recessive syndrome, also known as **APECED (Autoimmune Polyendocrinopathy, Candidiasis and Ectodermal Dysplasia)**, is caused by mutations in the AIRE gene (see Chapter 5). Families with **type 2 polyglandular syndromes** have adrenal failure together with thyroid and/or islet cell autoimmunity. **Type 3 polyendocrine disease** consists of the combination of thyroid autoimmunity with at least two other autoimmune disorders, particularly pernicious anaemia, IDDM and non-

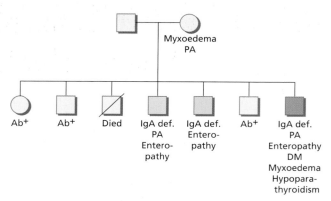

Fig. 15.8 A family study in type 3 autoimmune polyendocrinopathy. Ab+, Autoantibody positive but no clinical disease; DM, diabetes mellitus; IgA def., IgA deficiency; PA, pernicious anaemia.

endocrine immunological disorders such as IgA deficiency, autoimmune enteropathy or myasthenia gravis. Type 2 and 3 autoimmune syndromes are genetically heterogeneous, although both have been linked to the A1 B8 DR3 haplotype and tend to have a dominant pattern of inheritance (Fig. 15.8). An X-linked syndrome has also been described, characterised by diarrhoea, diabetes, hypothyroidism and eczema. This syndrome, known as **IPEX (Immune dysregulation, Polyendocrinopathy and X-linked Inheritance)** is caused by mutations in a gene encoding a transcription factor which is expressed at high levels in CD4 CD25 regulatory T cells.

There is a strong link between coeliac disease (section 14.4.2) and type 1A diabetes. Approximately 10% of patients with type 1 diabetes have tissue transglutaminase and/or endomysial IgA antibodies, and about half of these patients have histological evidence of coeliac disease on small bowel biopsy, which is usually clinically silent. There is overlap between the genetic predisposition to these two diseases, with the DR3, DQ2 haplotype being strongly associated with both.

FURTHER READING

See website: www.immunologyclinic.com

16 Haematological Diseases

16.1 Introduction

Since many of the components of the immune system circulate in blood, it is not surprising that there is some overlap between immunology and haematology. Malignancies of lymphocytes, namely leukaemias and lymphomas, are discussed in Chapter 6. In this chapter, those haematological diseases in which the immune response plays a pathogenic role will be considered, for example anaemia, thrombocytopenia, neutropenia or disordered blood clotting can all be due to **antibodies directed against components of blood**. In most cases, these antibodies are autoantibodies. However, disease also results from the stimulation of alloantibodies (isoimmune antibodies) by repeated blood transfusions or pregnancy (see Chapter 18). Direct activation of complement by erythrocytes and the role of the immune system in bone marrow failure (such as aplastic anaemia) are also discussed here.

The pathophysiology of anaemia (Fig. 16.1) is a good model for immune reductions in circulating cells in general, illustrating failure of production or excess destruction of any blood component.

16.1.1 Mechanisms of immune destruction

The immune system can destroy mature erythrocytes, plate-

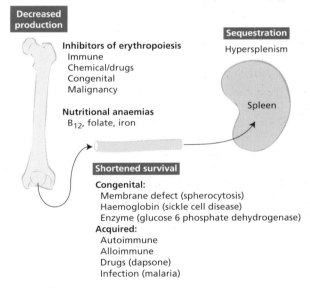

Fig. 16.1 The pathophysiology of anaemia.

lets and neutrophils as well as some haematological precursors in the bone marrow. Immune destruction of red cells is the best known and is used as the model below, though the **mechanisms are common** to all forms of destruction of cellular blood components resulting in cytopenias (Box 16.1).

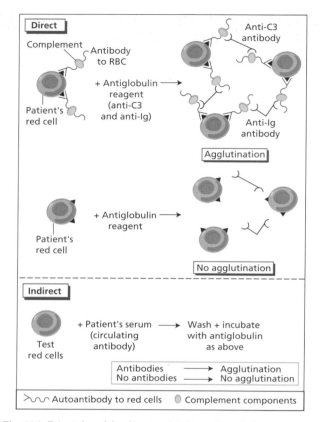

Fig. 16.3 Principles of the direct and indirect Coombs' tests.

BOX 16.1 MECHANISMS OF DESTRUCTION IN CYTOPENIAS

- Antibodies attach to antigen on cell surfaces prior to phago-cytosis in spleen—most common

- Complement-mediated lysis following antibody binding—less common

- Direct complement lysis without antibody involvement—rare

- Soluble immune complexes binding via CR1 (C3b) receptors (immune adherence)

- Soluble immune complexes binding via Fc receptors (innocent bystander destruction)

16.2 Autoimmune haemolytic anaemias

The common **causes** of anaemia are given in Fig. 16.1, which shows that the immune system is not often involved; nutritional deficiencies account for many more cases of anaemia than autoimmune processes. Autoimmune haemolytic anaemia (AIHA) is the commonest cause of shortened survival of red cells in Caucasians, though hereditary defects are more common in other racial groups.

AIHA may be **primary** (idiopathic, with no known cause) or **secondary** to pre-existing disease. Autoantibodies formed in the secondary cases do not appear to be any different, either serologically or immunochemically, from those in primary AIHA. Figure 16.2 shows the different types.

The **diagnosis** of AIHA depends on the demonstration of autoantibodies attached to the patient's red cells or free in the serum. The screening test used is the Coombs' test (Fig. 16.3); antibodies and complement components are detected on the surface of red cells by means of an antiglobulin

reagent. This is a mixture of antibodies that reacts with IgG, IgM or C3 but cannot distinguish between specific antibodies directed against red cells and immune complexes. In practice, the only immune complexes that are adsorbed sufficiently firmly to be a problem are drug–antibody complexes. Therefore, if the patient has signs of increasing haemolysis and no history of medication, a positive Coombs' test is good presumptive evidence that an AIHA is present. Specific antibodies to IgG, IgM and C3 can be used at different incubation temperatures to type the AIHA (Box 16.2) and antibodies eluted off the red cell surface to enable typing of their specificity.

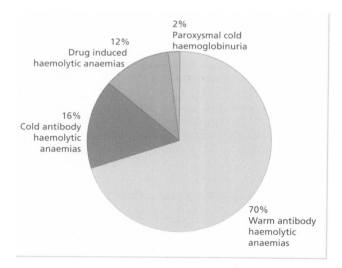

Fig. 16.2 Frequencies of different types of haemolytic anaemias.

BOX 16.2 ANTIBODIES IN AUTOIMMUNE HAEMOLYTIC ANAEMIA

- Warm reactive IgG autoantibodies, which are best detected at 37 °C

- Cold reactive IgM autoantibodies, which are detected at temperatures below 37 °C

- Drug-provoked immune haemolytic anaemias

- Complement-activating IgG of paroxysmal cold haemoglobulinuria (Fig. 16.4)

CASE 16.1 PRIMARY AUTOIMMUNE HAEMOLYTIC ANAEMIA

A 32-year-old man gradually noticed that he had 'yellow eyes' and dark urine, felt continually tired, and was short of breath when climbing stairs. He had no other symptoms; in particular, there was no itching, fever or bleeding, and he was not taking any drugs. On examination, he was anaemic and jaundiced but afebrile, with no palpable lymphadenopathy, hepatosplenomegaly, rash or arthropathy.

On investigation, his haemoglobin was very low at 54 g/l. The white cell count appeared raised (40 × 10⁹/l), but this was due to nucleated red cells being counted as leucocytes by the automated counter. The blood film showed gross polychromasia with nucleated red cells and spherocytes; the reticulocyte count was 9%. His serum bilirubin (47 mmol/l), aspartate transaminase (90 IU/l) and lactate dehydrogenase levels (5721 IU/l) were raised. Further

tests showed that his red cells had IgG and C3 on their surfaces by the direct Coombs' test. Serum contained warm non-specific autoantibodies (i.e. reactive with all the red cells in the test panel). Antinuclear antibodies and rheumatoid factor tests were negative and immunoglobulin levels were normal; there were no paraprotein bands in his serum or urine. Large amounts of urinary haemosiderin were detected.

A laboratory diagnosis of primary AIHA due to warm antibodies (leading to haemolysis and jaundice) was made. He failed to respond to high-dose corticosteroids and had a splenectomy 3 weeks later. Although impalpable, the spleen was twice the normal size; histology did not reveal a malignancy. He made a good post-operative recovery; his haemoglobin rose rapidly and the reticulocyte count fell.

16.2.1 Warm antibody haemolytic anaemias

The **warm antibody type** of AIHA (Table 16.1) affects all ages and both sexes, although most patients are over 30 years old. It is of varying severity and may be transient or persist for years. About one-half of the patients have idiopathic disease (Table 16.1), but in the remainder the anaemia is secondary to lymphoma or autoimmune disease, especially systemic lupus erythematosus (SLE) (see Fig. 16.4). The aetiology of primary idiopathic AIHA is unknown, although there are sporadic reports of familial occurrences of AIHA.

Red cells from AIHA patients are **direct Coombs' test positive**. The commonest reaction pattern (50%) is to find that the red cells have both IgG and C3 fixed on their surfaces and, in 40% of cases, only IgG is found. In the remaining 10%, complement alone is detected, nearly always in the

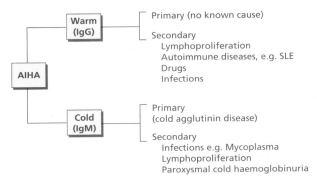

Fig. 16.4 Causes of different types of haemolytic anaemias.

form of C3d (see Chapter 1). The immunoglobulin is nearly always polyclonal, i.e. of mixed κ and λ light chain types.

Table 16.1 Comparative features of warm and cold autoimmune haemolytic anaemia (AIHA)

	Warm AIHA	Cold AIHA
Age (in years)	30+	60+
Cause of symptoms	Chronic haemolysis	Peripheral microvascular obstruction, e.g. Raynaud's phenomenon
Mechanism of anaemia	Opsonization and phagocytosis	Intravascular haemolysis related to cold
Jaundice	Common	Uncommon
Splenomegaly	Common	Uncommon
Underlying disease	Present in approx. 50%	Occasional
Response to steroids	Good	Poor
Response to splenectomy	50% of cases improve	Poor
Usual class of antibody + type of response	IgG — polyclonal	IgM — monoclonal/polyclonal
Commonest specificity of antibody	Usually non-specific	Anti-I antigen

Free autoantibodies can also be demonstrated in the serum of about one-third of patients by an indirect antiglobulin test (see Fig. 16.3). In most cases, the IgG class autoantibodies are non-agglutinating and therefore called 'incomplete' by haematologists. A positive test for free autoantibody is associated with more severe haemolysis (as in Case 16.1). If enzyme-treated cells are used, the sensitivity of the test is increased due to a reduction of surface charge, making the cells more 'agglutinable'.

Many of the antibodies can be **eluted** from the red cells' surfaces even if there is no free antibody in the serum. These polyclonal autoantibodies may have specificity against a particular red cell antigen or represent a mixture of antibodies against common erythrocyte surface antigens.

The commonest pathogenesis in warm antibody haemolytic anaemia is coating of red cells by opsonizing antibody alone or antibody and complement components (including C3b) followed by their removal from the circulation by **splenic macrophages** (Box 16.1).

Management consists of attempts to reduce antibody production and excessive red cell destruction. Corticosteroids are the mainstay of treatment and have reduced mortality considerably. Other immunosuppressive drugs, such as cyclophosphamide and azathioprine, have been used as steroid-sparing agents. Unfortunately, the condition tends to relapse when azathioprine is stopped.

Splenectomy is nearly always beneficial if steroids fail; as well as removing the site of phagocytosis, a source of autoantibody production is eliminated. This has to be balanced against the increased risk of infection (see section 3.5.1). Removal of B cells producing the autoantibodies is also achieved by Rituximab (Chapter 7) and is successful in 40% or so of AIHA patients, but at the cost of destroying all mature B cells and resulting transient antibody deficiency. *Blood transfusion is contraindicated unless anaemia is life threatening.*

16.2.2 Cold antibody haemolytic anaemias

Cold antibody haemolytic anaemias may be primary or secondary (Fig. 16.4). Patients with **cold haemagglutinin disease (CHAD)** present with a chronic haemolytic anaemia (anaemia, haemoglobinuria and jaundice) and severe Raynaud's phenomenon on exposure to cold (see Table 16.1). Idiopathic CHAD is the most common form and is a disorder of the elderly; secondary cases occasionally occur in association with non-Hodgkin's lymphoma, Mycoplasma pneumoniae infection or infectious mononucleosis. Rarely, a patient who has had 'idiopathic' CHAD for years develops a lymphoma.

The red cells become coated with IgM antibodies in the **patient's cold extremities**. As the blood warms up again, complement is activated and intravascular haemolysis results. This is one of few known examples of a direct haemolytic role of complement in vivo. Red cells from all patients with CHAD have detectable IgM on their surfaces at 4 °C; on warming, the antibody detaches from the erythrocyte surface, but fixed C3d can still be detected by a Coombs' test. The temperature between which the antibody reacts with the red cell antigens is termed the **thermal range**.

Free cold autoantibodies (**cold agglutinins**) are also present in the patient's serum. Ninety percent of pathological cold antibodies are specific for I antigen (Case 16.2). This antigen occurs on adult red cells and the 'i' antigen, by contrast, on cord blood cells. Eight percent of cold antibodies are anti-i; such cases are usually associated with infectious mononucleosis. In contrast to warm agglutinins (see Table 16.1), the cold antibodies found in idiopathic CHAD or in association with a lymphoma are monoclonal; those that develop after an infection are polyclonal. However, the amount of monoclonal antibody is usually far too small to be detectable as a paraprotein by serum electrophoresis.

CASE 16.2 COLD HAEMAGGLUTININ DISEASE

A 77-year-old man presented one winter with malaise and very cold hands and feet. He admitted to a tendency to bruise easily, and to passing dark urine in cold weather. He was not on any medication, and was a non-smoker. On examination, he had some bruising on the shins and was mildly jaundiced. His fingers and toes were cold, but not ischaemic. He had small but palpable lymph nodes in both axillae and groins but no hepatosplenomegaly.

His haemoglobin was low (100 g/l) and the blood film showed rouleaux formation (autoagglutination) and polychromasia; neutrophil, lymphocyte and platelet counts were normal. He had raised serum bilirubin and lactate dehydrogenase levels: serum folate and vitamin B_{12} measurements were normal. He had normal IgG (8.3 g/l) and IgA (1.2 g/l) levels and a slightly raised IgM (4.2 g/l); electrophoresis of serum and urine showed no paraprotein bands. He had a normal level of serum β_2- microglobulin. However, there were cold antibodies in his serum, which agglutinated red cells of 'I' specificity. A laboratory diagnosis of cold haemagglutinin disease leading to haemolysis and mild jaundice was made. He was advised to keep as warm as possible at all times. He has been seen regularly over the last 8 years but has not required active treatment or developed an overt lymphoid malignancy.

CASE 16.3 CEPHALOSPORIN-INDUCED HAEMOLYTIC ANAEMIA

A 72-year-old woman with osteoarthritis suffered acute haemolysis after her right hip was replaced. She had no evidence of splenomegaly and no lymphadenopathy to suggest an underlying malignancy. No explanation was found for the episode; warm and cold antibody tests were negative. She remained well until she had the other hip replaced 2 years later, when she again developed haemolysis soon after the anaesthetic. This time anaesthetic agents were suspected and she was tested for IgG antibodies to induction agents, although the mechanism of involvement in haemolysis was speculative. Unfortunately, this operation was not so successful and needed revision 7 months later; she haemolysed again, but this time the prophylactic antibiotic was suspected. Her serum was found to react with red cells coated with the cephalosporin used at the time of anaesthetic induction. She was advised that she had cephalosporin-induced haemolytic anaemia and to avoid this antibiotic in the future. She invested in a MediAlert bracelet to ensure that she was not given cephalosporins even if unconscious.

Treatment is usually unnecessary provided that the patient keeps the extremities warm. Steroid treatment and splenectomy are relatively ineffective since red cell destruction is predominantly intravascular. Treatment of an underlying lymphoma may stop the haemolysis, especially if Rituximab is used. Plasma exchange removes circulating IgM rapidly in severe cases.

16.2.3 Drug-induced autoimmune haemolytic anaemias

Drugs can provoke an AIHA (Case 16.3) by three mechanisms (Box 16.3). Not all patients with a positive Coombs' test develop overt haemolysis; *only those affected clinically need to have the drug withdrawn.*

16.2.4 Paroxysmal nocturnal haemoglobinuria

Paroxysmal nocturnal haemoglobinuria (PNH) is a rare disorder of stem cells in which a mutation in the PIG-A gene results in the **production of abnormal anchor protein (GPI)** in red cells, granulocytes and platelets. The haemolytic manifestations are due to failure of inhibition of ongoing complement activation on the surface of the abnormal erythrocytes. Although the name suggests that haemolysis occurs at night, it can occur at any time, intermittently, and particularly associated with intercurrent infections, surgery or immunization.

The proportion of abnormal cells in a given patient is **highly variable**. Some patients have fewer than 2% PNH clones, whereas others have over 90%. Patients with only a small proportion of abnormal cells may show no overt haemoglobinuria and yet develop chronic haemolytic anaemia. Some patients have a thrombotic tendency due to abnormal platelets, while others seem prone to infections, presumably due to defective neutrophil function.

The basic abnormalities lie in the cell membrane protein, GPI; abnormalities of this protein allow the alternate complement pathway to proceed once activated, resulting in lysis. This forms the basis of the Ham's test, in which lysis of the patient's red cells is produced by serum acidified to activate the alternate pathway. Normal red cells are protected by the presence of **two complement-inhibitory proteins** on their surface; these **are missing** in PNH.

Treatment of mild PNH is largely symptomatic but patients with severe PNH, particularly if associated with myelodysplasia, are good candidates for bone marrow transplantation.

16.2.5 Alloantibodies causing anaemia

Alloantibodies are, by definition, directed against antigens not found in the host (see Chapter 1). They can cause anaemia in only two situations: transfusion of incorrectly matched blood (see section 16.7); or in pregnancy, when maternal antibodies (IgG) cross the placenta and react with 'foreign' fetal red cell antigens (see Chapter 18).

16.3 Immune thrombocytopenia

Thrombocytopenia is defined as a blood platelet count of $< 150 \times 10^9/l$, though may not be symptomatic until the platelet count drops to $< 10 \times 10^9/l$ (Fig. 16.5). Thrombo-

BOX 16.3 MECHANISMS OF DRUG-INDUCED HAEMOLYTIC ANAEMIAS

- Most antibodies against drugs have specificity for rhesus antigens for an unknown reason, e.g. dapsone
- Drug may act as hapten after active or passive binding to the red cell; antibodies against the drug opsonize the red cells prior to phagocytosis
- Immune complex of drug and antibody, adsorbed on to red cells by immune adherence
- Some drugs trigger an AIHA indistinguishable from idiopathic warm AIHA

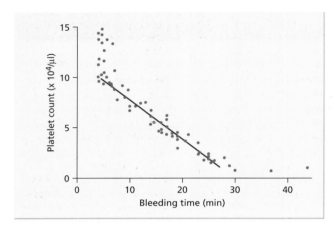

Fig. 16.5 Relevance of platelet level to bleeding time using platelets from normal individuals (from Harker and Slichter 1972).

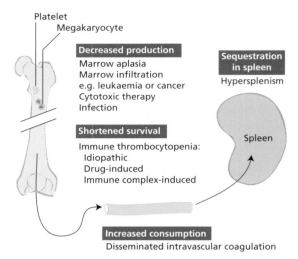

Fig. 16.6 Known causes of thrombocytopenia.

cytopenia may be caused by decreased production, shortened survival, increased consumption or sequestration in the spleen (Fig. 16.6), processes similar to those of anaemia. **Autoimmune thrombocytopenia** can also be considered in the same way as AIHA: idiopathic (Case 16.4) or secondary to autoimmune diseases (e.g. SLE), infection (e.g. HIV) or drugs (e.g. quinine). Unlike haemolytic anaemia, the antibodies are not temperature dependent. Autoantibodies are directed against platelet-specific antigens.

Immune thrombocytopenia (ITP) differs from thrombocytopenia due to circulating immune complexes with 'bystander involvement', when the antigen may be unrelated to platelets. **Bystander involvement** occurs in acute immune thrombocytopenia of childhood (which follows infection) and in some drug-induced thrombocytopenias, and involves Fc (IgG) receptors on platelets (Box 16.1). However, classic 'immune-complex' diseases other than SLE are rarely associated with thrombocytopenia, which suggests that circulating platelet-specific antibodies are probably responsible for low platelet counts in SLE.

Alloantibodies can also cause thrombocytopenias. Those provoked by pregnancy can cause neonatal thrombocytope-

nia (see Case 16.5), while those induced by transfusion cause post-transfusion purpura.

16.3.1 Immune thrombocytopenia

As with other idiopathic diseases, the *diagnosis is one of exclusion* of the known causes of thrombocytopenia (Fig. 16.6); low platelets are due to autoantibodies, though these are difficult to demonstrate by routinely available assays. The term 'immune thrombocytopenia' is applicable in adults and in *chronic* disease in children, where circulating **autoantibodies to platelets** have been shown to have platelet specificity.

Acute ITP is characterized by the rapid appearance of generalized purpura in a previously healthy child or, less commonly, adult. Large bruises follow minor trauma. Haemorrhagic bullae may occur in the mouth, epistaxis and conjunctival haemorrhages are common, and gastrointestinal haemorrhage and haematuria are less frequent. Other physical signs may be absent.

Acute ITP is the commonest form of **ITP in children** (Table 16.2), with a peak incidence about the age of 7. In over

---

CASE 16.4 IMMUNE THROMBOCYTOPENIA

A 29-year-old man presented with spontaneous bruising of his legs and arms. He had had three recent epistaxes but no other bleeding. He was not taking any drugs and had no risk factors for HIV. There were no physical signs apart from bruises and scattered petechiae on the legs. The spleen was not palpable. On investigation, he had a normal haemoglobin (138 g/l) and white cell count, but a low platelet count of 10×10^9/l (normal > 150×10^9/l). His erythrocyte sedimentation rate was 6 mm/h; direct Coombs' test was negative;

antinuclear and DNA-binding antibodies and rheumatoid factor were absent. His bone marrow contained an increased number of normal megakaryocytes but was otherwise normal. A diagnosis of immune thrombocytopenia was made and he was started on prednisolone. His platelet count rose rapidly over the next few days and the steroids were tailed off over 4 weeks. He relapsed 10 months later with further bruising, but again responded to a short course of oral steroids.

Table 16.2 Comparison of acute and chronic immune thrombocytopenia

	Acute	Chronic
Age of onset	Childhood	20–50 years
Sex	Both	F : M = 3 : 1
Preceding infection	Usual	Not associated
Bleeding	Sudden	Insidious
Platelets*	Low (≤ 20)	Variable (≤ 10–40)
Spontaneous resolution	Most patients	Rare
Duration	Few weeks	Months to years
Treatment	Nil usually	Corticosteroids ± splenectomy
Pathogenesis	Probably immune complexes	Specific antiplatelet antibodies

*× 10^9/l.

50% of the children it follows immunization or a common viral infection 1–3 weeks previously. Most children (85%) have a benign course, do not require treatment and recover spontaneously within 3 months. Treatment is reserved for life-threatening haemorrhage (such as cerebral haemorrhage), though this is extremely rare, as the platelets are functional and few are required to prevent severe haemorrhage (Fig. 16.5). *Fewer than 10% of children progress to chronic ITP.*

Chronic ITP usually has an insidious onset with minor bruising and scattered petechiae (Table 16.2). Episodes of bleeding may be separated by months or years, during which the platelet counts are normal. This is mainly a disorder of adults, affecting women more than men. As ITP can be a feature of HIV-related disease, this should be considered in the differential diagnosis, especially if there are other clinical features (see section 3.5.4). **Investigations** show a low platelet count, usually < 40 × 10^9/l, for more than 3 months. A blood film may show large platelets and minute platelet fragments. Bone marrow examination shows an increased number of megakaryocytes, suggesting that the thrombocytopenia is due to increased platelet destruction rather than decreased production (Fig. 16.6). The spleen is not enlarged.

Tests for platelet antibodies are of two types: the direct test detects IgG fixed on the patient's platelets (a platelet Coombs' test) and is positive in 90% of adult patients with chronic ITP. The remaining 10% may constitute a separate disease, since the bone marrow does not show increased megakaryocytopoiesis and the patients are refractory to therapy. Free serum antibodies with specificity for the platelet antigens, glycoprotein IIb/IIIa, can be assayed by an indirect test using a pool of normal donor platelets but are only positive in 30% of patients with chronic ITP. Neither test is sufficiently reliable for routine use and the *diagnosis is therefore by exclusion and finding increased megakaryocytes in the bone marrow.*

The **pathogenesis** of ITP has been well studied. The spleen is a major site of autoantibody synthesis. Platelets with IgG on their surfaces are sequestered in the red pulp of the spleen (Fig. 16.6), where circulating platelets with surface IgG are rapidly removed by phagocytosis. This has been shown with radiolabelled platelets sensitized with IgG, which are removed from the circulation in a few hours, compared with a normal half-life of a few days.

The object of **management** is to restore the platelet count to normal, but active therapy is not indicated unless there is acute bleeding. The vast majority of children recover spontaneously without sequelae. Adults whose platelet counts are between 40 and 100 × 10^9/l and who only have occasional bruising rarely require active treatment.

Children or adults with **active bleeding** require corticosteroids to prevent further destruction of platelets and about 60% of patients respond within 2 weeks. Corticosteroids may work by suppressing phagocytosis of antibody-coated platelets by macrophages in the spleen and liver. Patients who fail to respond, or who have a transient response but relapse into fresh bleeding after a month of steroids, may need splenectomy after intravenous immunoglobulin has raised the platelet count. **Splenectomy** removes both the major site of phagocytosis and that of autoantibody production and is successful in most patients. Intravenous immunoglobulin is useful in refractory patients. The infused IgG transiently blocks Fc (IgG) receptors on phagocytic cells and reduces platelet binding of autoantibodies by idiotypic neutralization. Cytotoxic drugs may be used in adults if these measures fail, or as second-line treatment in those unfit for splenectomy. Fulminant ITP has been treated successfully with plasmapheresis.

Pregnancy in women with ITP is usually uneventful, but the newborn may have neonatal thrombocytopenia. This is due to transplacental passage of IgG autoantibodies that then fix to fetal platelets. If bleeding or purpura develops, or the platelet count is very low, intravenous immunoglobulin can be given to raise the number of circulating platelets. Alternatively, the mother may receive intravenous immunoglobulin prior to delivery. In untreated infants, the platelet count gradually rises over the next 3 months as the maternal autoantibody is catabolized.

16.3.2 Drug-induced thrombocytopenia

The pathogenesis of drug-induced thrombocytopenia is similar to that of drug-induced autoimmune haemolytic anaemia (Box 16.3). Many drugs have been implicated, including quinine and *p*-aminosalicylic acid. There is clinical improvement and an increase in the platelet count when the drug is stopped.

16.3.3 Neonatal thrombocytopenia

Neonatal thrombocytopenia may be due to **antibodies that cross the placenta**. These may be autoantibodies in mothers with chronic ITP, or alloantibodies formed by the mother to paternal antigens present on fetal platelets. The immunopathology is similar to that of haemolytic disease of the newborn (see section 18.5.5). Several platelet iso-antigen systems are recognized; the most important is the HPA-1a system. Sera from women who have an obstetric history of a bruised or thrombocytopenic baby should always be tested against their husbands' platelets (Case 16.5). The treatment of an infant with 'neonatal alloimmune thrombocytopenia' is the same as those whose mothers have ITP.

16.4 Neutropenia

Neutropenia may be due to failure of production in or, rarely, export from the bone marrow (Fig. 16.7); alternatively, increased consumption or sequestration (usually in the spleen) can also cause neutropenia (Fig. 3.10). The traditional definition of neutropenia is $1.5 \times 10^9/l$, but *clinical effects are unusual unless the count drops below $0.5 \times 10^9/l$*.

Antibodies to neutrophils can cause syndromes which parallel AIHA and ITP, such as autoimmune neutropenia, al-

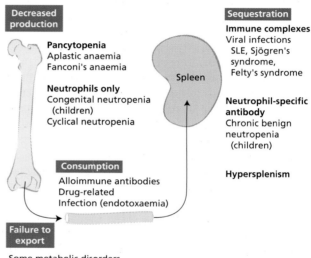

Fig. 16.7 Causes of neutropenia.

CASE 16.5 NEONATAL ALLOIMMUNE DISEASES

A 32-year-old woman undergoing a twin pregnancy had been given a blood transfusion for a post-partum haemorrhage in her first pregnancy 3 years earlier. The current pregnancy and delivery were normal and non-identical twin boys were born, both with Apgar scores of 10. Four hours later, both infants had extensive purpura on their abdomens, arms and legs but neither was jaundiced.

Twin 1 had a platelet count of $30 \times 10^9/l$ and his haemoglobin was 176 g/l. He did not become jaundiced and his platelet count gradually rose without treatment over several weeks. His platelet count was normal ($400 \times 10^9/l$) at 2 months.

Twin 2 had a platelet count of $46 \times 10^9/l$ and a normal haemoglobin (190 g/l). However, he rapidly developed anaemia (Hb 84 g/l) and jaundice (bilirubin 300 mmol/l) at 48 h. A Coombs' test was positive and his red cells were found to be group A, whereas his mother's cells were group O. In view of the rising serum bilirubin, an exchange transfusion was performed. Following this, his haemoglobin and platelet count returned to normal and he was discharged 6 days later with a platelet count of $213 \times 10^9/l$ and a haemoglobin of 132 g/l.

The mother's serum was found to contain IgG antibodies to the father's platelets and to some, but not all, of a panel of platelets from normal, unrelated donors. These antibodies were typed as specific anti-HPA-1a antibodies and had been provoked by the previous pregnancy and transfusion. These antibodies crossed the placenta to cause alloimmune thrombocytopenia in both twins. Twin 2 also had a red cell incompatibility and so needed an exchange transfusion to compensate for haemolysis. It is unusual for an ABO incompatibility to require an exchange transfusion (see section 18.5.5). His platelet count returned to normal more quickly than that of twin 1 because the antibodies to platelets were removed by the exchange.

loimmune neonatal neutropenia and drug-induced immune neutropenia. As for other blood components, neutropenia may be idiopathic or secondary to diseases such as SLE and other immune-complex diseases.

Autoimmune **antibodies to neutrophils** react with neutrophil antigens but are difficult to detect because the cells themselves rapidly ingest the complex formed by their membrane antigen and the autoantibody. Autoantibodies are difficult to distinguish from immune (IgG) complexes reacting with IgG Fc receptors.

Neutropenia secondary to SLE may be due to immune complexes or to antineutrophil IgG antibodies. **Felty's syndrome** describes a complex of neutropenia accompanied by splenomegaly, high-titre rheumatoid factor and rheumatoid arthritis (see section 10.4). There is increased granulocyte production by the bone marrow as well as increased granulocyte turnover. It is thought that neutrophils coated with IgG are sequestered in the spleen, eventually resulting in splenomegaly. However, splenectomy does not always cure the problem, suggesting that this mechanism operates in only some of the patients.

Antineutrophil antibodies have also been detected in **drug-induced neutropenia**; these antibodies appear to be autoantibodies, which disappear when the drug is discontinued.

Neonatal neutropenia due to allogeneic antibodies is an extremely rare but sometimes fatal syndrome; the mother produces IgG antibodies to neutrophil-specific antigens present on fetal neutrophils. Although these antibodies are commonly found in multiparous women, they rarely result in neonatal disease. These antibodies may also be responsible for some transfusion reactions (see section 16.7).

16.5 Haematopoietic progenitor cells

Aplastic anaemia is the term given to pancytopenia due to reduced numbers of pluripotent stem cells. It may be congenital (e.g. Fanconi's anaemia), secondary (to infection, drugs or thymoma) or, in 60% of cases, idiopathic (acquired with no known cause).

Suppression of erythropoiesis in the bone marrow involves **autoantibodies (IgG) to erythroblast progenitors or to erythropoietin**, excessive **suppression by autologous CD8+ T** lymphocytes, or both. The response to antilymphocyte globulin or ciclosporin in 50% of patients suggests variable aetiologies. Stem cell transplantation is the treatment of choice and the 5-year survival is > 90%. For those for whom there is no suitable donor, ciclosporin with antilymphocyte globulin offers 90% survival at 5 years. However, non-transplanted patients remain at risk of developing marrow malignancies in the longer term.

16.6 Immune disorders of coagulation

16.6.1 Primary antiphospholipid antibody syndrome

A stroke in a young person (under 50 years), recurrent fetal loss or recurrent thrombosis (arterial/venous) may indicate an underlying primary antiphospholipid antibody syndrome (see Table 16.3) (see Chapters 10 and 18). The vastly increased risk of cerebral thrombosis or embolism in these patients makes it important to measure these antibodies in all **young stroke patients** as well as those with major arterial or venous thrombosis (Fig. 16.8). Patients with high-

Table 16.3 Comparison of primary antiphospholipid antibody (APA) syndrome and systemic lupus erythematosus (SLE)

	Primary APA	SLE
Female : male	2 : 1	9 : 1
Age (years):		
range	20–60	15–60
mean	38	24
Antinuclear antibody	45%	> 90%
Antibodies to double-stranded DNA	Nil	80%
Antiphospholipid antibodies	100%	40%
Lupus anticoagulant	60%	10%

CASE 16.6 PRIMARY ANTIPHOSPHOLIPID ANTIBODY SYNDROME

A 28-year-old woman was admitted with a stroke due to a cerebral vascular thrombosis. She had had four spontaneous abortions in the past. She was a non-smoker. Cerebral angiography confirmed the thrombosis but showed normal vasculature otherwise. Haemoglobin, platelet and white cell counts were normal, as were her serum immunoglobulins, C3 and C4 levels. Antibodies to nuclei, extractable nuclear antigens and double-stranded DNA were negative, but she did have high-titre antiphospholipid antibodies. Coagulation tests showed a prolonged kaolin–cephalin clotting time which did not correct with normal plasma, i.e. lupus anticoagulant. A diagnosis of primary antiphospholipid antibody syndrome was made, so she received long-term anticoagulant therapy.

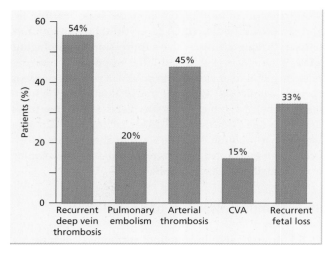

Fig. 16.8 Clinical presentations in the primary phospholipid antibody syndrome.

titre antiphospholipid antibodies alone (commonly called anticardiolipin antibodies as this is the major phospholipid involved) should be anticoagulated for life, since devastating, acute vasculopathy can occur, involving major vessels to vital organs.

16.6.2 Other antibodies to coagulation factors

Antibodies to circulating coagulation factors occur in treated haemophiliacs and in association with SLE and other autoimmune states. **Factor VIII antibodies** are the commonest and developed in 15% of patients with severe haemophilia treated with human factor VIII concentrates, although the increasing use of recombinant products has reduced this. Treatment with very high doses of intravenous immunoglobulin has been used successfully for patients with catastrophic bleeding. Factor VIII autoantibodies are also found in rare patients with SLE, or in elderly persons without overt underlying disease, in whom bleeding is difficult to stop.

Antibodies to the prothrombin converter complex (factors Xa, V, phospholipid and calcium) are found in up to 40% of patients with SLE, provided a sensitive assay is used. These are usually patients who have had thrombotic episodes or renal involvement. They have prolonged kaolin–cephalin clotting time and failure to correct the clotting defect with normal plasma implies that an antibody is present. Such an antibody is known as the **'lupus anticoagulant'**. It is paradoxical that this 'anticoagulant' usually results in thrombosis in vivo. These antibodies are distinct from those to cardiolipin with different specificities, although they usually occur together and have related immunopathologies (see Table 16.3). There is considerable overlap between the clini-

cal features associated with both the lupus anticoagulant and antiphospholipid antibodies.

16.7 Blood transfusion

Blood transfusion must be safe, i.e. immunologically compatible and free of infection (Box 16.4).

16.7.1 Principles of blood transfusion

The ABO red cell system is unique because **naturally occurring antibodies** (IgM) are found in human sera. For example, if group A blood was given to a group B patient whose blood contains natural anti-A antibodies, these antibodies would lyse the donated cells, causing a potentially fatal transfusion reaction. Blood is always matched for ABO antigens.

To prevent sensitization to rhesus antigens (and the risk of a subsequent transfusion reaction), donor and recipient are also tested for compatibility for the immunologically strongest Rhesus antigen, D antigen. Most minor red cell antigens occur only infrequently or are poorly immunogenic.

Matching for ABO and rhesus antigens alone should **prevent major incompatibilities**. However, recipients' sera are screened for rare pre-existing antibodies, produced as a result of a pregnancy or previous transfusion, which may destroy donor red cells. Transfusion reactions due to pre-existing antibodies can be fatal. A test panel of red cells, containing most antigens of known blood group systems, is used as well as cells from selected donors. Sera are screened for 'complete' (IgM) antibodies, which will agglutinate red cells in saline, and 'incomplete' antibodies (IgG), which are detectable by an indirect antiglobulin (Coombs') test. It is not necessary to identify donor antibodies because these are rapidly diluted on transfusion.

Despite these precautions, red cells are sometimes destroyed by a **haemolytic transfusion reaction** (Table 16.4). Unfortunately, *the commonest cause of a transfusion reaction is still a human error* either in handling blood samples, or mistaken patient identity. Haemolytic transfusion reactions due

---

BOX 16.4 STEPS TAKEN TO ENSURE THE SAFETY OF BLOOD FOR TRANSFUSION

- Screening the recipient's serum for antibodies that react with donor red cells

- Ensuring that the transfused red cells will not stimulate any unwanted antibodies in the recipient

- Screening all units of blood for hepatitis B antigen, antibodies to HIV and hepatitis C, and syphilis antigens

- Blood used for babies is also screened for antibodies to cytomegalovirus

Table 16.4 Potential complications of blood transfusion (fortunately rare)

Complication	Cause
Red cell destruction	ABO mismatch Antibodies to other red cell antigens previously undetected in recipient's plasma Boost of low-level antibody to significant level by transfusion
Febrile reactions (rarely anaphylaxis)	Anti-leucocyte antibodies Anti-platelet antibodies (e.g. HLA, HPA-1a) Anti-IgA antibodies in selective total IgA deficiency
Infection	Hepatitis C Non-A, non-B, non-C, hepatitis viruses Cytomegalovirus Malaria Human immunodeficiency virus

to ABO incompatibility usually result in massive haemolysis, haemoglobinuria, shock and disseminated intravascular coagulation. A mismatch due to rhesus incompatibility usually results in gradual haemolysis, which does not interfere with renal function, but the patient's haemoglobin fails to rise following transfusion.

Occasionally, transfusion reactions occur 5–10 days after transfusion. The delay is due to the time lag required for the production of antibodies by the patient. This alloimmune response means that the patient's own cells are negative in a direct Coombs' test, but the transfused cells are positive for IgG and complement. This type of **delayed transfusion reaction** occurs after multiple blood transfusions, such as those required in open-heart surgery or severe gastrointestinal bleeding.

16.7.2 Risks of blood transfusion

A variety of **blood-borne infections** can be transmitted by blood transfusion, though measures to screen donors and treat blood products with antiviral agents have reduced the risks considerably. Donors likely to have been exposed to malaria, hepatitis viruses or HIV are discouraged from giving blood. Together with increased screening, these measures have dramatically reduced transmitted infection in the last three decades (Fig. 16.9)—see Case 16.7.

Currently, whole blood is given rarely. Haemorrhage requires plasma expanders to maintain blood volumes and red cell concentrates to raise the haemoglobin. Concentrated platelets are used to prevent bleeding in marrow failure (aplastic anaemia, acute leukaemia); a failure to increase the

CASE 16.7 TRANSMISSION OF HEPATITIS C BY A BLOOD PRODUCT

David was diagnosed as having a common variable immune deficiency disorder aged 58 years, after developing bronchiectasis over the preceding 5 years. He had also suffered from episodes of urethritis, eventually found to be due to Ureaplasma urealytica (a common organism known to cause significant infections in antibody-deficient patients). He received 25 g of intravenous immunoglobulin at 3-weekly intervals, with regular monitoring of his liver function tests (6-weekly). In 1994, after 3 years of uneventful infusions, he developed raised alanine transaminase levels and rapidly became jaundiced. His serum was now positive for hepatitis C virus by polymerase chain reaction (HCV-PCR). He had iatrogenic hepatitis C.

He was admitted for assessment and the jaundice and liver enzyme levels reversed spontaneously; he received 6 million units of interferon (IFN)-α subcutaneously three times a week for 6 months. The PCR became negative within 4 weeks and has remained so over the next 12 years, as have his liver function tests.

This type of transmission of hepatitis C is thankfully very rare nowadays, since blood products are treated routinely with solvent: detergent or other methods to inactivate lipid-coated viruses. Such a patient would now receive Ribavirin with IFN-α, as the results of such treatment in blood transfusion-transmitted disease are superior.

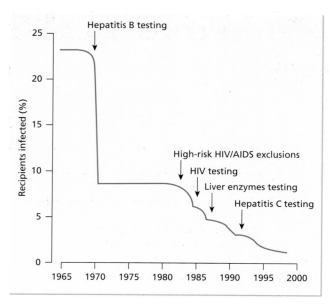

Fig. 16.9 Reduction of risk of hepatitis by multiple blood transfusions.

platelet count suggests destruction by recipient's alloantibodies and potential platelet donors and the recipient may have to be HLA class I matched. The advent of granulocyte–colony-stimulating factors (G-CSF) has made granulocyte transfusions largely unnecessary. **Plasma products** currently include immunoglobulin, fresh frozen plasma, factor VIII and albumin, though the last two are being replaced by recombinant products. Polyclonal immunoglobulin and fresh frozen plasma, however, will continue to be made from human blood and measures, such as solvent:detergent treatment against lipid-coated viruses and pasteurization, have improved the safety of these agents.

FURTHER READING

See website: www.immunologyclinic.com

CHAPTER 17

17 Neuroimmunology

17.1 Introduction

The central and peripheral nervous systems are not excluded from immune disease. The immune system participates actively in nervous tissue to counteract infection, and so, as elsewhere, cells can enter these tissues **in inflammation**. T and B lymphocytes, as well as macrophages, can invade inflamed nervous tissue. In such situations, intrathecal B cells are responsible for locally synthesized immunoglobulin found in the cerebrospinal fluid. T cells and macrophages, whilst protecting against infection, can also cause direct damage, as in chronic viral infection, postinfective states and demyelination.

The **blood–brain barrier** normally excludes intravascular proteins (including IgG) and this must be breached before extrathecal circulating autoantibodies reach the central or peripheral nervous systems. In this way, circulating autoantibodies are responsible for the pathogenesis of several antibody-mediated neuropathies, such as the Lambert–Eaton myasthenic syndrome (LEMS). This is an excellent example of the way in which an autoimmune pathogenesis has been proven by following clinical clues over many years (Box 17.1). Other autoimmune diseases selectively damage central or peripheral nervous tissue itself (e.g. multiple sclerosis and Guillain–Barré syndrome, respectively) or the muscle endplates (e.g. myasthenia gravis). On the other hand, involvement of nervous tissue may be part of a systemic disorder (e.g. systemic lupus erythematosus).

BOX 17.1 EVIDENCE FOR AUTOIMMUNE AETIOLOGY OF LAMBERT–EATON MYASTHENIA (LEMS)

1953 Clinical description of disease

1972 LEMS associated with other autoimmune diseases in patients

1984 Plasma exchange—successful therapy for affected patients

1987 Human plasma from patients causes characteristic changes (electrophysiological + electron-microscopical) in mice

1991 Autoantibodies to calcium channels in 20% of patients detected

1991 Autoantigen in small-cell cancer, found in 50% of LEMS patients

1994 Additional epitopes for antibodies to Ca^{2+} channels defined; now disease-specific antibodies in 100% of patients

1995 Randomized, placebo-controlled, cross-over study showed improved muscle strength with intravenous immunoglobulin therapy (immuno-modulation)

17.2 Infections

The incidence of meningitis in infants has been reduced dramatically by means of immunization against the encapsulated organisms that are the major causes of these diseases.

CASE 17.1   HAEMOPHILUS INFLUENZAE TYPE B MENINGITIS

Alice was a normal, full-term baby who was breast-fed and gained weight appropriately in the first 6 weeks of life. At 7 weeks she became acutely miserable, stopped feeding and her mother felt that she was very warm; when she took her temperature, it was 40 °C. In the surgery, the doctor found that she had neck stiffness and Alice then vomited all over the couch. There was no rash or bruising but the left eardrum was inflamed. Meningitis was suspected; the doctor gave Alice an intramuscular injection of penicillin and instructed her mother to take her straight to the hospital where the on-call paediatrician was waiting. The clinical diagnosis of meningitis was confirmed and blood and cerebrospinal fluid

(CSF) samples were taken immediately and intravenous antibiotics started. The CSF showed increased numbers of neutrophil leucocytes (131×10^6/l) and a few Gram-negative coccobacilli despite the initial dose of penicillin. Three days later these were shown to be Haemophilus influenzae and serotyping showed them to be Haemophilus influenzae type b. The full blood count showed a circulating neutrophilia (29×10^9/l), the C-reactive protein level was 230 mg/l. Alice made a rapid recovery with intravenous and subsequently oral antibiotics, with supportive management to ensure adequate ventilation and fluids. There were no long-term sequelae.

Even normal children under the age of 2 years are unable to make antibodies to the carbohydrate capsules of Haemophilus influenzae type b, Streptococcus pneumoniae or Neisseria meningitidis and these pathogens accounted for 90% of meningitis seen in children until the early 1990s. Since the introduction of new vaccines, in which these carbohydrate antigens have been coupled to protein carriers in order to provoke protective antibodies in infants (see section 7.7), the incidence of meningitis due to Haemophilus influenzae type b and Neisseria meningitides type C has fallen dramatically in many countries. However, **routine immunization** has only been shown to be effective after the age of 2 months and infants are susceptible until then (as in Case 17.1) if their mothers are not immune to provide protective IgG via the placenta. Such infections in immunized infants should now lead to suspicion of a primary immune deficiency.

Infections of the central nervous system (CNS), meningitis and encephalitis, are relatively uncommon in immunocompetent adults. Severe, unusual or recurrent brain infections should raise the possibility of an immune defect (see Chapter 3 and below).

This is exemplified in human immunodeficiency virus (HIV)-positive patients in whom opportunistic microorganisms—viruses, fungi, parasites or intracellular bacteria—may infect the CNS (Table 17.1). The signs of infections in **HIV-positive patients** may be modified; fever and meningism are often absent and CSF may contain few cells, little protein and no detectable antibodies to the organisms involved, making diagnosis more difficult before the routine use of polymerase chain reaction (PCR) to detect infective agents.

In addition, the causative virus, HIV, can itself infect the brain to produce a range of problems including **AIDS dementia**. Neurological abnormalities occur clinically in about 50% of HIV-infected adult patients and in many HIV-infect-

Table 17.1 Important neurological complications of human immunodeficiency virus (HIV) infection

---

Primary HIV infection
Dementia
Atypical meningitis
Myelopathy

Opportunistic infections
Cerebral toxoplasmosis
Meningitis—cryptococcal, tuberculous
Cytomegalovirus/herpes simplex virus encephalitis
Progressive multifocal leucoencephalopathy (papovavirus)
Cytomegalovirus retinitis

Tumours
Kaposi's sarcoma
B-cell lymphoma

---

ed children. Subclinical disease may be even more common, since up to 75% of brains of AIDS patients are found to be affected post-mortem. Pathological changes range from white matter pallor and mild lymphocytic infiltration to macrophage abnormalities (including multinucleate giant cells) associated with macrophage activation. Computed tomography (CT) may show cerebral atrophy.

Infections can result in damage even after the pathogen has been eliminated. **Parainfectious encephalitis** occurs some time following a childhood viral illness (rubella, measles, chicken pox). This is due to demyelination following bystander activation of T cells or molecular mimicry resulting in specific T cells mistaking myelin for virus (see section 5.5 in Chapter 5, Autoimmunity). Although the condition is usually self-limiting, permanent damage or death may result.

In contrast, **subacute sclerosing panencephalitis (SSPE)** is a rare, progressive disease of children, who present with insidious dementia. The disease follows measles infection several years earlier, and high levels of specific anti-measles antibody as well as measles virus are found in the brain, blood and CSF. The intrathecal IgG is not only oligoclonal but also can be absorbed out with measles virus itself. Since there is no obvious defect in the adaptive immune responses to measles virus, it is possible that such children have defective innate immunity and Toll-like receptors are under investigation, having been shown to be important in early protection against many viruses.

Progressive multifocal leucoencephalopathy is a rare demyelinating disease that can be induced by papovaviruses and typically occurs in immunosuppressed patients, such as those with AIDS or those receiving immunosuppressive treatment. The pathogenesis is unclear.

17.3 Demyelinating diseases of the central nervous system

17.3.1 Multiple sclerosis (MS)

MS is common in Caucasians, with a prevalence of 1 case per 2000 population (see Table 3.3). It is an **inflammatory disease of white matter** in the CNS. It is a hugely variable disease, in terms of disability, rate of progression of the disease and prognosis. The clinical diagnosis of MS can be difficult, as definite histopathological confirmation by biopsy is not done in life. The **clinical features** depend on the site of the pathological lesion in the brain, as in Case 17.2; many plaques are clinically silent. The rate of new lesions is

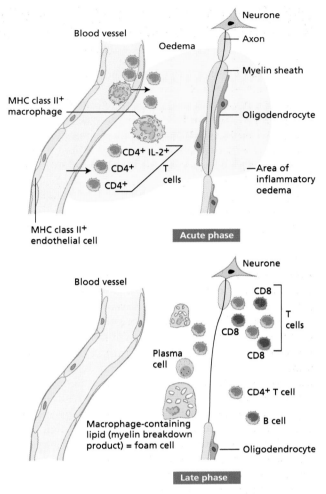

Fig. 17.1 Immunopathogenesis of demyelination.

CASE 17.2 MULTIPLE SCLEROSIS

A 38-year-old woman presented with tingling, numbness and clumsiness of both hands for 1 week, with a band of numbness from the umbilicus to the axillae. Six months earlier, following an upper respiratory tract infection, she had experienced a short episode of blurred vision which she put down to tiredness. She was now anxious because her maternal grandmother had suffered from multiple sclerosis (MS).

On neurological examination, she had absent abdominal reflexes with brisk tendon jerks and bilateral extensor plantar responses. Blood investigations were normal, including a full blood count, C-reactive protein, vitamin B_{12} and folate levels and syphilis serology. A lumbar puncture was carried out. The cerebrospinal fluid (CSF) investigation results are shown in Table 17.2. Oligoclonal IgG bands (see Fig. 19.8) are not found in normal CSF, but are found

in 90% of patients with MS; in the absence of clinical signs of infection, this test is almost diagnostic of MS (see Box 17.2).

The clinical diagnosis was multiple sclerosis; other possible diagnoses, such as neurosyphilis or subacute combined degeneration of the cord, were excluded.

Table 17.2 Cerebrospinal fluid investigations in Case 17.2, multiple sclerosis

Protein concentration	0.4 g/l (NR 0–0.4 g/l)
Red blood cells	None
Lymphocytes	$3 \times 10^6/l$ (NR $< 5 \times 10^6/l$)
IgG/albumin ratio	26% (NR 4–22%)
Isoelectric focusing	Oligoclonal bands present

unpredictable and also variable. Subgroups of MS depend on the rate of progression and recovery between attacks; relapsing and remitting MS is quite distinct from progressive disease.

Optic neuritis is a similar inflammatory, demyelinating disease of one or both optic nerves, with recovery in 75–90% of patients. An oligoclonal pattern of IgG is found in CSF from most patients with optic neuritis and nuclear magnetic resonance imaging (MRI) shows silent lesions elsewhere in the brain. It can be due to many causes, but approximately 50–80% of these patients will develop MS within 15 years, as in Case 17.2.

Clinical diagnosis of MS depends on evidence of at least two attacks separated in time and site of lesion, with exclusion of all other causes, as in Case 17.2. **Confirmatory tests** are required. Poor nerve conduction can be demonstrated by prolonged responses on evoked potential testing. MRI of the brain (Fig. 17.2) shows lesions in 90% of affected individuals but, like all imaging, is non-specific and can be unreliable, especially in the elderly.

The pathological lesion in MS, seen at post-mortem brain biopsy, is a 'plaque'; this is an area of the white matter in which myelin and oligodendrocytes are absent. Myelin is a protein–phospholipid material that surrounds axons in a multilayered, dense spiral. Myelin sheaths in the CNS are formed by compacted membranes of oligodendrocyte extensions. The integrity of the myelin sheaths depends on the maintenance of normal oligodendrocyte function. Axons without myelin sheaths are poor conductors of nerve impulses, resulting in a neurological deficit. In the early stages of a plaque, there is tissue oedema, apoptotic oligodendrocytes and infiltrating cells; lymphocytes and macrophages are seen around the venules in the area. B cells are involved in the local production of immunoglobulin, whilst others, including T cells and macrophages, are part of the acute inflammatory process (Fig. 17.1).

Routine examination of CSF is not enough. It is essential to look at the nature of the immunoglobulin (Box 17.2). Immunoglobulin present in the CSF may have been synthesized in

---

BOX 17.2 IMMUNOLOGICAL FINDINGS IN CEREBROSPINAL FLUID (CSF) FROM PATIENTS WITH DEFINITE MULTIPLE SCLEROSIS (MS)

Finding	Percentage of positive MS patients
Oligoclonal bands by isoelectric focusing	> 95
Increased CSF IgG index	70–80
Increased cell count	50
Raised IgG/albumin ratio	50

---

the CNS or passively transferred from the serum. The concentration of CSF IgG is best expressed in relation to another serum protein, not synthesized in the brain, as this level will indicate the integrity of the blood–CSF barrier. Most formulae are based on the ratio of IgG/albumin measured by the same technique (see section 19.4). Intracerebral synthesis of IgG will produce a rise in the IgG/albumin ratio. However, if the raised CSF IgG concentration is due to a 'leaking' blood–brain barrier, then the albumin content will be similarly elevated and the resulting IgG/albumin ratio will remain constant. The IgG synthesized in the brain is restricted in nature, has a narrow range of isoelectric points and appears as **typical oligoclonal bands** on isoelectric focusing (Fig. 19.8). This pattern is seen in over 95% of patients with MS, although it is not confined to MS. CSF from patients with cerebral infections, such as neurosyphilis or subacute sclerosing panencephalitis, shows a similar pattern, although such conditions rarely cause diagnostic difficulty.

The cause of MS is unknown, but **environmental and genetic factors** are important. Several epidemiological observations link MS to an exogenous environmental agent (Box 17.3), but extensive efforts to isolate a specific agent in MS have failed. There appears to be no single trigger. The

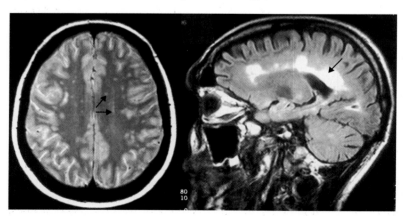

Fig. 17.2 MRI scan of MS plaques (from Axford & O'Callaghan, with permission).

BOX 17.3 EPIDEMIOLOGICAL OBSERVATIONS IN MULTIPLE SCLEROSIS (MS) THAT SUGGEST AN INFECTIVE ORGANISM MAY BE THE AETIOLOGICAL AGENT

- MS is a disease of temperate climates, with a well-recognized north/south gradient in the USA and Europe
- Migrants assume the risk of the region to which they migrate if they go before the age of 15; if they go later, they retain the risk associated with their country of origin
- Occasional epidemics of MS have occurred
- 40% of new clinical events follow viral infections
- Raised titres of CSF antibodies to measles virus in many MS patients

BUT

- CSF IgG from patients with MS react with a variety of viruses
- CSF IgG shows a variety of different idiotypes
- IgG shows different specificities and isoelectric points, even within plaques from the same brain
- No herpes simplex (HSV 1/2) Epstein–Barr virus (EBV), cytomegalovirus (CMV), varicella zoster virus (VZV), human herpes virus-6 or -7 or enteroviruses within plaques by PCR
- Using random peptide libraries, huge number of possible reactivities within a single IgG oligoclone (brain proteins, HSV, CMV and human papilloma virus sequences)

animal model of experimental autoimmune encephalitis in mice (EAE), induced by immunizing susceptible mice with myelin proteins, can be transferred to non-immunized animals by transfer of activated T cells reacting with small fragments of myelin proteins. These T cells, like those in affected humans, have restricted T-cell receptors (TCR); attempts to block these TCR in mice have been successful in limiting the progress of the relapsing and remitting disease (see section 7.8).

The precise immunopathogenesis of demyelination is not clear. Many inflammatory cells are present in the local lesions, known as plaques (see Fig. 17.1). Whether cells injure the oligodendrocytes directly or whether the damage results from viral or toxic agents remains controversial. New data suggest that **apoptosis of oligodendrocytes** may precede inflammation and demyelination. CD4 and CD8 T cells, with specificity for the human brain component, myelin basic protein, are present in blood and brains of patients with MS. Whereas previously CD4+ cells were thought to be most important, newer data favour **CD8 T cells** as the cause of oligodendrocyte death and CD4+ cells responsible for inflammation. However, the precise nature of the sensitizing process and the cytokines involved remain a mystery. Activated

macrophages are seen in close proximity to myelin-stripped axons and are probably involved too. Autoreactive T cells are found in healthy people but are activated only in patients with MS. Human CD4-regulatory T cells (CD4/CD25hi) can prevent activation and function of other T cells. Whereas the same numbers of CD4/CD25hi suppressor cells were found in healthy individuals and MS patients, those CD4/CD25hi from patients with MS were less able to inhibit specific activation of CD4/CD25⁻ cells, suggesting that impairment of these regulatory T cells may contribute to the breakdown of immune tolerance in patients with MS.

Genetic factors are important. MS is common in Caucasians, with a prevalence of 50 cases per 100 000 population (see Table 3.3). There is a well-documented association with HLA-DR2, DR1 and DQ1 antigens in northern Europeans and North Americans but the susceptibility of an individual will be **multi-factorial**, including environmental agent(s).

There is **no specific treatment** that will reverse demyelination, although each episode is usually associated with some recovery as the initial oedema subsides. Corticosteroids (intravenously in severe relapse) have been used in an acute attack to suppress the inflammatory response, but elimination of the inflammatory component does not stop disease progression. The efficacy of interferon (IFN)-β is controversial, as is the use of high-dose human intravenous immunoglobulin therapy; since both are expensive therapies, their use is limited. Copolymer 1 shows some promise. Targeted immunotherapy with humanized antibodies has proved successful. Natalizumab, a monoclonal antibody to $\alpha_4\beta_1$ integrin (VLA4) has been shown to be clinically effective. It is thought to act by preventing the entry of damaging cells into the white matter but serious side effects prevent its use. Humanized anti-CD25+ antibody (daclizumab) inhibits interleukin-2 signalling and looks promising in those MS patients with incomplete response to IFN-β therapy. In an open-label study, there was a 70% decrease in gadolinium contrast-enhancing lesions, compared with treatment with IFN-β alone. Trials of immune stimulation have been disappointing and IFN-γ made the disease worse.

The prognosis of MS depends on the subtype of disease. Overall, 20% have died 20 years after diagnosis and > 60% are significantly disabled.

17.4 Autoimmune diseases of the neuromuscular junction

17.4.1 Myasthenia gravis

Myasthenia gravis is an uncommon disease (prevalence 9 per 10^5 population) characterized by weakness and fatigue of voluntary muscles, including those of the eye (see Cases 17.3 and 5.2). The weakness results from impaired transmission from nerve to muscle at the neuromuscular junctions.

CASE 17.3 MYASTHENIA GRAVIS

A 67-year-old man, complaining of double vision, was found to have bilateral ptosis, covering most of the pupil on the right side and partially obscuring that on the left. The ptosis was worse in the evening and almost absent in the morning. He admitted to tiredness in the arms and legs on exercise, which recovered with resting. A clinical diagnosis of ocular myasthenia gravis was made. A Tensilon test, involving intravenous injection of edrophonium, a short-acting cholinesterase inhibitor to abolish the symptoms, was positive but electromyography was inconclusive.

His serum contained antibodies to thyroid microsomes and to acetylcholine receptors (see section 19.7). The patient improved on treatment with pyridostigmine, which prolongs the action of acetylcholine by inhibiting the breakdown.

This case is not typical of myasthenia gravis but demonstrates that myasthenia may affect mainly ocular muscles (although only 60% have detectable antibodies to acetylcholine receptors). Myasthenia gravis is more commonly a disease of young women, who present with increasing systemic muscle fatigue (see Case 5.2 in Chapter 5, Autoimmunity).

Neurotransmission is impaired by **autoantibodies to the acetylcholine receptors** in the postsynaptic membrane of the muscle (Fig. 17.3). These antibodies reduce the number of receptors, by complement-mediated lysis and accelerated internalization, and possibly by blocking the receptors. Myasthenia gravis is an autoimmune disease (see Box 17.4).

The **aetiology** of myasthenia gravis is unknown, although a dog model suggests infectious agents are involved in disease induction and HLA associations (HLA-B8 and HLA-DR3) raise the possibility of genetic susceptibility. At least

BOX 17.4 EVIDENCE THAT MYASTHENIA GRAVIS IS AN AUTOIMMUNE DISEASE

- Strong association with organ-specific autoimmune diseases, such as myxoedema or diabetes, in an individual patient
- Increased incidence of organ-specific autoimmune diseases in close family members
- Thymic abnormalities, including B cells forming follicles
- Occurrence of a transient form of MG in 10% of newborn babies of myasthenic mothers

four subgroups of patients are recognized (Table 17.3), suggesting different aetiologies. Myasthenia gravis may also be induced by d-penicillamine therapy but reverses on discontinuation of the drug. The idiotypes of the receptor antibodies provoked by d-penicillamine are very limited, in contrast to the wide heterogeneity seen in these antibodies in 'idiopathic' myasthenia gravis.

As in other autoimmune diseases, there are **hyperplastic thymic changes** (Table 17.3), which include prominent formation of lymphoid follicles, germinal centres, increased numbers of mononuclear and plasma cells; the latter are one source of receptor antibodies. Myoid cells, present in myasthenic thymus and thymoma, act as a source of antigen for the production of acetylcholine receptor antibodies and antigen-specific T cells. It is essential to check for underlying thymoma by CT scanning of the chest.

The receptor autoantibodies were discovered when a known neuromuscular toxin was injected into rabbits and caused both the production of circulating anti-acetylcholine antibodies and paralysis with neuromuscular block, similar to that found in myasthenia gravis. Such antibodies (see section 19.7) are **diagnostic** for myasthenia; nearly 90% of patients with systemic myasthenia have this antibody, whereas only 60% of patients with myasthenia confined to the ocular muscles are positive. Acetylcholine receptor antibodies of IgG class cross the placenta. However, only 10% of babies

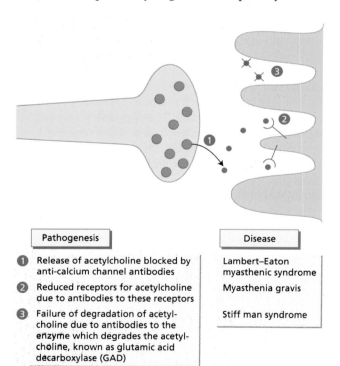

Pathogenesis	Disease
1 Release of acetylcholine blocked by anti-calcium channel antibodies	Lambert–Eaton myasthenic syndrome
2 Reduced receptors for acetylcholine due to antibodies to these receptors	Myasthenia gravis
3 Failure of degradation of acetylcholine due to antibodies to the enzyme which degrades the acetylcholine, known as glutamic acid decarboxylase (GAD)	Stiff man syndrome

Fig. 17.3 Impaired transmission from nerve to muscle at the neuromuscular junctions in myasthenia gravis and other muscle end-plate diseases.

Table 17.3 Heterogeneity of myasthenia gravis

	Young women	Older men	Thymoma	No antibody
Proportion of patients	40–50%	15–30%	15–20%	15%
Thymic changes	Hyperplasia	Atrophy	Tumour	Unknown
Ab titre to acetylcholine receptors	High	Low	Intermediate	None
Muscle weakness	Systemic	Systemic/ocular	Systemic	Systemic/ocular
Immunological therapy	Thymectomy (recover in 2 years) plus immune suppression	Prednisolone ± azathioprine	Thymectomy for tumour; if little improvement in weakness— use immune suppression	Prednisolone ± azathioprine
HLA associations	A1 B8 DR3	B7 DR2	None	None

of myasthenic mothers develop neonatal myasthenia, since the receptor antibodies are neutralized by fetal production of anti-idiotypic antibodies, presumably IgM.

Treatment of myasthenia gravis involves suppression of production of acetylcholine receptor antibodies (prednisolone and azathioprine) (see Table 17.3), as well as prevention of stimulation. Patients with severe myasthenia gravis respond well to plasmapheresis, which is done in conjunction with immunosuppression. Thymectomy in those with an enlarged thymus or thymoma (Fig. 17.4) removes not only some of the plasma cells producing the antibodies (see above), but also at least one source of antigen. These immunological approaches are in addition to conventional therapy with anticholinesterase drugs, as in Case 17.3.

17.4.2 Other autoimmune diseases of muscle end-plates

A similar **mechanism** of action by autoantibodies is seen in the Lambert–Eaton myasthenic syndrome, in which antibodies to calcium channels related to the release of acetylcholine from vesicles result in weakness (see Box 17.1). In contrast, the stiff man syndrome is caused by autoantibodies to the intracellular enzyme glutamic acid decarboxylase (GAD), which results in inability to relax muscles by breaking down the transmitter. This neurological syndrome is always associated with type 1 diabetes mellitus, in which such

antibodies are also pathogenic (see section 15.4.2 on diabetes mellitus and cross-reactive antibodies).

17.5 Immune-mediated neuropathies

Peripheral neuropathy can be a complication of some common immune-mediated diseases, such as rheumatoid arthritis or diabetes mellitus (Table 17.4), or a common feature of rare diseases, such as polyarteritis nodosa (see section 10.9) or amyloidosis (see section 9.7.3). Those known to be

Table 17.4 Common associations of peripheral neuropathies

	Percentage of patients who develop a peripheral neuropathy
Common conditions	
Rheumatoid arthritis	3
Diabetes mellitus	5–10
Myxoedema	1
Pernicious anaemia	1
Uncommon conditions	
Systemic vasculitis	40
Amyloid	10
Cryoglobulinaemia	10

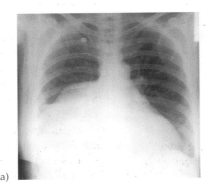
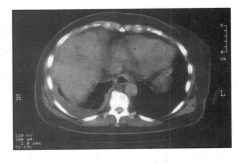

Fig. 17.4 X-ray and CT scan of chest in a patient with a thymoma and myasthenia gravis. (a) X-ray shows mass in right chest and pleural effusion. (b) CT scan shows this mass pushing heart and large vessels to left (and enlarged lymph nodes and a pleural effusion due to a chest infection).

(a)

(b)

Table 17.5 Immune-mediated peripheral neuropathies (with associated autoantibodies)

Acute	Chronic
Guillain–Barré syndrome (anti-GD1 antibodies)	Chronic inflammatory demyelinating polyneuropathies
Systemic vasculitis	Paraproteinaemic neuropathy (anti-MAG antibodies)
	Subacute sensory neuropathy (anti-Hu antibodies)
	Chronic multifocal motor neuropathy (anti-GM1 antibodies)
	Miller–Fisher syndrome (anti-GQ1 antibodies)

directly mediated by immune components, including paraproteins, are listed in Table 17.5.

17.5.1 Acute idiopathic polyneuritis (Guillain–Barré syndrome)

This is an uncommon disease of subacute onset in which the peripheral nervous system is infiltrated with lymphocytes and macrophages, and myelin is destroyed as a result.

Half the cases of this rare condition occur in relation to an infectious illness, often a diarrhoeal illness due to Campylobacter jejuni, as in Case 5.5 (in section 5.5), though 10% follow a surgical procedure and the rest are idiopathic. There is evidence to suggest that the **pathogenesis** involves the production of autoantibodies to peripheral nerve tissue gangliosides, triggered by infection (see Box 17.5). There is an increase in CSF protein, including IgG, which is often oligoclonal. Antibodies to known gangliosides such as GM1b can be demonstrated in 70% of patients.

Most patients improve within a few weeks of onset; their recovery is usually complete and therapy is avoided, as in Case 17.4. In severely affected patients, recovery times to unaided ventilation and walking are shortened considerably by the use of large doses of intravenous immunoglobulin (IVIG) given as soon as the diagnosis is made, as in Case 5.5. This has become the treatment of choice if **therapy** is needed.

> ### BOX 17.5 EVIDENCE FOR THE AUTOIMMUNE NATURE OF GUILLAIN–BARRÉ SYNDROME
>
> - Association with preceding infection
> - Cross-reactive epitopes between pathogen and autoantigen gangliosides
> - IgG and C1q deposited in nerves—seen on biopsies
> - Antiganglioside antibodies and antimyelin antibodies in serum
> - Correlation of antibodies with clinical disease course
> - Oligoclonal IgG in cerebrospinal fluid
> - Successful therapy with plasma exchange or intravenous immunoglobulin (immune modulation doses)

Plasma exchange has also been beneficial in severely affected patients when used within 48 h of start of symptoms.

17.5.2 Chronic inflammatory peripheral neuropathies

These several conditions differ from the Guillain–Barré syndrome in that they may be relapsing and remitting or have a progressive course. Patients are usually middle-aged and present gradually; the prevalence is around 30 per 10^5

CASE 17.4 GUILLAIN–BARRÉ SYNDROME

A 14-year-old boy awoke one morning 2 weeks after an episode of influenza with a mild weakness in his legs; his sceptical parents wondered if this was a ploy to avoid school but during the day he developed pain in his back and 'pins and needles' in his feet. He was considerably worse the next day and complained of weakness in his arms as well, and he was admitted to hospital that evening with suspected acute idiopathic inflammatory polyneuropathy.

Lumbar puncture showed no cells but a slightly raised protein level in the CSF. Peripheral nerve conduction studies the next day revealed demyelination, confirming a diagnosis of Guillain–Barré syndrome. Antibodies to ganglioside GD1 were present in his blood. His condition was by now stable and so he was not treated with high-dose intravenous immunoglobulin but monitored carefully; he made a complete recovery in 8 days.

CASE 17.5 MULTIFOCAL MOTOR NEUROPATHY

An 8-year-old boy presented with gradually increasing weakness in his arms. Leg weakness followed after 2 weeks and he experienced steady but slow downhill progression over 4 weeks. He had no consistent sensory symptoms. On examination, he was found to have a motor tetraparesis, most marked in the arms. Sensation was normal. Nerve conduction studies showed a demyelinating motor neuropathy in upper and lower limbs, with motor conduction velocities of 26 m/s. Antibodies to GM1 ganglioside were present in the serum, confirming the diagnosis of chronic multifocal motor

neuropathy. He was treated initially with prednisolone but this provoked further deterioration.

IVIG (2 g/kg body weight) was initially instituted every 8 weeks, with an initial excellent response after 5 days that gradually deteriorated after 4 weeks, returning to pretreatment levels by 8 weeks, in keeping with the half-life of IgG in the serum. This response to therapy was confirmed by a further infusion, after which changing the interval between infusions to 3 weeks and infusing IVIG (at a dose of 0.8 g/kg) resulted in sustained improvement.

Table 17.6 Paraneoplastic syndromes

Condition	Signs	Cancer	Autoantibodies to:
Cerebellar degeneration	Ataxia	Small cell lung cancer	Voltage gated calcium channels
Limbic encephalitis	Dementia	Small cell lung cancer	Voltage gated calcium channels
Paraneoplastic sensory neuropathy	Sensory loss and areflexia	Small cell lung cancer	Neuron antigen—Hu
Sensorimotor neuropathy	Mononeuritis multiplex	Cancer or vasculitis	
Paraproteinaemic polyneuropathies	Motor and sensory loss	Lymphoid malignancies	Myelin-associated glycoprotein

population. A history of a preceding illness is uncommon and the aetiology remains obscure. Sensory or motor symptoms or both are accompanied by **conduction block**. Some but not all patients have serum antibodies to gangliosides (see Table 17.5). **Treatment** with prednisone and/or plasma exchange is partially successful in some groups of patients. Regular infusions of IVIG are successful in some patients, but a trial of therapy is needed before embarking on long-term therapy.

17.5.3 Multifocal motor neuropathy

Patients with this condition have purely motor symptoms, which are usually symmetrical. **Autoantibodies** against **GM1 gangliosides** are found in many patients. The condition is exacerbated by steroid therapy, and intravenous immunoglobulin is now the treatment of choice since > 70% of patients respond to a trial of high-dose IVIG therapy. Maintenance therapy with immunoglobulin then enables them to live disability-free lives.

17.5.4 Monoclonal gammopathies

Sensory or motor neuropathies have been described in patients with monoclonal gammopathies. Twenty percent of patients with sensory neuropathies have monoclonal anti-

bodies to **myelin-associated glycoprotein (MAG)**—a major component of peripheral nerve (see Tables 17.5 and 17.6). These antibodies have been shown to cause demyelination in animals. Plasmapheresis, with or without immune suppression, is effective treatment. Peripheral neuropathy is also found in 10% of patients with cryoglobulinaemia (see section 11.6.3).

17.6 Paraneoplastic syndromes

There is a group of neurological conditions of the central and peripheral nervous systems that are associated with tumours. The neurological syndrome may predate an overt malignancy by many years, so it is always important to search for a resectable cancer, especially in the lung (Table 17.6).

17.7 Cerebral systemic lupus erythematosus

Up to 60% of patients with SLE suffer neuropsychiatric episodes at some time (see section 10.7). Most patients experience only mild but fluctuating symptoms. In some patients, spontaneous improvement occurs with time; others have irreversible changes. Cerebral thrombosis is not infrequent and is associated with antibodies to clotting factors and phospholipids (see section 16.6).

CASE 17.6 SYSTEMIC LUPUS ERYTHEMATOSUS

A 45-year-old woman presented with acute disorientation so severe that she was unable to dress herself. On neurological examination, there were no abnormal findings, and routine laboratory investigations, including examination of the urine, were normal. Nuclear MRI showed three frontal lobe lesions with the characteristic appearances of vasculitis, so a detailed search for a cause was undertaken.

A laboratory diagnosis of systemic lupus erythematosus (SLE) was made (Table 17.7). Prednisolone was given with a dramatic improvement in the patient's mental state; within a week she was able to dress herself, and 10 days after admission she was able to go home. Serological tests 9 months later showed only a weakly positive ANA at 1/160, a normal C3 level of 0.77 g/l, a low C4 level of 0.14 g/l, and persistent elevated DNA binding (68%).

Table 17.7 Investigations for Case 17.6, cerebral SLE

Antinuclear antibody (ANA)	Positive: 1/80
Antineutrophil cytoplasmic antibodies	Negative
dsDNA binding	High, 91% (normal < 30%)
DNA antibodies (IgG)	Positive on Crithidia luciliae (titre 1/120)
Serum IgG	16.5 g/l (NR 6.0–12.0)
C3	0.54 g/l (NR 0.65–1.25)
C4	0.03 g/l (NR 0.2–0.5)

Cerebral involvement is a clinical diagnosis. It can be the presenting feature of SLE in an otherwise undiagnosed patient, as in Case 17.6, but this is unusual. Serological tests are important, although there is no test that is specific for cerebral lupus.

FURTHER READING

See website: www.immunologyclinic.com

CHAPTER 18

18 Pregnancy

18.1 Introduction

In pregnancy, one-half of the transplantation antigens of the fetus are of paternal origin and, in an outbred species such as humans, these differ from those of the mother. The mother therefore carries a 'mismatched' fetus but, despite this, the fetus is not usually rejected. The reasons for this remain controversial and this chapter discusses the relationship between the local active recognition process (which allows successful implantation of the embryo and development of the placenta) and those systemic mechanisms which help maintain the pregnancy and prevent rejection. Protection against infection is also covered, as well as immunological disorders of pregnancy itself.

18.2 Immunological mechanisms in implantation and pregnancy

The mechanisms involved in implantation and maintenance of the fetus and placenta are complex, with the result that failure of one of these processes does not necessarily jeopardize this important process.

18.2.1 The role of the uterus

The uterus is *not* an immunologically privileged site (see Box 18.1). It is well vascularized, with a good lymphatic

> **BOX 18.1 EVIDENCE THAT THE UTERUS IS NOT AN IMMUNOLOGICALLY PRIVILEGED SITE**
>
> - T and B lymphoid cells are present in the healthy uterus and uterine cervix
> - Numbers of lymphocytes increase in the presence of local infection
> - Lymphoid infiltration is present in unexplained infertility
> - High numbers of CD4+ lymphocytes and macrophages in vaginal fluids in HIV and other sexually transmitted diseases
> - Free immunoglobulin molecules, particularly IgA and secretory IgA, in vaginal fluids

drainage, and can respond to infection and reject foreign tissue.

18.2.2 The role of the placenta

A successful pregnancy requires an influx of lymphoid cells for implantation.

The most abundant **lymphoid cell** population in human endometrium in the late luteal phase of the menstrual cycle and early pregnancy are granulated natural killer (NK) cells, which comprise around 75% of the total decidual cells. These uterine NK cells (uNK cells) proliferate and differentiate in the second half of the cycle and result in menstruation in the absence of an embryo.

In invading the decidua, to establish a pregnancy, the embryonic trophoblast cells interact with the proteins of the extracellular matrix of the maternal endometrium and break them down by secretion of metalloproteases. To control this invasion, the maternal tissue secretes transforming growth factors and tissue metalloprotease inhibitors. Furthermore, the decidua is colonized by maternal uNK cells, as well as macrophages and dendritic cells. These cells are responsible for local production of cytokines that promote or inhibit this trophoblastic invasion. In the process of implantation, these CD3+ CD56+ CD16− uNK cells play an important role by controlling the **invasion of extravillous trophoblast** into the spiral arteries of the decidua (see Fig. 18.1). The extravillous trophoblasts remodel these arteries by displacing the endothelium and destroying the muscularis, thereby increasing their bore to accommodate the increased blood flow to the placenta required by the fetus as it grows. In contrast, increased numbers of different cytolytic CD56+ CD16+ natural killer cells are found in endometrial tissue from recurrent miscarriage patients.

In the placenta, maternal blood is in direct contact with the villous trophoblast (Fig. 18.1). Extravillous trophoblast uniquely expresses **HLA-C, -E and -G MHC class I**, the latter differing from classical class I molecules in that they are of limited polymorphism. Their presence inhibits destruction by NK cells which normally attack cells that are not express-

ing self MHC. HLA-C, HLA-E and HLA-G molecules are all good ligands for NK cell receptors (see Box 18.2). These ligand–receptor pairs probably control the interaction of uNK cells with extravillous trophoblast cells. They are thought to play a role in the perturbation of pregnancy, pre-eclampsia, which is the major cause of maternal and fetal deaths in developed countries (see section 18.5.3). Classical MHC class I products, HLA-A and -B, involved in T-cell cytotoxicity, are not detected on the trophoblast; nor is there any MHC class II expression on trophoblast in humans.

In the past, the evidence suggested that the maternal immune system in pregnancy was biased away from TH1 inflammatory responses (potentially harmful to the fetus), by the release of TH2 cytokines (such as interleukin (IL)-4 and IL-10) from the placenta. Whilst good in theory, data

BOX 18.2 LIGAND:RECEPTOR PAIRS FOR UTERINE NK CELLS AND TROPHOBLAST ANTIGENS

HLA family	Distribution	Ligands on NK cells
HLA-G	Only on extravillous trophoblasts and epithelial cells of thymic medulla	LILRB1 ligand
HLA-C	Ubiquitous	KIR family
HLA-E	Ubiquitous	CD94–NKG2A/C

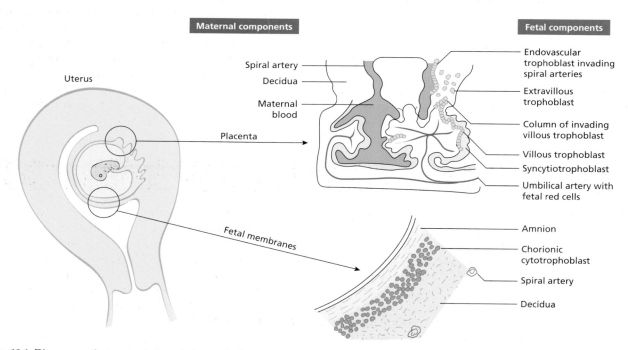

Fig. 18.1 Diagrammatic representation of placental relationships. (From Dr I. Sargent, University of Oxford, with permission.)

from knockout mice did not confirm this and recent data have thrown doubt on this paradigm, not least since the discovery of extended cytokine families and new molecules, as well as the cross-reactions of cytokine epitopes, cast doubt on past methods. The peri-implantation uterine NK cells are activated to produce high levels of inflammatory (TH1 type) **cytokines**, IL-18/IL-15, and monocytes to produce IL-12 in normal human pregnancies. IL-11, LIF and IL-1 have also been found to be important and others will no doubt be shown to play a role shortly.

On the other side of the coin, tumour necrosis factor (TNF)-α and interferon (IFN)-γ genes are up-regulated in placentas from abortion-prone mice, whereas injection of IL-10 prevents fetal death. Data from women with a history of recurrent fetal loss (see section 18.5.1) are more difficult to interpret, but increased production of TH1 cytokines suggests that the balance of cytokine production, locally and systemically, is important for both implantation and maintenance of the placenta. For example, the secretion of the crucial **vascular growth factor**, angiopoietin 2, is crucial for the development of placentas in both mice and humans and granulocyte/macrophage–colony-stimulating factor (GM CSF) is important in 'uterine priming' by seminal fluid.

18.3 Pregnancy and maternal infection

Human pregnancy has been associated with increased risk of infection. Infections with malaria, Toxoplasma or mycobacteria (tuberculosis and leprosy) are particularly common in developing countries, where malnutrition may be a major factor. Maternal infection is rare in developed countries, but Case 18.1 illustrates that the risk still persists. Listeria, toxoplasmosis and HIV are the most common infections, suggesting that there is **reduced TH1 cell activity** against intracellular pathogens during pregnancy. Pregnant women are advised to avoid unpasteurized dairy products and all women are checked antenatally for antibodies to sexually transmitted diseases.

Women should check their own **immunization status** for common viral infections (especially rubella, measles and polio) prior to pregnancy and avoid exposure to chickenpox if they are not immune. The more severe risks to the fetus are discussed below.

18.4 Protection of the fetus and neonate against infection

The fetus and neonate are susceptible to both bacterial and viral infections by transplacental transfer and during vaginal delivery. The extent and nature of the infection depend on the immune maturity of the fetus at the time of infection. This, in turn, depends on the gestational age of the fetus (Table 18.1).

18.4.1 Development of fetal immune responses

The fetus becomes partially immunocompetent early in **intrauterine life** (Table 18.1), e.g. intrauterine infection with rubella virus provokes the production of fetal IgM antibodies against the virus as early as week 11. However, *T-cell development is slow* and this may account for the particular susceptibility of the fetus to viruses and intracellular bacteria. Plenty of T cells are detectable early in gestational life and T-cell numbers in blood are much higher at birth than in adults. However, their functional capacity develops late in fetal life, is still reduced at birth and increases in early life to reach adult levels in the first 2 months.

At birth, although CD4$^+$ cell numbers are high and IL-2 production is normal, production of other important cytokines, IFN-γ, TNF and TH2 cytokines, is low. Cytotoxic T-cell function is only one-third of that of adults and natural killer cell cytolysis is reduced also. These findings may account for the severity of neonatal infections with herpes simplex virus, cytomegalovirus, Listeria and Toxoplasma. In the neonate, cytotoxic T-cell lysis is reduced, as is production of IFN-γ (see Table 18.1). Listeria, a facultative in-

CASE 18.1 A MOTHER INFECTED WITH LISTERIA

A 22-year-old primagravida planned to stay on a small-holding in France for the last 3 months of the pregnancy. She had been well, apart from morning sickness during the first 4 weeks of gestation. In France, she had been drinking fresh unpasteurized milk and eating home-made cheeses for 3 weeks when she developed fever, vomiting and diarrhoea followed by headache, myalgia and low back pain which persisted for 5 days. Four weeks later, at 28 weeks' gestation, she went into premature labour and a still-born, jaundiced child was delivered after 36 h. At the baby's

post mortem, there was evidence of hepatitis, purulent pneumonia, conjunctivitis and meningitis. Listeria monocytogenes was cultured from several sites and a diagnosis of fatal neonatal Listeria monocytogenes infection was made. The organism was sensitive to ampicillin and gentamycin and since there was no longer a teratogenic risk (the pregnancy being over), the mother was given a 4-week course of both antibiotics in case organisms were silently sequestered in her deep tissues.

Table 18.1 Development of immune responsiveness in the fetus

Gestational age (weeks)	Immune development*	
4	Blood centre with macrophages in the yolk sac	
6	Complement synthesis detected	
6	NK cells present in liver	
6–7	Thymic epithelium develops	
7	Lymphocytes and macrophages in blood	
7–9	Lymphocytes in thymus: CD3$^+$, 4$^+$, 8$^+$, TCR$^+$	
11	Serum IgM detectable in infection (e.g. rubella)	
	Mitogen responsiveness of thymocytes	
12–14	Neutrophil leucocytes in blood	
13	B cells in bone marrow	
14	Mitogen responsiveness of peripheral lymphocytes	
17	Endogenous IgG in serum—in infection only	
20	Alloreactivity detected	
Term:	B cells	Normal numbers but immature, i.e. CD5$^+$; CD27$^-$
	Antibodies	IgM to proteins but not to carbohydrate antigens
	Complement**	Classical 90% and alternative 60%, both of adult levels
		C8 and C9 only 20% of adult
	Cytokines	IL-2 production normal
		IFN-γ, TNF only 20% of adult levels
		TH2 cytokines also very low
	Lymphocyte function	T cells higher numbers than adult levels, but immature functionality
		Poor T-cell help for B cells—low CD40 ligand levels
		Cytotoxic T cells—only 30–60% of adult levels
		NK cell activity normal numbers, with > 50% being good cytokine producers (CD56^{++}); reduced NK cytolysis
	Neutrophils	Normal numbers but reduced stores, adhesion and migration

* NK, Natural killer; IL-2, interleukin 2; IFN-γ, interferon-γ.
**Particularly marked in pre-term babies.

tracellular bacterium, is killed as a result of CD8$^+$ cytotoxic T cells recognizing listerial antigen and MHC class I antigens on the surface of the infected histiocyte or hepatocyte. With reduced cytotoxic T cells and TH1 cytokine production, the fetus is more susceptible to intracellular and viral infections than the mother, as in Case 18.1.

The fetus is protected against bacterial infection by active transfer of **maternal IgG** across the placenta (see below). Fortunately, neutrophil leucocytes and macrophages are fully competent and plentiful in the circulation within a few days of birth.

18.4.2 Placental transfer of IgG

IgG is transferred by means of specific receptors on the trophoblast for the Fc region of IgG (see section 1.2.4 and Fig. 7.18). Transfer begins at about 12 weeks, but most of the maternal immunoglobulin is transferred after 32 weeks of intrauterine life. Extremely premature babies therefore lack

circulating maternal IgG at birth (Fig. 3.3) and are susceptible to infection (Fig. 18.2).

Infants with poor fetal growth also have lower levels of IgG at birth, due to poor placental transfer. Infants of very low birth weight (< 1.5 g) have a high prevalence (up to 20%) of late-onset infections related to invasive procedures, with an infection-related mortality of 5–10%. Such infections are bacterial (involving staphylococci, enterococci, Klebsiella and Pseudomonas) and are notably those infections against which antibodies play an important protective role. Intravenous immunoglobulin (IVIG) infusions (0.5 g/kg per week) have been shown to reduce late-onset infections (like that in Case 18.2) in placebo-controlled studies in the USA. IVIG is not used routinely in the UK, since the rate of serious late-onset infections is < 1%; this is probably due to avoidance of invasive procedures whenever possible.

In a full-term baby, the serum level of IgG in the neonate is equivalent to that of the mother, due to transfer of maternal IgG. However, there is little active neonatal synthesis of IgG

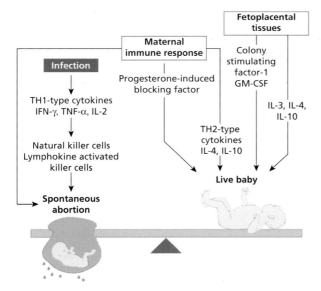

Fig. 18.2 Competing immune mechanisms to prevent infection and spontaneous abortion in fetal life.

or IgA at this stage. The result is a fall in the IgG level as the maternal IgG is catabolized. The half-life of IgG is 3–4 weeks, resulting in a period of relative IgG deficiency in the blood ('**physiological trough**') between 3 and 6 months.

The gradual increase of IgG thereafter is associated with expression of CD40 ligand on an increasing number of T cells and **isotype switching** from IgM to IgG and IgA production by the infant. The immaturity of B cells at birth, i.e. their CD5+ nature, results in low-affinity antibody production and the provision of the molecules involved in **somatic hypermutation** (as well as switching) results in the maturation of antibody production to high-affinity antibodies. This is accomplished by 2 months of age when routine immunizations with protein antigens begin. IgG level rises to approach adult levels by the age of 4 years (see Fig. 3.3), by

which time antibodies to carbohydrate antigens can be produced too. Replacement immunoglobulin is not needed in the physiological trough unless the child suffers from serious recurrent infections that are not preventable with prophylactic antibiotics (see section 3.2.2).

18.4.3 Immunological value of breast-feeding

The **anti-infective properties** of breast-feeding have been established for many years. An array of factors in breast milk helps to reduce the incidence of neonatal infections (Table 18.2). The principal immunoglobulin in human colostrum and breast milk is secretory IgA, which is resistant to the proteolytic effects of enzymes in the neonatal gut. The protective role of IgA includes virus neutralization, bactericidal activity and aggregation of antigen and prevention of bacterial adherence to epithelial cells. There is no evidence that significant amounts of these antibodies can be absorbed from the human neonatal gut and provide systemic protection, in contrast to other mammals.

The **cells in milk** are important in phagocytosis and their phagocytic ability is equal to that of blood leucocytes. There is evidence that protection against infection is provided by the macrophages in breast milk. Necrotizing enterocolitis

Table 18.2 Protective factors in breast milk

IgA—mainly secretory IgA resists digestion in fetal gut. These antibodies include those against bacteria and viruses

Cells—macrophages, polymorphonuclear leucocytes, lymphocytes

Complement components may be involved in opsonization by alternate pathway

Lysozyme can attack bacterial cell walls

Lactoperoxidase—antistreptococcal agent

Lactoferrin inhibits growth of bacteria

CASE 18.2 HYPOGAMMAGLOBULINAEMIA OF PREMATURITY

A normal infant girl was delivered by caesarean section at 30 weeks of gestation as her 35-year-old primagravida mother had severe pre-eclampsia. The infant weighed 0.75 kg and had no obvious congenital abnormalities and respiration was established quickly. In view of her young gestational age, cord blood immunoglobulin measurements and amniotic fluid lecithin/sphingomyelin ratio were obtained. Her gestational age was actually 26 weeks; her serum IgG level was 0.1 g/l (NR at birth is equivalent to that of the mother, i.e. 7.2–19.0 g/l). A diagnosis of hypogammaglobulinaemia of prematurity was made.

Nutritional support was given and an intravascular catheter inserted to enable blood sampling. On day 10, the infant developed apnoea, bradycardia and abdominal distension. Investigations showed a neutrophilia and raised C-reactive protein (CRP) and blood cultures grew Staphylococcus aureus. Intravenous antibiotic therapy was started for this neonatal staphylococcal infection; IVIG therapy was considered too, but the infant made a good recovery and was discharged after 8 weeks (rather than on day 14 as hoped).

is caused by bacterial penetration of the gut and occurs in infants with poor local defences; the condition is relatively uncommon in breast-fed infants.

Immunocompetent **lymphocytes** are present in human milk and, although there is no evidence that these react against the neonate in a harmful way, CD4+ cells will carry HIV in an HIV+ mother. *Transmission of HIV from mother to baby* has been documented in this way. Breast-feeding by HIV+ mothers is therefore discouraged in developed countries, although this is inappropriate in areas of malnutrition. With the introduction of human milk banks, the effect of sterilization (for safe storage) is important. Freezing milk reduces the number of viable cells, while autoclaving and pasteurization destroy some antibodies as well as the cells, although the nutritional properties are unaffected by these processes.

18.5 Disorders of pregnancy

Some diseases, such as recurrent abortions, pre-eclampsia or alloimmunization, are disorders of pregnancy itself. Diseases not restricted to pregnancy may also have profound effects on the pregnant woman and her baby.

18.5.1 Recurrent abortions

About 20% of all pregnancies abort spontaneously and *two-thirds of fetuses are lost even before the woman realizes that she is pregnant*. Many factors cause abortion: these include infections, congenital defects, endocrine abnormalities and autoimmune states, such as systemic lupus erythematosus (SLE) (see section 10.7) and the antiphospholipid syndrome (see section 16.6.1). *Only 10% of women probably have an immunological cause* for such abortions. Whilst suppression of specific maternal immune responses to fetal paternal antigens would be a convenient explanation for the survival of the fetus, there is little evidence to support this.

The most important role for the immunology laboratory is to exclude SLE (see Cases 18.3 and 18.4) and the antiphospholipid syndrome (see Case 16.6). The role of **anticardiolipin and antiphospholipid antibodies** in recurrent abortions has become clearer in recent years, although there is still a good deal of confusion. The overall prevalence of IgG and IgM antiphospholipid antibodies in healthy women varies from 2 to 7%. Only high-titre IgG antibodies are associated with recurrent fetal loss. Since 85% of women with these antibodies will have a normal pregnancy, screening women prior to pregnancy is not cost-effective. However, those who present with two or more spontaneous abortions and are found to have high-titre IgG antibodies are most at risk of further fetal loss, so these women are treated with aspirin and low-dose heparin in pregnancy. Steroids are reserved for those with evidence of SLE. The role of intravenous immunoglobulin remains to be proven by randomized controlled trial.

There is now a strong body of evidence (several clinical trials and a meta-analysis) that suggests that immunotherapy, i.e. *immunization* of the woman with her partner's lymphocytes in an attempt to suppress specific cell-mediated immunity, is *not successful in > 90%* of women with recurrent abortions. In many countries this has been abandoned anyway, due to the risks of transmissible diseases.

18.5.2 Outcome of pregnancy in systemic lupus erythematosus

SLE (see sections 10.7 and 11.5.4) is predominantly a disease of young women who may want to have children. There is no evidence that women with lupus are subfertile, although there is undoubtedly **increased fetal loss** (abortion > 10 weeks of gestation/stillbirth).

Human placental explants cultured in sera from untreated, non-pregnant women with SLE/APS demonstrated a significant **decrease in the trophoblastic cell proliferation** rate and an **increase in apoptosis** compared with non-pregnant women and those with treated SLE/APS, suggesting a role for serum antibodies in the pathogenesis of failed pregnancy. Furthermore, drugs used in the treatment of SLE can affect the fetus very early in pregnancy. It is therefore important to control the disease preconception in order to achieve a better outcome for mother and baby.

CASE 18.3 RECURRENT SPONTANEOUS ABORTION

A 32-year-old woman, who had had three previous spontaneous miscarriages in the first trimester, sought advice from a specialist obstetrician. There was no history of infections in these pregnancies. Examination of the fetal products had not been done but there was no family history of genetic disease or recurrent fetal loss in close female relatives. She had been extremely well but she and her husband were anxious. She had no obvious rash, arthritis or bruising and appeared to have a normal uterus and cervix.

Blood tests were negative for cardiolipin, thyroid and antinuclear autoantibodies, and CRP and immunoglobulin measurements were normal. She was advised that she had no underlying cause for the recurrent abortions and that the chance of a successful pregnancy was 30%; she delivered a healthy, live female infant 11 months later.

CASE 18.4 SYSTEMIC LUPUS ERYTHEMATOSUS

A 19-year-old girl had been diagnosed as having SLE 15 months earlier, following presentation with arthritis in her hands, a rash (livido reticularis) on her arms and considerable spontaneous bruising. She had had antinuclear antibodies of 1/320, C3 of 450 mg/l, C4 of 70 mg/l and a platelet count of 54×10^9/l at that time. Renal function was normal but she had both low-titre anticardiolipin antibodies and a lupus anticoagulant, though no antibodies to double-stranded DNA (dsDNA) at presentation. She consulted an obstetrician at 16 weeks into an unexpected pregnancy whilst in disease remission and on 5 mg of prednisolone daily; she had taken the message about possible difficulties in achieving a pregnancy

too literally! She was seen every 2 weeks throughout the pregnancy to monitor activity of the SLE; regular full blood counts, C3, C4, creatinine, anticardiolipin and dsDNA antibody measurements were done as well as urine and blood pressure monitoring. These tests were unchanged throughout the pregnancy. A live, normal, male infant was delivered uneventfully by caesarean section at 38 weeks in view of her low platelet count. In the puerperium she had a mild exacerbation of her arthritis and rash for 6 weeks but without proteinuria, increase in serum creatinine or DNA antibodies. The infant remained well.

Women with SLE have a **70% rate of successful** pregnancies, although 1–2% of mothers with the Ro antibody will have infants with congenital heart block. Successful pregnancies are often complicated by pre-eclampsia, intra-uterine growth retardation and prematurity.

Fetal loss has been associated with the presence of antiphospholipid antibodies and/or lupus anticoagulant, an antibody to the activated clotting factor X (see section 16.6.2). Patients with these antibodies are treated with low-dose aspirin to reduce platelet aggregation. Although high doses of intravenous immunoglobulin are sometimes used to reduce autoantibody levels prophylactically during pregnancy in APS women, this can exacerbate the disease in those with SLE. In patients whose lupus presents in pregnancy, both the morbidity risk to the mother and mortality risk to the fetus are greatly increased.

Women with other rheumatic diseases unrelated to pregnancy may become pregnant and require close medical supervision (Fig. 18.3).

18.5.3 Pre-eclampsia

Pre-eclampsia is a **disease of implantation**, in which the symptoms are expressed late in pregnancy once the complications of placental ischaemia due to poor implantation are apparent. The precise aetiology of pre-eclampsia is unknown, but inadequate trophoblast invasion and a failure to modify the structure of the spiral arteries result in an inadequate blood supply and hence placental ischaemia, leading to fetal anoxia. The maternal syndrome, characterized by hypertension, oedema and proteinuria, results from systemic maternal endothelial damage and inflammation caused by factors released into the maternal circulation from the **ischaemic placenta**.

Studies suggest that abnormal production of placental cytokines, growth factors and metalloproteinase inhibitors (see Fig. 18.1) results in deranged vasculature of the placenta. Pre-eclampsia is more **common in primagravida**; in contrast, those women previously sensitized to human an-

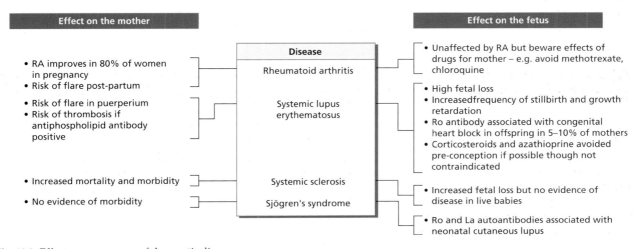

Fig. 18.3 Effects on pregnancy of rheumatic diseases.

tigens (including HLA) by previous pregnancies with the same partner have a lower incidence of pre-eclampsia. It has been suggested that specific exposure to the paternal HLA-C, -E and -G antigens by maternal uNK cells enables better invasion of trophoblast cells for implantation.

18.5.4 Alloimmunization

Alloimmunization (sensitization) of a woman against **fetal antigens** can occur when fetal red cells pass into the mother's circulation. This happens at delivery and even following minor uterine events during pregnancy. These antibodies then cross the placenta to react with fetal erythrocytes. The opsonized fetal red cells are sequestrated and destroyed by macrophages in the fetal spleen and liver, resulting in **haemolytic disease of the newborn**.

The commonest cause of haemolytic disease of the newborn (HDN) remains **rhesus incompatibility** between mother and fetus. Routine blood grouping of all antenatal women and their spouses detects those rhesus D-negative women who may be at risk. HDN is now preventable by administration of anti-D antibodies antenatally and immediately after delivery, by destroying any rhesus-positive fetal cells and preventing the mother from becoming sensitized. HND may also be due to ABO incompatibility, but this is rarely severe enough to require an exchange transfusion at birth, probably because ABO antigens are less well developed in the fetus than rhesus antigens.

Alloimmunization with fetal platelets may induce the mother to produce specific **antiplatelet antibodies** (see Chapter 16). The placental transfer of such antibodies results in **alloimmune neonatal thrombocytopenic purpura**; this is uncommon (1 : 1000 births), as the antigen to which these antibodies are directed (HPA-1a) is common in the general population and so most mothers are positive for the antigen and do not produce antibodies. This condition should be distinguished from idiopathic thrombocytopenic purpura (ITP), in which the mother has circulating autoantibodies to her own platelets (see below). *The risk of severe intracerebral bleeding in either infant is extremely rare, as the function of the platelets is not reduced.*

Maternal antibodies to the histocompatibility antigens of her fetus are commonly found; they are weak in the first pregnancy but become stronger with successive pregnancies. There is *no* evidence that these antibodies, which are often IgG and thus cross the placenta, are detrimental to the fetus.

18.5.5 Organ-specific autoimmune diseases in pregnancy

The mother and/or fetus can be affected by an organ-specific autoimmune disease in pregnancy (Fig. 18.4). **Haemolytic anaemia** can worsen during pregnancy, probably due to raised levels of hormones; the fetus may be affected by immunological complications of the pregnancy such as anoxia (Fig. 18.4).

In those autoimmune disorders associated with **circulating IgG autoantibodies**, these antibodies may directly damage the fetus once they have crossed the placenta, as in Case 18.5 (see also Table 5.2). However, this may be infrequent, as in the 10% of babies born to myasthenic mothers (see section 17.4.1).

In **ITP** the mother has thrombocytopenia due to circulating autoantibodies to her own platelets. It is rare for this to cause problems at delivery but, if so, prompt treatment with high-dose IVIG will result in a rapid rise in platelets. Autoantibodies cross the placenta, to induce neonatal thrombocytopenia in 50% of infants. Testing of the mother's and the baby's platelets will detect platelet-bound antibody. If this

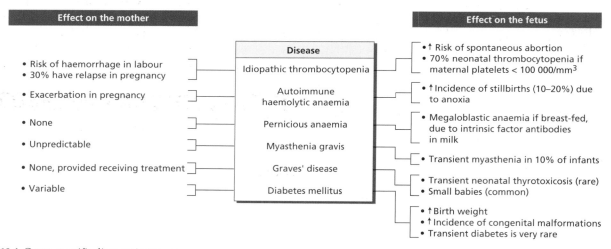

Fig. 18.4 Organ-specific diseases in pregnancy.

CASE 18.5 TRANSIENT NEONATAL GRAVES' DISEASE

A 32-year-old primagravida was seen in the obstetric clinic at 16 weeks of gestation, having suffered from severe morning sickness until the 14th week. She was now complaining of heat intolerance, weight loss, palpitations and fatigue. There was no past history of thyroid disease and no family history. On examination she had a marked tachycardia, was thin and there was a bruit over the thyroid. Thyroid function tests showed undetectable thyroid-stimulating hormone (TSH) and high levels of free T3 and T4. Levels of autoantibodies to thyroid microsomes were extremely high (1/400 000) and antibodies to TSH receptors revealed that she had

Graves' disease. She was treated with carbimazole and the dose was kept to a minimum to keep the T3 in the high-normal range. Surgery was not required.

As the level of TSH receptor antibodies was still high at 36 weeks, it was no surprise when the cord blood from a female infant with normal-sized thyroid delivered at 37 weeks, was found to have high T3 and T4 levels and positive TSH receptor antibodies. The neonatologist judged that no treatment was required and the parents were reassured that neonatal Graves' disease is transient. At 3 months the baby had normal thyroid function.

is present on platelets from both individuals, they are autoimmune as in ITP, or if restricted to the neonate, they are alloimmune (see above). The management of immune neonatal thrombocytopenia is discussed in Chapter 16. A similar mechanism has been detected in which antineutrophil antibodies cause neonatal neutropenia, but this is extremely rare.

18.6 Clinical relevance of antibodies to reproductive components

18.6.1 Antibodies to hormones

Antibodies against reproductive hormones are able to block their action in achieving a successful pregnancy. If immunization using such hormones can provoke adequate titres of neutralizing antibodies in sexually mature individuals, the vaccinee becomes infertile for the duration of these antibodies. Unlike anti-tumour vaccines, which aim to provoke a cytotoxic T-lymphocyte (CTL) response, it would be highly undesirable for a **contraceptive vaccine** to stimulate T cells other than those required for T-cell help for antibody production.

To date, no contraceptive vaccines have been licensed, but phase II trials in women have been partially successful with potent vaccines to human chorionic gonadotrophin, which act post-fertilization in prevention and curtailment of implantation (see Box 18.3). Vaccines against follicle-stimulating hormone for use in men have been tested in male monkeys, but have not been sufficiently immunogenic and have failed to result in aspermia.

BOX 18.3 PROGRESS IN HUMAN CONTRACEPTIVE VACCINES

Success with hCG (part human/part ovine), conjugated to toxoid, plus potent approved adjuvants

- provokes high-titre neutralizing antibodies in 80% of recipients
- successful in prevention of pregnancies in these women
- vaccination is safe and reversible

But antibody production not always optimal; T cell induced oophoritis

18.6.2 Antibodies to sperm

Fertilization is reduced or inhibited by antibodies present on the sperm surface; such antibodies are produced by the male after sterilization or by plasma cells in the female genital tract. Attempts to remove bound antibodies from sperm have been largely unsuccessful. Microinjection of such compromised sperm directly into the oocyte cytoplasm has been shown to overcome this and to increase fertilization rates. Anti-sperm antibodies can be detected in specialist andrology laboratories and are no longer part of a routine clinical laboratory repertoire.

FURTHER READING

See website: www.immunologyclinic.com

CHAPTER 19

19 Techniques in Clinical Immunology

19.1 Introduction

Laboratory tests can be graded according to their value in the care of patients. Some tests are **essential** for diagnosis or monitoring, some are **useful** in subclassifying disorders with varying complications or outcomes, and others are of current **research** interest, but may provide added diagnostic insight in future. Unfortunately, tests are **useless** if requested in inappropriate circumstances and this applies particularly to uncritical requests such as 'autoantibody screens'. Nobody highlighted the problem better than the late Dr Richard Asher over 50 years ago (Box 19.1).

Laboratory tests differ in their sensitivity and specificity (Fig. 19.1). For optimal results, the cut-off point for any assay — the point above which results are considered positive — is set so that virtually no diseased patients are test-negative (false-negative results) and the fewest possible individuals without the disease are test-positive (false-positive results). The **sensitivity** of a test is defined as the propor-

---

BOX 19.1 WHY DOES A CLINICIAN ORDER A TEST?

- I order this test because if it agrees with my opinion I will believe it, and if it does not I shall disbelieve it

- I do not understand this test and am uncertain of the normal figure, but it is the fashion to order it

- When my chief asks if you have done this or that test I like to say yes, so I order as many tests as I can to avoid being caught out

- I have no clear idea what I am looking for, but in ordering this test I feel in a vague way (like Mr Micawber) that something might turn up

- I order this test because I want to convince the patient there is nothing wrong, and I don't think he will believe me without a test

Asher R (1954) Straight and crooked thinking in medicine. *Br Med J* **ii**, 460–2.

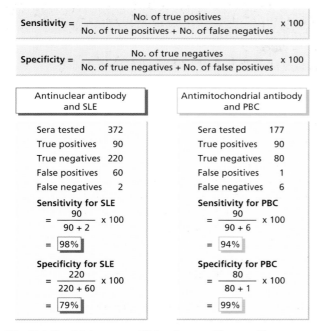

$$\text{Sensitivity} = \frac{\text{No. of true positives}}{\text{No. of true positives} + \text{No. of false negatives}} \times 100$$

$$\text{Specificity} = \frac{\text{No. of true negatives}}{\text{No. of true negatives} + \text{No. of false positives}} \times 100$$

Antinuclear antibody and SLE

Sera tested	372
True positives	90
True negatives	220
False positives	60
False negatives	2

Sensitivity for SLE

$$= \frac{90}{90 + 2} \times 100$$

$$= \boxed{98\%}$$

Specificity for SLE

$$= \frac{220}{220 + 60} \times 100$$

$$= \boxed{79\%}$$

Antimitochondrial antibody and PBC

Sera tested	177
True positives	90
True negatives	80
False positives	1
False negatives	6

Sensitivity for PBC

$$= \frac{90}{90 + 6} \times 100$$

$$= \boxed{94\%}$$

Specificity for PBC

$$= \frac{80}{80 + 1} \times 100$$

$$= \boxed{99\%}$$

Fig. 19.1 Sensitivity vs. specificity of assays illustrated by antinuclear antibody testing for systemic lupus erythematosus (SLE) and antimitochondrial antibody (AMA) testing for primary biliary cirrhosis (PBC).

tion of diseased individuals in whom the test is positive. A negative result of a test which is very sensitive can be used to exclude the relevant disease ('rule-out'). Test results should be negative both in healthy people and in individuals with different diseases but similar clinical features. The **specificity** of a test is the proportion of individuals without a given disease in whom the test is negative. A positive test is then virtually restricted to the disease in question ('rule-in') and tests of high specificity, such as antimitochondrial antibody (AMA) (Fig. 19.1), are used to confirm the clinical diagnosis.

Of the assays described in this chapter, some are quantitative, others are qualitative. Quantitative assays usually produce precise results. In general, such assays can be automated and international reference preparations are available to standardize results. Qualitative assays provide answers of normal/abnormal or positive/negative type. They can involve considerable technical expertise and interpretation of results can be subjective.

All laboratories strive to ensure quality and accuracy of results. **Quality assurance** (QA) is achieved by internal quality control (QC) of assays and participation in External Quality Assessment Schemes (EQAS), which may be organized on a regional, national or international basis.

19.2 Polyclonal and monoclonal antisera used in clinical immunology laboratories

Antisera used in laboratory tests are usually raised in animals by injection of the relevant antigen. Animals respond by making **polyclonal antibodies**, i.e. the resultant sera contain mixtures of antibodies from different B-cell clones. The antibodies all react with the relevant antigen but vary in the precise nature of their variable regions.

In contrast, **monoclonal antibodies** are the product of a single cell and its progeny and are therefore identical throughout their variable and constant regions; they react only with one determinant (epitope) on a given antigen. Spleen cell suspensions from immunized mice contain numerous secreting B cells from different clones recognizing different epitopes. These B cells are fused with a non-secreting myeloma cell line to form hybrids that have the antibody-producing capacity of the parent B cell and the immortality of the malignant plasma cell. Hybrid cells are then selected and cloned (Fig. 19.2). Large-scale culture can provide considerable quantities of such antibodies, which are pure and precise in their reactivity.

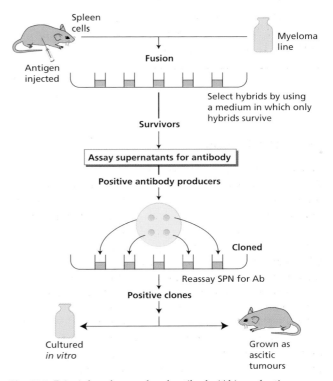

Fig. 19.2 Principles of monoclonal antibody (Ab) production. SPN, Supernatants.

19.3 Measurement of immunoglobulins and other specific proteins

Serum immunoglobulin measurements are essential in patients with repeated or severe infections and those with myeloma and some other lymphoproliferative disorders. They are sometimes useful in the differential diagnosis of hypergammaglobulinaemic states (Table 19.1).

The classical techniques used for measurement involve immune-complex formation. At low concentrations, these immune complexes remain in suspension as fine particles which can disperse a beam of light. Light dispersion can be measured using machines such as a centrifugal analyser, in which ultracentrifugation speeds complex formation. For a constant antibody concentration, the amount of light scatter is proportional to the concentration of the antigen. The method is rapid and suitable for automation; precise results can be obtained in 1–2 h from venepuncture.

For some proteins, machine-compatible reagents may not be available. Under these circumstances, laboratories may use the single radial immunodiffusion (RID) technique originally described by Mancini. Both RID and centrifugal analysis can be used for measurement of many proteins in serum, amniotic fluid, cerebrospinal fluid, saliva and gastrointestinal juice. They include a range of immune reactants, acute-phase proteins, transport proteins, coagulation proteins and 'tumour markers'. Standard preparations are used, which have been calibrated against international WHO standards. *Each hospital laboratory determines its own reference range for each protein* and this will vary according to the method and antisera used and the ethnic origin of the group. Reference ranges of most proteins also vary with age, especially in children, but 95% of the 'normal' population will fall within that range.

Table 19.1 Examples* of major polyclonal elevations in immunoglobulin levels

Immunoglobulin	Example
IgM	Primary biliary cirrhosis
IgA	Alcoholic liver disease
IgG	Primary Sjögren's syndrome
	HIV infection
	Systemic lupus erythematosus
Mixed isotypes	Tuberculosis
	Hepatic cirrhosis
	Chronic bacterial infections/occult abscesses

*But not sufficiently specific to be of diagnostic value in individual patients.

19.4 Qualitative investigation of immunoglobulins

19.4.1 Serum

It is essential that sera sent for immunoglobulin quantification on adults be screened by serum **protein electrophoresis** for the presence of paraproteins (monoclonal bands). A wet membrane or gel is stretched across an electrophoresis tank, and filter-paper wicks provide a continuous buffer phase. Serum samples are applied to the surface on the cathodal side and an electric current is passed through the membrane or gel for about 45 min. It is then removed and the protein bands visualized with an appropriate dye (Fig. 19.3). A normal serum is always run with the test specimens for comparison and quality control.

Discrete monoclonal (M) bands can appear anywhere along the strip and must be investigated further. False-positive bands, which are not due to immunoglobulin, may be caused by haemoglobin (in a haemolysed sample), fibrinogen (in plasma or an incompletely clotted specimen) or ag-

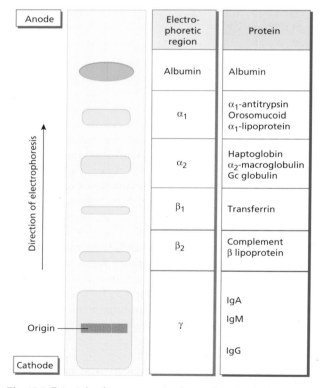

Fig. 19.3 Principle of serum protein electrophoresis. At the pH of routine electrophoresis (pH 8.6), serum proteins carry a net negative charge and migrate towards the anode. Some weakly charged proteins, such as immunoglobulins, are carried back towards the cathode by the flow of buffer.

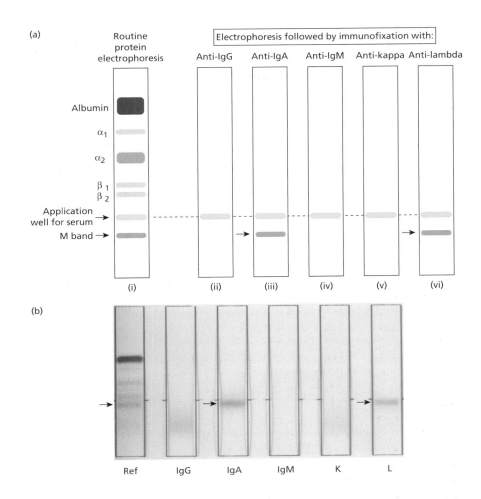

Fig. 19.4 Typing an M band by immunofixation. In this schematic example (a), the M band found on electrophoresis (i) is identified as an IgA (type λ) as shown on the actual fixation gel (b).

gregated IgG (in a stored specimen). It is therefore important to send fresh clotted blood specimens for this test.

When an M band is found on electrophoresis, the nature of the band must be determined by immunofixation. Several samples of test serum are first electrophoresed on agar gel (Fig. 19.4). Specific antisera to IgG, IgA, IgM and κ and λ light chains are then applied to the electrophoresed samples by soaking strips of cellulose acetate membrane in the individual antisera and laying these strips on the surface of the gel. Precipitation (i.e. immunofixation) of the M protein is achieved by incubating the gel and antisera for about 2 h. Unfixed (non-precipitated) protein is washed from the gel and the 'fixed' bands are stained.

In the absence of a heavy-chain abnormality, an abnormal reaction with antisera specific for light chains alone suggests that the M band is due to free monoclonal light chains or, very rarely, an IgD or IgE paraprotein. An abnormal reaction with a heavy-chain antiserum alone suggests a rare, heavy-chain disease (see Chapter 6).

Individual M bands can be quantified by a machine called a densitometer; this measures the intensity of stain taken up by each band and produces a tracing corresponding to the electrophoretic strip (Fig. 19.5). The proportion attributable to the monoclonal protein is expressed as a percentage of the whole tracing and converted to absolute terms (g/l) by reference to the total serum protein concentration. Scanning densitometry is the only reliable method for measuring paraprotein concentration, particularly for serial monitoring or

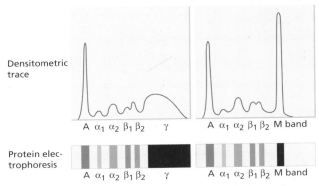

Fig. 19.5 Densitometric analysis of protein electrophoresis for quantification of an M band. A, Albumin.

in samples containing large amounts of non-paraprotein immunoglobulins.

Gross elevations of the immunoglobulin levels indicate the need to measure the relative serum viscosity (RSV); this is the time taken for a given volume of serum to pass through a narrow capillary tube, relative to water. RSV is normally 1.4–1.8. Symptoms of hyperviscosity (see Case 6.9) usually develop when the RSV value exceeds 4.0.

Provided the serum is fresh, a heavy deposit of protein at the origin in serum electrophoresis may indicate the presence of **cryoglobulins**. Cryoglobulins are immunoglobulins that form precipitates, gels or even crystals in the cold. The severity of the symptoms (see Case 11.7 and section 11.6.3) depends on the cryoprotein concentration and the temperature at which cryoprecipitation occurs. If cryoglobulins are suspected clinically, a fresh specimen of blood must be taken directly into a warmed container (37 °C) and delivered warm (37 °C) to the laboratory; it is allowed to clot at 37 °C and also separated at 37 °C. Aliquots of separated serum are kept at 4 °C for 24 h or longer. Centrifugation and washing of any resultant precipitate must be done at 4 °C. The precipitate is redissolved by warming back to 37 °C and then analysed for its constituent proteins by immunofixation at 37 °C.

19.4.2 Urine

Analysis of urine is essential in suspected myeloma or any condition in which a serum M band has been found, in hypogammaglobulinaemia of unknown cause and in amyloidosis.

Normal immunoglobulin synthesis is accompanied by production of excessive amounts of free polyclonal light chains (see section 6.6). These are excreted into the urine, where they can be detected in minute amounts in everyone. Patients with renal damage excrete larger quantities of polyclonal free light chains in the urine.

Free monoclonal light chains (Bence-Jones proteins) cannot be detected by routine measurement of total urinary protein or urine dipstick testing. The only reliable test for suspected 'Bence-Jones proteinuria' consists of three stages:
- concentration of urine;
- electrophoresis to demonstrate the presence of an M band; and
- immunofixation to confirm that the monoclonal band is composed of either monoclonal κ or λ free light chains.

The excretion of a whole paraprotein by a damaged kidney may give a false-positive result, unless the free light-chain nature of the M band is confirmed or the serum paraprotein is run alongside for identification.

19.4.3 Cerebrospinal fluid

IgG and albumin concentrations in cerebrospinal fluid (CSF)

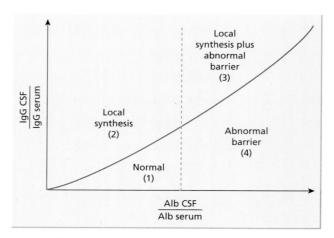

Fig. 19.6 Cerebrospinal fluid (CSF) IgG index. The y axis shows increasing values for the quotient of IgG in CSF: IgG in serum, and the x axis shows increasing values for the quotient of albumin in CSF: albumin in serum. The four areas signify: (1) normal; (2) local synthesis (normal barrier function); (3) local synthesis plus abnormal barrier function; (4) barrier function abnormal (not local synthesis).

can be measured. Since albumin is not synthesized in the brain, the relationship between IgG and albumin—the CSF IgG index—gives an indirect indication of how much CSF IgG has been synthesized by lymphocytes inside the brain (Fig. 19.6). In contrast to serum, the IgG in CSF is often of a restricted nature and forms **oligoclonal bands**, i.e. there are two or more discrete bands rather than a diffuse increase. Oligoclonal bands cannot be detected by routine electrophoresis of unconcentrated CSF and the degree of concentration needed (80-fold) to make bands visible induces artefacts. The most satisfactory method is isoelectric focusing and immunofixation with an enzyme-labelled antiserum to IgG (Fig. 19.7). This is an essential test in the investigation of demyelinating disorders such as multiple sclerosis (see Case 17.2).

19.5 Investigation of complement and immune complex disorders

Assays for complement in the serum are divided into those assays which recognize the antigenic nature of the individual complement components, and those which measure functional activity, such as cell lysis.

19.5.1 Assays for individual components

Immunochemical measurements of C3 and C4 are the most useful assays. International reference preparations and reliable automated methods are widely available. Measurements of other components can be done but are rarely

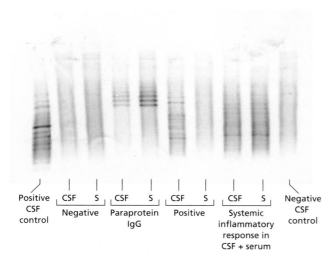

Fig. 19.7 Oligoclonal bands of IgG detected in cerebrospinal fluid (CSF). Isoelectric focusing separates proteins within a pH gradient according to their acidic or basic nature. The proteins are then transferred to a nitrocellulose membrane by blotting and the nitrocellulose immunofixed with an antiserum to IgG to show the IgG-specific bands. The pattern is interpreted by comparing paired samples of CSF and serum (S). A positive test is one where oligoclonal IgG bands are found in CSF but not in serum.

needed, except in patients with suspected genetic deficiencies and abnormal functional assays. C1 inhibitor must be measured if hereditary angioedema is suspected (see Case 11.5 and section 11.6.1).

Low levels of complement components are more relevant clinically than high levels. As all complement components can act as acute-phase reactants, rates of synthesis rise in any inflammatory condition.

To understand complement changes in disease, it is useful to consider complement components in three groups (Fig. 19.8):

- early components of the classical pathway;
- early components of the alternate pathway; and
- late components common to both pathways.

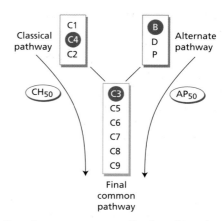

Fig. 19.8 Complement components distributed into three groups (see text). Ringed components are those measured as representatives of the groups. Functional integrity of the classical and alternate pathways is measured by CH_{50} and AP_{50} assays (see text).

In practice (Table 19.2), low C4 and C3 but normal Factor B levels suggest that activation of the classical pathway alone has occurred; if C4, C3 and Factor B levels are low, the alternate pathway is probably also activated, either via the feedback loop (see Chapter 1) or by simultaneous activation. Normal C4 levels with low C3 and Factor B concentrations provide evidence of activation of the alternate pathway alone.

Serial measurements of C3 and C4 are useful in monitoring disease activity or treatment in patients with some forms of glomerulonephritis, systemic lupus erythematosus (SLE) and vasculitis. If low initially, they often return to normal in remission (see Chapters 9 and 10). Routine complement tests are of little value in other acute and chronic inflammatory diseases.

19.5.2 Detection of complement breakdown products

Even if complement levels are normal, consumption may

Table 19.2 Interpretation of complement changes in disease

C4	C3	Factor B	Activation pathway	Examples
↓	↓	N	Classical pathway	Systemic lupus erythematosus (SLE); vasculitis
↓	↓	↓	Classical and alternate pathways	Gram-negative bacteraemia Some cases of SLE
N	↓	↓	Alternate pathway	C3 NeF autoantibody
↓	N	N	Classical pathway to C4 and C2 only	Hereditary angioedema (C1 inhibitor deficiency)
↑	↑	↑	Increased synthesis of components	Acute and chronic inflammation

be recognized by measuring 'breakdown' or activation products of the pathway. This is helpful in endotoxic shock, where alternate pathway activation of C3 is suspected. The electrophoretic mobility of native C3 and that of its cleavage products (e.g. C3c and C3dg) are different. Other activation products, such as C3a, C5a, C1r/C1s complex and C5b-9 complex, can also be measured for research purposes but are not used routinely.

19.5.3 C3 nephritic factor

C3 nephritic factor (C3 NeF) is an autoantibody to activated C3 which stabilizes the alternate pathway C3 convertase and allows further C3 breakdown (see Chapter 9). C3 NeF is suspected in patients in whom an unexplained low C3 level is found; these are usually patients with kidney disease or recurrent infections. It is detected by incubation of the patient's serum with normal serum; this allows the C3 nephritic factor in patient's serum to break down C3 in the normal serum.

19.5.4 Functional assays

Functional assays are essential if a genetic defect of complement is suspected but are not helpful in other conditions.

The commonest assay used in routine laboratories is the CH_{50} **assay** (total haemolytic complement) (Fig. 19.8). This estimates the quantity of serum required (as a complement source) to produce haemolysis of 50% of a standard quantity of sensitized red blood cells. Patients' sera are always titrated against a standard serum. A similar functional assay of the alternate complement pathway is also available. Provided that specimens reach the laboratory promptly, these assays are sensitive and reliable.

19.5.5 Assays for immune complexes

Immune complexes are involved in the pathogenesis of tissue lesions in a variety of human diseases. In all conditions where an immune-complex aetiology is suspected, **direct analysis of tissue biopsies** should be done. Biopsy specimens for direct immunofluorescent examination must not be fixed, but delivered directly to the laboratory on ice by arrangement. They are then snap-frozen and sliced; sections are well washed in saline to reduce background staining, before incubation with the appropriate conjugated antiserum. A parallel section is also stained with haematoxylin and eosin to show the morphology of the specimen. The technique is commonly used for renal (Chapter 9) and skin (Chapter 11) biopsies and is very useful in diagnosis. Indications are given in the relevant clinical chapters.

Tests for circulating immune complexes in serum are not available in most hospitals, which is appropriate in our view: such tests are variable, the problem of standardization is considerable and external quality assessment is non-existent.

19.6 Antibodies to microbial antigens

The detection of antibodies to microorganisms has been used in the **diagnosis of infection** for many years. The presence of circulating antibody indicates only that the antigen has been met previously. For diagnosis of an acute infection, a significant rise in antibody titre (usually fourfold) must be demonstrated in paired sera taken 2 weeks apart. If an immediate answer is required, the presence of a high-titre, specific IgM antibody implies a primary response (see Chapter 1).

Detection of antimicrobial antibodies is also an essential part of the **investigation of immune deficiency**. The ability to produce specific antibodies against defined antigens is the most sensitive method of detecting abnormalities of antibody production (see section 3.2). Such antibodies are usually detected by enzyme-linked immunosorbent assays (ELISA) (see below) and reported in International Units if there is an international standard, or arbitrary units if no standard is available. Antibodies to Streptococcus pneumoniae are found in most normal adult subjects, but not in those individuals with primary antibody deficiency (see Chapter 3). Antibodies to common viral antigens are also useful if there is a history of viral exposure. Similarly, if the patient has been immunized, it is useful to look for antibodies to tetanus toxoid, diphtheria toxoid and polio virus. If antibody levels are low, the patient is test-immunized with the appropriate killed antigen and the response re-evaluated 4–6 weeks later (Table 19.3 and Cases 3.2 and 3.3).

19.7 Detection of autoantibodies

19.7.1 In serum

The detection of circulating autoantibodies commonly involves four methods: immunofluorescence, radioimmunoassay (RIA), enzyme-linked immunoassay and countercurrent electrophoresis. Each type of assay system has its own snags. Immunofluorescence is the least sensitive of these techniques, and depends on subjective interpretation by an experienced observer. RIAs require expensive reagents, facilities for γ and β counting of radioisotopes and facilities for handling and disposal of radioactive waste. ELISAs avoid the problems of radioisotope handling and disposal but also require specialized equipment. Countercurrent electrophoresis is easy and cheap but relatively insensitive.

Indirect immunofluorescence

This is used for the detection of many serum autoantibodies (Tables 19.4 and 19.5). Animal tissue can be used when the

Table 19.3 The use of test immunization to assess antibody production in a patient with recurrent infections

Antibody specificity	Preimmunization	Postimmunization	
		4 weeks	Reference range
Pneumococcal polysaccharide			
Total IgG	4	8	80–100 IU/ml
IgG1	< 1	2	30–80 IU/ml
IgG2	< 1	< 1	45–100 IU/ml
Tetanus toxoid	< 0.01	7.6	>0.85 IU/ml

Pneumococcal antibodies are shown in arbitrary units. Tetanus antibodies are shown in international units per millilitre. The patient, a 38-year-old man, has responded well to test immunization with tetanus toxoid but shows no response to Pneumovax. He has a defect in specific antibody production (see Chapter 3).

Table 19.4 Indirect immunofluorescent tests for commoner non-organ-specific autoantibodies

Autoantibody	Typical substrate	Staining pattern	Main clinical relevance
Antinuclear antibody (ANA)	Human cell line (HEp2) or rat liver	All nuclei	Screening test for systemic rheumatic diseases
Centromere	Human cell line (HEp2)	Centromere of human chromosomes	Limited systemic sclerosis (CREST syndrome)
Smooth-muscle antibody (SMA)	Rat stomach, liver and kidney	Smooth muscle, i.e. muscularis mucosa, muscle of intergastric glands and arterial tunica media	Chronic active hepatitis Non-specific liver damage (weak)
Antimitochondrial antibody (AMA)	Rat kidney, liver and stomach	All mitochondria (esp. distal renal tubules)	Primary biliary cirrhosis
Endomysial antibody	Monkey oesophagus	Sarcolemma of smooth-muscle fibrils	Coeliac disease; dermatitis herpetiformis
Antineutrophil cytoplasmic antibody (ANCA)	Human neutrophils	Cytoplasmic (cANCA)	Wegener's granulomatosis; microscopic polyarteritis
		Perinuclear (pANCA)	Many forms of vasculitis

Table 19.5 Indirect immunofluorescent tests for commoner organ-specific autoantibodies

Autoantibody	Typical substrate	Staining pattern	Major clinical relevance (Case ref.)
Gastric parietal cell antibody	Rat stomach	Parietal cells only	Pernicious anaemia (Case 14.1)
Adrenal antibody	Human adrenal	Adrenal cortical cells	Idiopathic Addison's disease (Case 15.5)
Pancreatic islet cell antibody	Human pancreas	β-cells of pancreatic islet	Insulin-dependent diabetes (Case 15.4)
Skin antibodies	Human skin or guinea-pig lip	Intra-epidermal intercellular cement	Pemphigus vulgaris (Case 11.4)
		Epidermal basement membrane	Bullous pemphigoid

substrate contains antigens common to human and animal tissue, but some autoantigens are restricted to human tissue or human cell lines. Tissues are snap-frozen and sections are cut at − 20 °C on a cryostat.

The patient's serum is incubated with the substrate for 30 min. The unbound proteins are then washed off before a second antibody, with a visible tag (usually fluorescein), is added. This reacts with those serum immunoglobulins which have combined with antigens in the substrate. The site of antibody fixation can then be visualized by fluorescent microscopy (Fig. 19.9).

An autoantibody is defined by the **staining pattern** seen on a given substrate (Tables 19.4 and 19.5); only patterns of proven clinical significance are reported. Where relevant, a positive serum is titrated to determine the strength of the antibody. The results are expressed as a titre or in International Units if a known standard has been used for comparison. Most laboratories use an IgG-specific second antibody, because this class of autoantibody is clinically significant; autoantibodies of other isotypes are of very limited importance. The staining pattern for antinuclear antibodies (ANAs) can be clinically useful by suggesting possible diagnoses (Box 19.2), but is never diagnostic. In SLE, about 5% of patients were previously said to have ANA-negative lupus. Such patients had anti-Ro antibodies instead (Table 19.9), which cannot be detected on animal tissues. The use of human cells as substrate allows anti-Ro antibodies to be de-

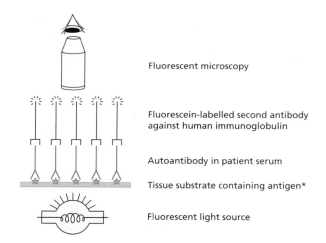

Fig. 19.9 Indirect immunofluorescence.

tected on ANA screening: as a result, ANA-negative lupus is much rarer (about 1%). Although several autoantibodies can be detected simultaneously by using a composite block of tissues, only tests relevant to the clinical problem should be requested. *Requests for uncritical 'autoantibody screens' are discouraged* (Box 19.1).

Interpretation of the results depends on the class and titre of the antibody and the age and sex of the patient. The elderly, especially women, are prone to develop autoanti-

---

BOX 19.2 PATTERNS OF NUCLEAR STAINING FOR ANTINUCLEAR ANTIBODIES (ANAS) ARE USEFUL BUT NOT DIAGNOSTIC

Pattern	Appearance	Disease association
Homogeneous (diffuse)		Common pattern
Rim of nucleus (peripheral; annular)		SLE
Nucleolar		SLE
Speckled		SLE Sjögren's syndrome Mixed connective tissue disease
Centromere (dividing cells only)		Limited systemic sclerosis (CREST syndrome)

SLE, Systemic lupus erythematosus.

bodies in the absence of clinical autoimmune disease. In contrast, high-titre autoantibodies in a child or young adult suggest that overt disease may appear later. The ANA test is an example of a test which is sensitive but not specific (see Fig. 19.1). The mere presence of ANA does not equate with autoimmune disease and certainly not with SLE, but by using an appropriate cut-off point, a negative ANA is strong screening evidence against the diagnosis. Using human cell lines, over 98% of patients with SLE will be ANA positive, but the false-positive rate will also be about 5–10%. Because of the high rate of false positives and the relatively low incidence of SLE in the population (see Table 3.3), a positive result is more likely to be a false positive rather than a true positive, unless patients are carefully selected for this test.

Radioimmunoassay and enzyme-linked immunosorbent assays (Fig. 19.10)

These are extremely sensitive methods of detecting autoantibodies in low concentration. Some RIAs for detecting autoantibodies are listed in Table 19.6. The techniques are used in other branches of pathology, for example for hormone assays.

Tests for **antibodies to double-stranded DNA (dsDNA)** are essential if SLE is suspected. They are detected by a variety of methods; those commonly used involve enzyme-labelled DNA or ^{125}I-DNA. Positive results usually indicate SLE or chronic active hepatitis. The dsDNA does gradually dissociate to single-stranded DNA, and it is important to look closely at control binding values for each run to determine the cut-off point for significant positivity. A fluorescent test, using the organism Crithidia luciliae, is specific for dsDNA, but rather insensitive, in that only 60% of SLE patients' sera react. The problem of standardization is helped by the availability of a WHO international standard for anti-dsDNA.

Snake venom toxin—α-bungarotoxin—binds strongly to acetylcholine receptors in human skeletal muscle extract. This has been exploited to provide a RIA for **acetylcholine receptor (AChR) antibodies**. Purified α-bungarotoxin is labelled with radioiodine and then complexed with human muscle extract. AChR antibodies react with this antigenic

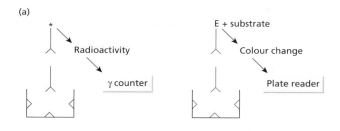

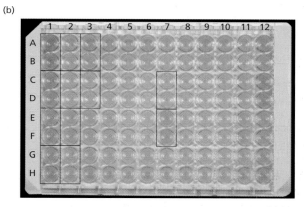

Fig. 19.10 (a) Principle of radioimmunoassay vs. enzyme-linked immunosorbent assay (ELISA). E, Enzyme-labelled antibody which binds to human IgG. *Radioisotopically labelled antibody which binds to human IgG. (b) An ELISA assay plate. In this example, anti-cardiolipin antibodies are being measured. Wells 1AB, 1CD, 1EF, 1GH, 2AB and 2CD contain duplicate samples of standard anticardiolipin antibody activity ranging from highest (1AB) to lowest (2CD). Wells 2EF, 2GH, 3AB and 3CD contain duplicates of known positive and negative quality control samples. Remaining wells contain test sera tested in duplicate. Wells 7CD contain a negative patient serum while wells 7EF contain a strong positive serum sample.

material and can be precipitated with an antiserum to human immunoglobulin. It is a sensitive assay; about 90% of patients with systemic myasthenia gravis are positive (see section 17.4), and there are few false positives. This test is

Table 19.6 Some autoantibodies detected by radioimmunoassay

Antibody	Method	Result	Clinical relevance
Double-stranded DNA antibody	^{125}I-DNA—direct binding	Percent of binding or IU/ml	Systemic lupus erythematosus (see Chapter 10) Chronic active hepatitis (see Chapter 14)
Acetylcholine receptor antibody	Direct binding of ^{125}I α-bungarotoxin complexed with acetylcholine	Binding reported as fmol/l of specific antibody receptors from cultured cell lines	Myasthenia gravis (see Chapter 17)

Table 19.7 Some autoantibodies detected by enzyme-linked immunosorbent assay (ELISA)

Antibody	Target autoantigen	Clinical relevance
Thyroid microsomal antibody	Thyroid peroxidase	Autoimmune thyroid disease (Chapter 15)
Mitochondrial (M2) antibody	E2 pyruvate dehydrogenase complex	Primary biliary cirrhosis (Chapter 14)
Glomerular basement membrane antibody	C terminal end of type IV collagen	Goodpasture's syndrome (Chapter 9) Antiglomerular basement membrane nephritis (Chapter 9)
Antineutrophil cytoplasmic antibody cANCA pANCA	Proteinase 3 Myeloperoxidase	Wegener's granulomatosis (Chapters 9 and 13) Microscopic polyarteritis (Chapter 9)
Double-stranded DNA antibody	dsDNA	Systemic lupus erythematosus (Chapter 10)
Phospholipid antibody	Cardiolipin	Primary phospholipid antibody syndrome (Chapter 16) Systemic lupus erythematosus

essential for diagnosis and useful in monitoring immunotherapy in myasthenia gravis.

Enzymes can also be used as labels instead of radioisotopes: the tests are then known as enzyme-linked immunosorbent assays, or ELISAs. In general, they are more sensitive but less specific (see Fig. 19.1) than RIA. Because the problem of handling and disposal of radioisotopes is avoided, their 'green' credentials mean ELISAs are used increasingly in immunoassays (Table 19.7). For example, although countercurrent electrophoresis (see below) remains the 'gold standard' for detecting and identifying antibodies to extractable nuclear antigens, automated ELISA assays using pure, recombinant antigens may become the method of choice.

Countercurrent immunoelectrophoresis

Countercurrent immunoelectrophoresis (CIE) involves electrophoresis of antigens and antibodies towards each other.

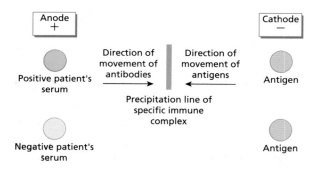

Fig. 19.11 Countercurrent immunoelectrophoresis.

At the appropriate pH, relatively acidic antigens will move rapidly towards the anode and the antibodies towards the cathode, maintaining their original concentrations. If the patient's serum contains a relevant antibody, a precipitin line is formed between the wells (Fig. 19.11). CIE is most commonly used for screening test sera for antibodies against 'extractable nuclear antigens' (ENA).

The antigen specificity of positive sera can then be confirmed by a further CIE run or by the Ouchterlony method (see Fig. 19.13 below). Reference sera containing antibodies of known ENA specificity are available. The antigen extract is placed in the central well, surrounded by the positive test serum and prototype sera of known specificity. Test and prototype sera are placed in adjacent wells: a reaction of identity indicates that the sera have the same antigen specificity. Patients' sera often contain antibodies against more than one ENA. Each antibody specificity is usually found only in small subsets of patients with rheumatic disorders and is diagnostically useful (Table 19.8). CIE is increasingly being replaced by automated ELISA assays using pure, recombinant antigens as targets.

19.7.2 Biopsy material

Immunohistochemical examination of biopsy specimens of damaged or normal tissue may reveal deposits of immunoglobulins caused by antibodies reacting with an organ or tissue-specific antigens. This approach is especially important in the diagnosis of antiglomerular basement antibody disease (Chapter 9) and the bullous skin disorders (Chapter 11). Biopsies must be handled as outlined in section 19.5.5.

Table 19.8 Antibodies to different components of extractable nuclear antigens (ENA)

Antigen	Molecular target	Clinical relevance*
'Smith' (Sm)	Common core proteins of U1, U2, U4, U5, U6 — s RNPs	Alone or with RNP antibody — a subset of SLE (20%)
Ribonucleoprotein (RNP)	U1 — s RNP	High titre — mixed connective tissue disease (100%)
Ro (SS-A)	60-kDa small RNP-binding Ro RNAs	Neonatal lupus and congenital heart block Subacute cutaneous lupus
La (SS-B)	Transcription terminator of Ro RNAs	Primary Sjögren's syndrome
Scl-70	Topoisomerase I	Systemic sclerosis (20%)
Jo-1	Histidyl-transfer RNA synthetase	Myositis, arthritis — often with pulmonary fibrosis

*Figures in parentheses show percentage of patients in disease category who have demonstrable antibody. U, Uridine rich; s RNP, nuclear ribonucleoproteins.

19.8 Tests for allergy and hypersensitivity

Some antibodies to non-invasive antigens result in immune damage ('hypersensitivity'). The type of test used depends on whether the damage is predominantly an IgE-mediated (type I) mechanism or an immune-complex-mediated (type III) mechanism involving IgM or IgG antibodies.

In atopic disorders, such as allergic rhinitis or extrinsic asthma (see Chapter 4), skin-prick testing can be useful. Provocation tests, by nasal, bronchial or oral challenge, are the most clinically relevant type of test but are potentially hazardous. These tests are discussed in Chapter 4; this chapter concentrates on laboratory tests only.

19.8.1 Antigen-specific IgE antibodies

The RAST (radioallergosorbent technique) test (Fig. 19.12) enables **antigen-specific IgE antibodies** to be measured. Here, the antigen is coupled to a solid phase such as cellulose; only IgE antibodies reactive against this particular antigen are detected by means of an antibody specific for the ε heavy chain. *RAST results correlate well with skin-prick tests but are expensive and of limited clinical value.* They should be used only if skin tests are contraindicated or unhelpful. This includes very young children, those with severe dermatitis, those dependent on medicines which modify skin reactivity, such as antihistamines, and those in whom a severe reaction is pos-

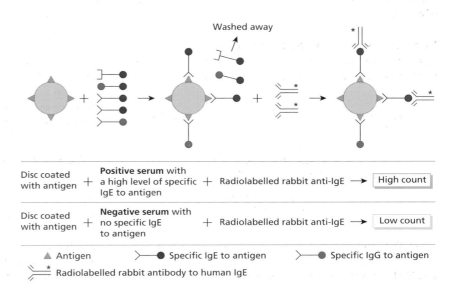

Disc coated with antigen	+	**Positive serum** with a high level of specific IgE to antigen	+ Radiolabelled rabbit anti-IgE →	High count
Disc coated with antigen	+	**Negative serum** with no specific IgE to antigen	+ Radiolabelled rabbit anti-IgE →	Low count

▲ Antigen   ⊱● Specific IgE to antigen   ⊱● Specific IgG to antigen

⫽* Radiolabelled rabbit antibody to human IgE

Fig. 19.12 Principle of measurement of antigen-specific IgE antibodies.

sible, such as wasp venom anaphylaxis. Allergen-specific IgE levels are reported quantitatively as arbitrary units/ml or semiquantitatively as RAST classes 0–6, where 0 is negative, 1 is borderline, 2 and 3 are positive to a degree, and 4–6 are increasingly strongly positive. The ease with which RASTs can be performed must not be allowed to overexaggerate their value in the assessment of allergic patients.

19.8.2 Total serum IgE

Measurement of total serum IgE is useful in the UK only in patients in whom parasite infestation is suspected, and is of little value in the differentiation between IgE- and non-IgE-mediated disorders (see Chapter 4). This is usually performed by RIA or enzyme immunoassay, since the normal level of IgE in the serum is extremely low (< 120 IU/ml). This test is expensive and of little clinical value.

19.8.3 Precipitating antibodies

Precipitating antibodies to specific antigens are usually IgM or IgG. The investigation of the extrinsic allergic alveolitides (see Chapter 13) requires testing for such antibodies. Precipitation tests are done by the Ouchterlony method; this is insensitive but cheap compared with immunoassay. Extracts of the relevant antigens are placed in the outside wells (Fig. 19.13) with the patient's serum in the centre. After several days, the plate is examined for precipitates formed by antibodies complexed with the given antigen. Some of the commonly used antigens (Fig. 19.13) are available commercially and a national external quality assurance scheme has been established in the UK. Where an unusual substance is suspected as the cause of a patient's symptoms, a simple

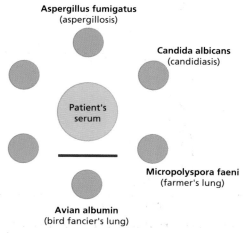

Fig. 19.13 Detection of precipitating antibodies in extrinsic allergic alveolitis. The patient has precipitating antibodies to avian albumin, suggesting possible bird fanciers' lung.

extract of that substance can be used as the antigen in a precipitation test.

19.9 Assessment of lymphocytes

Two types of test are used to assess cells:
- the quantification of different types of cells; and
- in vitro assays of their individual functions.

19.9.1 Quantification of lymphocytes

The study of lymphocyte populations was made possible when it was shown that they expressed different cell surface markers. Quantification of T and B lymphocyte subpopulations is essential in immunodeficiency (see Chapter 3) and certain lymphoproliferative diseases (see Chapter 6). The number of circulating $CD4^+$ T lymphocytes (Chapter 3) is a strong prognostic factor in HIV infection and used as a surrogate marker for assessing progress of the disease and the need for, and response to, anti-HIV therapy. National and international quality assessment schemes are in operation.

All estimations must be done on fresh anticoagulated blood, preferably after prior consultation with the immunology laboratory. Monoclonal antibodies are used to identify human peripheral blood B and T lymphocytes. These antisera recognize CD antigens (see Chapter 1) expressed characteristically, but not uniquely, by cells of a certain lineage and at certain stages of their differentiation. Cells are identified and counted by an automated fluorescence-activated cell scanner — or **flow cytometer** — which measures the fluorescence generated by each labelled cell. Aliquots of whole blood are incubated with appropriately labelled monoclonal antibodies. Cells are aspirated into the machine and surrounded by sheath fluid, which forces the cells to flow through the chamber in single file past a laser beam and light sensors. Light emitted by the excited fluorescent dye on the cell surface is detected by the sensors and analysed by on-board computer software. The instrument can be fitted with detectors for a number of different fluorescent dyes — 'double' or 'triple' labelling.

Cell populations vary in size and granularity. These properties can be used to define the cell population of interest in a suspension of mixed cells or whole blood, prior to analysis by monoclonal antibodies. Specified limits on cell size and granularity can be used to 'gate' the cell population, ensuring that further analysis is confined to these cells (Fig. 19.14). The data are then displayed as a series of profile histograms (Fig. 19.15), with the fluorescent intensity generated by the monoclonal antibody shown on the horizontal axis and the number of cells on the vertical axis. If double-labelling is used, a dot plot of individual cells can be obtained, where the intensity of fluorescence of one dye is plotted against the intensity of fluorescence of the other (Fig. 19.16). The pro-

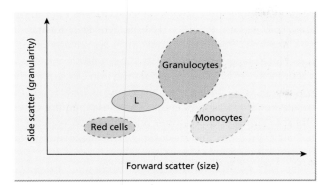

Fig. 19.14 'Gating' of cell populations. A cell population is analysed for forward and side (90%) scatter. Each cell is quantified in this way and represented by a dot on the graph (a dot plot). Each cell population forms a discrete cluster of dots. One such cluster, e.g. lymphocytes (L), can be selected, i.e. 'gated', for further analysis with fluorescent markers, while other cell clusters (---) are ignored.

portions of cells reactive with both antibodies, either one, or neither is shown by the intensity of the dots, and quantitative results are generated by the machine's computer. Results should always be expressed in absolute numbers and this is best achieved by gating lymphocytes using a combination of CD45 and side-scattering before identifying individual lymphocyte populations—the single platform approach—rather than by multiplying the percentage lymphocyte sub-population from flow cytometry by the lymphocyte number derived from the haematology analyser— the dual platform approach. Although flow cytometers are expensive, results are obtained quickly and easily by experienced users, and results are very accurate due to the vast numbers of cells that are counted.

It should be noted that values for lymphocyte subsets in children differ significantly from those in normal adults and vary significantly with age, especially in the first 12 months of life.

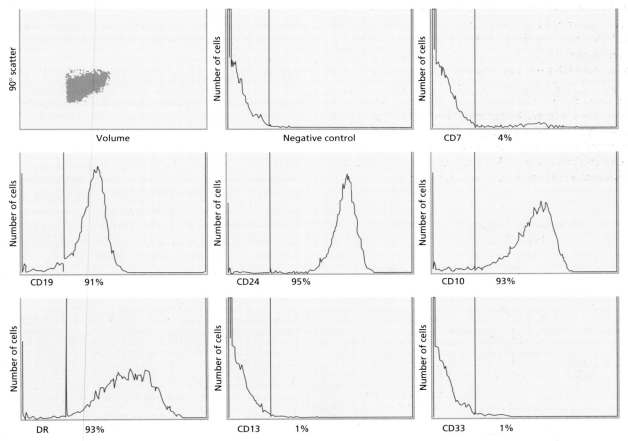

Fig. 19.15 Histograms of immunofluorescent staining of bone marrow cells in a case of acute lymphoblastic leukaemia. The *x* axis represents fluorescence intensity, the *y* axis the number of cells. The percentage of positive cells is based on a cursor set for the negative control. The gated population (blasts) is shown in the dot plot (top left). These blasts are CD19+, CD24+, CD10+, HLA class II.

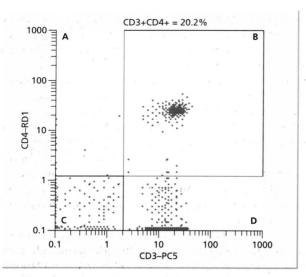

Fig. 19.16 Dual-colour immunofluorescence. A cell preparation has been incubated with two different monoclonal antibodies (MAb) conjugated to different fluorescent dyes (PC5 and RD1): one is anti-CD3; the other is anti-CD4. Lymphocytes in quadrant C stain with neither monoclonal (CD3⁻CD4⁻), while those in quadrant B stain with both (CD3⁺CD4⁺). Cells in A stain only with anti-CD4 (very few) and those in D only with CD3.

19.9.2 Functional tests

In vitro tests of lymphocyte function should be performed only if the clinical features suggest abnormal cell-mediated immunity. These assays are therefore only essential in suspected T-cell immunodeficiencies and prior discussion with the laboratory is essential.

These tests can be done using either whole blood or separated lymphocytes. Either way, fresh anticoagulated blood is required as viable cells are tested. When lymphocytes are activated by certain substances, a few small resting lym-

phocytes respond by changing into blast cells over a few days. This process is called **lymphocyte transformation** (see Chapter 1). Stimulating substances are usually of four types (Table 19.9). The proliferative response is measured by radioactive thymidine incorporation into DNA or by the expression of cell-surface markers, such as CD69, found on activated cells after a few hours. These tests require tissue culture facilities and are time-consuming and expensive. The batch variability and lack of standards make interpretation difficult without rigorous controls.

It is possible to measure a large number of soluble or intracellular cytokines, interleukins, surface adhesion molecules or receptors and their messenger RNAs. Such assays are readily available and non-invasive but, as yet, must be considered as research investigations, not as assays of proven clinical value in any disorder.

19.10 Assessment of neutrophils and monocytes

19.10.1 Neutrophil and monocyte quantification

Absolute numbers of these cells can easily be calculated from the total and differential white blood cell counts.

19.10.2 Functional tests

Tests of neutrophil function are essential in patients with recurrent or severe staphylococcal or fungal infections. Neutrophils can be separated from whole blood using a sedimentation method and their functional properties broken down into a series of key steps (Fig. 19.17).

The surface proteins which mediate **adhesion** of neutrophils to vascular endothelium are the β_2-integrin family (see Chapter 1). These proteins have a common β chain (CD18) which combines with different α chains (CD11a, CD11b and CD11c) to form heterodimers including leuco-

Table 19.9 Tests of T-lymphocyte activation pathways

Stimulating agent	Example	Activation pathway	Specificity of response	Need for prior exposure
Antigen	Purified protein derivative (PPD) of tuberculosis	TcR	Specific	Yes
Plant mitogen	Phytohaemagglutinin (PHA)		Non-specific	No
Monoclonal antibody	Anti-CD3	TcR/CD3 complex	Non-specific	No
Phorbol ester and calcium ionophore	Phorbol myristate acetate (PMA) and ionomycin	Signal transduction pathway distal to TcR/CD3 complex	Non-specific	No

TcR, T-cell receptor.

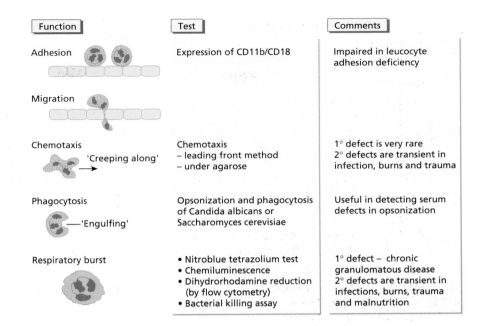

Function	Test	Comments
Adhesion	Expression of CD11b/CD18	Impaired in leucocyte adhesion deficiency
Migration		
Chemotaxis 'Creeping along'	Chemotaxis – leading front method – under agarose	1° defect is very rare 2° defects are transient in infection, burns and trauma
Phagocytosis 'Engulfing'	Opsonization and phagocytosis of Candida albicans or Saccharomyces cerevisiae	Useful in detecting serum defects in opsonization
Respiratory burst	• Nitroblue tetrazolium test • Chemiluminescence • Dihydrorhodamine reduction (by flow cytometry) • Bacterial killing assay	1° defect – chronic granulomatous disease 2° defects are transient in infections, burns, trauma and malnutrition

Fig. 19.17 Key steps in neutrophil function with relevant laboratory tests.

cyte function antigen 1 (LFA-1: CD11a/CD18) and complement receptor 3 (CR3: CD11b/CD18). In leucocyte adhesion deficiency, there is a genetic defect of CD18 with non-functional receptors preventing normal neutrophil adhesion to vascular endothelium. These markers are variably expressed on neutrophils, though detection of CD18 is reliable and absence of this marker is significant.

Chemotaxis is the purposeful movement of cells towards an attractant, usually the synthetic peptide f-Met-Leu-Phe. The ability of the patient's serum to generate chemotactic factors can be tested by incubating fresh serum with endotoxin. In the leading front type of assay, the cells to be tested are separated from the chemotactic stimulus by a Millipore membrane. After incubation, the filter membrane is removed, fixed and stained. The distance that cells have migrated through the filter towards the stimulus can be measured using a conventional light microscope. Chemotaxis is not used routinely but can be helpful as a research assay.

Phagocytosis is the ingestion of foreign material. Ingestion can be determined by incubation of phagocytic cells with inert particles, such as latex beads, or yeasts or bacteria. Intracellular particles or bacteria can be seen microscopically. Cross-over studies using normal controls allow the testing of the patient's cells for their ability to phagocytose particles opsonized with normal serum, while the patient's serum is tested for its ability to opsonize particles for ingestion by normal neutrophils. These are still research assays.

Intracellular enzyme activity accompanying the '**respiratory burst**' can be measured by bacterial killing. A standard intracellular killing assay involves incubation of leucocytes with viable organisms, such as Staphylococcus aureus. Fol-

lowing incubation, the cells are washed and centrifuged to remove extracellular organisms. Bacteria ingested but not killed are then cultured by lysing the cells with distilled water to release ingested bacteria onto nutrient agar. Provided that phagocytosis is normal, the number of viable organisms inversely reflects the degree of intracellular killing.

The **nitroblue tetrazolium (NBT) test** measures the ability of phagocytic cells to ingest and reduce this soluble yellow dye to an intracellular blue crystal. Separated neutrophils are added to a solution containing NBT and stimulated with endotoxin. The cells can be viewed microscopically to count the number of polymorphs containing blue crystals. This is an easy screening test, widely available and essential for the exclusion of chronic granulomatous disease (see section 3.4 and Case 3.5). The granulocyte respiratory burst can also be measured by **dihydrorhodamine (DHR) reduction**. Activation of granulocytes loaded with DHR generates reactive oxygen intermediates which react with DHR, and the resulting increase in fluorescence can be measured by flow cytometry. In the X-linked form of chronic granulomatous disease, carriers demonstrate two-cell populations, one reacting with DHR, the other not, whereas neutrophils from affected boys are unable to react with DHR (see section 3.4).

19.11 Recombinant DNA technology in clinical immunology

Advances in molecular biology have important implications for diagnosis and treatment of immunological diseases.

19.11.1 DNA analysis

In molecular pathology, known unique segments of nucleic acid sequences are used as DNA probes to determine the presence of complementary sequences of DNA (or RNA) in patient samples. The target DNA is composed of thousands of nucleotide bases and the reactivity of the probe, a single strand of DNA, with its complementary target — **DNA hybridization** — is the most specific intermolecular interaction known between biological macromolecules.

Nucleic acids remain intact in fresh-frozen as well as formalin-fixed, paraffin-embedded tissues. In the technique of **in situ hybridization**, DNA probes are applied directly on to the tissue sections on microscope slides. The principle is essentially similar to other DNA hybridization techniques, except that tissue sections must first undergo deparaffinization and proteolytic digestion to expose intracellular nucleic acid targets.

Restriction endonucleases are enzymes that cleave DNA at sites specifically related to the nucleotide sequences. The use of enzymes of different specificities allows a DNA fragment containing a particular gene to be cut out from the rest of the DNA molecule. In the **Southern blotting technique** (Fig. 19.18), fragments of DNA cleaved by a restriction endonuclease are electrophoresed on agarose gel, smaller fragments migrating further than larger fragments. Among these fragments will be one containing the gene of interest. Alkali denaturation of the DNA fragments uncoils them so that the resulting single-stranded DNA will hybridize with complementary pieces of DNA after transfer to a special nitrocellulose filter. Blotting the gel with the nitrocellulose filter fixes the DNA fragments at the same positions that they occupied after electrophoresis. A radiolabelled 'probe' containing DNA known to be complementary to the DNA of interest will hybridize to it and the fragment can then be identified by autoradiography of the nitrocellulose filter. The **Northern blotting technique** uses the same principle to transfer RNA, instead of DNA, from gel to blot.

In many genetic disorders, the defect is not known and production of gene-specific probes is not feasible. In these cases, however, the disease-producing gene may be closely linked to the recognition site of a particular restriction endonuclease. Scattered throughout the human genome are harmless variations in DNA sequences which may produce new restriction endonuclease sites or remove pre-existing ones. The fragments of DNA produced by a particular restriction enzyme will therefore be of differing lengths in different people. These are called **restriction fragment length polymorphisms (RFLP)** and are inherited in a simple Mendelian fashion. RFLPs provide a potentially large number of linkage markers for tracing disease-producing genes in families, without knowing anything about the gene itself.

These methods have been largely superseded by a major advance in recombinant DNA technology called the **polymerase chain reaction (PCR)**, a method for dramatic amplification of target DNA prior to cleavage with a restriction enzyme (Fig. 19.19). Complementary oligonucleotide primers from either end of the target DNA are added to the denatured sample along with a heat-resistant DNA polymerase. If the target sequence is present, the primers anneal to it and provide a starting-point for the polymerase to begin the synthesis of second-strand DNA. The newly synthesized double-stranded DNA is then denatured by heating and exposed again to the polymerase enzyme at a lower temperature. In this way, newly synthesized molecules and original DNA can reassociate with the primer and act as templates for further rounds of DNA synthesis. After completing about 30 cycles, which takes 2–3 h in an automated procedure, the specific target sequence is amplified over one-millionfold. This powerful and sensitive technique can detect a specific

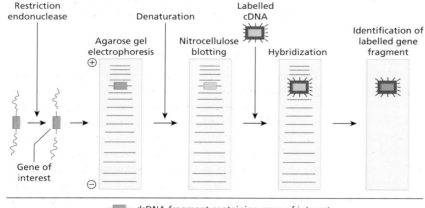

Fig. 19.18 Gene mapping by the Southern blotting technique. (See text for explanation.)

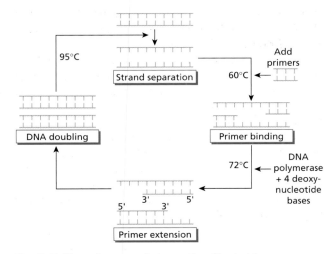

Fig. 19.19 The polymerase chain reaction. (See text for explanation.)

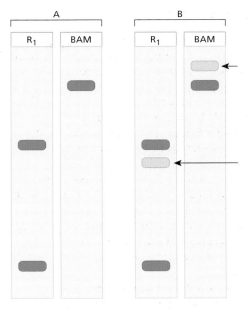

Fig. 19.20 TcR gene rearrangement studies by Southern blotting. DNA was digested with the enzymes Eco R1 (R1) and Bam H1 (Bam). The control (A) shows germline bands for both enzymes, but in a patient with lymphoma (B) the bands are rearranged (arrowed).

DNA sequence from a single cell (e.g. lymphocyte, sperm), fixed pathological specimens and dried blood spots. The disadvantage is that contamination of the reaction mixture with traces of DNA from another source will lead to false-positive results.

19.11.2 Diagnostic implications

Recombinant DNA technology has led to a major change in methodology for tissue typing (see below) and provides precise **diagnosis of genetic disease**, including prenatally using tissue obtained by chorionic villus sampling, fetoscopy or amniocentesis. It can also detect preclinical cases of autosomal dominant disorders of late onset, and female carriers of X-linked conditions, including some types of congenital immunodeficiency (see Chapter 3). PCR has proved of particular value in the rapid diagnosis of infectious diseases and in immunogenetic studies. One example is the detection of the HIV genome in patients who cannot be determined to be HIV-positive by conventional means, such as infants born to HIV-infected mothers. The great sensitivity of PCR and its ease of use with multiple patient samples allows the identification of critical human or viral DNA sequences that would be impossible to detect by other means.

Gene rearrangement studies are used increasingly to analyse the origin of potentially malignant lymphocytes that lack conventional T- and B-cell markers. The normal maturation of lymphocytes is associated with somatic gene rearrangements (see Chapter 1) of immunoglobulin heavy and light chain complexes in B cells and of TcR gene complexes in T cells. Gene rearrangements are random and so the structure of the rearranged genes varies from one cell to another.

Clonal expansion of a neoplastic cell results in identical rearrangements for all cells in the clone. By Southern blotting, it is possible to identify a clonal population and distinguish it from a polyclonal proliferation. This technique can detect monoclonality when clonal cells account for 5% or fewer of the cell population.

TcR gene rearrangements are the most definitive, non-morphological approach for the diagnosis of T-cell malignancies (Fig. 19.20). Prior to this approach, diagnosis based on morphology and immunophenotyping with monoclonal antibodies often failed to detect monoclonality.

19.11.3 Genomics and microarrays

Traditional disease classification is based mainly on morphological, histological, biochemical or immunological criteria. However, classification at the level of gene expression provides a potentially more accurate tool for diagnosis and treatment. DNA microarray technology is an extremely powerful tool for analysing the expression of up to 30 000 genes (i.e. the genome) and investigating the underlying disease mechanisms, biomarkers and therapeutic targets of many human diseases. The difficult part is making sense of the vast amounts of data generated. DNA microarrays are small, solid supports, usually glass microscope slides, silicon chips or nylon membranes, onto which DNA sequences from different genes are attached at fixed locations. The microarray exploits the ability of a given mRNA molecule to bind specifically (i.e. hybridize) to the DNA template from which it originated. In a single experiment, the expression level of thousands of genes within tissues or cells can be determined by computer analysis of the amount of mRNA bound to the spots on the microarray, so generating a profile of gene expression in that cell. By tagging the mRNA from control or diseased cells or samples with differently coloured (green or red) fluorescent labels, sophisticated computer analysis of the pattern can determine the ratio of red-to-green fluorescent intensity at each spot on the array. Determining the level at which a certain gene is expressed is called **microarray expression analysis** and the arrays used are called expression chips. If a gene is over-expressed in a certain disease, then more sample cDNA will hybridize to the spot compared with control cDNA and the spot will fluoresce red with greater intensity than it will fluoresce green. Expression chips can be used in understanding disease mechanisms by identifying new genes involved in pathogenesis of autoimmune or allergic disorders and in developing new treatments (Fig. 19.21). For instance, if a certain gene is overexpressed in a disease, expression chips can be used to determine if a new drug reduces this overexpression and modifies progression of the disease. Gene expression patterns can be used as 'fingerprints' to distinguish between different forms of the diseases, most commonly in tumour classification but with increasing applications elsewhere.

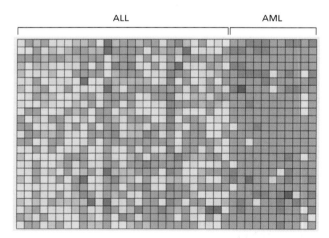

Fig. 19.21 An example of a microarray chip showing genes distinguishing acute lymphoblastic leukaemia (ALL) from acute myeloid leukaemia (AML). Twenty-five genes are shown, each row corresponding to a different gene and each column corresponding to expression levels in different samples. Expression levels greater than the mean are shaded in red and those below the mean are shaded in blue. Reprinted with permission from Golub TR *et al.* Science 1999; 286:531–7. Copyright 1999.

19.12 Histocompatibility testing

There are many histocompatibility antigens on leucocytes and other cells, but those of the human leucocyte antigen (HLA) system are the most important (see Chapter 1). These antigens are present on all tissues of the body, but their high concentration on peripheral blood lymphocytes enables immunogenetic studies to be carried out easily on these cells. Unlike the ABO system for red cells, there are no spontaneously occurring anti-HLA antibodies. Serological typing reagents are antibodies produced as a result of immunization during transfusion or in pregnancy, i.e. alloantibodies.

The commonly used test to detect **MHC class I antigens** is a serological one—the microlymphocytotoxicity test. Viable lymphocytes are prepared on density gradients as described. Aliquots of patients' cells are then mixed with the various typing sera in separate wells, and complement (usually normal rabbit serum) is added. Following incubation at 37 °C, cells recognized by the antibody are killed by complement-mediated lysis. If most (> 90%) of the cells in a well are killed, those cells carried the relevant HLA antigen recognized by the typing antibody in that well.

The application of molecular techniques to tissue typing has led to a fundamental change in methodology for **MHC class II typing**. These techniques have several advantages over serotyping (Table 19.10). Initially, Southern blotting techniques were used to allow identification of RFLPs (see section 19.11.1) which correlate with known serological (HLA-DR/DQ) and cellular (HLA-DW) defined specificities. At present, however, the majority of HLA typing centres use enzymatic amplification of a particular locus of HLA-DR/DQ class II genes using the PCR and subsequent analysis of the product with radiolabelled probes specific for a particular gene sequence (sequence-specific oligonucleotides).

These tests are available only in specialized centres where immunogenetic studies are essential for organ and bone

Table 19.10 Advantages of DNA typing over serological techniques

- Better correlation with clinical outcomes in transplantation
- Additional information on genetic variations
- Homozygosity can be confirmed
- Less subjectivity in data interpretation
- Easier to perform
- DNA samples transported easily between laboratories
- Not dependent on viability and type of lymphocyte
- DNA probes can be synthesized cheaply or regenerated
- Continuous screening for serotyping alloantisera unnecessary
- DNA typing can be performed in economical batches

marrow transplantation. They are time-consuming and expensive and require considerable skill and experience to interpret the results. Prior consultation is essential and fresh, anticoagulated whole blood must be sent direct to the laboratory. HLA typing for HLA-B27 is useful in patients with suspected ankylosing spondylitis. The use of HLA typing in other diseases remains speculative and of research interest only.

FURTHER READING

See website: www.immunologyclinic.com

Clinical Immunology and Allergy on the World Wide Web

A selection of web addresses dealing with immunological topics

Basic science

Immunogenetics

www.ebi.ac.uk/imgt/index.html
Comprehensive database of the HLA system, immunoglobulins and T-cell receptors covering nomenclature and sequence information from Leiden University provided by the European Bioinformatics Institute.

CD antigens

http://mpr.nci.nih.gov/prow
Structured reviews of various protein families. Of particular immunological interest is the list of human cell-surface molecules assigned a CD number (up to CD339 as of October 2005) by international workshops on leucocyte differentiation antigens.

Cytokines

www.copewithcytokines.de/cope.cgi
Up-to-date survey of literature on cytokines, including potential therapeutic implications. Encyclopaedia of cytokines linked to fully integrated dictionaries on angiogenesis, apoptosis, chemokines, etc.

Macrophage homepage

http://www.macrophages.com
Lists freely accessible sources related to macrophages and immunology, for professionals From Institute for Molecular Bioscience at the University of Queensland.

Clinical topics

Allergy information and resources

http://www.allergy-network.co.uk
Database of current developments in allergy.

Web page of the Division of Allergy, Immunology and Transplantation of the National Institute of Health, USA

http://www.niaid.nih.gov/research/daithtm
Provides succinct summaries of recent workshops and expert reports on a variety of topics in clinical immunology and allergy.

AIDS knowledge base

http://www.aidsinfo.nih.gov
Provides comprehensive coverage of medical aspects of HIV infection, including immunopathogenesis, HIV clinical trials and anti-retroviral drugs from the University of South California.

The Immunology Link

http://www.immunologylink.com/
Features comprehensive lists of links to immunology associations, journals and databases. The alphabetical list of murine gene knockouts represents excellent value.

Organizations which promote the science and practice of immunology

American Academy of Allergy, Asthma and Immunology

http://www.aaaai.org/

British Society for Immunology

http://www.immunology.org

British Society for Histocompatibility and Immunogenetics

http://www.bshi.org.uk/

French Society for Immunology

http://www.inserm.fr/sfi

British Society for Allergy and Clinical Immunology
www.bsaci.org

European Society for Immunodeficiencies
http://www.esid.org

Clinical Immunology Society
http://www.clinimmsoc.org

European Federation of Immunological Societies
http://www.efis.org

MCQs

The following MCQs are based on the content of each chapter. Answers are given on pp. 344–6.

Online version
Visit:
www.immunologyclinic.com
to attempt these MCQs online and to see full feedback on your answers.

CHAPTER 1 Basic Components: Structure and Function

1 **Which cells are known to be involved in the initial presentation of antigen to T lymphocytes?**
   a Dendritic cells
   b Plasma cells
   c Neutrophil polymorphonuclear leucocytes
   d Erythrocytes
   e Platelets

2 **Which of the following cells are thought to be of monocyte–macrophage lineage?**
   a 'Veiled' cells of lymph
   b Follicular dendritic cells of lymph nodes
   c Kupffer cells in liver
   d Histiocytes in tissues
   e All of the above

3 **B cells cannot produce specific IgG antibodies without T-cell help via which ligands?**
   a CD3
   b TCR
   c CD40L
   d ICOS
   e CD11

4 **Which of the following cells produce IgE?**
   a Mast cells
   b Eosinophils
   c Basophils
   d T lymphocytes
   e Plasma cells

5 **A helper T lymphocyte is known to recognize which of the following on a presenting cell?**
   a HLA class I antigen
   b HLA class II antigen
   c Whole antigen
   d CD8 antigen
   e Surface immunoglobulin

6 **Endotoxin activates which complement pathway?**
   a Classical
   b Alternate
   c Mannan binding
   d Final lytic
   e All of the above

7 **Which of the following statements about the alternate pathway are true?**
   a Properdin forms part of the C5 convertase
   b It is phylogenetically older than the classical pathway
   c It can be activated by bacterial cell walls
   d There is a positive feedback loop
   e All of the above

8 **Which of the following cells are not phagocytic?**
   a Macrophages
   b Histiocytes
   c Monocytes
   d Neutrophil polymorphonuclear leucocytes
   e Plasma cells

9 **Type I hypersensitivity classically involves which of the following?**
   a IgM
   b IgD
   c Macrophages
   d IgE
   e Histiocytes

10 **Type III hypersensitivity reactions are the direct result of interaction between which of the following?**
   a Sensitized T lymphocytes and antigen
   b Pre-formed antibodies and antigen
   c Mast cells and antigen
   d Plasma cells and antigen
   e Histiocytes and antigen

11 **Mature dendritic cells have which of the following markers?**
   a Adhesion molecules, e.g. ICAM-1

329

b Cytokine receptors, e.g. IL-12

c Co-stimulatory molecules, e.g. CD80

d None of the above

e All of the above

12 **Opsonization is the process involved in which one of the following immune functions?**

a Peptides are engulfed by macrophages and digested

b IgE antibody is produced

c Foreign particles are coated in specific IgG and/or complement C3

d Complement lysis

e Immune complexes are attached to erythrocytes for transport to the liver

13 **Which of the following cytokines act as chemoattractants for eosinophils?**

a IL-5

b C5a

c RANTES

d IL-10

e IFN-γ

14 **Endothelial cells are believed to play a key role in the physiological regulation of IgG turnover through one of the following:**

a Production of endothelium-derived relaxing factor

b Endothelin

c Prostacyclin

d Expression of E-selectin

e Expression of FcRn

15 **Regulatory T cells are defined by a characteristic phenotype. Which one of the following is it?**

a CD8$^+$,CD25$^+$

b CD4$^+$,CD25$^+$

c CD4$^+$,CD69$^+$

d CD8$^+$,CD69$^+$

e CD4$^+$,CD28$^+$

16 **Which one of the following represents the main outcome of signal transduction via Toll-like receptors?**

a Interleukin-10 secretion

b Complement consumption

c Natural killer cell activation

d Pro-inflammatory cytokine secretion

e Immunoglobulin production

CHAPTER 2 Infection

1 **Which of the following are phagocytic cells?**

a Polymorphonuclear leucocytes

b B lymphocytes

c T lymphocytes

d Macrophages

e Kupffer cells

2 **Which of the following statements about rheumatic fever are true?**

a It is a complication of β-haemolytic streptococcal infection

b It only affects the elderly

c It complicates 3% of acute sore throats

d It shows evidence of genetic susceptibility

e It is caused by immediate hypersensitivity to streptococci

3 **Epstein–Barr virus is known to be implicated in the following conditions:**

a Infectious mononucleosis

b Carcinoma of the oesophagus

c Chronic lymphatic leukaemia

d Burkitt's lymphoma

e Hepatoma

4 **In infectious mononucleosis, the 'atypical lymphocytes' are predominantly suppressor/cytotoxic T cells. True/false**

5 **Which of the following predispose to superficial Candida albicans infection?**

a Pregnancy

b Lymphoma

c Diabetes mellitus

d Drug addiction

e Broad-spectrum antibiotics

6 **Antigenic variation refers to the ability of certain microorganisms to change their surface antigenic structures. True/false**

7 **Which of the following microorganisms uses antigenic variation as a major means of evading host defences?**

a Streptococcus pneumoniae

b Influenza A virus

c Borrelia recurrentis

d Mycobacterium tuberculosis

e Trypanosomes

8 **Latent infection of the trigeminal ganglion is characteristic of herpes simplex virus. True/false**

9 **The following survival mechanisms occur commonly in parasitic infections:**

a Immunosuppression

b Antigenic disguise

c Antigenic variation

d Premunition

e Resistance to macrophage killing

10 **IgE antibodies play a role in protection against helminth infection. True/false**

11 **Which of the following statements regarding superantigens are true?**

a Superantigens activate large numbers of B cells

b Staphylococcal toxic shock syndrome is an example of superantigen-associated disease c Superantigens are presented by antigen-presenting cells in an identical manner to conventional antigens

d Superantigen-associated diseases are characterized by markedly elevated circulating levels of pro-inflammatory cytokines

e In humans, a superantigen reacts with approximately 1 in 50 T cells

12 The human immunodeficiency virus interacts with the following cell-surface molecules to gain entry into cells of the immune system:

a CD4
b CD19
c The chemokine receptors CXCR4 and CCR5
d CD8
e CD25

13 Interferon-γ is a powerful macrophage activating factor.
True/false

14 The cytokine profile of a helper T cell (TH1 or TH2) is an important determinant of host immunity. Which of the following statements regarding the cytokine profile of various diseases are true?

a Cutaneous leishmaniasis is associated with a predominant TH2 profile

b Visceral leishmaniasis is associated with a predominant TH1 profile

c Tuberculoid leprosy is associated with a predominant TH1 profile

d Lepromatous leprosy is associated with a predominant TH2 profile

15 Which one of the following molecules is a receptor for the SARS-Coronavirus?

a CD21
b ACE-2
c CXCR 5
d HLA B53
e ICAM-1

16 Which one of the following cytokines is predominantly responsible for driving eosinophil production?

a IL-1
b IL-2
c IL-3
d IL-4
e IL-5

17 The main cell type infected by Epstein–Barr virus is:

a T cells
b Natural killer cells
c B cells
d Macrophages
e Kupffer cells

18 The release of one of the following cytokines during the in vivo immune response to infection with Mycobacterium tuberculosis has been used to develop immunodiagnostic assays for the diagnosis of latent TB. Which one is it?

a IL-7
b IL-8
c IL-10
d Interferon gamma
e TNF

CHAPTER 3 Immunodeficiency

1 Primary immunodeficiencies are commoner than secondary causes of immunodeficiency. Which statement is true?

a This statement is only true for adults
b This statement is true at all ages
c This statement is totally untrue for all ages
d Secondary immune deficiencies are rarely due to drugs
e Vegetarians are particularly at risk of immune suppression

2 The most frequently diagnosed form of specific primary immunodeficiency is:

a Severe combined immunodeficiency
b X-linked agammaglobulinaemia
c Chronic granulomatous disease
d Selective IgA deficiency
e DiGeorge anomaly

3 Which of the following is most pertinent to healthy individuals with selective IgA deficiency?

a All can be considered to be normal without risk of infections

b They are more likely to develop heart disease than those with normal IgA levels

c Will always have a high risk of HIV infection

d They have a high risk of a serious bacterial infection every year

e They have a higher risk of developing an organ-specific autoimmune disease than the general population

4 Which of the following is most pertinent to common variable immune deficiency disorders?

a Always presents before the age of 10 years
b Is due to a single gene defect on the X chromosome
c Affects 1 in 500 of the population
d Is treated by replacement immunoglobulin, intravenously or subcutaneously
e Is complicated in the long term by a high risk of malignancy

5 Transient hypogammaglobulinaemia of infancy usually:

a Occurs at 1–2 months of age
b Is more pronounced in premature babies
c Is due to placental absorption of IgG
d Is linked with autoimmune disease in later life
e Involves all three major immunoglobulin classes

6 Replacement therapy for hypogammaglobulinaemia consists mainly of:
   a IgG
   b IgA
   c IgM
   d IgD
   e IgE

7 Which of the following is the primary defect in chronic granulomatous disease?
   a Neutrophil production in the bone marrow
   b Neutrophil chemotaxis
   c Neutrophil intracellular killing of organisms
   d Opsonization
   e Cytotoxic T-cell activity

8 Which of the following is most commonly associated with secondary antibody deficiency in Europe?
   a Protein–energy malnutrition
   b Multiple myeloma
   c Non-Hodgkin's lymphoma
   d HIV infection
   e Hodgkin's disease

9 One of the following is a cellular co-receptor for HIV:
   a CD8 antigen
   b CD21 antigen
   c CD69 antigen
   d CXCR4 antigen
   e FAS ligand

10 Which one of the following clinical features is not usually associated with HIV infection?
   a A glandular fever-like illness
   b Persistent generalized lymphadenopathy
   c Cardiac failure
   d 'Slim disease'
   e Presenile dementia

11 Which one of the following is a proven route of transmission of HIV?
   a Swimming pools
   b Mosquitoes
   c Shared bathroom facilities
   d Semen
   e Bed bugs

CHAPTER 4 Anaphylaxis and Allergy

1 Which of the following diseases usually occur in 'atopic' individuals?
   a Anaphylactoid reactions
   b Hay fever
   c Asthma
   d Urticaria
   e Atopic eczema

2 Systemic anaphylaxis can be caused by:
   a Wasp venom
   b ACE inhibitors
   c Penicillin
   d Aspirin
   e Latex

3 Which of the following statements about food allergy are correct?
   a In children, it is often due to cow's milk
   b It can be diagnosed confidently by skin-prick testing
   c Migraine is a common presenting feature
   d Diagnosis may require food elimination and challenge
   e Most children will 'grow out' of nut allergy by the age of 11 years

4 Which of the following are true statements about atopic eczema?
   a It commonly begins in infancy
   b Superadded herpes simplex infection is a serious complication
   c The serum IgE level is normally raised
   d The skin lesions are typically itchy
   e Treatment with systemic steroids is rarely necessary

5 Which of the following commonly cause seasonal allergic rhinitis?
   a Tree pollen
   b House dust mite
   c Grass pollen
   d Fungal spores
   e Cat fur

6 Which of the following statements about penicillin allergy are true?
   a Anaphylaxis to penicillin occurs in 1–2% of those taking the drug
   b Reactions occur only in those with a previous history of penicillin allergy
   c A severe reaction is more likely with parenteral penicillin than with oral penicillin
   d A negative skin-prick test indicates a low risk of a reaction

7 Which of the following are true statements about chronic urticaria?
   a By definition, it must be present for at least 3 weeks
   b It is commonly due to urticarial vasculitis
   c It can be triggered by IgE antibodies to aspirin
   d It can be associated with autoantibodies to $Fc_\varepsilon RI$
   e Systemic steroids are usually required to suppress attacks.

8 Hyposensitization (specific allergen immunotherapy) is of proven benefit in the following conditions:
   a Peanut allergy
   b House dust mite allergy
   c Wasp venom hypersensitivity

d Coeliac disease

e Latex anaphylaxis

9 Asthma is characterized by which of the following?

a Response to cyclosporin therapy in severe disease

b Reversible airways obstruction

c TH2 cells in bronchoalveolar lavage fluid

d Affects 5% of the population

e Is diagnosed routinely by use of RAST

10 In patients with allergies to cats or dogs, removal of the pet from the home typically leads to reduction of the allergen load within what period of time?

a 1–2 days

b 1–2 weeks

c 1–2 months

d 6–12 months

e Never

CHAPTER 5 Autoimmunity

1 Which one of the following statements is true? Autoimmune diseases:

a Affect about 1 person in every 1000

b Are more common in women

c Tend to begin in childhood

d Are an inevitable consequence of autoimmune responses

e Are usually curable with immunosuppression

2 Which one of the following statements is true?

a The thymus controls peripheral tolerance of T cells

b No self-reactive T cells can be found in healthy normal subjects

c Naive T cells need more than one signal in order to become activated

d B-cell tolerance is more important than T-cell tolerance in the prevention of autoimmunity

e Class II MHC molecules are expressed on most cells

3 Which one of the following is NOT true? Tolerance can break down:

a Following administration of an immunological adjuvant

b After IL-2 treatment

c By a process of molecular mimicry

d After surgical removal of the thymus in the first year of life in humans

e If there is abnormal expression of the AIRE gene in the thymus

4 Which one of the following is NOT true? Autoimmune diseases:

a Can cluster within families

b Are often associated with particular HLA alleles

c Are usually mediated by type I hypersensitivity

d May occur in humans or animals with inherited defects in apoptosis

e May occur in inherited complement deficiencies

5 Which one of these statements regarding genetic defects of the immune system is NOT true?

a Fas deficiency in humans causes lymphadenopathy and thrombocytopenia

b C1q deficiency is associated with systemic lupus erythematosus

c Mutations of the AIRE gene are associated with endocrine autoimmunity

d Over-expression of TNF-α in transgenic mice is associated with inflammatory arthritis

e CD40 ligand deficiency in humans is associated with primary biliary cirrhosis

6 Which one of the following is NOT a well-defined autoantigen

a Mitochondrial pyruvate dehydrogenase

b The TSH receptor

c Acetylcholine receptor

d Topoisomerase I

e Creatine kinase

CHAPTER 6 Lymphoproliferative Disorders

1 Most cases of acute leukaemia in children are:

a T-cell ALL

b B-cell ALL

c Hairy cell leukaemia

d Common pre-B-cell ALL

e Histiocytic ALL

2 Acute leukaemias may be associated with which of the following symptoms?

a Bleeding

b Bruising

c Tiredness

d None of the above

e All of the above

3 The following surface marker results were obtained with lymphocytes from a 21-year-old man with a lymphocytosis of 16 × 109/l.

Percentages of peripheral lymphocytes reactive with antisera to

κ	λ	CD19	CD11c	CD3	CD56 (NK cells)
6	4	10	0	81	9

Which is the most likely diagnosis?

a Early chronic lymphocytic leukaemia

b Sézary syndrome

c Infectious mononucleosis

d Non-Hodgkin's lymphoma

e Acute lymphoblastic leukaemia

4 Chronic B-cell lymphocytic leukaemia is commonly associated with which feature?
   a Invariable rapid demise
   b A slow but progressive course
   c Overwhelming bleeding
   d Hepatitis
   e Thymoma

5 The type of leukaemia most likely to have skin involvement is:
   a Acute leukaemia
   b Hairy cell leukaemia
   c Plasma cell leukaemia
   d Chronic lymphocytic leukaemia (common type)
   e Sézary syndrome

6 Low serum levels of all major immunoglobulin classes are often a feature of which of these diseases?
   a Multiple myeloma
   b Benign paraproteinaemia
   c Waldenström's macroglobulinaemia
   d Infectious mononucleosis
   e Non-Hodgkin's lymphoma

7 Bence-Jones proteins are:
   a Fragments of transferrin
   b Polyclonal free light chains
   c Monoclonal free light chains
   d β2-microglobulins
   e Prostaglandins

8 Waldenström's macroglobulinaemia patients frequently develop which of the following?
   a Meningitis
   b Duodenal ulcer
   c Hyperviscosity syndrome
   d Non-Hodgkin's lymphoma
   e Multiple myeloma

9 Which one of the following studies is essential for the diagnosis of all B-cell tumours?
   a Gene rearrangement studies
   b CT scanning of the thorax for a thymoma
   c Bone marrow examination
   d Analysis of urine for protein
   e X-ray of the skull

10 Which of the following statements about patients with monoclonal serum bands is true?
   a All will develop a lymphoid malignancy within 3 years
   b All should be followed up once a year, with quantification of the band and examination of the urine
   c All should have a skull X-ray
   d > 90% will have frank myeloma
   e Only those with renal failure will need urine examination for monoclonal free light chains

CHAPTER 7 Immune Manipulation

1 Which of the following agents are known to be immunosuppressive?
   a Levamisole
   b Corticosteroids
   c Azathioprine
   d Cyclosporin
   e Total lymphoid irradiation

2 Corticosteroids cause a profound lymphocytosis within 2 h of administration.
   True/false

3 Which of the following statements about azathioprine is true?
   a It is inactive until metabolized
   b It can affect all dividing cells
   c It suppresses B cells directly to prevent antibody production
   d It can cause severe bone marrow suppression
   e It is effective in patients with liver failure

4 Organ transplant recipients are at increased risk of developing Epstein–Barr virus-associated lymphoma.
   True/false

5 Intravenous immunoglobulin is increasingly used as a therapeutic agent in autoimmune/inflammatory disease. In which of the following diseases have its beneficial effects been shown in randomized trials?
   a Chronic fatigue syndrome (postviral fatigue)
   b Kawasaki's disease
   c Guillain–Barré syndrome
   d Dermatomyositis
   e Rheumatoid arthritis

6 Plasmapheresis is the treatment of choice in the emergency management of severe hyperviscosity syndrome.
   True/false

7 Which of the following statements about interferon-α are true?
   a It is useful in chronic hepatitis B infection
   b It induces differentiation of natural killer cells
   c It suppresses natural killer activity
   d Genetically engineered recombinant interferon-α is available
   e It is therapeutically useful in hairy cell leukaemia

8 Freund's complete adjuvant is used to boost antibody responses in humans.
   True/false

9 Which of the following are live vaccines?
   a Oral polio
   b Diphtheria
   c Tetanus
   d BCG
   e Hepatitis B

10 In the UK, immunization schedules are routinely started at the age of 12 months.
True/false

11 The risk of brain damage following pertussis immunization is 2.5 times greater than that from natural whooping cough infection.
True/false

12 Patients with hyposplenism are at risk from pneumococcal infection.
True/false

13 In mice, direct intramuscular injection of plasmids containing mycobacterial DNA evokes protective immunity.
True/false

14 The immunosuppressive action of mycophenolate mofetil therapy is mediated via inhibition of one of the following enzymes:
a Thiopurine methyl transferase
b Adenosine deaminase
c Purine nuceloside phosphorylase
d Inosine monophosphate dehydrogenase
e Xanthine oxidase

15 Treatment with anti-TNF is associated clinically with a significantly increased risk of one of the following infections:
a Tuberculosis
b Influenza
c Enteroviral diarrhoea
d Glandular fever
e Pneumococcal meningitis

16 Which one of the following immunoglobulin classes forms the main constituent of pooled intravenous immunoglobulin?
a IgG
b IgA
c IgM
d IgD
e IgE

CHAPTER 8 Transplantation

1 Which of the following sets of antigens are important in relation to successful renal grafting?
a MHC class II antigens
b Lewis red cell antigens
c Rhesus red cell antigens
d Sex antigens (products of X and Y chromosomes)
e ABO red cell antigens

2 The major human histocompatibility complex is on chromosome 17.
True/false

3 Which of the following factors may indicate renal graft rejection?

a Fever
b Increase in serum IgG level
c Tender graft
d Rise in urine volume
e Rise in creatinine

4 Cytomegalovirus infection is often associated with a rejection episode in renal transplantation.
True/false

5 Which of the following conditions are accepted indications for bone marrow transplantation?
a Acute leukaemia in remission
b Chronic lymphocytic leukaemia
c Severe combined immunodeficiency
d CD40 ligand deficiency
e Osteosarcoma

6 HLA-DR (MHC II) incompatibility is a contraindication to bone marrow grafting without T-cell depletion.
True/false

7 Which of the following statements regarding graft-versus-host disease (GVHD) are true?
a Occurs in only a minority of patients receiving allogeneic bone marrow transplants
b May occur mildly following bone marrow transplantation between HLA-identical siblings
c May occur following unirradiated blood transfusion in babies with severe combined immune deficiency
d Is preventable by depleting T cells from donor bone marrow
e Clinically involves the skin, liver and intestine

8 Primate recipients of xenografts do not require immunosuppressive treatment.
True/false

9 Allogeneic bone marrow transplantation may lead to prolonged remission of rheumatoid arthritis.
True/false

10 Which of the following statements regarding immunological and haematological reconstitution following bone marrow transplantation are true?
a The rate of granulocyte recovery is faster than that of lymphocytes
b T-cell function returns to normal 6–12 weeks following transplantation
c Recovery of B-cell function may be protracted
d The overall pace of immunological recovery is slower in recipients of HLA-incompatible bone marrow
e Immune reconstitution is delayed in recipients who develop severe graft-versus-host disease

11 Which one of the following microorganisms is the causative agent for Kaposi's sarcoma?
a Cytomegalovirus
b Human immunodeficiency virus
c Human herpes virus-6
d Human herpes virus-8

e West Nile virus

12 Which one of the following cell types is most important in the rejection of allogeneic transplants?
a CD4⁺ T cells
b Mast cells
c Natural Killer cells
d B cells
e Neutrophils

CHAPTER 9 Kidney Diseases

1 In which of the following types of glomerulonephritis is the serum C3 level characteristically low?
a Early acute poststreptococcal nephritis
b Active systemic lupus erythematosus nephritis
c Minimal-change nephropathy
d IgA nephropathy
e Membranoproliferative glomerulonephritis (type II)
f Membranous nephropathy

2 Which of the following is the commonest cause of the nephrotic syndrome in children?
a Henoch–Schönlein nephritis
b Minimal-change nephropathy
c Membranoproliferative glomerulonephritis
d Acute poststreptococcal glomerulonephritis
e IgA nephropathy

3 Which of the following histological terms means an increase in the number of cells within the glomerular tuft?
a Focal
b Crescentic
c Membranous
d Segmental
e Proliferative

4 Which of the following conditions typically lead to rapidly progressive glomerulonephritis?
a Goodpasture's syndrome
b Membranous glomerulonephritis
c Henoch–Schönlein nephritis
d Membranoproliferative glomerulonephritis
e ANCA-associated glomerulonephritis

5 Direct immunofluorescent examination of a renal biopsy shows linear deposition of IgG along the glomerular basement membrane. Which one of the following is the most likely diagnosis?
a Minimal-change nephropathy
b Membranous nephropathy
c Membranoproliferative glomerulonephritis
d Amyloid disease
e Anti-GBM nephritis
f IgA nephropathy

6 In acute poststreptococcal glomerulonephritis, which of the following statements are true?
a It only occurs following upper respiratory tract infection
b It typically follows within 5 days of streptococcal infection
c The anti-DNAse B titre is a better indicator of streptococcal skin sepsis than the ASO titre
d It is consistently associated with a low C3 level in the early phase
e The clinical course is usually one of complete recovery

7 Which of the following statements about glomerulonephritis are true?
a Minimal change nephropathy is most common in children under the age of 10 years
b Membranous nephropathy is linked to HLA-DR3
c In Goodpasture's syndrome, pulmonary haemorrhage is more common in smokers
d IgA nephropathy is a cause of < 1% of renal failure
e Glomerulonephritis nearly always recurs clinically in the allografted kidney

8 Which of the following statements about C3 NeF are correct?
a C3 NeF is produced by the kidneys
b C3 NeF is an IgG class autoantibody
c C3 NeF is characteristic of membranoproliferative glomerulonephritis (type II)
d C3 NeF causes the characteristic renal damage
e C3 NeF may be transferred across the placenta into the fetal circulation

9 Following cadaveric renal transplantation, which one of the following conditions is most likely to be associated with recurrence of glomerulonephritis in the allograft?
a Minimal-change nephropathy
b Membranoproliferative glomerulonephritis (type II)
c Henoch–Schönlein nephritis
d Polycystic disease
e Poststreptococcal glomerulonephritis

10 Antibodies to neutrophil cytoplasmic antigens are characteristically found in which of the following conditions?
a Pauci-immune crescentic glomerulonephritis
b Goodpasture's syndrome
c Amyloidosis
d Wegener's granulomatosis
e IgA nephropathy

CHAPTER 10 Joints and Muscles

1 With regard to rheumatoid factor, which one of the following statements are true?
a Rheumatoid factor is an acute-phase protein

b A positive rheumatoid factor is diagnostic of rheumatoid arthritis

c A positive rheumatoid factor suggests a poor prognosis in rheumatoid arthritis

d Rheumatoid factor is an autoantibody directed against the Fab region of IgG

e About 1% of healthy normal people have rheumatoid factor in the peripheral blood

2 Which of the following statements about rheumatoid arthritis are true?

a Most patients progress to complete disability

b Oral corticosteroids form the basis of drug therapy

c Parvovirus B-19 is the causative agent

d Always responds to plasma exchange therapy

e Serum C-reactive protein measurement is a useful measure of joint inflammation

3 Which of the following is associated with ankylosing spondylitis?

a Serum antinuclear antibodies

b Rheumatoid factor in the serum

c HLA-B27

d Female sex

e Chronic uveitis

4 Which of the following is a common feature of Reiter's disease?

a Age greater than 60 years

b Acute uveitis

c Orchitis

d Raised DNA-binding activity in serum

e The pathergy phenomenon

5 Which of the following is least likely to be present in patients with systemic lupus erythematosus (SLE)?

a A raised serum IgE level

b Antibodies to double-stranded DNA

c Decreased C3 and C4 levels

d A 'positive' VDRL

e Antibodies to platelets

6 Infliximab is of no clinical benefit in which of the following conditions?

a Behçet's syndrome

b Ankylosing spondylitis

c Psoriasis

d Juvenile idiopathic arthritis

e Multiple sclerosis

7 Which of the following statements about diagnostic tests is true?

a Antinuclear antibodies are usually present in polyarteritis nodosa

b Raised CRP levels are usually present in active SLE

c The presence of antibodies to RNP and Sm is strongly suggestive of SLE

d 75% of patients with giant cell arteritis have ANCA antibodies

e Anti-CCP antibodies are strongly associated with Sjögren's syndrome

CHAPTER 11 Skin Diseases

1 Which one of the following statements about the skin is untrue?

a Langerhans cells are intra-epidermal antigen-presenting cells

b Keratinocytes can produce a variety of chemokines

c CLA-positive T cells recirculate to the skin

d Ultraviolet radiation enhances immune responses in the skin

e Keratinocyte turnover is increased in psoriasis

2 Which one of the following statements about cryoglobulins is correct?

a Samples for cryoglobulin detection must be stored on ice before they reach the laboratory

b Types I cryoglobulins are associated with hepatitis C infection

c Mixed cryoglobulinaemia can be associated with a vasculitic illness

d Cryoglobulins are always monoclonal immunoglobulins

e Symptoms are invariably worse in the cold

3 Which one of the following statements about allergic contact dermatitis is untrue?

a The best diagnostic test for the triggering antigen is intradermal prick testing

b Type IV hypersensitivity plays a major role in the pathogenesis

c The triggering antigen is often a low molecular weight molecule which becomes attached to skin proteins

d Sensitization to an allergen usually takes at least 7 days

e Nickel in jewellery is a common cause

4 Which one of the following statements about hereditary angioedema is correct?

a A normal C4 concentration during an episode of angioedema excludes a diagnosis of hereditary angioedema

b Urticaria is a recognized feature

c Laryngeal oedema does not occur

d Inheritance follows an X-linked pattern

e Treatment is with antihistamines

5 Which one of the following statements about bullous skin disease is untrue?

a Dermatitis herpetiformis is associated with granular deposits of IgA in dermal papillae

b Pemphigus is associated with antibodies to desmosomal proteins

c Pemphigoid is associated with antibodies to type VII collagen

d Biopsies for diagnosis should be taken from perilesional skin

e High-dose corticosteroids can be life-saving in pemphigus

6 **Which one of the following statements about discoid lupus erythematosus is correct?**

a The skin lesions rarely, if ever, scar

b Only about 20% of patients have antibodies to dsDNA

c The lupus band test typically shows granular deposits of immunoglobulin at the dermoepidermal junction of unaffected skin

d Systemic involvement is rare

e Anti-Ro antibodies are a characteristic feature

7 **Which one of the following clinical features is not a common feature of limited systemic sclerosis (CREST)?**

a Raynaud's phenomenon

b Oesophageal dysfunction

c Pulmonary fibrosis

d Sclerodactyly

e Telangiectasia

8 **Circulating autoantibodies to skin-specific antigens may be diagnostically helpful in which one of the following conditions?**

a Pemphigus

b Vitiligo

c Allergic contact dermatitis

d Subacute cutaneous lupus erythematosus

e Dermatitis herpetiformis

CHAPTER 12 Eye Diseases

1 **Which one of the following statements about conjunctivitis is untrue?**

a Atopic keratoconjunctivitis is an ocular equivalent of atopic dermatitis

b In infective conjunctivitis, lymphoid follicles may form in the conjunctiva

c Conjunctivitis due to Chlamydia trachomatis is a major global cause of blindness

d Conjunctivitis in patients with antibody deficiency is often caused by Haemophilus influenzae

e Conjunctivitis is a rare feature of Reiter's syndrome

2 **Which one of the following is normally avascular?**

a The iris

b The conjunctiva

c The retina

d The cornea

e The pinna

3 **Which one of the following is not usually associated with uveitis?**

a Pauciarticular arthritis in children

b Sarcoidosis

c Ankylosing spondylitis

d Rheumatoid arthritis

e Behçet's disease

4 **Which one of the following statements about immunological disease of the eye is true?**

a Epstein–Barr virus is a major cause of eye disease in patients with HIV infection

b Scleritis is a benign condition which usually resolves without treatment

c Sympathetic ophthalmia is a common and serious consequence of penetrating eye injury

d Children with juvenile chronic arthritis require assessment by an ophthalmologist

e Matching for MHC antigens between graft and recipient is required for successful corneal transplantation

CHAPTER 13 Chest Diseases

1 **Recurrent bacterial pneumonia is unlikely to complicate:**

a Complement C3 deficiency

b Hypogammaglobulinaemia

c Secondary immunodeficiency

d Splenectomy

e Prolonged immunosuppression following transplantation

2 **Which one of the following statements regarding sarcoidosis is untrue?**

a The disease is characteristically associated with a negative Mantoux test

b Hypercalcaemia reflects increased vitamin D synthesis

c Acute sarcoidosis usually requires treatment with corticosteroids

d Uveitis may occur in chronic disease

e Hilar lymphadenopathy is a common feature

3 **Which one of the following statements regarding extrinsic allergic alveolitis is untrue?**

a Extrinsic allergic alveolitis is characteristically caused by exposure to an organic dust

b Symptoms typically occur about 1–2 h after exposure to the triggering antigen

c Both Type III and Type IV hypersensitivity mechanisms occur in this disorder

d Chronic disease may lead to pulmonary fibrosis

e Caged birds are the commonest cause in the UK

4 **Which one of the following statements about bronchial eosinophilia due to Aspergillus fumigatus is true?**

a Patients usually have chronic asthma

b The fungus is nearly always seen on chest X-ray

c Serum IgA levels are often raised

d Precipitating antibodies to Aspergillus fumigatus are rarely found e Basophils are frequently found in mucus plugs

5 Which one of the following statements regarding vasculitis is untrue?

a Intravenous immunoglobulin is beneficial in the treatment of Kawasaki disease

b Wegener's granulomatosis is usually treated with cyclophosphamide and corticosteroids

c Pulmonary vasculitis may present with lung haemorrhage

d Takayasu's arteritis typically produces microaneurysms in middle-sized arteries

e Churg–Strauss syndrome is associated with asthma

6 Which one of the following cell types is not typically found in a granuloma?

a T lymphocyte
b B lymphocyte
c Macrophage
d Epithelioid cell
e Giant cells

7 Which one of the following statements about idiopathic pulmonary fibrosis is true?

a Haemoptysis is the most common presenting symptom

b Antineutrophil cytoplasmic antibodies are positive in 90% of patients at presentation

c Ground glass shadowing is found on CT scanning in most patients

d A good response to corticosteroids is found in around 40% of patients

e Lung transplantation is effective in selected patients

CHAPTER 14 Gastrointestinal and Liver Diseases

1 Which of the following are characteristically expressed by the main population of intra-epithelial lymphocytes?

a CD 19
b CD 103
c CD 4
d CD 8
e MAdCAM-1

2 Where are M cells found in the intestine?

a Interacting with intra-epithelial lymphocytes
b In the lamina propria
c In follicle-associated epithelium
d In the dome area of Peyer's patches
e In the sinusoids of mesenteric lymph nodes

3 Which of the following statements about intrinsic factor antibodies are correct?

a They are found in less than 40% of patients with pernicious anaemia

b They are found in about 25% of patients with iron-deficiency anaemia

c They are more frequently found in gastric juice than serum

d They are more often binding (type II) than blocking (type I)

e They are helpful in the diagnosis of pernicious anaemia

4 Which of the following statements about gastric parietal cell antibodies are true?

a Found more frequently in gastric juice than in serum
b They are diagnostic of pernicious anaemia
c They are best considered a screening test for pernicious anaemia
d They inhibit absorption of vitamin B_{12} in the ileum
e They are usually of IgM isotype

5 Match the following autoantigens with the typical disease association.

a Endomysium
b Actin
c Pyruvate dehydrogenase
d Tissue transglutaminase
e H+ K+ ATPase

i Primary biliary cirrhosis
ii Coeliac disease
iii Autoimmune hepatitis
iv Atrophic gastritis type A
v Crohn's disease

6 Which of the following are correct statements regarding coeliac disease?

a There is a strong association with HLA-DQ2
b There is a strong association with HLA-B27
c It is diagnosed from the finding of increased faecal fat excretion
d It may be complicated by intestinal lymphoma
e It affects only boys

7 Which of the following statements about hepatitis B are correct?

a It is more common in warm countries than in cold countries
b If occurring in neonates, it will usually lead to a carrier state
c It is common in male homosexuals
d It has an incubation period of about 30 days
e It is accompanied by an increased risk of hepatocellular carcinoma

8 Which of the following are correct statements about hepatitis A?

a In developed countries, it is mainly a disease of the young
b It has an incubation period of about 100 days
c It is spread by the faecal–oral route
d It is associated with HLA-B8, -DR3
e It is best diagnosed by finding IgM-specific antibody to hepatitis A

9 Which of the following statements about hepatitis C are correct?

a It is commonly spread by the enteric route

b The incubation period is about 50 days

c It is characterized clinically by mild disease

d It frequently progresses to chronic hepatitis

e It can be effectively prevented by vaccination

10 **Which of these statements are true? Antimitochondrial antibodies:**

a Are found in about two-thirds of patients with primary biliary cirrhosis

b Are found in some patients with chronic active hepatitis

c Are known to be directly responsible for bile duct damage

d Are often accompanied by a rise in serum IgM in patients with PBC

e Are directed against pyruvate dehydrogenase

CHAPTER 15 Endocrinology and Diabetes

1 **The pathogenic antibody in Graves' disease has specificity for which one of the following?**

a Nuclei

b Thyroid microsomes

c Thyroglobulin

d Thyroid-stimulating hormone (TSH) receptors

e TSH

2 **The most useful routine autoantibody test in suspected autoimmune thyroid disease is that to:**

a Nuclei

b TSH receptors

c Thyroid peroxidase

d TSH

e Thyroglobulin

3 **Children with insulin-dependent diabetes mellitus usually have serum antibodies to which one of the following autoantigens at presentation?**

a Pancreatic islet cells

b Thyroid microsomes

c Gastric parietal cells

d Nuclei

e IgG molecules

4 **Which one of the following conditions is not associated with idiopathic Addison's disease?**

a Autoimmune ovarian failure

b Idiopathic hypoparathyroidism

c Mucocutaneous candidiasis

d Hyperparathyroidism

e Pernicious anaemia

5 **The Autoimmune Polyendocrinopathy, Candidiasis and Ectodermal Dysplasia (APECED) syndrome is associated with mutations in which gene?**

a HLA-DR3

b CMC

c AIRE

d CTLA-4

e ADA

CHAPTER 16 Haematological Diseases

1 **The commonest cause of anaemia is which of the following?**

a Autoimmune haemolytic anaemia

b Non-Hodgkin's lymphoma

c B_{12} deficiency

d Iron deficiency

e Drug-induced haemolysis

2 **The typical autoantibodies in warm autoimmune haemolytic anaemia are which of the following?**

a Polyclonal IgG

b Polyclonal IgM

c Monoclonal IgG

d Monoclonal IgM

e Of anti-I specificity

3 **Pathogenic mechanisms in immune thrombocytopenia are known to include:**

a IgA antibodies directed against megakaryocytes

b Complement lysis of platelets intravascularly

c Opsonization of platelets by IgG antibodies

d Phagocytosis of platelets by neutrophils intravascularly

e Phagocytosis of megakaryocytes in the spleen

4 **Cold haemagglutinin diseases (CHADs) are associated with which one of the following features?**

a Young patients

b Common complication of SLE

c Good response to oral steroids

d 50% of patients respond to splenectomy

e Associated with monoclonal/polyclonal IgM antibodies

5 **Which one of the following statements about red cell antibodies is true?**

a Transfusion reactions are always due to red cell incompatibility

b The ABO system is the only common red cell system with naturally occurring antibodies

c Naturally occurring antibodies to red cells are IgG in nature

d Only IgA antibodies are provoked by rhesus antigens

e Blood for routine transfusion requires to be matched at the HLA loci

6 **The commonest cause of thrombocytopenia in children is:**

a Aplastic anaemia

b Leukaemia

c Iron deficiency

d Infection

e Mismatched blood transfusion

7 Hypersplenism is one cause of which of the following?
  a Anaemia
  b Neutropenia
  c Thrombocytopenia
  d All of the above
  e None of the above

8 Which one of the following is not a cause of neutropenia?
  a Failure of production of stem cells
  b Vitamin B_{12} deficiency
  c Splenomegaly
  d Antineutrophil antibodies
  e Immune complexes

9 The primary antiphospholipid antibodies are not associated with which one of the following?
  a Arterial thrombosis
  b Recurrent fetal loss
  c Systemic lupus erythematosus
  d Patients aged > 60 years
  e Syphilis

10 Which one of the following statements about the treatment of immune thrombocytopenia (ITP) is not true?
  a Children with acute ITP always require treatment
  b Splenectomy is successful second line therapy in > 75% of patients
  c Corticosteroids are the mainstay of therapy in patients with active bleeding
  d Intravenous immunoglobulin therapy may be helpful if steroids do not work
  e Intravenous immunoglobulin therapy is useful in pregnant women with ITP

CHAPTER 17 Neuroimmunology

1 Which of the following is the single, most useful laboratory test to diagnose multiple sclerosis?
  a IgG level in serum
  b Positive ANA in serum
  c IgG : albumin ratio in CSF
  d Increased CSF cell count
  e Isoelectric focussing of cerebrospinal fluid

2 Interferon-β therapy has been shown to be effective in reducing rate of relapse in which group of patients with multiple sclerosis?
  a All
  b None
  c Relapsing and remitting group
  d Those with major disabilities
  e Those in whom IVIG has failed

3 What proportion of patients with myasthenia gravis have thymic hyperplasia?
  a None
  b 100%
  c 10%
  d 90%
  e 40%

4 Which one of these forms of therapy is not useful in treatment of myasthenia gravis?
  a Anticholinesterases
  b Immune suppression
  c Plasma exchange
  d Thymectomy
  e Vitamin B_{12}

5 Antibodies to gangliosides in patients with Guillain–Barré syndrome:
  a Are found in most patients
  b Are a guide to using IVIG therapy
  c Have specificity for MAG antigens
  d Have specificity for GD1 gangliosides
  e Are indicative of associated thyroid disease

6 Intravenous immunoglobulin is the first treatment of choice for patients with which one of the following?
  a Guillain–Barré syndrome
  b Meningitis
  c Paraproteinaemic neuropathy
  d Mononeuritis multiplex
  e Multiple sclerosis

7 A patient with a small paraprotein in the serum may have which of the following features in association with the paraprotein?
  a Clinical peripheral neuropathy
  b Hyperviscosity of the blood
  c Renal tubular failure
  d Skeletal lytic lesions
  e All of the above

8 Which of the following investigations maybe helpful in cerebral systemic lupus erythematosus (SLE)?
  a Antinuclear antibodies
  b Antineuronal antibodies
  c C3 levels in serum
  d C3 levels in CSF
  e Immune complex levels in CSF

9 Useful therapies in MS patients include which of the following?
  a Monoclonal antibodies to integrins
  b Monoclonal antibodies to CD25
  c Corticosteroids
  d Co-polymer 1 (Glatiramer)
  e All of the above

10 Which of the following observations in multiple sclerosis (MS) are true?
  a 40% of new clinical events follow viral infections
  b Occasional epidemics of MS have occurred
  c MS is a disease of temperate climates

d There are many antibodies with differing isotopes in a single MS plaque

e All of the above

CHAPTER 18 Pregnancy

1 **Which one of the following statements about immune responses in the human uterus/cervix is true?**

a It is an immunologically privileged site

b Is never infiltrated by T or B lymphocytes

c Has no lymphatic drainage

d Contains specialised NK cells

e Provides an environment free of pathogenic organisms

2 **Which one of the following statement about immunoglobulin in fetal and neonatal humans is untrue?**

a Maternal IgG is placentally transferred from 32 to 40 weeks of gestation

b IgM is the first Ig to be made in the fetus

c Transfer of maternal IgG across the placenta is an active process

d All maternal IgG has been catabolized in a normal infant by 3 weeks of life

e Breast milk IgA is absorbed by the infant's small intestine

3 **Which one of the following statements about haemolytic disease of the newborn is true?**

a Most commonly due to ABO red cell antibodies

b Most commonly due to rhesus red cell antibodies

c Prevented by passive antibodies to HLA antigens

d Most commonly due to HLA antigens

e Treated with corticosteroids

4 **Which of the following immunologically mediated diseases characteristically improve during pregnancy?**

a Thyrotoxicosis

b SLE

c Autoimmune haemolytic anaemia

d None

e All

5 **The protective effects of breast milk are known to be associated with which one of the following?**

a IgM antibodies

b NK cells

c Mast cells

d CD4 T cells

e Secretory IgA antibodies

6 **Recurrent abortions are known to be associated with which of the following maternal findings?**

a Autoantibodies to Ro

b Autoantibodies to thyroid microsomes

c Anticardiolipin antibodies

d Antibodies to ABO red cell antigens

e Cytotoxic T cells to paternal HLA antigens

7 **HLA-G antigens are:**

a Ubiquitous

b Classical MHC class I antigens

c Invariant

d Large molecules

e Recognized by cytotoxic T cells

8 **A successful pregnancy is thought to be associated with:**

a A strong maternal TH1 response to paternal antigens

b Failure to respond to paternal HLA antigens

c Protection provided by pre-existing antibodies to EBV

d Local production of cytokines in the placenta

e Antibodies to fetal neutrophils preventing destruction of the trophoblast

9 **Which one of the following statements concerning the phospholipid syndrome in pregnancy are true?**

a 95% of pregnant women with antiphospholipid antibodies will suffer a miscarriage

b Immunosuppression is used to reduce the level of antibody titres to achieve a successful pregnancy

c Infants of mothers with antiphospholipid antibodies have congenital heart block

d Mothers with antiphospholipid antibodies suffer from malignant hypertension

e Women with a history of serious thrombotic episodes and high levels of antiphospholipid antibodies are treated with aspirin and low-dose heparin in pregnancy

10 **Which one of the following is true of an infant with alloimmune neonatal thrombocytopenia?**

a There is a 50% chance of severe cerebral bleeding

b Exchange transfusion is always indicated

c The infant should be treated for at least 9 months

d Is common due to recognition of HLA antigens on the fetal platelets

e Is due to recognition of a rare paternal platelet antigen on fetal platelets

CHAPTER 19 Techniques in Clinical Immunology

1 **Which of the following specimens should be sent for immunological investigation of a possible myeloma?**

a Heparinized blood

b Clotted blood

c Sputum

d Jejunal juice

e Urine

2 **Put these tests for autoantibody detection in order of increasing sensitivity, starting with the least sensitive.**

a Enzyme-linked immunosorbent assay

b Haemagglutination

   c Radioimmunoassay

   d Indirect immunofluorescence

   e Immunoprecipitation

3 **Which is the quickest method for measuring serum immunoglobulin levels accurately?**

   a Immunoelectrophoresis

   b Nephelometry

   c Radioimmunoassay

   d Serum protein electrophoresis

   e Radial immunodiffusion

4 **The method of choice for measuring antigen-specific IgE in the serum is:**

   a Radial immunodiffusion

   b Serum protein electrophoresis

   c Indirect immunofluorescence

   d Countercurrent electrophoresis

   e Enzyme-linked immunosorbent assay

5 **An antinuclear antibody assay is which of the following?**

   a Sensitive but not specific

   b Sensitive and specific

   c Specific but not sensitive

   d Neither specific nor sensitive

6 **An antinuclear antibody (ANA) of which isotype is generally most significant in active SLE?**

   a IgA

   b IgD

   c IgE

   d IgG

   e IgM

7 **The polymerase chain reaction is a method for which of the following?**

   a Amplification of DNA

   b Concentration of Bence-Jones protein

   c Identification of oligoclonal banding

   d Amplification of lymphocyte transformation responses

   e Neutralization of RNA polymerization

8 **Which of the following are functional tests of neutrophils?**

   a NBT test

   b Lymphocyte transformation

   c Bacterial killing

   d Complement activation

   e Pneumococcal antibody levels

9 **Which one of the following is the most common lymphocyte type in peripheral blood?**

   a NK cells

   b B cells (kappa chain)

   c CD8$^+$ cells

   d CD3$^+$ cells

   e CD4$^+$ cells

10 **An M band on protein electrophoresis indicates which of the following?**

   a A raised serum IgM level

   b A raised monocyte count

   c Mitochondrial antibody of M2 type

   d A paraprotein requiring further investigation

   e Microsomal antibodies (thyroid peroxidase antibodies)

MCQ Answers

For detailed feedback on your answers please go to the MCQs section of our website at: www.immunologyclinic.com. Cases and images are also available on our website—www.immunologyclinic.com

Chapter 1
1 a
2 e
3 c ,d
4 e
5 b
6 b
7 e
8 e
9 d
10 b
11 e
12 c
13 c
14 e
15 b
16 d

Chapter 2
1 a,d,e
2 a,d
3 a,d
4 True
5 a,b,c,d,e
6 True
7 b,c,e
8 True
9 a,b,c,d,e
10 True
11 b,d,e
12 a,c
13 True
14 c,d
15 b
16 e

17 c
18 d

Chapter 3
1 c
2 d
3 e
4 d
5 b
6 a
7 c
8 b
9 d
10 c
11 d

Chapter 4
1 b,c,e
2 a,c,e
3 a,d
4 a,b,c,d,e
5 a,c,d
6 c,d
7 d
8 c
9 a,b,c,d
10 d

Chapter 5
1 b
2 c
3 d
4 c
5 e
6 e

Chapter 6
1 d
2 e
3 c

4 b
5 e
6 a
7 c
8 c
9 c
10 b

Chapter 7
1 c,d,e
2 False
3 a,b,d
4 True
5 b,c,d
6 True
7 a,b,d,e
8 False
9 a,d
10 False
11 False
12 True
13 True
14 d
15 a
16 a

Chapter 8
1 a,e
2 False
3 a,c,e
4 True
5 a,c,d
6 True
7 b,c,d,e
8 False
9 True
10 a,c,d,e
11 d
12 a

Chapter 9
1 a,b,e
2 b
3 e
4 a,e
5 e
6 c,d,e
7 a,b,c
8 b,c,e
9 b
10 a,d

Chapter 10
1 c
2 e
3 c
4 b
5 a
6 e
7 c

Chapter 11
1 d
2 c
3 a
4 a
5 c
6 d
7 c
8 a

Chapter 12
1 e
2 d
3 d
4 d

Chapter 13
1 d
2 c
3 b
4 a
5 d
6 b
7 e

Chapter 14
1 b,d
2 c
3 c,e
4 c
5 a, ii; b, iii; c, i; d, ii; e, iv
6 a,d
7 a,b,c,e
8 a,c,e
9 b,c,d
10 b,d,e

Chapter 15
1 d
2 c
3 a
4 d
5 c

Chapter 16
1 d
2 a
3 c
4 e
5 b
6 d
7 d
8 b
9 d
10 a

Chapter 17
1 e
2 c
3 e
4 e
5 d
6 a
7 a
8 a
9 e
10 e

Chapter 18
1 d
2 d
3 b
4 d
5 e
6 c
7 c
8 d
9 e
10 e

Chapter 19
1 b,e
2 e,d,b,c,a
3 b
4 e
5 a
6 d
7 a
8 a,c
9 d
10 d

Index

'hygiene hypothesis', helminth infections 51
hyper-IgE: recurrent infection syndrome **68**
hyper-IgM syndromes 57
hypersensitivity
   fungal infection 48
   techniques, clinical immunology 317–18
   tests 317–18
hypersensitivity, immediate, allergy 78–9
hypersensitivity mechanisms, autoimmune disease 107–8, **108**
hypersensitivity reactions
   immune system 27–9, *28*, **29**
   parasitic infection 51
hypocalcaemia, autoimmune disease 97
hypogammaglobulinaemia of prematurity, pregnancy 301
hyposensitization (specific allergen immunotherapy) 81
hypothyroidism 268–9

idiopathic Addison's disease 272–3
idiopathic interstitial pneumonias (IIPs) 234–6
idiopathic pulmonary fibrosis (IPF) 234, 235–6
idiopathic thyroid atrophy (myxoedema) 268–9
idiotypic determinant 8
IF *see* intrinsic factor antibodies
IgA
   deficiency 58–60
   nephropathy 159–60, *160*
   secretory *8*, 242
   significance 10–11
IgD, significance 10–11
IgE, significance 10–11
IgG
   placental transfer 300–1
   significance 10–11
IgM pentamer (MW 800 kDA), schematic representation *8*
IgM, significance 10–11
IHD *see* ischaemic heart disease
IIPs *see* idiopathic interstitial pneumonias
IL-12 receptor deficiency 69
immediate hypersensitivity, allergy 78–9
immune complex disorders, techniques, clinical immunology 310–12
immune complexes
   rheumatoid arthritis *182*
   techniques, clinical immunology 312
Immune dysregulation, Polyendocrinopathy and X-linked Inheritance (IPEX) 274
immune manipulation 125–42
   cancer immunotherapy 141–2

immune potentiation 132–5
immunization against infection 137–41
immunosuppression 125–32
IVIG 135–6
monoclonal antibodies 136–7
novel approaches to autoimmune disease 142
psychological factors 137
immune-mediated arthritis 180
immune-mediated neuropathies **293**, 293–5, **294**
immune potentiation 132–5
immune reactions, bacterial antigens 44
immune responses
   bacterial infection 43–4
   bystander damage 40–1, 43–4, 48
   factors influencing **3**, 26
   microorganisms *35*
   mycobacterial infection *45*, 45–7
   overview *35*
   parts 1–2
   phases 2
   physiological outcomes 26–7
   protozoal infection 48–50
   viral infection 37–8, *38*, 40–1
   viral strategies to avoid 39–40, **40**
immune system
   bone marrow 31
   hypersensitivity reactions 27–9, *28*, **29**
   lymphatic network 31, *31*
   organization overview 29–32
   thymus 30–1
   tissue damage 27–9
immune thrombocytopenia (ITP) 279–82
   acute/chronic **281**
   causes *280*
immunization 137–41
   see also vaccines
   contraindications **140**
   infection 137–41
   oral tolerance 142
   passive 140
   routine **139**, 139–40
   splenectomy 139–40
   theoretical basis 137–8
   travellers 140
   whooping cough 139
immunodeficiency 52–77
   age influence 53
   combined primary T- and B-cell immunodeficiencies 61–5
   CVIDs 57–60
   infection 52–3, *53*
   primary *52*
   primary antibody deficiencies 53–61
   primary defects in non-specific immunity 65–70

SCID 61–5, **63**
   secondary *52*, 70–7
immunofluorescence *207*, *320*
   ALL *319*
immunofluorescence, indirect 312–15, **313**, *314*
immunoglobulin genes 8–9, *9*
immunoglobulin, intravenous, Kawasaki's disease 135
immunoglobulin replacement therapy 61
immunoglobulins
   classes *7*
   functions *7*
   isotypes 10–11
   measurement *308*, 308
   protein electrophoresis 308–10
   qualitative investigation 308–10
   structure *7*, 7–8
immunomodulation by IVIG 135–6
immunosuppression 125–32
   drugs 125–9, *126*
immunosuppression of T- and B-cell responses, helminth infections 51
immunosurveillance, cancer 142
immunotherapy, cancer 141–2
impaired cell-mediated immunity 36
indirect immunofluorescence 312–15, **313**, *314*
infection 33–51
   autoimmunity 106
   bacterial 41–4
   conjunctival 219
   factors influencing **33**
   fungal 47–8
   and the gut 244
   helminth 50–1
   immunization 137–41
   immunodeficiency 52–3, *53*
   immunosuppressed host 76–7, *77*
   macrophages 34–5, *35*, 48–9, 50
   mechanical barriers 34, *34*
   mycobacterial 45–7
   neuroimmunology 287–9
   non-specific resistance 34–5
   opportunistic 76–7, *77*
   parasitic 48–51
   pregnancy 299–302
   protozoal 48–50
   renal transplantation *150*
   resistance, normal 34–6
   skin diseases 202
   specific resistance 35–6
   viral 36–41
infectious mononucleosis ('glandular fever') 36
infertility 273–4
inflammation 16, 18, 27